Holistic Nursing
A Handbook for Practice
Third Edition

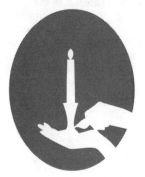

Barbara Montgomery Dossey, RN, MS, HNC, FAAN
Director
Holistic Nursing Consultants
Santa Fe, New Mexico

Lynn Keegan, RN, PhD, HNC, FAAN
Director
Holistic Nursing Consultants
Port Angeles, Washington and Temple, Texas
Formerly, Associate Professor
University of Texas Health Science Center
School of Nursing
San Antonio, Texas

Cathie E. Guzzetta, RN, PhD, FAAN
Nursing Research Consultant
Children's Medical Center of Dallas and Parkland
Health & Hospital Systems
Director
Holistic Nursing Consultants
Dallas, Texas

Endorsed by the American Holistic Nurses' Association

An Aspen Publication®
Aspen Publishers, Inc.
Gaithersburg, Maryland
2000

The author has made every effort to ensure the accuracy of the information herein. However, appropriate information sources should be consulted, especially for new or unfamiliar procedures. It is the responsibility of every practitioner to evaluate the appropriateness of a particular opinion in the context of actual clinical situations and with due considerations to new developments. The author, editors, and the publisher cannot be held responsible for any typographical or other errors found in this book.

Library of Congress Cataloging-in-Publication Data

Holistic nursing: a handbook for practice/Barbara Montgomery Dossey
. . . [et al.]. — 3rd ed.
p. cm.
Includes bibliographical references and index.
ISBN 0-8342-1629-9
1. Holistic nursing Handbooks, manuals, etc. I. Dossey, Barbara
Montgomery. II. American Holistic Nurses' Association.
[DNLM: 1. Holistic Nursing. WY 86.5 H732 1999]
RT42.H65 1999
610.73—dc21
DNLM/DLC
for Library of Congress
99-27912
CIP

Orders: (800) 638-8437
Customer Service: (800) 234-1660

About Aspen Publishers • For more than 35 years, Aspen has been a leading professional publisher in a variety of disciplines. Aspen's vast information resources are available in both print and electronic formats. We are committed to providing the highest quality information available in the most appropriate format for our customers. Visit Aspen's Internet site for more information resources, directories, articles, and a searchable version of Aspen's full catalog, including the most recent publications:
http://www.aspenpublishers.com
Aspen Publishers, Inc. • The hallmark of quality in publishing
Member of the worldwide Wolters Kluwer group.

Editorial Services: Ruth Bloom
Library of Congress Catalog Card Number: 99-27912
ISBN: 0-8342-1629-9

Printed in the United States of America

1 2 3 4 5

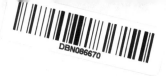

*Nursing is an art; and if it is to be made
    an art,
it requires as exclusive a devotion, as hard
    a preparation, as any painter's or
    sculptor's work;
for what is the having to do with dead
    canvas or cold marble,
compared with having to do with the living
    spirit—the temple of God's spirit?
It is one of the Fine Arts;
I had almost said,
    the finest of Fine Arts.*

Florence Nightingale

To Our Colleagues in Nursing:

When a nurse
Encounters another
Something happens
What occurs
Is never a neutral event

A pulse taken
Words exchanged
A touch
A healing moment
Two persons
Are never
The same

Table of Contents

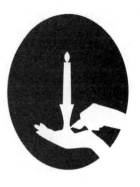

Visions of Healing

Contributors

Jeanne Anselmo, RN, BSN
Holistic Nurse Consultant
Co-Director
Holistic Nursing Associates
Bayside, New York

Genevieve M. Bartol, RN, EdD, HNC
Professor Emeritus
University of North Carolina at
   Greensboro
School of Nursing
Greensboro, North Carolina

Margaret A. Burkhardt, RN, PhD, CS,
   HNC, FNP
Associate Professor
West Virginia University
School of Nursing
Charleston, West Virginia
Family Nurse Practitioner
Gulf Family Practice
Sophia, West Virginia

Nancy F. Courts, RN, PhD, NCC
Chair and Associate Professor
Adult Health Division
University of North Carolina at
   Greensboro
School of Nursing
Greensboro, North Carolina

Barbara Montgomery Dossey, RN,
   MS, HNC, FAAN
Director
Holistic Nursing Consultants
Santa Fe, New Mexico

Joan C. Engebretson, RN, DrPH, CS,
   HNC
Associate Professor
University of Texas Houston Health
   Science Center
School of Nursing—Target Populations
Houston, Texas

Noreen Cavan Frisch, RN, PhD,
   HNC, FAAN
Chair and Professor
Department of Nursing
Cleveland State University
Cleveland, Ohio

H. Lea Barbato Gaydos, RN, PhD, CS,
   HNC
Director and Faculty
Holistic Nursing Studies
Beth-El College of Nursing and Health
   Science
University of Colorado at Colorado
   Springs
Colorado Springs, Colorado

Cathie E. Guzzetta, RN, PhD, FAAN
Nursing Research Consultant
Children's Medical Center of Dallas and
    Parkland Health & Hospital Systems
Director
Holistic Nursing Consultants
Dallas, Texas

**Judith A. Headley, RN, PhD, CS,
AOCN**
Assistant Professor
University of Texas Houston Health
    Science Center
School of Nursing
Houston, Texas

**Dorothea Hover-Kramer, RN, EdD,
CNS**
Director
Behavioral Health Consultants
Poway, California

Mary Gail Nagai Jacobson, RN, MSN
Community Health Consultant
San Marcos, Texas

Lynn Keegan, RN, PhD, HNC, FAAN
Director
Holistic Nursing Consultants
Port Angeles, Washington and Temple,
    Texas
Formerly, Associate Professor
University of Texas Health Science Center
School of Nursing
San Antonio, Texas

Leslie Gooding Kolkmeier, RN, MEd
Private Practice
Celeste, Texas

Susan Luck, RN, MA, HNC
Holistic Health Educator
Holistic Nurse Consultant
Director
Nutrition Education
Biodoron Immunology Center
Miami, Florida
Co-Director
Holistic Nursing Associates
New York, New York

E. Jane Martin, RN, CS, PhD, FAAN
Dean and Professor
West Virginia University
School of Nursing
Morgantown, West Virginia

**Maggie McKivergin, RN, MS, CNS,
HNC**
Holistic Nurse Consultant
Nurse Coordinator
Center for Alternative Health Care
    Practitioners, Inc.
Charleston, West Virginia

Melodie Olson, RN, PhD
Associate Professor
Medical University of South Carolina
College of Nursing
Charleston, South Carolina

Sue Popkess-Vawter, RN, PhD
Professor
University of Kansas
School of Nursing
Kansas City, Kansas

Pamela J. Potter, RN, MA, MSN, CS
Holistic Nurse Therapist
Wisdom Tree Resources for Healing
New Haven, Connecticut

Janet F. Quinn, RN, PhD, FAAN
Associate Professor
University of Colorado Health Sciences
    Center
School of Nursing
Denver, Colorado

Lynn Rew, RN,C, EdD, HNC, FAAN
Professor
The University of Texas at Austin
School of Nursing
Austin, Texas

Beryl H. Cricket Rose, RN, MEd, MSN
Nursing Supervisor
City of Austin Health and Human Services
Rosewood-Zaragosa Community Health
    Clinic
Austin, Texas

Sharon Scandrett-Hibdon, RN, PhD, CS, FNP, HNC
Adjunct Professor
Texas Woman's University
Groff Clinic Assoc.
Pilot Point, Texas

Bonney Gulino Schaub, RN, MS, CS
Co-Director New York Psychosynthesis
   Institute
Clinical Specialist
Adult Psychiatric Mental Health Nursing
Director
Clinical Imagery and Meditation
   Certificate Program
New York, New York and Huntington,
   New York
Co-Director
Holistic Nursing Associates
New York, New York

Eleanor A. Schuster, RN, DNSc, HNC
Professor
Florida Atlantic University
College of Nursing
Boca Raton, Florida

Karilee Halo Shames, RN, PhD, HNC
Assistant Professor
Florida Atlantic University
College of Nursing
Boca Raton, Florida

Victoria E. Slater, RN, PhD, CHTP/I, HNC
Private Practitioner
Energetic Healing
Clarksville, Tennessee

Eileen M. Stuart-Shor, RN, MS, CS
Nurse Practitioner, Preventive Cardiology
Roxbury Health Center
Adjunct Faculty
Graduate Program in Health Sciences
Simmons College
Consultant
WellCare Associates for Integrative
   Health
Boston, Massachusetts

Jean Watson, RN, PhD, HNC, FAAN
Distinguished Professor of Nursing
Founder
Center for Human Caring
Endowed Chair on Caring Science
University of Colorado
Health Sciences Center
School of Nursing
Denver, Colorado

Carol L. Wells-Federman, RN, MEd, MS, CS
Director, Pain Management Program
Arnold Pain Center
Division of Pain Medicine
Beth Israel Deaconess Medical Center
Associate in Anesthesia
Harvard Medical School
Boston, Massachusetts
Nurse Practitioner, Pain Medicine
DartmouthHitchcock Manchester
Manchester, New Hampshire

Patty Wooten, RN, BSN
Nurse Humorist
President
Jest For the Health of It!
Santa Cruz, California

Christine A. Wynd, RN, PhD, CNAA
Professor
The University of Akron
College of Nursing
Akron, Ohio

Reviewers

Gayle Acton, RN, PhD
Assistant Professor
The University of Texas at Austin
School of Nursing
Austin, Texas

Karen Ahijevych, RN, PhD
Assistant Professor
Ohio State University
College of Nursing
Columbus, Ohio

Elizabeth Ann Manhart Barrett, RN, PhD, FAAN
Professor
Hunter College of the City University of New York
Coordinator
Center for Nursing Research
Hunter-Bellevue School of Nursing
New York, New York

Tom Barron
Software Developer
Nashville, Tennessee

Ruth Benor, RGN, RM, RNT, M.BAFATT
Lecturer in Palliative Nursing and Integrative Care
Medford, New Jersey

Ramita Bonadonna, RN, MSN
Psychiatric Consultation Liaison Nurse
Medical University of South Carolina
Charleston, South Carolina

Anne Boykin, RN, PhD
Dean and Professor
College of Nursing
Adult and Community Nursing
Florida Atlantic University
Boca Raton, Florida

Megan McInnis Burk, RN, MS
Co-ordinator of Complementary Care Program
Areba Casriel Institute
New York, New York

Margaret A. Burkhardt, RN, PhD, CS, HNC, FNP
Associate Professor
West Virginia University
School of Nursing
Charleston, West Virginia
Family Nurse Practitioner
Gulf Family Practice
Sophia, West Virginia

Elizabeth Florentino Buselli, RN, CS, PhD
Clinical Nurse Specialist/Consultant
Cardiovascular Nursing
Wellcare Associates for Integrative Health
Boston, Massachusetts

Karyn Buxman, RN, MSN
Professional Speaker
President HumoRx
Hannibal, Missouri

Ruth Rosnick Carlson, RN, MNS
Instructor
University of Akron
College of Nursing
Akron, Ohio

Angela P. Clark, RN, PhD, CS, FAAN
Associate Professor
The University of Texas at Austin
School of Nursing
Austin, Texas

Horace W. Crater, PhD
Professor of Physics
The University of Tennessee Space
    Institute
Tullahoma, Tennessee

Dona Donato, LPCMHS, CHTP/I
Healing Touch Practitioner/Instructor
Psychotherapist
Memphis, Tennessee

Suzanne Doscher, RN, MS
Associate Professor
Medical University of South Carolina
College of Nursing
Charleston, South Carolina

Carol Eckert, BFA, MA
Associate Professor of Art
Austin Peay State University
Clarksville, Tennessee

Dezra J. Eichhorn, RN, MS, CNS
Adult Psychiatric—Mental Health
Trauma Psychosocial Clinical Nurse
    Specialist
Parkland Health & Hospital System
Dallas, Texas

Jill Eichhorn, PhD
Adjunct Instructor
Austin Peay State University
Clarksville, Tennessee

Cyndi Ellis-Stoll, RN, MSN
Perioperative Clinical Nurse Specialist
Via Christie St. Joseph's Medical Center
Wichita, Kansas

Noreen Cavan Frisch, RN, PhD, HNC, FAAN
Chair and Professor
Cleveland State University
Department of Nursing
Cleveland, Ohio

Patricia George, RN, MSN
Certified Gerontological Nurse
    Practitioner
Southern West Viriginia Clinic
Beckley, West Virginia

Mary Gail Nagai Jacobson, RN, MSN
Community Health Consultant
San Marcos, Texas

Bonnie Johnson, RN, MS, HNC, CHTP/I
Choices for Healing, A Holistic Nursing
    Practice
Nashville, Tennessee

Dorothy M. Johnson, RN, EdD
Assistant Professor
West Virginia University
School of Nursing
Department of Health Systems
Morgantown, West Virginia

Jane H. Kelley, RN, PhD
Professor and Director
MSN Nurse Executive Track
University of Mississippi Medical Center
School of Nursing
Jackson, Mississippi

Leslie Gooding Kolkmeier, RN, MEd
Private Practice
Celeste, Texas

Kathleen Lagana, RN, PCNS, PhD
Assistant Professor
University of Colorado at Colorado
    Springs
Coordinator
Childbearing Family Nursing
Colorado Springs, Colorado

Judy Lane, RN, MS
Nurse Practitioner
Sausalito, California

Dorothy Larkin, RN, MA, CS
Instructor
College of New Rochelle
Graduate Program in Holistic Nursing
New Rochelle, New York

Phyllis Mabbett, RN, PhD
Director
Center for Behavioral Health
Scripps Mercy Hospital System
Encinitas, California

Carol Lynn Mandle, RN, PhD, CS
Associate Professor
Boston College
Chestnut Hill, Massachusetts
Co-Director
Medical Symptom Reduction Clinic
    Program
Mind-Body Medical Institute
Beth Israel Deaconess Medical Center
Harvard Medical School
Boston, Massachusetts

Janet Mason, RN, MSN, LMT
Instructor
Mental Health Nursing
Albuquerque Technical Vocational
    Institute Community College
Albuquerque, New Mexico

Doris Milton, RN, PhD
Coeditor, *Alternative Therapies in Health
    and Medicine*
Faculty
Arizona State University and University of
    Phoenix
Phoenix, Arizona

Eloise Monzillo, RN, PhD, CNS
Private Practice
Verona, New Jersey

**Gail C. Mornhinweg, RN, PhD, ARNP,
CS**
Professor
Adult Primary Care
University of Louisville
Louisville, Kentucky

**Mary Elizabeth O'Brien, RN, PhD,
FAAN**
Professor
The Catholic University of America
School of Nursing
Washington, DC

Dorothy A. Otto, RN, MSN, EdD
Associate Professor
University of Texas-Houston Health
    Science Center
School of Nursing
Houston, Texas

Marilyn E. Parker, RN, PhD
Professor and Associate Dean
Florida Atlantic University
College of Nursing
Boca Raton, Florida

Lynn Rew, RN,C, EdD, HNC, FAAN
Professor
The University of Texas at Austin
School of Nursing
Austin, Texas

Tracy A. Riley, RN, MSN, CS
Instructor
University of Akron
College of Nursing
Clinical Nurse Specialist
Akron General Medical Center
Akron, Ohio

Vera Robinson, RN, EdD
Professor Emeritus
California State University at Fullerton
Aurora, Colorado

Richard Schaub, PhD
Co-Director
New York Psychosynthesis Institute
New York, New York

Carole Schoffstall, RN, PhD
Dean
Beth-El College of Nursing and Health
    Sciences
University of Colorado at Colorado Springs
Colorado Springs, Colorado

Karilee Halo Shames, RN, PhD, HNC
Assistant Professor
Florida Atlantic University
College of Nursing
Boca Raton, Florida

Mary K. Shannahan, RN, PhD
Associate Professor
Florida State University
Tallahassee, Florida

Aron Skrypeck, DOM, RN, MSN
Independent Practice/Psychiatric Nursing
    and Oriental Medicine
Wisdom Tree Resources for Healing
New Haven, Connecticut

David Squire, LCSW
Clinical Director
Center for Learning and Growth
Poway, California

J. Carole Taxis, RN, MSN
Instructor
The University of Texas at Austin
School of Nursing
Austin, Texas

Elias Vasquez, RN, PhD, NNP
Director
Neonatal Nurse Practitioner Program
Neonatal Substance Abuse
Assistant Professor
The University of Texas Houston Health
    Science Center
School of Nursing
Houston, Texas

Marty Wachter-Downey, RN, MS, CCRN, HNC
Assistant Professor
Boise State University
Department of Nursing—Target
    Populations
Boise, Idaho

Denise C. Webster, RN, PhD, CS
Professor
University of Colorado Health Sciences
    Center
School of Nursing—Target Populations
Denver, Colorado

Pamela O. Werstlein, RN, PhD, CFNP, LPC
Assistant Professor
University of North Carolina at
    Greensboro
School of Nursing
Greensboro, North Carolina

Gerald R. White, PhD
President, CEO
GRTW Inc.
Houston, Texas

Dina Wilson, RN, MSN
Instructor
Johnson County Community College
Department of Nursing
Overland Park, Kansas

Deborah Wolf, PhD
Psychotherapist/Lecturer
New York, New York

Foreword

The third edition of *Holistic Nursing: A Handbook for Practice*, while building upon the seminal work from the first two editions, takes a quantum leap forward. Indeed, this third edition becomes the blueprint for holistic nursing for the next era in nursing's history, unveiling the latest and most contemporary thinking in the field.

In this edition, the world renowned authors and contributors are no longer anticipating new breakthroughs for the twenty-first century; rather they are explicating them, developing and enveloping them within the most comprehensive approaches in body-mind-spirit nursing and its intersection with complementary–alternative modalities—all congruent with transpersonal human caring and healing. Thus, this latest work stands alone as *the* model for education and practice of holistic nursing.

What is also noteworthy in this edition is the organization of the content around the five core, consensus values for holistic nursing: Holistic Philosophy and Education; Holistic Ethics, Theories and Research; Holistic Nurse Self-Care; Holistic Communication, Therapeutic Environment, and Cultural Diversity; and Holistic Caring Process. Such an arrangement offers a coherent framework, whereby integrative praxis is made explicit, manifesting the oneness of knowing-being-doing as much as the oneness of being human, as much as the oneness of the art-science-technology of caring and healing practices.

The culmination of the exquisite artistry of holistic practices is further informed by the newly revised AHNA Standards of Holistic Nursing Practice from the American Holistic Nurses' Association, as well as the North American Nursing Diagnosis Association. Such a strong intellectual foundation offers students, practicing nurses, faculty, and researchers alike a special epistemologic framework for the field of holistic nursing, at both the general and advanced educational and practice levels.

By providing both an advanced orientation and advanced knowledge, this work continues to move holistic nursing beyond the exclusive Westernized modern medical/nursing focus, beyond the functional techniques and subspecialist knowledge, toward higher and deeper levels of commitment, compassion, love, and caring in the service of human health and healing. Thus, postmodern nursing and Era III thinking converge and come alive.

These postmodern advances awaken the sacred feminine energy, necessary for, and consistent with, holistic nursing and transpersonal caring and healing.[1] Thus, this work helps to transform our views of what it means to be human, to be whole, and to sustain caring and wholeness within the dynamic, yin–yang unity of unbroken wholeness among individuals, environment, and nature.

These breakthroughs include notions of an expanding human consciousness, intentionality, energetic healing, and spirituality, dimensions that transcend time and space to affect health and healing outcomes. These breakthroughs include psychophysiology of body-mind-spirit, values, holistic ethics, and new meanings of human potential.

As holistic nursing experts, these authors are committed to the fullest actualization of nursing, both ancient and futuristic. They practice what they teach in ways that integrate and translate the latest postmodern thinking into concrete nursing actions, processes, and artistic acts of caring and healing. In so doing, they bring new meaning to wholeness; they help us to understand the "critical" nature of healing practices contained within the latest standards of professional care.

A consequence of this work is that the self of each nurse is invited, if not reminded, into self-care and self-healing, as essentials toward authentic living of holistic practices. Thus, translating one's own expanded consciousness toward greater use of the transpersonal self help to transform both self and system in the process.

The authors both guide and challenge the reader at every level toward more authenticity and integrative use of self whereby holistic nursing becomes

- a paradigm case for all of nursing's caring–healing practices

- an integrative practice model for personal–professional coherence and integrity
- an ontologic and epistemologic model for both living out and creating additional nursing knowledge, theory, and advanced practices

In summary, the third edition of this pace-setting book expands and grounds holistic knowledge and practice through its handbook approach. It invites nurses and nursing alike to remember and reintegrate past, present, and future as one, as it assists in translating holistic caring theory into concrete healing modalities framed by national professional standards. The result: a new pathway whereby nursing's caring–healing competencies and transpersonal self dimensions are made visible and explicit for theory, practice, education, research, and life itself. This work transcends centuries and paradigms, while generating new traditions and standards of excellence that will project nursing into the mid-2000s.

Jean Watson, RN, PhD, HNC, FAAN
Distinguished Professor of Nursing
Founder, Center for Human Caring
Endowed Chair in Caring Science
University of Colorado
Health Sciences Center
School of Nursing
Denver, Colorado

NOTE

1. J. Watson, *Postmodern Nursing and Beyond.* (UK: Churchill-Livingston/Harcourt-Brace, 1999).

Preface

The American Holistic Nurses' Association (AHNA) has joined with the authors and contributors of *Holistic Nursing: A Handbook for Practice* to develop further the knowledge base for holistic nursing and delineate the essence of contemporary nursing. The purpose of this book is threefold: (1) to expand an understanding of healing and the nurse as an instrument of healing; (2) to explore the unity and relatedness of nurses, clients, and others; and (3) to develop caring–healing interventions to strengthen the whole person.

This book guides nurses in the art and science of holistic nursing and healing. It also assists nurses in their challenging roles of bringing healing to the forefront of health care and helping to shape health care reform. Because of public demand for alternative medicine, the National Institutes of Health (NIH) created in 1992 the Office of Alternative Medicine (OAM). In 1999, the OAM was elevated to a freestanding center status. The OAM, recently renamed the National Center for Complementary and Alternative Medicine (NCCAM), is now able to fund its own research grants without partnering with other institutes. The NCCAM is evaluating therapies that capitalize dramatically on bodymind and transpersonal therapies. More and more research findings are revealing that these therapies not only work and are extremely safe, but are also cost-effective. Among these therapies are relaxation, imagery, biofeedback, meditation, hypnosis, therapeutic touch, expressive therapies (e.g., art, dance, music), and spiritual healing. As nurses, we must become aware of research findings that can help integrate these modalities into mainstream medicine. At the present time, they should, in general, be considered complements to orthodox medical treatments and not a replacement for them. We advocate a "both/and" instead of an "either/or" approach in interfacing these healing modalities with contemporary medical and surgical therapies.

In the third edition of this book, we have further developed body-mind-spirit and transpersonal therapies and translated healing into action or the "knowing-doing-being" of healing. Six new chapters have been added to expand our exploration of the dynamics of healing and holism: spirituality and health, energetic healing, nurse as an instrument of healing, therapeutic communication, and cultural diversity and care. We challenge nurses to explore the following three questions:

1. What do you know about the meaning of healing?
2. What can you do each day to facilitate healing in yourself?
3. How can you be an instrument of healing and a nurse healer?

Healing is a lifelong journey into understanding the wholeness of human existence. Along this journey, our lives mesh with those of clients, families, and colleagues, where moments of new meaning and insight emerge in the midst of crisis. Healing occurs when we help clients, families, others, and ourselves embrace what is feared most. It occurs when we seek harmony and balance. Healing is learning how to open what has been closed so that we can expand our inner potentials. It is the fullest expression of oneself that is demonstrated by the light and shadow and the male and female principles that reside within each of us. It is accessing what we have forgotten about connections, unity, and interdependence. With a new awareness of these interrelationships, healing becomes possible, and the experience of the nurse as an instrument of healing and as a nurse healer becomes actualized. A *nurse healer* is one who facilitates another person's growth toward wholeness (body-mind-spirit) or who assists another with recovery from illness or transition to peaceful death. Healing is not just curing symptoms. Rather, it is the exquisite blending of technology with caring, love, compassion, and creativity.

This holistic approach is developed by incorporating ideas of perennial philosophy, natural systems theory, and the holistic caring process. The information presented within *Holistic Nursing: A Handbook for Practice* may be of additional interest to the nurse because it incorporates the following:

- American Holistic Nurses' Association Standards of Holistic Nursing Practice
- nursing diagnoses established by the North American Nursing Diagnosis Association
- guidelines for integrating holistic interventions divided into four areas: before, at the beginning, during, and at the close of the session

- both basic and advanced strategies for integrating complementary and alternative interventions
- client case studies in the acute care and outpatient settings
- research and directions for future research

As we have explored new meanings of healing in our work and lives, we have interwoven the many diverse threads of knowledge from nursing as well as from other disciplines. This has engendered a more vivid, dynamic, and diverse understanding about the nature of holism, healing, and its implications for nursing. Allow yourself to explore ideas of healing as they are first developed in a Vision of Healing before each chapter. Each chapter begins with Nurse Healer Objectives to direct your learning to the theoretical, clinical, and personal domains. Each chapter has a glossary of definitions for easy reference. The term *patient* is used for acute care settings and the term *client* is used in the outpatient settings. With both the patient and the client, we view persons as co-participants in all phases of care. The challenge is to integrate all concepts in this text in clinical practice and daily life. As clinicians, authors, educators, and researchers, we have successfully used these holistic concepts and interventions from the critical care unit and home health to the classroom. Each chapter ends with Directions for Future Research specific to each topic. This section presents suggested research questions that are timely and in need of scientific exploration in nursing. In concluding each chapter, Nurse Healer Reflections are offered to nurture and spark a special self-reflective experience of body-mind-spirit and the inward journey toward self-discovery and healing.

This book is organized by the five core values contained within the newly revised American Holistic Nurses' Association Standards of Holistic Nursing Practice which are as follows:

Core Value I: Holistic Philosophy and
               Education
Core Value II: Holistic Ethics, Theories,
               and Research
Core Value III: Holistic Nurse Self-Care
Core Value IV: Holistic Communication,
               Therapeutic Environment,
               and Cultural Diversity
Core Value V: Holistic Caring Process

Core Value I presents the philosophic concepts that explore what occurs when the nurse honors, acknowledges, and deepens the understanding of inner knowledge and wisdom. It lays the foundation for understanding transpersonal human caring and psychophysiology of bodymind healing. It also provides insight into how people create change and sustain these new health behavior changes related to wellness, values clarification, and motivation theory. Spirituality and energetic healing are also developed to expand further one's understanding and practice of holism.

Core Value II addresses holistic ethics in both personal and professional arenas. Holistic nursing theorists and theories are developed to guide holistic nursing practice. Guidelines for holistic research are also explored to help nurses provide care consistent with research findings and other sound evidence.

Core Value III develops and explores the concepts of therapeutic presence and the qualities and characteristics of becoming an instrument of healing. It expands on the integrated theory supporting relationship-centered care.

Core Value IV explores therapeutic communication and the art and skills of helping. The necessary steps in creating an external as well as an internal healing environment are expanded to help nurses recognize that each person's environment includes everything surrounding the individual, both the external and the internal, as well as patterns not yet understood. Concepts related to cultural diversity are presented so that the nurse can recognize each person as a whole body-mind-spirit being. This helps to develop a mutually, co-created plan of care that addresses the cultural background, health beliefs, sexual orientation, values, and preferences of each unique individual.

Core Value V expands the nursing process to the holistic caring process. This is a six-part circular process: assessment, patterns/problems/needs, outcomes, therapeutic care plan, implementation, and evaluation. Nine human response patterns are used to guide holistic assessment and to identify clients' problems/patterns/needs. Self-assessments and complementary and alternative strategies are developed to expand concepts relevant to healing and reaching human potential. Specific areas covered are cognitive therapy, self-reflection, nutrition counseling, movement and exercise, laughter, play and humor, relaxation, imagery, music, touch, relationships, death and grief counseling, weight management counseling, smoking cessation counseling, addictions and recovering counseling, and incest/child sexual abuse and violence counseling.

Our book is intended for students, clinicians, educators, and researchers who desire to expand their knowledge of holism, healing, and spirituality. The philosophic and conceptual frameworks are beginner, intermediate, and advanced. Therefore, the reader can approach this book as a guide for learning basic content or for exploring advanced concepts. The specific "how to" for implementing holistic interventions into clinical practice are divided into both basic and advanced levels. Some advanced interventions may require additional training that can be obtained in practicums under mentors or in elective or continuing education courses. Each chapter also presents case studies that illustrate how to use and integrate the interventions into clinical practice.

Holistic Nursing: A Handbook for Practice challenges nurses to explore the inward journey toward self-transformation and to identify the growing capacity for change and healing. This exploration creates the synergy and the rebirth of a compassionate power to heal ourselves and to facilitate healing within others. This inner healing allows us to return to our roots of nursing where healer and healing have always been understood and to carry Florence Nightingale's vision of health and healing into the new millennium. As she said, "My work is my must." By her shining example, she invites each of us to find and know our "must" and to explore our own meaning, purpose, and spirituality.[1]

The radical changes necessary in health care reform are occurring rapidly. Change has always been the rule in health care. These changes provide us with a greater opportunity to integrate caring and healing into our work, research, and lives. It is up to us to help determine what these new changes will be. We challenge you to capture your essence and to emerge as true healers in this twenty-first century. Best wishes to you in your healing work and life.

Barbara Montgomery Dossey
Lynn Keegan
Cathie E. Guzzetta

NOTE

1. B.M. Dossey, *Florence Nightingale: Mystic, Visionary, Healer* (Springhouse, PA: Springhouse Corporation, 1999).

For more information on the American Holistic Nurses' Association and the AHNA continuing education programs and home study courses, contact:
   American Holistic Nurses' Association
   2733 East Lakin Drive, Suite #2
   Flagstaff, AZ 86004
   Telephone: 800-278-AHNA or 520-526-2196
   Fax: (520) 526-2752
   E-Mail: AHNA-flag@flaglink.com

For information on the holistic nursing certification examination, contact:
   American Holistic Nurses' Certification Corporation
   P. O. Box 845
   Clarkdale, AZ 86324
   Telephone: 877-284-0998
   Fax: (520) 634-5441

For information on the *AHNA Core Curriculum for Holistic Nursing* (study guide for the holistic nursing certification examination), contact:
   Aspen Publishers, Inc.
   200 Orchard Ridge Drive
   Gaithersburg, MD 20878
   Telephone: 800-638-8453 or 301-417-7500

Acknowledgments

Our book flows out of the larger questions that have been raised for us in the health or illness of clients/patients, the professional community with which we have worked, and our families and friends with whom we live and play.

We celebrate with our colleagues in nursing as we explore new meanings of healing in our work and life, as we acknowledge what we have done well, and as we anticipate what we must do better. We honor the work of our colleague and dear friend Leslie Kolkmeier who was our co-author on the first and second editions of this book.

Special thanks are due to Bob Howard, formerly Acquisitions Editor at Aspen Publishers, and Mary Ann Langdon, Senior Development Editor, who helped us keep our goals in sight and believed in the project; to Ruth Bloom, Managing Editor—Books, for her attention to editorial details; to Laura Smith, Book Production Manager, for logo, book design, and production details; and to Gail Martin, for helping us keep our writing clear.

Most of all, for their understanding, encouragement, and love in seeing us through one more book, we thank our families—Larry Dossey; Gerald, Catherine, and Genevieve Keegan; Philip, Angela, and Philip C. Guzzetta—who share our interconnectedness.

CORE VALUE I

Holistic Philosophy and Education

VISION OF HEALING

Exploring Life's Meaning

What do you tell yourself about your state of health? Is your health excellent, good, fair, or poor? Over the last few years, the answers that people give to this simple question have become better predictors of who will live or die over the next decade than in-depth physical examinations or extensive laboratory tests. This question is a way of asking what our health means to us—what it represents or symbolizes in our thoughts and imagination.[1]

What does it mean to be human? What is meaning? Why should we seek out meaning? What do we do with it? How do we keep it? Phenomenology is a philosophy that is mainly interested in these "phenomenal" questions.[2]

Meanings are individual and personal. They have relevance to the person's experiences, events, expectations, belief systems, and core values. Within each person's story are meanings about the past and present life story, as well as beliefs about future events that can be explored in a healing journey. Within the story, one looks at patterns, insights, and broad relationships to find or seek out the meanings. Only when some meaning is clear can an experience become a paradigm experience. Meaningless experiences are seldom retained to form a foundation for future reference.

Meaning becomes apparent as differences, contrasts, novelty, and heterogeneity—and is necessary for the healthy function of human beings. We seek out meaning because our lives are fuller and richer when life means something positive for us. Take away the important meaning of our lives, and it is not worth living. The more we understand about meaning in life, the more we are able to empower ourselves to recognize more effective ways to cope with life and to learn more effective methods of working on life issues. In doing this, we create richer meaning in our daily lives. This attention to meaning allows us to be more effective with others as we guide them in searching for the meanings in their lives.

The meanings that a person attaches to symptoms or illness are probably the most important factors in the journey through a life crisis. Human beings can view illness from at least eight frames of reference: (1) illness as challenge, (2) illness as enemy, (3) illness as punishment, (4) illness as weakness, (5) illness as relief, (6) illness as strategy, (7) illness as irreparable loss or damage, and (8) illness as value.[3]

When we believe meaning is absent, our bodies become bored; bored bodies become the spawning ground for depression, disease, and death. Failure of meaning has become a cliché. Professions, personal lives, even entire cultures are said to suffer from a breakdown of meaning. Although at times it seems that meaning may be absent from our lives and our universe, in fact, such a thing is not possible, even in theory. Our existence is awash with meaning, and we must choose our meanings. The choices are crucial. Nowhere is this more important or apparent than in health and illness. It is clear from the wealth of scientific

3

data that it is impossible to separate the bio-logic parts from the psychologic, sociologic, and spiritual part of our being. The importance of meaning can no longer be ignored, for it is directly linked with mind modulation of all body systems that influence states of wellness or illness. Because meanings and emotions go hand in hand, is it strange that the meanings we perceive could affect the body? Or that the body could affect our emotions and our meanings? These connections are so intimate that we must think of bodymind as a single integrated unit. What are the lessons here? How can we put meaning in our life?[4]

- *We need simply to pay more attention to the meanings we perceive in life. This is easy to say, but difficult to do. It is much easier to concentrate on the cholesterol level, blood pressure, diet, vitamin intake, body weight, and the annual physical examination than to concentrate on meanings in life. If we really believed that we could die not only from heart failure, but also from "meaning failure," perhaps we would be more attentive to the meanings we create in our lives.*
- *Wellness and illness are vastly more complex than we have heretofore believed. Wellness is not a matter of simply covering the bases physically, for we know that there is no clear separation of the physical and the mental. This recognition*

places much more responsibility on each individual and less on the physician for one's health. No prescriptions can be written for meaning; each of us has to attend to our own meanings in the way that is best for us. Routinely, we need to assess and evaluate our human potentials to keep meaning in our life.

- *We need to be leery of anyone who proclaims that any particular problem is "all physical" or "all mental." These simplistic statements are indefensible in modern medical science. Those who make such claims cannot even tell us what it is they mean by "the physical" or "the mental," for the dividing line between them has become increasingly thin.*
- *We need to recognize the good news here—positive perceptions and meanings can actually increase the level of our health, all other factors being equal. They can be as therapeutic as a medication or a surgical procedure.*
- *We need to recognize science for the information that it can give us and understand that the true meaning of wellness and life is in our evolving process of expanding our awareness and potentials.*
- *We need to realize that meanings matter. When the time comes for your next annual physical examination, keep this fact in mind: It is not just the body that needs the checkup; one's personal life meanings need checkups from time to time, too.*

NOTES

1. L. Dossey, What Does Illness Mean? *Alternative Therapies* 1, no. 3 (1995): 6–10.
2. P. Munhall, *Revisioning Phenomenology: Nursing and Health Science Research* (New York: National League for Nursing Press, 1994).
3. Z.J. Lipowski, Physical Illness, the Individual and the Coping Process, *Psychiatric Medicine* 1 (1970): 90.
4. L. Dossey, *Meaning and Medicine: A Doctor's Tales of Breakthrough and Healing* (New York: Bantam Books, 1991).

Chapter 1

Holistic Nursing Practice

Barbara Montgomery Dossey and Cathie E. Guzzetta

NURSE HEALER OBJECTIVES

Theoretical

- Synthesize the concepts of natural systems theory.
- Compare and contrast the allopathic and holistic models of health care.
- Describe the components of the bio-psycho-social-spiritual model.
- Describe the practice and standards of holistic nursing.
- Compare and contrast the different eras of medicine.
- Discuss the activities of the National Center for Complementary and Alternative Medicine.

Clinical

- Explore two ways to integrate a natural systems view into your clinical practice.
- Determine if you use a bio-psycho-social-spiritual model to guide your clinical practice.
- Integrate the Standards of Holistic Nursing Practice established by the American Holistic Nurses' Association (AHNA) into clinical practice, education, and research.
- Integrate complementary and alternative therapies into clinical practice.

Personal

- Integrate complementary and alternative therapies into your daily life to enhance your well-being.
- Develop short- and long-term goals related to increasing your commitment to the holistic developmental process.

DEFINITIONS

Allopathic/Traditional Therapies: invasive and noninvasive medical or surgical procedures, including the administration of medications, in diagnosis and treatment.

Caring–Healing Interventions: nontraditional therapies that can interface with traditional medical and surgical therapies, sometimes used as complements to conventional treatments; also called alternative/complementary/integrative therapies or interventions.

Source: Definitions Copyright © 1988, American Holistic Nurses' Association. Permission is given to duplicate this document for teaching purposes by an educational institution. Written consent is required for duplication by an author or publisher. AHNA, 2733 E. Lakin Drive, Suite 2, Flagstaff, AZ 86004-2130; telephone 520-526-2196; http://www.ahna.org.

Cultural Competence: the ability to deliver health care with knowledge of and sensitivity to cultural factors that influence the health behavior of the person.

Healing: the return toward the natural state of integrity and wholeness of an individual; the process of bringing together aspects of one's self, body-mind-spirit, at a deep level of inner knowing in a way that leads toward integration and balance, with each aspect having equal importance and value; can lead to more complex levels of personal understanding and meaning; may be synchronous, but is not synonymous with curing.

Healing Process: a continual journey of changing and evolving of one's self through life; the awareness of patterns that support or are challenges/barriers to health and healing; may be done alone or in a healing community.

Health Promotion: activities and preventive measures such as immunizations, fitness/exercise programs, breast self-examination, appropriate nutrition, relaxation, stress management, social support, prayer, meditation, healing rituals, cultural practices, and promoting environmental health and safety.

Holistic Caring Process: a circular process that involves six steps that may occur simultaneously. These parts are assessment, patterns/problems/needs, outcomes, therapeutic care plan, implementation, and evaluation.

Holistic Communication: a free flow of verbal and nonverbal interchange between and among people and significant beings, such as pets, nature, and God/Life Force/Absolute/Transcendent, that explores meaning and ideas in a way intended to produce mutual understanding and growth.

Human Caring Process: the moral state in which the holistic nurse brings her or his whole self to a relationship with the whole self of another person and other significant beings, thus reinforcing the meaning and experience of oneness and unity.

Intention: the conscious awareness of creating an image of a person's spiritual essence and wholeness experienced as a "sacred space" of inner calm; a volitional act of love.

Intuition: the perceived knowing of things and events without the conscious use of rational processes; the use of all the senses to receive information.

Nurse As an Instrument of Healing: a nurse who creates a healing space within herself or himself that can enhance the opportunity for another to feel safe and bring into alignment that which has been painful and out of harmony; one who shares the authenticity of unconditional presence that helps to remove the barriers to the healing process.

Patterns/Problems/Needs: a person's actual and potential life processes related to health, wellness, disease, or illness which may or may not facilitate well-being.

Person: an individual, client, patient, family member, support person, or community member who has the opportunity to engage in interaction with a holistic nurse.

Person-Centered Care: the condition of trust in which holistic care can be given and received: the human caring process in which the holistic nurse gives full attention and intention to the whole self of a person, not merely to the presenting symptoms, illness, crisis, or tasks to be accomplished; the reinforcement of the person's meaning and experience of communion and unity.

Presence: the core essential in healing; a way of approaching an individual that respects and honors her or his essence; a way of relating that reflects a quality of *being with* and *in collaboration with* rather than *doing to*; a way of entering into a shared experience (or field of consciousness) that promotes healing potentials and an experience of well-being.

Spirituality: a unifying force of a person; the essence of being that permeates all of life and is manifested in one's being, knowing, and doing; the interconnectedness with self, others, nature, and God/Life Force/Absolute/Transcendent.

Standards of Practice: a group of statements describing the level of care expected from a holistic nurse.

HOLISM

Natural Systems Theory

Derived primarily from the work of von Bertalanffy,[1] natural systems theory provides a way of comprehending the interconnectedness of natural structures in the universe. The theory is complex, but has relevance for the health care professions (Figure 1–1). In brief, natural structures vary in size from the level of subatomic particles (i.e., quarks) to the universe, but each possesses specific characteristics within a structure and is governed by similar principles of organization. Therefore, a change

in any one part of the hierarchy affects all other parts. Changes are occurring in all levels simultaneously; for example, the ripple effect of a pebble thrown in a body of water changes the surface while simultaneously changing the air surface above and the water surface below. As with a kaleidoscope, a slight turn changes the whole configuration.

The traditional biomedical Western view of disease usually begins at the systems level and stops at the molecule level (see Figure 1–1). From the more precise perspective of the natural systems approach, however, disease can originate in a disturbance at any level from the subatomic to the suprapersonal, and it may result when a force disturbs or disrupts the structure of the natural systems themselves. The goal of health care is to decrease the many different disturbances and stressors caused by a person's illness. These disturbances also have an impact on the family's routine. As the ill person and the family strive to reweave the social fabric of their lives and achieve more harmonious interaction, this moving balance affects all the components of the natural systems hierarchy.

A key characteristic of the hierarchy of natural systems is information flow.[2] Regardless of the point at which it originates, information spreads up and down the components of the hierarchy. Information flow has a domino effect as it affects the whole system. The magnitude of the problems that a disturbance at one level may cause and its impact on the whole hierarchy are clear in any study of the overpopulation of the planet. The result of overpopulation is depletion of natural resources and chaos associated with too many people living in disharmony.

Holism and natural systems theory have important implications for clients' and nurses' views of health and disease, even though medicine's technologic, allopathic focus remains strong today. Those who advocate the allopathic method combat dis-

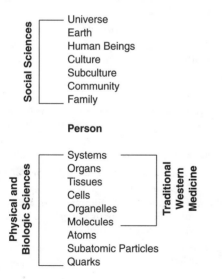

Figure 1–1 Patterns of Natural Systems Components

ease with techniques that produce effects different from those produced by the disease; those who advocate the holistic model assert that consciousness is real and is related to all matters of health and illness. Table 1–1 provides a comparison of the allopathic and holistic models.

Bio-Psycho-Social-Spiritual Model

The most comprehensive model available to guide mainstream health care is the bio-psycho-social-spiritual model. In this holistic model, all disease has a psychosomatic component, and biologic, psychologic, social, and spiritual factors always contribute to a patient's symptoms, disease, or illness.[3] The spiritual dimension in the bio-psycho-social-spiritual model incorporates spirituality in a broad context: values, meaning, and purpose in life. It reflects the human traits of caring, love, honesty, wisdom, and imagination. The concept of spirit implies a quality of transcendence, a guiding force, or something outside the self and beyond the individual

Table 1–1 Assumptions of Allopathic and Holistic Models of Care

Allopathic Model	Holistic Model
Treatment of symptoms	Search for patterns, causes
Specialized	Integrated; concerned with the whole patient
Emphasis on efficiency	Emphasis on human values
Professional should be emotionally neutral	Professional's caring is a component of healing
Pain and disease are wholly negative	Pain and disease may be valuable signals of internal conflicts
Primary intervention with drugs, surgery	Minimal intervention with appropriate technology, complemented with a range of noninvasive techniques (psychotechnologies, diet, exercise)
Body seen as a machine in good or bad repair	Body seen as a dynamic system, a complex energy field within fields (family, workplace, environment, culture, life history)
Disease or disability seen as an entity	Disease or disability seen as a process
Emphasis on eliminating symptoms and disease	Emphasis on achieving maximum bodymind health
Patient is dependent	Patient is autonomous
Professional is authority	Professional is therapeutic partner
Body and mind are separate; psychosomatic illnesses seen as mental; may refer (patient) to psychiatrist	Bodymind perspective, psychosomatic illness is the province of all health care professionals
Mind is secondary factor in organic illness	Mind is primary or co-equal factor in all illness
Placebo effect is evidence of power of suggestion	Placebo effect is evidence of mind's role in disease and healing
Primary reliance on quantitative information (charts, tests, and dates)	Primary reliance on qualitative information, including patient reports and professional's intuition; quantitative data an adjunct
"Prevention" seen as largely environmental; vitamins, rest, exercise, immunization, not smoking	"Prevention" synonymous with wholeness: in work, relationships, goals, body-mind-spirit

Source: Reprinted with permission from M. Ferguson, *Aquarian Conspiracy: Personal and Social Transformation in Our Time*, rev. ed., pp. 246–248, © 1987, J.P. Tarcher.

nurse or client. It may reflect a belief in the existence of a higher power or a guiding spirit. To some, spirit may suggest a purely mystical feeling or a flowing dynamic quality of unity. It is undefinable, yet it is a vital force profoundly felt by the individual. The human spirit can make the difference between life and death, as well as wellness and illness.

As shown in Figure 1–2, each component of the bio-psycho-social-spiritual model is interdependent and interrelated. It is necessary to address all these components to achieve optimal therapeutic results. Regardless of the illness involved, the technology developed, or the therapy used, the bio-psycho-social-spiritual model provides the major overall road map in caring for the whole patient and in meeting the mandates of the Joint Commission on Accreditation of Healthcare Organizations. For example, the Patient Bill of Rights states that

care of the patient must include consideration of the psychosocial, spiritual, and cultural variables that influence the perception of illness. The provision of patient care reflects consideration of the patient as an individual with personal value and belief systems that impact upon his/her attitude and response to the care that is provided by the organization.[4]

HOLISTIC NURSING

Two major challenges in nursing have emerged in the twenty-first century. The first is to integrate the concepts of technology, mind, and spirit into nursing practice; the second is to create and integrate models for health care that guide the healing of self and others. Holistic nursing is the most complete way to conceptualize and prac-

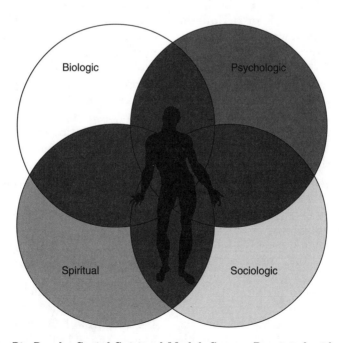

Figure 1–2 The Bio-Psycho-Social-Spiritual Model. *Source:* Reprinted with permission from C.E. Guzzetta and B.M. Dossey, *Cardiovascular Nursing: Holistic Practice*, p. 6, © 1992, Mosby Year Book.

tice professional nursing. The AHNA description of holistic nursing and holism appears in Appendix 1–A.[5] (See the Resource List at the end of the chapter for AHNA's address.)

Standards of Holistic Nursing Practice

The AHNA Standards of Holistic Nursing Practice define and establish the scope of holistic practice and describe the level of care expected from a holistic nurse (Appendix 1–A).[6] These standards have been recently revised as a result of a sophisticated research study on the professional knowledge, activities, and skills required to practice holistic nursing on a day-to-day basis. Over a 3-year period, an AHNA Task Force gathered data from the professional literature; educational and clinical programs; academic, clinical, and research content experts; and a representative sample of AHNA's membership. The data were used to develop the Inventory of Professional Activities and Knowledge of a Holistic Nurse (IPAKHN). After it was revised based on recommendations from the National League for Nursing,[7] the IPAKHN was sent to the AHNA membership with a request that they prioritize holistic nursing activities and knowledge. Thus, the data-gathering process captured the "real" world or the core concepts of holistic nursing based on the consensus of nearly 700 people.

The blueprint or framework of the Standards made it possible to develop the *Core Curriculum for Holistic Nursing,*[8] which delineates the fundamental knowledge, competencies, theories, and research for holistic nursing. In turn, the current edition of this book as well as *Essential Readings in Holistic Nursing*[9] were developed to expand and augment the knowledge of the *Core Curriculum;* all three can be used as major references in teaching holistic nursing as well as in preparing for AHNA's holistic nursing certification exam. The

AHNA's certification examination also originated in the blueprint of the Standards. It provides a yardstick by which to measure and confirm that certain individuals are competent to practice holistic nursing as defined by the AHNA. Nurses who pass the examination earn the distinction of certification in holistic nursing and can use the initials HNC (i.e., holistic nurse certified) after their name, along with those of their other credentials.

The revised AHNA Standards of Holistic Nursing Practice now reflect five core values of holistic nursing, each of which has an accompanying description and standard-of-practice action statements (Figure 1–3). The Standards are to be used in conjunction with the American Nurses' Association Standards of Practice and the standards of the specific specialty in which holistic nurses practice. They are to be implemented in one's personal life, clinical and private practice, education, research, and community service. Depending on the setting or area of practice, however, holistic nurses may or may not use all of the action statements.

The Standards describe a diversity of nursing activities in which holistic nurses are engaged. They are based on the philosophy that nursing is an art and a science whose primary purpose is to provide services that enable individuals, families, and communities to achieve their inherent wholeness. The concepts embodied in the Standards incorporate a sensitive balance between art and science, intuitive and analytic skills, and the ability to understand the interconnectedness of the body, mind, and spirit.

ERAS OF MEDICINE

Three eras of medicine currently are operational in Western biomedicine (Figure 1–4 and Table 1–2).[10] Era I medicine began to take shape in the 1860s when medicine was striving to become increasingly scientific. The underlying assumption of this ap-

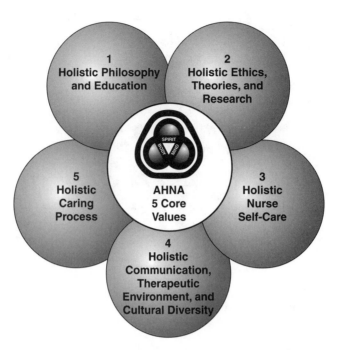

Figure 1-3 The Five Core Values Embodied in the Standards of Holistic Nursing Practice of the American Holistic Nurses' Association (AHNA). *Source:* Copyright © American Holistic Nurses' Association (AHNA).

proach is that health and illness are completely physical in nature. The focus is on combining drugs, medical treatments, and technology. A person's consciousness is considered a by-product of the chemical, anatomic, and physiologic aspects of the brain and is not considered a major factor in the origins of health or disease.

In the 1950s, Era II therapies began to emerge. These therapies reflect the growing awareness that the actions of a person's mind or consciousness—thoughts, emotions, beliefs, meaning, and attitudes—exert important effects on the behavior of the person's physical body. In both Era I and Era II, a person's consciousness is said to be "local" in nature, that is, confined to a specific location in space (the body itself) and in time (the present moment and a single lifetime).

Era III, the newest and most advanced era, originated in science. Consciousness is said to be nonlocal in that it is not bound to individual bodies. The minds of individuals are spread throughout space and time; they are infinite, immortal, omnipresent, and, ultimately, one. Era III therapies involve any therapy in which the effects of consciousness create bridges between different persons, as with distant healing, intercessory prayer, shamanic healing, so-called miracles, and certain emotions (e.g., love, empathy, compassion). Era III approaches involve transpersonal experiences of being. They raise a person above control at a day-to-day, material level to an experience outside his or her local self.

"Doing" and "Being" Therapies

Holistic nurses use both "doing" and "being" therapies (Figure 1–5). Doing therapies include almost all forms of modern medicine, such as medications, procedures, di-

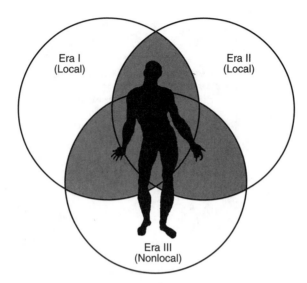

Figure 1–4 Eras of Medicine. *Source:* Adapted with permission from L. Dossey, *Reinventing Medicine: Beyond Mind-Body to a New Era of Healing,* Copyright © 1999, Harper San Francisco.

etary manipulations, radiation, and acupuncture. In contrast, being therapies do not employ things, but use states of consciousness, such as imagery, prayer, meditation, and quiet contemplation, as well as the presence and intention of the nurse. These techniques are therapeutic because of the power of the psyche to affect the body. They may be either directed or nondirected.[11] A person who uses a directed mental strategy attaches a specific outcome, such as the regression of disease or the normalization of the blood pressure, to the imagery, for example. In a nondirected approach, the person images the best outcome for the situation, but does not try to direct the situation or assign a specific outcome to the strategy. This reliance on the inherent intelligence within one's self to come forth is a way of acknowledging the intrinsic wisdom and self-correcting capacity from within.

It is obvious that Era I medicine uses "doing" therapies that are highly directed in their approach. It employs things, such as medications, for a specific goal. Era II medicine is a classic bodymind approach that does not require the use of things, with the exception of biofeedback instrumentation to increase awareness of bodymind connections. It employs "being" therapies that can be directed or nondirected, depending on the mental strategies selected (e.g., relaxation or meditation). Era III medicine is similar in this regard. It requires a willingness to become aware, moment by moment, of what is true for our inner and outer experience. It is actually a "not doing" so that we can become conscious of releasing, emptying, trusting, and acknowledging that we have done our best, regardless of the outcome. As the therapeutic potential of the mind becomes increasingly clear, all therapies and all people are seen to have a transcendent quality. The minds of all people, including families, friends, and the health care team, both those in close proximity and those at a distance, flow together in a collective as they work to create healing and health.

Table 1–2 Eras of Medicine

	Era I	Era II	Era III
Space-Time Characteristic	Local	Local	Nonlocal
Synonym	Mechanical, material, or physical medicine	Mindbody medicine	Nonlocal or transpersonal medicine
Description	Causal, deterministic, describable by classical concepts of space-time and matter-energy. Mind not a factor; "mind" a result of brain mechanisms.	Mind a major factor in healing *within* the single person. Mind has causal power; is thus not fully explainable by classical concepts in physics. Includes but goes beyond Era I.	Mind a factor in healing both *within* and *between* persons. Mind not completely localized to points in space (brains or bodies) or time (present moment or single lifetimes). Mind is unbounded and infinite in space and time—thus omnipresent, eternal, and ultimately unitary or one. Healing at a distance is possible. Not describable by classical concepts of space-time or matter-energy.
Examples	Any form of therapy focusing solely on the effects of *things* on the body is an Era I approach—including techniques such as acupuncture and homeopathy, the use of herbs, etc. Almost all forms of "modern" medicine—drugs, surgery, irradiation, CPR, etc.—are included.	Any therapy emphasizing the effects of consciousness solely within the individual body is an Era II approach. Psychoneuroimmunology, counseling, hypnosis, biofeedback, relaxation therapies, and most types of imagery-based "alternative" therapies are included.	Any therapy in which effects of consciousness bridge between different persons is an Era III approach. All forms of distant healing, intercessory prayer, some types of shamanic healing, diagnosis at a distance, telesomatic events, and probably noncontact therapeutic touch are included.

Source: Reprinted with permission from L. Dossey, *Reinventing Medicine: Beyond Mind-Body to a New Era of Healing,* copyright © 1999, Harper San Francisco.

Rational vs. Paradoxical Healing

All healing experiences or activities can be arranged along a continuum from the rational domain to the paradoxical domain.[12] The degree of doing and being involved determines these domains (Figure 1–6). Rational healing experiences include those therapies or events that make sense to our linear, intellectual thought processes, whereas paradoxical healing experiences include healing events that may seem absurd or contradictory but are, in fact, true.

"Doing" therapies fall into the rational healing category. Based on science, these strategies conform to our world view of common sense notions. Often, the professional can follow an algorithm, which dictates a step-by-step approach. Examples of rational healing include surgery, irradiation, medications, exercise, and diet.

On the other hand, "being" therapies fall into the paradoxical healing category, because they frequently happen without a scientific explanation. In psychological counseling, for example, a breakthrough is

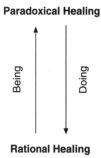

Paradoxical Healing

Being   Doing

Rational Healing

Figure 1–5 "Being" and "Doing" Therapies. *Source:* Reprinted with permission from L. Dossey, *Meaning and Medicine: A Doctor's Tales of Breakthrough and Healing*, p. 204, © 1991, Bantam Books.

a paradox. When a patient has a psychologic breakthrough, it is clear that there is a new meaning for the person; there are no clearly delineated steps leading to the breakthrough, however. Such an event is called a breakthrough for the very reason that it is unpredictable—thus, the paradox.

Biofeedback also involves a paradox. The best way to reduce blood pressure or muscle tension, or to increase peripheral blood flow, for example, is to give up trying and to learn how to be. Individuals can enter into a state of "being" or passive volition in which they let these physiologic states change in the desired direction. Similarly, the phenomenon of placebo is a paradox (see Chapter 9). If an individual has just a little discomfort, a placebo does not work very well. The more pain a person has, however, the more dramatic the response to a placebo medication can be. In addition, a person who does not know that the medication is a placebo responds best. This is referred to as the "paradox of success through ignorance."

Prayer and faith fall into the domain of paradox, because there is no rational scientific explanation for their effectiveness. Scientific studies are being conducted, however.[13] In a prayer study done by Byrd, for example, 5 to 7 people prayed each day

in Protestant and Catholic prayer groups across the United States for each of 201 patients with acute myocardial infarction.[14] Those in a control group of 192 patients with acute myocardial infarction were not prayed for, although they received the same medical care as the prayed-for group. In this 10-month randomized, prospective double-blind study, the following significant events occurred:

1. Patients in the prayed-for group were five times less likely than were those in the control group to require antibiotics (3 patients compared to 16 patients).
2. They were three times less likely to develop pulmonary edema (6 patients compared to 18 patients).
3. None of the prayed-for group required endotracheal intubation, although 12

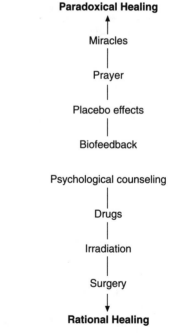

Paradoxical Healing

Miracles

Prayer

Placebo effects

Biofeedback

Psychological counseling

Drugs

Irradiation

Surgery

Rational Healing

Figure 1–6 Continuum of Rational and Paradoxical Healing. *Source:* Reprinted with permission from L. Dossey, *Meaning and Medicine: A Doctor's Tales of Breakthrough and Healing*, p. 205, © 1991, Bantam Books.

in the control group required mechanical ventilatory support.

4. Fewer patients in the prayed-for group died (although the difference was not statistically significant).

This study is an example of a nonlocal phenomenon, an Era III approach, because it involves the conscious effort of people praying for others at a distance.

"Miracle cures" also are paradoxical, because there is no scientific mechanism to explain them.[15] Every nurse has known, heard of, or read about a patient who had a severe illness that had been confirmed by laboratory evidence, but disappeared after the patient adopted a "being" approach. Some say that it was the natural course of the illness; some die, and some live. At shrines such as Lourdes in France and Medjugorje in Yugoslavia, however, people who experience a miracle cure are said to be totally immersed in a being state. They do not try to make anything happen. When interviewed, these people report experiencing a different sense of space and time; the flow of time as past, present, and future becomes an "eternal now." Birth and death take on new meaning and are not seen as a beginning and an end. These people go into the self and explore the "not I" to become empty so that they can understand the meaning of illness or present situations.

Complementary and Alternative Therapies

Also called unconventional or integrative therapies, complementary and alternative therapies traditionally have been defined as those interventions neither taught widely in medical schools nor generally available in U.S. hospitals.[16] More recently, it has been suggested that complementary and alternative therapies be defined as a broad set of health care practices (i.e., already available to the public) that are not readily integrated into the

dominant health care model because they challenge diverse societal beliefs and practices (cultural, economic, scientific, medical, and educational).[17]

In 1992, the National Institutes of Health (NIH) created the Office of Alternative Medicine (OAM) to evaluate alternative therapies.[18] The 1993 OAM research budget was $2 million. In 1998, the OAM was raised to the status of a freestanding center, the National Center for Complementary and Alternative Medicine (NCCAM) with a budget of $50 million (see Resource List for NCCAM's address).

One of the reasons for the NCCAM's creation was the federal government's recognition that U.S. citizens are pursuing complementary and alternative methods of health care with unprecedented enthusiasm. It has been estimated that 40 percent of all U.S. adults use some form of complementary and alternative therapies.[19,20] Between 1990 and 1997, the total number of visits to complementary and alternative practitioners increased nearly 50 percent, from 425 million visits to 629 million visits; by 1997, it exceeded the total number of visits to primary care physicians in the United States. Recent estimates for out-of-pocket expenditures for complementary and alternative care now range from $27 billion to $34 billion.[21]

One of the most disturbing trends is that patients are not disclosing to their allopathic physicians more than 60 percent of the complementary and alternative therapies used, thus creating a "don't ask, don't tell" scenario.[22] This finding also may help explain why many allopathic physicians believe that the controversy over alternative measures is a tempest in a teapot; they simply are unaware of what their patients are doing. In addition, skeptics frequently charge that persons interested in complementary and alternative medicine are poorly educated and, thus, easily misled. Researchers have found the opposite to be true. Consumers of complementary and alternative therapies tend to be well educated and to hold a holistic orientation, believing in the importance of body, mind, and spirit in health.[23,24]

The development of the NCCAM makes it possible to move beyond the personal testimonials, anecdotes, and the skepticism surrounding complementary and alternative therapies. One of the major missions of this center is to determine which of these therapies are safe, beneficial, and cost-effective and which are not. Because it charts a legitimate scientific course for the field and confirms that such research has merit, the creation of the NCCAM represents the single most important event in the evolution of the complementary and alternative therapies field. It authorizes practitioners and scientists to use the tools of rigorous science to demonstrate whether complementary and alternative therapies actually have the potential to change the clinical course and outcomes of an illness.[25] Nurses have the opportunity to play a major role in the future direction and investigation of many of these complementary and alternative interventions.

Defining the domain of complementary and alternative therapies was one of the first objectives of the NCCAM. Based on consensus of practitioners and clinicians, seven categories of complementary and alternative therapies were identified in (Exhibit 1–1).[26] Also within this exhibit are highlighted the therapies most frequently used by holistic nurses, according to the data collected from the AHNA's 3-year IPAKHN study discussed earlier. The category of mind/body therapies (ranging from biofeedback, guided imagery, hypnotherapy, meditation, music therapy, and relaxation to prayer) is predominant in the

---

Exhibit 1–1 Complementary and Alternative Therapies

Classification of the National Center for Complementary and Alternative Medicine (NCCAM)

I. Alternative Systems of Medical Practice

Health care ranging from self-care according to folk principles, to care rendered in an organized health care system based on alternative traditions or practices.

Acupuncture*
Anthroposophically extended medicine
Ayurveda
Community-based health care practices
Environmental medicine
Homeopathic medicine
Latin American rural practices
Native American practices
Natural products
Naturopathic medicine
Past life therapy
Shamanism
Tibetan medicine
Traditional oriental medicine

II. Bioelectromagnetic Applications

The study of how living organisms interact with electromagnetic (EM) fields.

Blue light treatment and artificial lighting
Electroacupuncture
Electromagnetic fields
Electrostimulation and neuromagnetic stimulation devices
Magnetoresonance spectroscopy

III. Diet, Nutrition, Lifestyle Changes

The knowledge of how to prevent illness, maintain health, and reverse the effects of chronic disease through dietary or nutritional intervention.

Changes in lifestyle*
Diet†
Gerson therapy
Macrobiotics
Megavitamins
Nutritional supplements

continues

Exhibit 1-1 continued

IV. Herbal Medicine

Employing plant and plant products from folk medicine traditions for pharmacologic use.

Echinacea (purple cornflower)
Ginger rhizome
Ginkgo biloba extract
Ginseng root
Wild chrysanthemum flower
Witch hazel
Yellowdock

V. Manual Healing

Using touch and manipulation with the hands as a diagnostic and therapeutic tool.

Acupressure*
Alexander technique
Biofield therapeutics
Chiropractic medicine
Feldenkrais method
Massage therapy*
Osteopathy
Reflexology*
Rolfing®
Therapeutic touch*
Trager method
Zone therapy

VI. Mind/Body Control

Exploring the mind's capacity to affect the body, based on traditional medical systems that make use of the interconnectedness of mind and body.

Art therapy*
Biofeedback*
Counseling*,†
Dance therapy
Guided imagery*
Humor therapy*
Hypnotherapy
Meditation*
Music therapy*
Prayer*
Psychotherapy
Relaxation techniques*
Support groups*
Yoga

VII. Pharmacologic and Biologic Treatments

Drugs and vaccines not yet accepted by mainstream medicine.

Antioxidizing agents
Cell treatment
Chelation therapy
Metabolic therapy
Oxidizing agents (ozone, hydrogen peroxide)

Additional Interventions Frequently Used by Holistic Nurses†

Aromatherapy
Autogenics
Breathing exercises
Cognitive therapy
Exercise and movement
Goal setting and contracting
Healing presence
Healing touch modalities
Holistic self-assessments
Journaling
Nutrition counseling
Play therapy
Self-care interventions
Self-reflection
Smoking cessation
Weight management

Source: Reprinted from B.M. Berman and D.B. Larson, Co-chairs, Editorial Review Board: *Alternative Medicine: Expanding Medical Horizons.* A Report to the National Institutes of Health on Alternative Medical Systems and Practices in the United States (Washington, DC: U.S. Government Printing Office, 1994).

*Frequently used interventions in holistic nursing practice. From B. Dossey, et al., Evolving a Blueprint for Certification: Inventory of Professional Activities and Knowledge of a Holistic Nurse, *Journal of Holistic Nursing* 16, no. 1 (1998):33–56.

†Used to provide support to those experiencing situations such as addictions, death, grief, unhealthy environments, sexual abuse, and violence; to promote wellness; and to resolve relationship and lifestyle issues.

holistic nursing domain, undoubtedly because these therapies have the potential to
affect the body-mind-spirit. To date, the
NIH has funded dozens of studies to evaluate such therapies as acupressure, massage therapy, electrochemical treatments,
hypnosis, music therapy, guided imagery,
biofeedback, prayer, antioxidants, and
herbs.

In addition, the NCCAM has funded 13
complementary and alternative medicine
research centers (Table 1–3). Each research
center focuses on specific chronic health
conditions and is responsible for evaluating
the effectiveness and safety of complementary and alternative treatments in their specialty area. The research centers establish
mechanisms by which promising comple-

Table 1–3 Research Centers To Evaluate Complementary and Alternative Therapies

Research Center	Objectives	Specialty
Center for Addiction and Alternative Medicine Research (University of Minnesota Medical School and Hennepin County Medical Center, Minneapolis)	To investigate the use, applicability, and effectiveness of selected alternative modalities in the treatment of addiction, as well as the health and psychologic complications of substance abuse	Addictions
Complementary and Alternative Medicine Program at Stanford (Stanford University, Palo Alto, CA)	To provide a mechanism to evaluate systematically the effectiveness of selective alternative medicine therapies for enhancing functional capacity and quality of life while decreasing physical disability and frailty in elders; provide technical help to alternative medicine practitioners for objective assessment of alternative medicine therapies; promote the understanding of alternative medicine to enhance physical functioning of elders; and disseminate responsible information regarding alternative medicine	Aging
Center for Alternative Medicine Research in Asthma and Immunology (University of California, Davis)	To identify potential treatments and develop protocols to evaluate the efficacy of alternative medicine practices in the treatment of asthma; to facilitate the exchange of pertinent information, development of educational forums, and communications with health care professionals and the general public regarding alternative approaches and research findings	Asthma, allergy, and immunology
University of Michigan Complementary and Alternative Medicine Research Center for Cardiovascular Diseases (University of Michigan, Ann Arbor)	Newly funded	Cardiovascular diseases
University of Texas Center for Alternative Medicine (University of Texas Health Science Center, Houston)	To evaluate the efficacy of biopharmacologic–herbal therapies for cancer prevention and treatment	Cancer

continues

Table 1–3 continued

Research Center	Objectives	Specialty
Consortial Center for Chiropractic Research (Palmer Center for Chiropractic Research, Davenport, IA)	To examine the potential effectiveness and validity of chiropractic health care	Chiropractic
Center for Alternative Medicine Research (Beth Israel Hospital, Deaconess Medical Center, Harvard Medical School, Boston, MA)	To investigate complementary and alternative therapies as they apply to common chronic medical conditions (e.g., low back pain and ischemic heart disease)	General medical conditions
Bastyr University AIDS Research Center (Bastyr University, Bothell, WA)	To describe forms and patterns of the use of alternative medical therapies for the treatment of patients with human immunodeficiency virus (HIV) infection and acquired immune deficiency syndrome (AIDS); evaluate the effectiveness of alternative therapies for the treatment of HIV/AIDS from five program areas of alternative medicine: nutrition, traditional and ethnomedicine, energetic therapies, pharmacologic and biologic therapies, and bioelectromagnetic medicine	HIV/AIDS
University of Virginia Center for the Study of Complementary and Alternative Therapies (University of Virginia, School of Nursing, Charlottesville)	To establish a mechanism that stimulates research in complementary and alternative therapies for pain management, including the evaluation of the effectiveness, safety, and cost of selected therapies	Pain
Center for Alternative Medicine Pain Research and Evaluation (University of Maryland School of Medicine, Baltimore)	To promote scientific research on a variety of complementary and alternative medicine practices for the treatment of pain	Pain
Program in Integrative Medicine (University of Arizona, Health Sciences Center, Tucson)	Newly funded	Pediatric conditions
Center for Research in Complementary and Alternative Medicine for Stroke and Neurological Disorders (Kessler Institute for Rehabilitation, West Orange, NJ)	To examine the potential effectiveness and validity of alternative medicine therapies as applied to the rehabilitation of stroke and related medical conditions	Stroke and neurologic conditions
Center for Complementary and Alternative Medicine Research in Women's Health (Columbia University, New York)	To conduct collaborative research in high-priority areas of women's health	Women's health issues

mentary and alternative research ideas can be reviewed, developed, and executed in a scientifically rigorous manner. As a result of these investigative studies, many of the so-called complementary and alternative therapies are likely to be found ineffective. Some will be shown to be worthless or actually harmful. Others, however, will almost certainly be validated as genuinely effective, safe, and relatively inexpensive when compared to conventional modalities.

The ultimate goal of the complementary and alternative therapies movement is not to supplant modern medicine with alternatives, but rather to integrate validated alternative approaches with the best of current conventional medical practices. For example, cancer treatment appears to be a particularly fertile area in which to investigate the best combination of conventional modalities (i.e., surgery, radiation, and chemotherapy) and alternative strategies (i.e., nutrition, vitamins, exercise, group support, visual imagery, and relaxation) to enhance bio-psycho-social-spiritual outcomes.[27] Thus, complementary and alternative therapies must be considered adjuncts to conventional medical and surgical treatments rather than replacements for them.

Complementary and alternative therapies expand the strategies that nurses can employ independently to provide holistic, body-mind-spirit care. For centuries, nurses have largely kept the spirit of caring and healing alive in Western cultures, while medical science has sought a physical answer for every question. The caring–healing paradigm is at the very root of professional nursing practice. The modern nurse healer is a hybrid of scientific skill and spiritual commitment who understands that healing is much more than curing disease. Such nurses understand that they do not heal *disease* (i.e., the pathophysiologic breakdown of the body); rather, they facilitate healing in the *person with an illness* who not only has disease, but also is struggling with the human experience of that disease in terms of its symptoms, suffering, and consequences to find the wholeness embodied in the experience.[28] Many of the complementary and alternative practitioners have been taught both to attend competently to the physical illness and suffering that accompany disease and to provide patients with the understanding, meaning,

and self-care strategies that they need to deal with their condition.[29]

Although many patients cannot be—or choose not to be—cured, they all are in need of healing. Even during devastating illness, crisis, and death, healing can take place, and growth toward wholeness can occur.[30] This caring–healing paradigm opens an exciting new frontier to nurses who are willing to pursue knowledge, expertise, and research in complementary and alternative modalities. By integrating complementary and alternative therapies into traditional clinical environments, these nurses will bring true healing to the forefront of health care.[31]

RELATIONSHIP-CENTERED CARE

In 1994, the Pew Health Professions Commission published its report on relationship-centered care. This report serves as a guideline for addressing the bio-psycho-social-spiritual dimensions of individuals in integrating caring, healing, and holism into health care.[32] The guidelines are based on the tenet that relationships and interactions among people constitute the foundation for all therapeutic activities.

The three components of relationship-centered care include the patient–practitioner relationship (Table 1–4), the community–practitioner relationship (Table 1–5), and the practitioner–practitioner relationship (Table 1–6). Each of these interrelated relationships is essential within a reformed system of health care, and each involves a unique set of tasks and responsibilities that address self-awareness, knowledge, values, and skills.

Patient–Practitioner Relationship

In a patient–practitioner relationship, the practitioner incorporates comprehensive biotechnologic care as well as psycho-social-spiritual care. Active collaboration with the patient and family in the decision-

Table 1–4 Patient–Practitioner Relationship: Areas of Knowledge, Skills, and Values

Area	Knowledge	Skills	Values
Self-awareness	Knowledge of self Understanding self as a resource to others	Reflect on self and work	Importance of self-awareness, self-care, self-growth
Patient experience of health and illness	Role of family, culture, community in development Multiple components of health Multiple threats and contributors to health as dimensions of one reality	Recognize patient's life story and its meaning View health and illness as part of human development	Appreciation of the patient as a whole person Appreciation of the patient's life story and the meaning of the health-illness condition
Developing and maintaining caring relationships	Understanding of threats to the integrity of the relationship (e.g., power inequalities) Understanding of potential for conflict and abuse	Attend fully to the patient Accept and respond to distress in patient and self Respond to moral and ethical challenges Facilitate hope, trust, and faith	Respect for patient's dignity, uniqueness, and integrity (mind-body-spirit unity) Respect for self-determination Respect for person's own power and self-healing processes
Effective communication	Elements of effective communication	Listen Impart information Learn Facilitate the learning of others Promote and accept patient's emotions	Importance of being open and nonjudgmental

Source: Pew Health Professions Commission at the Center for the Health Professions, University of California, San Francisco, 1388 Sutter Street, Suite 805, San Francisco, California 94109, (415) 476-8181.

making process, promotion of health, and prevention of stress and illness within the family are also part of the relationship. A successful relationship involves active listening and effective communication; integration of the elements of caring, healing, values, and ethics to enhance and preserve the dignity and integrity of the patient and family; and a reduction of the power inequalities in the relationship with regard to race, sex, education, occupation, and socioeconomic status.

To work effectively within the patient–practitioner relationship, the practitioner must develop specific knowledge, skills, and values (see Table 1–4), including expanding self-awareness, understanding the patient's experience of health and illness, developing and maintaining caring relationships with patients, and communicating clearly and effectively.[33]

Community–Practitioner Relationship

The patient and his or her family simultaneously belong to many types of communities, such as the immediate family, relatives,

Table 1-5 Community–Practitioner Relationship: Areas of Knowledge, Skills, and Values

Area	Knowledge	Skills	Values
Meaning of community	Various models of community Myths and misperceptions about community Perspectives from the social sciences, humanities, and systems theory Dynamic change—demographic, political, industrial	Learn continuously Participate actively in community development and dialogue	Respect for the integrity of the community Respect for cultural diversity
Multiple contributors to health within the community	History of community, land use, migration, occupations, and their effect on health Physical, social, and occupational environments and their effects on health External and internal forces influencing community health	Critically assess the relationship of health care providers to community health Assess community and environmental health Assess implications of community policy affecting health	Affirmation of relevance of all determinants of health Affirmation of the value of health policy in community services Recognition of the presence of values that are destructive to health
Developing and maintaining community relationships	History of practitioner–community relationships Isolation of the health care community from the community-at-large	Communicate ideas Listen openly Empower others Learn Facilitate the learning of others Participate appropriately in community development and activism	Importance of being open-minded Honesty regarding the limits of health science Responsibility to contribute health expertise
Effective community-based care	Various types of care, both formal and informal Effects of institutional scale on care Positive effects of continuity of care	Collaborate with other individuals and organizations Work as member of a team or healing community Implement change strategies	Respect for community leadership Commitment to work for change

Source: Pew Health Professions Commission at the Center for the Health Professions, University of California, San Francisco, 1388 Sutter Street, Suite 805, San Francisco, California 94109, (415) 476-8181.

friends, co-workers, neighborhoods, religious and community organizations, and the hospital community. Practitioners must be sensitive to the impact of these various communities on patients and foster the collaborative activities of these communities as they interact with the patient and family.

The restraints or barriers within each community that block the patient's healing must be identified and improved to promote the patient's health and well-being.

The knowledge, skills, and values needed by practitioners to participate effectively in and work with various commu-

Table 1-6 Practitioner-Practitioner Relationship: Areas of Knowledge, Skills, and Values

Area	Knowledge	Skills	Values
Self-awareness	Knowledge of self	Reflect on self and needs Learn continuously	Importance of self-awareness
Traditions of knowledge in health professions	Healing approaches of various professions Healing approaches across cultures Historical power inequities across professions	Derive meaning from others' work Learn from experience within healing community	Affirmation and value of diversity
Building teams and communities	Perspectives on team-building from the social sciences	Communicate effectively Listen openly Learn cooperatively	Affirmation of mission Affirmation of diversity
Working dynamics of teams, groups, and organizations	Perspectives on team dynamics from the social sciences	Share responsibility responsibly Collaborate with others Work cooperatively Resolve conflicts	Openness to others' ideas Humility Mutual trust, empathy, support Capacity for grace

Source: Pew Health Professions Commission at the Center for the Health Professions, University of California, San Francisco, 1388 Sutter Street, Suite 805, San Francisco, California 94109, (415) 476-8181.

nities, as summarized in Table 1–5, include understanding the meaning of the community, recognizing the multiple contributors to health and illness within the community, developing and maintaining relationships with the community, and working collaboratively with other individuals and organizations to establish effective community-based care.[34]

Practitioner–Practitioner Relationship

Providing holistic care to patients and families can never take place in isolation, for it involves many diverse practitioner–practitioner relationships. Collaborative relationships entail shared planning and action toward common goals with joint responsibility for outcomes.[35] There is a difference, however, between multidisciplinary care and interdisciplinary care. Multidisciplinary care consists of the sequential provision of discipline-specific health care by various individuals. Interdisciplinary care, however, also includes

coordination, joint decision making, communication, shared responsibility, and shared authority.[36]

Because the cornerstone of all therapeutic and healing endeavors depends on the quality of the relationships formed among the practitioners caring for the patient, it is necessary for all practitioners to understand and respect one another's roles. Conventional and alternative practitioners need to learn about the diversity of therapeutic and healing modalities that they each use. In addition, conventional practitioners must be willing to integrate complementary and alternative practitioners and their therapies in practice (i.e., acupuncture, herbs, aromatherapy, touch therapies, music therapy, folk healers). Such integration requires learning about the experiences of different healers, being open to the potential benefits of different modalities, and valuing cultural diversity. Ultimately, the effectiveness of collaboration among practitioners depends on their ability to share problem solving, goal setting, and decision making within a trusting, collegial, and caring environment. Practitioners must work interdependently rather than autonomously, with each assuming responsibility and accountability for patient care. To form a practitioner–practitioner relationship requires the knowledge, skills, and values shown in Table 1–6, including developing self-awareness; understanding the diverse knowledge base and skills of different practitioners; developing teams and communities; and understanding the working dynamics of groups, teams, and organizations that can provide resource services for the patient and family.[37]

CONCLUSION

Holism embodies the view that an individual is an integrated whole, independent of and greater than the sum of the parts. Natural systems theory provides the understanding of the interconnectedness of natural structures in the universe, while the biopsycho-social-spiritual model serves as a guide to practice. With these frameworks, the goal of holistic nursing is to enhance the healing of the whole person from birth to death.[38] The new AHNA Standards of Holistic Nursing Practice define the ways to accomplish this goal, describing the scope of holistic practice and the level of care expected from a holistic nurse. Nurses can reduce the devastating effects of crisis and illness of individuals by using these frameworks and Standards to provide care to the whole person.

DIRECTIONS FOR FUTURE RESEARCH

1. Examine complementary and alternative therapies in nursing that can facilitate healing and determine which ones are effective for which conditions.
2. Contrast the value that patients and their families attach to healing modalities with the value that nurses attach to them.
3. Investigate anticipated or actual solutions or complications that result from complementary and alternative therapies.

NURSE HEALER REFLECTIONS

After reading this chapter, the nurse healer will be able to answer or begin a process of answering the following questions:

- How do I define holism?
- What holistic processes are in need of further development in my personal and professional life?
- When I use the words *Guiding Force, Higher Power, God,* or *Absolute,* what kind of link with a universal wholeness do I experience?

NOTES

1. L. von Bertalanffy, *General Systems Theory* (New York: George Braziller, 1972).
2. E. Lazlo, *The Systems View of the World* (New York: George Braziller, 1968).
3. B. Dossey, *American Holistic Nurses' Association Core Curriculum for Holistic Nursing* (Gaithersburg, MD: Aspen Publishers, 1997).
4. Patient Rights, *Accreditation Manual for Hospitals* (Oakbrook Terrace, IL: Joint Commission on Accreditation of Healthcare Organizations, Suppl., 1992).
5. American Holistic Nurses' Association, Description of Holistic Nursing, working description, January 1994; revised, 1998.
6. American Holistic Nurses' Association, American Holistic Nurses' Association Standards of Holistic Nursing Practice (Flagstaff, AZ: AHNA, 1998).

7. B. Dossey et al., Evolving a Blueprint for Certification: Inventory of Professional Activities and Knowledge of a Holistic Nurse, *Journal of Holistic Nursing* 16, no. 1 (1998):33–56.

8. B. Dossey, *Core Curriculum for Holistic Nursing.*

9. C.E. Guzzetta, *Essential Readings in Holistic Nursing* (Gaithersburg, MD: Aspen, 1998).

10. L. Dossey, *Reinventing Medicine: Beyond Mind-Body To a New Era of Healing* (San Francisco: Harper San Francisco, 1999).

11. L. Dossey, *Meaning and Medicine: A Doctor's Tales of Breakthrough and Healing* (New York: Bantam Books, 1991).

12. L. Dossey, *Healing Words: The Power of Prayer and the Practice of Medicine* (San Francisco: Harper San Francisco, 1993).

13. L. Dossey, *Be Careful What You Pray For: You Just Might Get It* (San Francisco: Harper, 1997).

14. R. Byrd, Positive Effects of Intercessory Prayer in a Coronary Care Unit Population, *Southern Medical Journal* 81 (1988):826.

15. L. Dossey, Cancelled Funerals: A Look at Miracle Cures, *Alternative Therapies in Health and Medicine* 4, no. 2 (1998):10–19.

16. D.M. Eisenberg et al., Unconventional Medicine in the United States: Prevalence, Costs, and Patterns of Use, *New England Journal of Medicine* 328, no. 4 (1993):246–252.

17. D.P. Eskinazi, Factors That Shape Alternative Medicine, *Journal of the American Medical Association* 280, no. 18 (1998):1621–1623.

18. C. Marwick, Alternative Therapies Studies Moves into New Phase, *Journal of the American Medical Association* 268, no. 21 (1992):3040.

19. D.M. Eisenberg et al., Trends in Alternative Medicine Use in the United States, 1990–1997, *Journal of the American Medical Association* 280, no. 18 (1998):1569–1575.

20. J. Astin, Why Patients Use Alternative Medicine: Results of a National Study, *Journal of the American Medical Association* 279, no. 19 (1998):1548–1553.

21. Eisenberg et al., Trends in Alternative Medicine Use, 1573.

22. Eisenberg et al., Trends in Alternative Medicine Use, 1575.

23. Eisenberg et al., Trends in Alternative Medicine Use, 1571.

24. Astin, Why Patients Use Alternative Medicine, 1553.

25. P.B. Fontanarosa and G.D. Lundberg, Alternative Medicine Meets Science, *Journal of the American Medical Association* 280, no. 18 (1998):1618–1619.

26. B.M. Berman and D.B. Larson, Cochairs, Editorial Review Board: Alternative Medicine: Expanding Medical Horizons. A report to the National Institutes of Health on alternative medical systems and practices in the United States (Washington, DC: U.S. Government Printing Office, 1994).

27. C.E. Guzzetta, Alternative Therapies: What's All the Fuss? *Nurse Investigator* 3, no. 2 (Summer, 1996):1–2.

28. C.E. Guzzetta, *Essential Readings in Holistic Nursing* (Gaithersburg, MD: Aspen Publishers, 1998).

29. W.B. Jonas, Alternative Medicine—Learning from the Past, Examining the Present, Advancing the Future, *Journal of the American Medical Association* 280, no. 18 (1998):1616–1617.

30. M.A. Chulay et al., *AACN Handbook of Critical Care Nursing* (Stamford, CT: Appleton & Lange, 1997).

31. D. Milton and S.D. Benjamin, *Complementary & Alternative Therapies: An Implementation Guide to Integrative Health Care* (Chicago: AHA Press, 1999).

32. Pew–Fetzer Task Force on Advancing Psychosocial Health Education, *Health Professions Education and Relationship-Centered Care* (San Francisco: Pew Health Professions Commission and the Fetzer Institute, 1994).

33. Pew–Fetzer Task Force, *Health Professions Education and Relationship-Centered Care.*

34. Pew–Fetzer Task Force, *Health Professions Education and Relationship-Centered Care.*

35. L.L. Lindeke and D.E. Block, Maintaining Professional Integrity in the Midst of Interdisciplinary Collaboration, *Nursing Outlook* 46 (1998):213–218.

36. Pew Health Professions Commission, California Primary Care Consortium, *Interdisciplinary Collaborative Teams in Primary Care: A Model Curriculum and Resource Guide* (San Francisco: Center for the Health Professions, University of California, 1995).

37. Pew–Fetzer Task Force, *Health Professions Education and Relationship-Centered Care.*

38. B.M. Dossey, *Florence Nightingale: Mystic, Visionary, Healer,* (Springhouse, PA: Springhouse Publishing, 1999).

RESOURCE LIST

American Holistic Nurses' Association
2733 E. Lakin Drive, Suite 2
Flagstaff, AZ 86004-2130
Telephone: 520-526-2196
Web site at http://www.ahna.org

National Center for Complementary and Alternative Medicine Clearinghouse
P.O. Box 8218
Silver Spring, MD 20907-8218
Toll-free telephone: 1-888-644-6226
Fax: 301-495-4957
Web site at http://altmed.od.nih.gov

American Holistic Nurses' Association (AHNA) Standards of Holistic Nursing Practice

AHNA Holistic Nursing Description

Guidelines

Interventions Most Frequently Used in Holistic Nursing Practice
(See Exhibit 1–1, pp. 16–17)

AHNA Holistic Nursing Practice Definitions (See Definitions, Chapter 1, pp. 5–6)

Summary of Core Values (See each Core Value Statement)

AHNA Standards of Holistic Nursing Practice

Core Value I.   Holistic Philosophy and Education

Core Value II.   Holistic Ethics, Theories, and Research

Core Value III.   Holistic Nurse Self-Care

Core Value IV.   Holistic Communication, Therapeutic Environment, and Cultural Diversity

Core Value V.   Holistic Caring Process

Note: To obtain a copy of AHNA Standards of Holistic Nursing Practice in the above format, contact AHNA at the address below.

AHNA HOLISTIC NURSING DESCRIPTION

Holistic nursing embraces all nursing which has enhancement of healing the whole person from birth to death as its goal. Holistic nursing recognizes that there are two views regarding holism: that holism involves identifying the interrelationships of the bio-psycho-social-spiritual dimensions of the person, recognizing that the whole is greater than the sum of its parts; and that holism involves understanding the individual as a unitary whole in mutual process with the environment. Holistic nursing responds to both views, believing that the goals of nursing can be achieved within either framework.

To facilitate the healing process and for nurses to become therapeutic partners with individuals, families, and communities, holistic nursing practice draws on nursing knowledge, theories, research, expertise, intuition, and creativity. Holistic nursing practice encourages peer review of professional practice in various clinical settings and integrates knowledge of current professional standards, laws, and regulations governing nursing practice.

Practicing holistic nursing requires nurses to integrate self-care in their lives. Self-responsibility leads the nurse to greater awareness of the interconnectedness with self, others, nature, and God/Life Force/Absolute/Transcendent. This awareness further enhances the nurses' understanding of all individuals and their relationships to the human and global community, and permits nurses to use this awareness to facilitate the healing process.

GUIDELINES

The AHNA Standards of Holistic Nursing Practice:

- are used in conjunction with the American Nurses' Association Standards of Practice and the specific specialty standards where holistic nurses practice.
- contain 5 core values that are followed by a description and standards of practice action statements. Depending on the setting or area of practice, holistic nurses may or may not use all of these action statements.
- draw on modalities derived from a number of explanatory models, of which biomedicine is only one model.
- reflect the diverse nursing activities in which holistic nurses are engaged.
- serve holistic nurses in personal life, clinical and private practice, education, research, and community service.

CORE VALUE I. HOLISTIC PHILOSOPHY AND EDUCATION

Holistic Philosophy

Holistic nurses develop and expand their conceptual framework and overall philosophy in the art and science of holistic nursing to model, practice, teach, and conduct research in the most effective manner possible.

Standards of Practice

Holistic nurses:

- recognize the person's capacity for self-healing and the importance of supporting the natural development and unfolding of that capacity.
- support, share, and recognize expertise and competency in holistic nursing practice that is used in many diverse clinical and community settings.
- participate in person-centered care by being a partner, coach, and mentor who actively listens and supports others in reaching personal goals.
- focus on strategies to bring harmony, unity, and healing to the nursing profession.

- communicate with traditional health care practitioners about appropriate referrals to other holistic practitioners when needed.
- interact with professional organizations in a leadership or membership capacity at local, state, national, and international levels to further expand the knowledge and practice of holistic nursing and awareness of holistic health issues.

Holistic Education

Holistic nurses acquire and maintain current knowledge and competency in holistic nursing practice.

Standards of Practice

Holistic nurses:

- participate in activities of continuing education and related fields that have relevance to holistic nursing practice.
- identify areas of knowledge from nursing and various fields such as biomedicine, epidemiology, behavioral medicine, cultural and social theories.
- continually develop and standardize holistic nursing guidelines, protocols and practice to promote competency in holistic nursing practice and assure quality of care to individuals.
- use the results of quality care activities to initiate change in holistic nursing practice.
- may seek certification in holistic nursing as one means of advancing the philosophy and practice of holistic nursing.

CORE VALUE II. HOLISTIC ETHICS, THEORIES, AND RESEARCH

Holistic Ethics

Holistic nurses hold to a professional ethic of caring and healing that seeks to preserve wholeness and dignity of self, students, colleagues, and the person who is receiving care in all practice settings, be it in health promotion, birthing centers, acute or chronic care facilities, end-of-life centers, and in homes.

Standards of Practice

Holistic nurses:

- identify the ethics of caring and its contribution to unity of self, others, nature, and God/Life Force/Absolute/Transcendent as central to holistic nursing practice.
- integrate the standards of holistic nursing practice with applicable state laws and regulations governing nursing practice.
- engage in activities that respect, nurture, and enhance the integral relationship with the earth, and advocate for the well-being of the global community's economy, education, and social justice.
- advocate for the rights of patients to have educated choices into their plan of care.
- participate in peer evaluation to ensure knowledge and competency in holistic nursing practice.
- protect the personal privacy and confidentiality of individuals, especially with health care agencies and managed care organizations.

Holistic Theories

Holistic nurses recognize that holistic nursing theories provide the framework for all aspects of holistic nursing practice and transformational leadership.

Standards of Practice

Holistic nurses:

- strive to use nursing theories to develop holistic nursing practice and transformational leadership.

- interpret, use, and document information relevant to a person's care according to a theoretical framework.

Holistic Nursing and Related Research

Holistic nurses provide care and guidance to persons through nursing interventions and holistic therapies consistent with research findings and other sound evidence.

Standards of Practice

Holistic nurses:

- use available research and evidence from different explanatory models to mutually create a plan of care with a person.
- use expert clinical judgment to select appropriate interventions.
- discuss holistic application to clinical situations where rigorous research has not been done.
- create an environment conducive to systematic inquiry into healing and health issues by engaging in research or supporting and utilizing the research of others.
- disseminate research findings at meetings and through publications to further develop the foundation and practice of holistic nursing.
- provide consultation services on holistic nursing interventions to persons and communities based on research.

CORE VALUE III. HOLISTIC NURSE SELF-CARE

Holistic Nurse Self-Care

Holistic nurses engage in self-care and further develop their own personal awareness as being an instrument of healing to better serve self and others.

Standards of Practice

Holistic nurses:

- recognize that a person's body-mind-spirit has healing capacities that can be enhanced and supported through self-care practices.
- identify and integrate self-care strategies to enhance their physical, psychological, sociological, and spiritual well-being.
- recognize and address at-risk health patterns and begin the process of change.
- consciously cultivate awareness and understanding about the deeper meaning, purpose, inner strengths, and connections with self, others, nature, and God/Life Force/Absolute/Transcendent.
- use clear intention to care for self and to seek a sense of balance, harmony, and joy in daily life.
- participate in the evolutionary holistic process with the understanding that crisis creates opportunity in any setting.

CORE VALUE IV. HOLISTIC COMMUNICATION, THERAPEUTIC ENVIRONMENT, AND CULTURAL DIVERSITY

Holistic Communication

Holistic nurses engage in holistic communication to ensure that each person experiences the presence of the nurse as authentic and sincere; there is an atmosphere of shared humanness that includes a sense of connectedness and attention reflecting the individual's uniqueness.

Standards of Practice

Holistic nurses:

- develop an awareness of the most frequently encountered challenges to holistic communication.

- increase therapeutic and cultural competence skills to enhance their effectiveness through listening to themselves and others.
- explore with each person those strategies that can assist her/him, as desired, to understand the deeper meaning, purpose, inner strengths, and connections with self, others, nature, and God/Life Force/Absolute/ Transcendent.
- recognize that holistic communication and awareness of individuals is a continuously evolving multi-level exchange that offers itself through dreams, images, symbols, sensations, meditations, and prayers.
- respect the person's health trajectory which may be incongruent with conventional wisdom.

Therapeutic Environment

Holistic nurses recognize that each person's environment includes everything that surrounds the individual, both the external and internal (physical, mental, emotional, and spiritual), as well as patterns not yet understood.

Standards of Practice

Holistic nurses:

- promote environments conducive to experiencing healing, wholeness and harmony, and care for the person in as healthy an environment as possible.
- work toward creating organizations that value sacred space and environments that enhance healing.
- integrate holistic principles, standards, policies, and procedures in relation to environmental safety and emergency preparedness.
- recognize that the well-being of the ecosystem of the planet is a prior determining condition for the well-being of the human.

- promote social networks and social environments where healing can take place.

Cultural Diversity

Holistic nurses recognize each person as a whole being of body-mind-spirit and mutually create a plan of care consistent with cultural backgrounds, health beliefs, sexual orientation, values, and preferences.

Standards of Practice

Holistic nurses:

- assess and incorporate the person's cultural practices, values, beliefs, meaning of health, illness, and risk behaviors in care and health education.
- use appropriate community resources and experts to extend their understanding of different cultures.
- assess for discriminatory practices and change as necessary.
- identify discriminatory health care practices as they impact the person and engage in effective nondiscriminatory practices.

CORE VALUE V. HOLISTIC CARING PROCESS

Assessment

Each person is assessed holistically using appropriate traditional and holistic methods while the uniqueness of the person is honored.

Standards of Practice

Holistic nurses:

- use an assessment process including appropriate traditional and holistic methods to systematically gather information.
- value all types of knowing including intuition when gathering data from a

person and validate this intuitive knowledge with the person when appropriate.

Patterns/Problems/Needs

Each person's actual and potential patterns/problems/needs and life processes related to health, wellness, disease, or illness which may or may not facilitate well-being are identified and prioritized.

Standards of Practice

Holistic nurses:

- assist the person to access inner wisdom that can provide opportunities to enhance and support growth, development, and movement toward health and well-being.
- collect data and collaborate with the person and health care team members as appropriate to identify and record a list of actual and potential patterns/problems/needs.
- use collected data to formulate an etiology of the person's identified actual or potential patterns/problems/needs.
- make referrals to other holistic practitioners or traditional therapist when appropriate.

Outcomes

Each person's actual or potential patterns/problems/needs have appropriate outcomes specified.

Standards of Practice

Holistic nurses:

- honor the person in all phases of her/his healing process regardless of expectations or outcomes.
- identify and partner with the person to specify measurable outcomes and realistic goals.

Therapeutic Care Plan

Each person engages with the holistic nurse to mutually create an appropriate plan of care that focuses on health promotion, recovery, restoration, or peaceful dying so that the person is as independent as possible.

Standards of Practice

Holistic nurses:

- partner with the person in a mutual decision process to create a health care plan for each pattern/problem/need or opportunity to enhance health and well-being.
- help a person identify areas for education to make decisions about life choices in a conscious, informed manner that empowers the person to maintain her/his uniqueness and independence.
- offer self-assessment tools, word associations, storytelling, dreams, journals as appropriate.
- use skills of cultural competence and communicate acceptance of the person's values, belief, culture, religion, and socioeconomic background.
- assist the person in recognizing at-risk patterns/problems/needs for potential or existing health situations (e.g., personal habits, personal and family health history, age-related risk factors), and also assist in recognizing opportunities to enhance well-being.
- engage the person in problem-solving dialogue in relation to living with changes secondary to illness and treatment.

Implementation

Each person's plan of holistic care is prioritized and holistic nursing interventions are implemented accordingly.

Standards of Practice

Holistic nurses:

- implement the mutually created plan of care within the context of assisting the person toward the higher potential of health and well-being.
- support and promote the person's capacity for the highest level of participation and problem solving in the plan of care and collaborate with other health team members when appropriate.
- use holistic nursing skills in implementing care including cultural competency and all ways of knowing.
- advocate that the person's plan, choices, and unique healing journey be honored.
- provide care which is clear about and respectful of the economic parameters of practice, balancing justice with compassion.

Evaluation

Each person's responses to holistic care are regularly and systematically evaluated and the continuing holistic nature of the healing process is recognized and honored.

Standards of Practice

Holistic nurses:

- collaborate with the person and with other health care team members when appropriate in evaluating holistic outcomes.
- explore with the person her/his understanding of the cause of any significant deviation between the responses and the expected outcomes.
- mutually create with the person and other team members a revised plan if needed.

VISION OF HEALING

The Transpersonal Self

The act of synchronizing mind and body is not a random technique that someone created for self-improvement. Rather, it is a basic principle of the human experience: the integration of body, mind, and spirit. In exploring the foundations for healing self and facilitating healing in others, we nurses mature and exercise our human capacity to go beyond individual identity and evolve to our highest potential—the transpersonal self. Understanding the dimensions of the transpersonal self is a major force in our ability to enhance healing in our self and others. Yet, knowing states of the transpersonal self is not an end point, but a continuing, never ending process.

Throughout history, there has been a quest and universal need to understand why there is human life and what happens after death. This body of knowledge is perennial philosophy—philosophia perennis. Roots of perennial philosophy are found in all traditional lore, from the most primitive to the most highly developed cultures. The three major elements of perennial philosophy are

1. the metaphysics that recognizes a divine reality substantial to the world of things and lives and minds
2. the psychology that finds in the soul something similar to, or even identical with, divine reality

3. the ethics that places the human being's final end in the knowledge of the immanent and transcendent ground of all being—the thing is immemorial and universal[1]

In the writings of perennial philosophy, human beings are described as part of a whole, a part of the totality of the universe. In perennial philosophy, there are many levels of human consciousness, which are referred to as the Great Chain of Being. These levels begin with a physical level and move up to emotional, mental, existential, spiritual, and other levels. In different versions of the Great Chain, the levels of consciousness range in number from 3 to 20 or more. In order to reach wholeness, humans must understand the relationship of self with the universe and their existential identity; that is, we must come to terms with the finite nature of existence, accept our ego limitations, and be willing to face things as they appear in our life without denying that they exist.

Each level in the Great Chain transcends, but includes, its predecessor(s).[2] Each higher level contains functions, capacities, or structures not found on a lower level. The higher level does not violate the principles of the lower level; it simply is not exclusively bound to or explainable by them. All levels are available to us if we allow openness at each level. A person's wholeness and healing are determined by awareness of all levels. Absolute Spirit is that which transcends everything and includes everything.

As nurses reflect on the inner dimension of self and ways of being, this conscious journey toward wholeness evolves toward self-transcendence. Early in our personal ego development, self-consciousness arises as essential for healthy human development. As the self continues to develop and mature, however, different self-concepts, identities, and life experiences lead toward the conscious journey of inner understanding. The psyche has many layers of consciousness. As one moves more inward, seeking inner knowledge along with personal understanding, one experiences the Absolute that is composed of higher ordered wholes and integrations. Basic structures of the psyche are not replaced, but become part of the larger unity. The ultimate part of the journey is awakening, or enlightenment to the knowledge that one is part of the whole.

NOTES

1. A. Huxley, *The Perennial Philosophy* (New York: Harper Colophon Books, 1945), vii.

2. K. Wilbur, *Quantum Questions* (Boston: Shambhala Publications, 1984), 15–16.

Chapter 2

Transpersonal Human Caring and Healing

Janet F. Quinn

NURSE HEALER OBJECTIVES

Theoretical

- Define transpersonal human caring.
- Define healing.
- Compare and contrast the processes of healing and curing.
- Discuss the nature of "right relationship" as it relates to healing.

Clinical

- Apply the elements of a "caring occasion" to facilitate healing.
- Describe examples of healing at the body, mind, and spirit levels of human experience that you have observed in practice.
- Begin to imagine how your own clinical practice setting might evolve to become a true healing health care system.

Personal

- Imagine what right relationship would look like and feel like when it is applied to something you want to heal in yourself.

Portions of this chapter have been published as: J. Quinn, Healing: A Model for an Integrative Health Care System, *Advanced Practice Nursing Quarterly* 3, no. 1 (1997):1–7, by permission of Aspen Publishers.

- Identify ways in which you can create your own healing environment.
- Explore and celebrate an area of personal woundedness that has healed and has made you a better nurse.

DEFINITIONS

Healing: the emergence of right relationship at one or more levels of the body-mind-spirit system.[1]

Healing System: a true health care system in which people can receive adequate, nontoxic, and noninvasive assistance in maintaining wellness and in healing for body, mind, and spirit, together with the most sophisticated, aggressive curing technologies that are available.

Human Caring: the moral ideal of nursing in which the nurse brings his or her whole self into relationship with the whole self of the patient/client to protect the vulnerability and preserve the humanity and dignity of the one cared for.[2]

Right Relationship: a process of connection among or between parts of the whole that increases energy, coherence, and creativity in the whole body-mind-spirit system.

Transpersonal: that which transcends the limits and boundaries of individual ego identities and possibilities to include acknowledgment and appreciation of something greater. Transpersonal may refer to consciousness; intrapersonal dynamics; interpersonal relationships; and lived experiences of connection, unity, and oneness with the larger environment, cosmos, or Spirit.

THEORY AND RESEARCH

Within the discipline of nursing, there is widespread acceptance of the concept of caring as central to practice. There is no widespread consensus as to what caring is, however. Morse and her colleagues reported that five basic conceptualizations or perspectives on caring can be identified in the nursing literature: (1) caring as a human trait, (2) caring as a moral imperative or ideal, (3) caring as an affect, (4) caring as an interpersonal relationship, and (5) caring as a therapeutic intervention.[3]

The term *transpersonal human caring* is most often associated with Jean Watson's theory of nursing as the art and science of human caring. Watson defined human caring as the moral ideal of nursing in which the relationship between the whole self of the nurse and the whole self of the patient/client protects the vulnerability and preserves the humanity and dignity of the patient/client.[4] This emphasis on the whole self, the whole person of both nurse and patient, requires the addition of the term *transpersonal* in Watson's framework and in the discussion of human caring as it relates to holistic nursing practice. Within a transpersonal perspective, people are more than the body physical and the mind as contained in that body. A transpersonal perspective acknowledges that all people are body, mind, and spirit or soul, and that interactions between people engage each of these aspects of the self. A nurse with a transpersonal perspective recognizes that this is a fact of human interaction, not an optional event. A holistic nurse recognizes, as Watson suggested, that there is something beyond the personal, separate selves

of the nurse and the patient involved in the act of caring.

When nurses enter into caring–healing relationships with patients, bringing with them an acknowledgment and appreciation of the body, mind, and spirit dimensions of their own human existence, they are engaged in a transpersonal human caring process. In this type of relationship, they know themselves to be interconnected with the patient and with the larger environment and cosmos. They know that they are walking on sacred ground when they walk this path with their patients, and they recognize that neither will be the same afterward. For that moment, they are joined with the other who is patient, or client, and so become part of something larger than either alone. In this transpersonal healing process, they are each changed.[5]

Watson called these healing encounters "caring occasions" and suggested that they actually transcend the bounds of space and time. The field of consciousness created in and through the caring–healing relationship has the potential to continue healing the patient long after the physical separation of nurse and patient. Moreover, the nurse, following engagement in a true caring occasion, will also continue to benefit from the mutual process. When nurses are able to engage their full, caring selves in the art of nursing, it is energizing and satisfying. Today's nurses risk far more burnout due to the difficulty in finding the time to care with their whole selves in systems that do not value caring than they do from the often assumed cause of burnout, which is caring too much.

HEALING: THE GOAL OF HOLISTIC NURSING

While caring is the context for holistic nursing, healing is the goal. The origin of the word *heal* is the Anglo-Saxon word *haelan*, which means to be or to become whole. Defining what it means to be or become whole is a challenging task. For example, is wholeness a goal, an end point that is something to work toward, but rarely achieved? Is wholeness a state of perfection of body-mind-spirit? Is wholeness something that people either have or do not have, something that people can obtain and hold on to or something that comes and goes? Is it a state or a process? Is wholeness dependent on the structure and functioning of the body? Can one ever be *not* whole, that is, can one ever be other than wholly who/what one is at any point in space and time? If one cannot be *not* whole, then how is it possible to talk about becoming whole? Each holistic nurse should spend some time thinking about what this means to her or him, because a nurse's perspective on wholeness will influence everything that she or he does.

Healing As the Emergence of Right Relationship

Wholeness is frequently described as harmony of body, mind, and spirit, while harmony is defined as an ordered or aesthetically pleasing set of relationships among the elements of the whole. This simple definition illustrates the implications of associating harmony with healing. First, wholeness involves more than the intactness of physical structure and function, or the status of isolated parts of a person. Second, if healing is about harmony, it is necessary to expand the ways of knowing about healing to include the aesthetic as well as the scientific.

Synonyms for the word *harmony* include unity, integrity, connection, reconciliation, congruence, and cohesion. Taken together, these terms begin to suggest that wholeness is not necessarily a state of any kind, but a process that is fundamentally about relationship. Wholeness is about the relationship of the parts of a system to one another and to the larger systems of which

they are a part. When the great theoretical physicist David Bohm was asked, "How can anything become more whole if everything is already part of the indivisible wholeness of the implicit order of the universe?" he responded with one word. "Coherence," he said, creating no doubt that wholeness was not about adding and subtracting parts, but about how those parts related to each other.[6] Increasing the wholeness of a system is about establishing a pattern of relationships among its elements that is more and more coherent.

Healing, if it is a process of being or becoming whole, must be an emerging pattern of relationships among the elements of the whole person that leads to greater integrity, connection, and cohesion of the whole system. This pattern of relationships can be called right relationship.[7] Thus, healing is the emergence of right relationship at or between or among any and all levels of the human experience. It is a process rather than a state. It is dynamic, and it always affects the whole person, no matter at what level the shift actually occurs. Key to an understanding of the effects of a shift into right relationship at any level are theories about how systems, particularly living systems, work. The new sciences are "known collectively as the sciences of complexity, including general systems theory (Bertalanffy, Weiss), cybernetics (Wiener), non-equilibrium thermodynamics (Prigogine), cellular automata theory (von Neumann), catastrophe theory (Thom), autopoietic system theory (Maturana and Varela), dynamic systems theory (Shaw, Abraham), and chaos theories, among others."[8] Within a systems perspective, human beings are "holons,"[9] that is, simultaneously autonomous wholes and parts of larger wholes. Each holon is embedded in an "irreversible hierarchy of increasing wholeness, increasing holism, increasing unity and integration."[10]

Several principles related to the nature of systems are fundamental to all these theories and have direct implications for the understanding of healing. The first and most basic is that a system is more than and different from the sum of its parts. It is "more than" its parts because the pattern of relationships among the parts of the whole gives the system its own unique identity. "A pattern of organization (is) a configuration of relationships characteristic of a particular system."[11]

A second principle is that a change in the part always leads to a change in the whole. Because human beings are living systems governed by these principles, any shift, no matter how small or at what level it appears to occur, will always affect the whole body-mind-spirit. Furthermore, because every person is simultaneously a part of the larger whole of family, society, the ecosystem, and the universe, a change in an individual body-mind-spirit leads to a change in all of these as well. This awareness is, of course, part of the teaching of virtually every spiritual tradition, and it affirms that nurses' individual healing work matters to far more than just the nurses.

The third principle that relates directly to healing is that the nature of the change in the whole cannot be predicted by the nature of the change in the part. "The new state [of a system] is decided neither by initial conditions in the system nor by changes in the critical values of environmental parameters; when a dynamic system is fundamentally destabilized, it acts indeterminately."[12]

Human beings as living systems are self-organizing systems, capable of, indeed, striving toward order, self-transcendence, and transformation. "We are beginning to recognize the creative unfolding of life in forms of ever-increasing diversity and complexity as an inherent characteristic of all living systems."[13] Thus the healing process itself is inherent within the person. This urge toward healing, toward right relationship, when manifested, may be thought of as the "haelan effect."[14]

In the context of these principles, right relationship is not a moral judgment, a statement about right and wrong, good or bad. Rather, it is a way of understanding a particular quality of pattern and organization. The inherent tendency of any living system, as part of the evolutionary process, is toward actualizing its "deep structure"[15] (i.e., an acorn "wants" to actualize its inherent tree nature). The consequence of not being in right relationship is the tendency toward "self-dissolution."[16] Right relationship may be thought of as any pattern of organization within the system that supports, encourages, allows, or generates actualization and self-transcendence—at any or all levels. Thus, consistent with the tendencies inherent in all living systems healing, the emergence of right relationship, at any level, body, mind, or spirit

- increases coherence of the whole body-mind-spirit
- decreases disorder in the whole body-mind-spirit
- maximizes free energy in the whole body-mind-spirit
- maximizes freedom, autonomy, choice in the whole body-mind-spirit
- increases the capacity for creative unfolding of the whole body-mind-spirit

Because of its inherently creative nature, true healing is always a process of emergence into something new, rather than a simple return to prior states of being. Holistic nurses do not limit the focus of their care to recovery alone, but rather expand their focus to helping patients integrate their illness experience and transcend their former selves toward new patterns of self-actualization. This is the growth process of nature. Nightingale's statement that the goal is to put the patient in the best condition so that nature can act on him may refer to this natural, forward-moving tendency toward wholeness.[17]

Healing as the emergence of right relationship may occur at any level of the body-mind-spirit. For example, when an organ is transplanted, the emergence of right relationship between the new organ and the surrounding cells and tissues of the recipient's body-mind-spirit signals healing. If that right relationship does not occur, if the cells of the new organ do not become integrated into the existing body-mind-spirit, if rejection rather than acceptance happens, then the patient may die from a lack of right relationship, healing, at the cellular level. When broken bones knit together or when the edges of a wound begin to approximate, right relationship is emerging at the physical level. Each of these emerging right relationships has an impact on the whole, as noted earlier.

The effects on the whole person of a shift toward right relationship at the emotional level are evident in a moment of forgiveness or a release of a long-held resentment. At such a time, the way in which a person stands in relationship to an event and/or a person from the past changes. The letting-go of resentment carries with it an often overwhelming release of energy for new growth and an expanded consciousness. The body-mind-spirit of one who is experiencing forgiveness moves toward integration and transcendence of previous patterns and forms. Forgiveness of one's self or another has profound effects at every level of being.

Sometimes right relationship emerges at the spiritual level before it manifests itself anywhere else. In moments of deep love; of gratitude or of the sudden awareness that they are not alone, but are connected to everything and everyone else in the cosmos, individuals have come into right relationship with the transcendent dimensions of life—God, the One, Ultimate Reality, the Ground of being. The language is not as important as the recognition of change. Those who have this experience are more whole, more coherent, more free to become who they are most deeply meant to be, more healed.

Healing vs. Curing

Healing and curing are different processes. Curing is the elimination of the signs and symptoms of disease, which may or may not correspond to the end of the patient's disease or distress. The diagnosis and cure of disease provide the focus of modern health care (sickness–cure) system. This is not a wrong focus, only an incomplete one. When it is estimated that 85 percent of health problems are either self-limiting or chronic, it becomes clear that something in addition to a focus on the curing of diseases is required. That something is healing, which is different from curing in several key ways.

Healing may occur without curing. The person dying of acquired immune deficiency syndrome (AIDS) who reconciles with his parents after a long separation is healing. The person who has become quadriplegic and uses this as an opportunity to recommit to living a life of meaning and service is healing. The mother of young children who consents to radical, invasive surgery for an otherwise incurable cancer is healing by coming into a new relationship with the disease and making choices based on her commitment to live for her children. The surgery may not cure her disease, but the choice to undergo the surgery is a healing choice. Curing is almost always focused on the person as a physical entity, a body. If the body cannot be fixed, if the physical disease state or state of disability cannot be cured, then there is "nothing more we can do for you." Healing is multidimensional. It can occur at the physical level, but it can also occur at each of the other levels of the human system—emotion, mind, and spirit.

Curing may or may not be possible, but healing is always possible. Many of the diseases of our time are, in fact, not curable, and people who are living with chronic illnesses of the immune system and cardiovascular systems make up a large percentage of the caseload of any primary care provider. In contrast, because healing is the emergence of right relationship at any or all levels of the human system, it can happen even when there is no possibility for physical cure. The potential for healing exists within every human being by the very fact of the human multidimensional, self-reflective nature. Indeed, for some people, the very fact that they are facing an incurable disease or situation provides enough instability in the system to catalyze tremendous healing shifts, an "escape to a higher order" in the language of Prigogine's model of dissipative structures.[18]

Although curing follows a usual or predictable path, healing is always creative and unpredictable in both process and outcome. In textbooks on curing, the events that will be probable parts of recovery and the time line are described, and the actual progress of the patient is measured against these referents. The misapplication of this information is growing more and more apparent as patients in the modern sickness–cure system are being told exactly how many days of care they are permitted for cure to occur. The nature and the direction of a healing change cannot be predicted, however. Furthermore, because the direction of healing is always toward self-transcendence, something new is emerging, and the whole that was before becomes a part of the new, larger (or deeper) whole. This unidirectional unfolding toward increasing complexity and diversity is also, of course, a fundamental premise of the Science of Unitary Human Beings first proposed by Rogers in 1970.[19] The end point of a healing process cannot be predicted ahead of time. It can only be observed as it emerges.

Death is seen as a failure in the sickness–cure system, but a natural process in the healing system. Death is seen as the enemy, that which is to be avoided at all costs, even at the expense of the humanity and personhood of the one being treated in the sickness–cure system. The increasingly widespread use of "living wills"—formal, legal documents that are required to allow death without the heroic battle waged in sickness–cure institutions—provides abundant evidence of this observation. Rather than being a failure, however, death is part of the natural unfolding of the life process. All living systems eventually die. In some spiritual traditions, death itself is viewed as the ultimate healing, since it releases the eternal soul from the limitations, pain, and suffering of embodiment. This, of course, is a matter of individual belief.

Healing As an Outcome

Healing as a process of emergence does not lend itself to the type of outcome measurement usually applied to curing. It is one thing to evaluate whether the signs and symptoms of disease are still present. It is quite another to determine if there has been a shift at any level of this person's body-mind-spirit. Carper outlined four "patterns of knowing" for nursing: empirics, personal, ethical, and aesthetic.[20] Each of these ways of knowing is valid, according to Carper, but only empirical knowing is widely used and accepted as such.

The knowledge about people gained through the use of empirics—the data gathered through the five senses and their extensions by technology—is unquestionably abundant and important. Tools constructed to elicit information about quality of life, lifestyle, spiritual well-being, and other aspects of life can provide glimpses into healing, to be sure, but they cannot tell the whole story, nor can they be used as "outcome" measures (e.g., what the measures "should" show, what the patient "should" be feeling by this day).

To know if healing is actually happening, more than empirical knowing is necessary. Because the nature of healing is creative and unpredictable, often the best instrument for determining whether healing is happening is the subjective knowing of both patient and nurse. Most nurses have had the experience of participating in a healing moment, a caring occasion. In these moments with patients, there is often a felt sense of awe, reverence, and wonder. Nurses intuitively know that they are standing on holy ground, that they are in the presence of something sacred. It is a body sensation, a chill or a surge of energy. The nurse looks at the patient, the patient looks at the nurse, and they both know. There may be no words, no description, just knowing. Neither may even be able to name what the healing was, what shifted, but they trust that it is real.

Journal keeping is a powerful way for people to keep track of their own healing. Over time, content may shift, new awareness may arise, dreams may become vivid and clear, and as they see their own written words, they realize that they have changed, that they are more whole, more themselves, perhaps expanded in consciousness. This is healing, and the nurse can participate in this process by encouraging the patient to keep a journal and to share it. Sometimes it is through the aesthetic route that healing becomes apparent. Using paper and crayon, patients may draw the shift from despair to hope or fear to peace. Music and movement may become the means through which patients/clients communicate the progress of their healing, the quality of their wholeness.

None of these indicators of healing can be predicted. They cannot be put into a formula to determine length of stay or number of office visits allowed. They are valid and important indicators nevertheless. It may be that, just as nurses have come to accept the definition of pain as being what the patient says it is, they will come to see that healing is happening when the patient (or their intuitive knowing) says it is. This, of course, presents a problem in a system that is increasingly moving to managed care and outcome prediction. It is here that ho-

listic nurses have the opportunity, even the responsibility, to help to define outcome in a way that preserves the wholeness of patients and does not allow their "progress" to be reduced to the behavior of the body physical.[21]

THE HEALER

"It is often thought that medicine is the curative process. It is no such thing; medicine is the surgery of functions as surgery proper is that of limbs and organs. Neither can do anything but remove obstructions; neither can cure. Nature alone cures."[22] This same perspective applies to healing.

Healing is completely unique and creative, and may not be coerced, manipulated, or controlled, even by the one healing. The nurse healer is a facilitator of this process, a sort of midwife, but is not the one doing the healing. Nor is the locus of the healing an isolated part of the patient (i.e., the "mind" or the "spirit"). All healing emerges from within the totality of the unique body-mind-spirit of the patient, sometimes with the assistance of therapeutic interventions, but not because of them. Therapeutics (drugs, surgery, complementary therapies) may be necessary for the patient to be cured or healed, but they are not sufficient causes. Every nurse has cared for patients who "should have" gotten better, but did not, as well as patients who "should have" died, but went on to live long, healthy lives.

The assumption that the patient accomplishes all healing and curing does not mean that the patient controls all healing and curing. The causes of illness and cure are so complex and multifaceted that no simple statement of cause and effect is appropriate to describe either. Nurses can participate knowledgeably in the healing process, formulating a healing intention and doing what they believe is best in this situation, but the outcome of that process remains a mystery. At least part of the healing process will always be mystery unfolding. Suggesting otherwise to patients may contribute to their sense of failure when they are unable to cure themselves of disease. True caring is a moral commitment to protect the vulnerability of another, not add to it.

A TRUE HEALING HEALTH CARE SYSTEM

As noted previously, the current health care system focuses almost exclusively on the curing process, thus making it more akin to a sickness–cure system. While necessary and excellent in its own right, this system is incomplete. The use of new tools of care, including alternative, holistic, or complementary therapies, without a fundamental shift in the philosophy of care with which they are used, will not transform the sickness–cure system into a true, healing health care system, however. This error of confusing the tools of care with the philosophy of care may lead to serious consequences for both health care practitioners and their patients.

The fundamental orientation of a holistic practitioner is toward an appreciation of and attention to the wholeness and uniqueness of every person. Holistic nurses remember that, in effect, there is nothing that is not holistic. There is no intervention that does not affect the whole body-mind-spirit of the patient, because the body-mind-spirit is integral and cannot be divided. There are natural versus non-natural modalities, for example, but both affect the whole body-mind-spirit. There are invasive and noninvasive interventions, but both affect the whole body-mind-spirit. There are interventions that start in the body (e.g., medications, surgery, exercise, movement therapy), the mind (e.g., autogenic training, hypnotherapy, guided imagery), or the spirit (e.g., meditation, prayer, gratitude practice, loving kindness). None of these interventions is inherently more "holistic" than the other, however, because all roads

lead to the body-mind-spirit; all interventions affect the whole.

For this reason, simply adding new tools of care will not transform the sickness–cure system. The way in which practitioners use the tools available, whether the tools are conventional or complementary, and their willingness to become a midwife to nature rather than the hero of success stories make the care holistic or integrative. The true health care system will emerge when both curing and healing processes are equally valued, sought after, and facilitated for all, and when the full range of curing, caring, and healing modalities is available to all. Holistic nurses have a key role to play in facilitating this level of change in the existing systems.

Integration of the Masculine and the Feminine

The Western sickness–care system is characterized almost exclusively by attributes usually ascribed to the masculine principle and usually carried by men. This is a natural consequence of the fact that men have been the principal creators of that system and continue to be the dominant culture of the system. These attributes are extremely useful in the treatment of acute injury and disease, but without the attributes usually ascribed to the feminine principle, they provide an incomplete foundation for a true, integrative healing health care system.

Table 2–1 suggests another perspective on these different attributes. A perspective that sees the goal as "getting the job done" can be associated with the sickness–cure model, while one that focuses on "holding sacred space" can facilitate healing of the whole body-mind-spirit.[23]

Nurse As Healing Environment

One of the most powerful tools for healing is the presence of the nurse in the

Table 2-1 Ways of Being with People Seeking Help

"Getting the Job Done"	*"Holding Sacred Space"*
Authority vested in the external "expert"	Authority vested in the individual client(s)
Source of healing: what the expert provides	Source of healing: the body-mind-spirit of the client(s)
Gathering, collecting, taking in information	Receiving information
Problem solving/fixing	Life unfolding/facilitating
Making "something" happen, where "something" is • defined by the external "expert" • defined ahead of time • meeting the goal	Allowing "something" to happen, where "something" is • defined mutually • defined in the moment • emergence of mystery
Directing/taking over to make it happen	Guiding/helping to allow it to happen
Doing to or for	Being with
Leading	Walking with
Power over	Power with
Expert is accountable and responsible for outcome	Facilitator is accountable and responsible for competent practice
Failure is the nonachievement of predetermined outcome	Failure is giving up on the unfolding process

patient's environment. In fact, the nurse has the greatest impact of all the elements in the patient's environment. Simply by virtue of the role, a nurse has all the ritual power of the shaman of other cultures. The nurse is guardian of the patient's journey through illness and healing; the keeper and bestower of information, medicines, and treatments; the mediator of the system, and the comings and goings of others in the system.

In a model of the universe that includes the nonlocal nature of consciousness[24] or the possibility for the existence of a human energy field that extends beyond the skin,[25] the nurse is not simply part of the patient's environment, but rather the nurse *is* the patient's environment.[26] As Newman noted, "In the case of a nurse interacting with a patient, the energy fields of the two interact and form a new pattern of inter-penetration, spirit within spirit."[27]

The healing environment of the patient may increase to the maximum when the nurse intentionally shifts consciousness into a centered or meditative state. The interconnectedness of the energy fields of the nurse and the patient can facilitate relaxation, rest, or healing in the patient.[28] When a nurse is centered in the present moment and has the intention to be a healing environment, he or she may carry this intention in the energy field and manifest it in the voice, the eyes, and the quality of touching. Nurses should ask themselves:

- Do patients hear in my voice that I care? That I have time for them? That they are safe with me?
- What is the quality of my facial expression? Of my eyes? Do they communicate care and compassion, or are they perfunctory and distant? Does the patient feel seen by me, or over-

looked? If the eyes are the windows of the soul, what is my soul saying to the soul of my patient? What is the patient's soul saying?

- Am I focused on the task at hand and simply touching the patient to get the job done? Or does my touch convey care, support, nurture, and competence? Does my touch communicate that I know I am touching this person's spirit as I contact his or her skin, because where else is the spirit located but in the body? Do I speak of love and kindness and respect through my hands?

Learning how to shift consciousness into a healing state is a basic skill for the holistic nurse. Nurses are not simply separate selves "doing to" the patient, but an integral part of the patient's environment, "being with" them on the healing journey. The quality of the energy with which the patient is interacting is part of what nurses attend to, and this means attending to their own state of consciousness and well-being before, during, and after their interactions with patients. Thus, taking time for themselves to learn and practice relaxation, meditation, centering, or other self-care strategies becomes essential in this model. Nurses are not being selfish by taking this time. They are recognizing that unless they are energized, relaxed, and centered, they will be trying to give what they do not have to give. This results in less than optimal care for the patients and burnout for the nurses.

THE WOUNDED HEALER

Everyone is wounded. Life does not allow anyone to slide under its radar and escape its trials. Thus, being wounded is not optional. What individuals do with their wounding is optional, however. When nurses do the work of healing that their own

woundedness requires, they have the capacity to become "wounded healers" for others. The wounded healer is not a healer because he or she is perfect, whole, and finished with life's growing pains. No, the wounded healer is a healer precisely because he or she knows deeply and personally the need for ongoing healing, caring, and wholeness. Having undertaken to become healed themselves, wounded healers are unafraid of the healing journey and are most courageous companions on the healing journey of others. They know the territory of healing from the inside and can guide others at one moment and console them the next, for the journey is always shifting.

Conversely, wounded healers know their limitations and can identify when a given patient is touching them in a place that is still unhealed. Instead of rejecting the patient because they are unconscious of this reality, wounded healers make sure that another staff member is assigned to the patient so that the patient's care will not be compromised by their inability to provide a caring presence.

The more nurses become healed and whole themselves, the more they have to offer their patients. As they grow and develop in self-love and compassion, their well of compassion and mercy for others expands. Frances Vaughan, a transpersonal psychologist, put it this way: "Healing happens more easily through us when we allow it to happen in us. In this way the wounded healer who, at the existential level, identifies with the pain and suffering of those he or she attempts to heal, becomes the healed healer who, being grounded in emptiness and compassion, can facilitate healing more effectively."[29]

As nurses heal, they become more and more aware of the sacred trust that is granted to them when they are privileged to participate in another person's healing journey. They accept the privilege and its demands and responsibilities willingly, because the wounded healer always wants to give something back.

CONCLUSION

Transpersonal human caring provides the context for holistic nurses to facilitate healing, the emergence of right relationship, in patients and clients. Through the use of centering and intentionality, the holistic nurse may become a healing environment and participate in the creation of a true, healing health care system that integrates both masculine and feminine attributes. "Holding sacred space" for healing is an additional skill of the holistic nurse, not replacing "getting the job (of curing) done," but adding to it. The nurse, as a wounded healer, recognizes that people are on their own healing journeys, but they may assist each other as personal healing evolves.

DIRECTIONS FOR FUTURE RESEARCH

1. Collect personal stories and narratives that provide exemplars of "caring occasions."

2. Conduct interviews with patients who see themselves as healing, even in the absence of curing, to search for patterns that may facilitate this shift for other patients.
3. Explore the relationship between job satisfaction in nurses and the practice of centering and holding sacred space.

NURSE HEALER REFLECTIONS

After reading this chapter, the nurse healer will be able to answer or begin a process of answering the following questions:

- How do I feel when I am engaged in a "caring occasion"?
- How do I know when healing is happening in my patients? In myself?
- What gives me true joy and peace in my practice as a holistic nurse, and how can I create more of that?
- What wounds have I consciously healed in my life, and what are the gifts of those wounds that help to make me a better nurse?

NOTES

1. J. Watson, *Nursing: Human Science and Human Care* (New York: National League for Nursing Press, 1988), 54.

2. J. Quinn, On Healing, Wholeness and the Haelan Effect, *Nursing and Health Care* 10, no. 10 (1989):553–556.

3. J. Morse et al., Concepts of Caring and Caring as a Concept, *Advances in Nursing Science* 13, no. 1 (1990):1–14.

4. Watson, *Nursing: Human Science and Human Care*, 59.

5. J. Ercums, Nursing's Caring Paradigm: A Story of Mutuality and Transcendent Healing, *Alternative and Complementary Therapies* 4, no. 1 (1998): 68–72.

6. D. Bohm, response to a question raised at the International Transpersonal Association meeting, Prague, Czechoslovakia, 1992.

7. Quinn, On Healing, Wholeness and the Haelan Effect, 553.

8. K. Wilber, *Sex, Ecology and Spirituality: The Spirit of Evolution* (Boston: Shambhala, 1996), 14.

9. A. Koestler, *The Ghost in the Machine* (New York: Random House, 1976).

10. K. Wilber, *The Marriage of Sense and Soul* (New York: Random House, 1998), 67.

11. F. Capra, *The Web of Life* (New York: Anchor Books, 1996), 80.

12. E. Lazlo, *Evolution, the Grand Synthesis* (Boston: Shambhala, 1987), 36.

13. Capra, *The Web of Life*, 222.

14. Quinn, On Healing, Wholeness and the Haelan Effect, 554.

15. Wilber, *Sex, Ecology and Spirituality*, 40.

16. Wilber, *Sex, Ecology and Spirituality*, 44.

17. D. Wardell and J. Engebretson, Professional Evolution, *Journal of Holistic Nursing* 16, no. 1 (1998): 64.

18. I. Prigogine, *Order Out of Chaos* (New York: Bantam Books, 1984).

19. M. Rogers, *An Introduction to the Theoretical Basis of Nursing* (Philadelphia: F.A. Davis, 1970).

20. B. Carper, Fundamental Patterns of Knowing, *Advances in Nursing Science* 1, no. 1 (1978):13–23.

21. Wardell and Engebretson, Professional Evolution.

22. F. Nightingale, *Notes on Nursing: What It Is and What It Is Not* (New York: Dover Press, 1969), 133.

23. J. Quinn, Holding Sacred Space: The Nurse as Healing Environment, *Holistic Nursing Practice* 6, no. 4 (1992):26–36

24. L. Dossey, *Healing Words* (San Francisco: Harper San Francisco, 1993), 43.

25. M. Rogers, Nursing: Science of Unitary, Irreducible, Human Beings: Update 1990, in *Visions of Rogers Science-based Nursing*, ed. E.A.M. Barrett (New York: National League for Nursing, 1990).

26. Quinn, Holding Sacred Space.

27. M. Newman, The Spirit of Nursing, *Holistic Nursing Practice* 3, no. 3 (1989): 6.

28. Quinn, Holding Sacred Space.

29. F. Vaughan, *The Inward Arc* (Boston: Shambhala, 1985), 70.

SUGGESTED READING

Capik, L. The Watson Theory of Human Care applied to ASPO/Lamaze perinatal education, *Journal of Perinatal Education* 6, no. 1 (1997):43-7.

Colbath, J. Holistic health options for women, *Critical Care Nursing Clinics of North America* 9, no. 4 (1997):589-99.

Gabrielson, A. Patient-centered care in the OR: is this possible? *Canadian Operating Room Nursing Journal*, 15, no.1 (1997):8-10.

Greer, T. Making connections, *Nursing* 27, no. 12 (1997):48-9.

Hartrick, G. Relational capacity: the foundation for interpersonal nursing practice, *Journal of Advanced Nursing* 26, no.3 (1997):523-8.

Leininger, M. Founder's focus: alternative to what? Generic vs. Professional caring, treatments, and healing modes, *Journal of Transcultural Nursing* 9, no. 19 (1997):37.

Pearson, A., Borbasi, S., Walsh, K. Practicing nursing therapeutically through acting as a skilled companion on the illness journey, *Advanced Practice Nursing Quarterly* 3, no. 1 (1997):46-52.

Sherwood, G. Patterns of caring: the healing connection of interpersonal harmony, *International Journal for Human Caring* 1, no. 1 (1997):30-8.

Smucker, C. Nursing, healing and spirituality, *Complementary Therapies in Nursing & Midwifery* 4, no. 4: (1998):95-7.

Taliaferro, D. Healing relationships: building effective teams, *Seminars in Perioperative Nursing* 7, no. 2 (1998):122-7.

Ward, S. Caring and healing in the 21st century, *MCN, American Journal of Maternal Child Nursing* 23, no. 4 (1998):210-5.

Webster, D. Caring for the caregiver: expanding ways of knowing through experiments in self-care, *Advanced Practice Nursing Quarterly* 3, no. 1 (1997):66-75

Williams, S. Caring in patient-focused care: the relationship of patients' perceptions of holistic nurse caring to their levels of anxiety, *Holistic Nursing Practice* 11, no. 3 (1997):61-8.

VISION OF HEALING

Reawakening the Spirit in Daily Life

Individuals who are said to possess "psychologic hardiness" have certain characteristics referred to as the three Cs.[1] First, these individuals feel open to change and are willing to take risks. They see life as a series of challenges rather than problems, and they seem to thrive on challenges. Second, these individuals feel a commitment to family, friends, and goals. Third, they have a sense of personal power and control over life and perceive their body-mind-spirit as an integrative unit. Hardiness characteristics not only apply to staying healthy, but also they have tremendous potential for adapting to more effective health promotion strategies if chronic illness is present.

These hardiness characteristics assist us in learning more about our human potentials. Change implies flexibility and suggests that lifestyle habits do not have to be permanent. It is wise to experiment, to try new ways of relating with friends, family, and colleagues, as well as with new healthier behaviors. Changing detrimental or risky habits is essential for well-being. The more we choose effective lifestyle patterns, the better we learn the change process. Changing and taking risks are important parts of life. Often, when people do not change, they conclude that they do not have the willpower to change. Rather than willpower, we should think in terms of "skillpower," which implies new information and skills that lead to long-lasting changes in lifestyle patterns. The more we risk at changing lifestyle, the more consistently we select positive changes because the fear of changing is lessened.[2]

Hardiness characteristics help us experience a sense of meaning and purpose in our work. "Work spirit" is related to increased effectiveness, productivity, and individual satisfaction, which contribute to positive results in the workplace. It is also directly related to the degree of responsibility that one is willing to take to change the course of one's life. Work spirit grows when associated with self-knowledge about maximizing human potentials through self-care modalities such as exercise, nutrition, play, relaxation, and stress management strategies. Work spirit also involves selflessness, that is, being unself-consciously engrossed in the outcome of work tasks and projects rather than worrying about others' perceptions of the way those tasks and projects are done. People with work spirit have abundant energy and always appear to be "on a roll" or "in a flow state." They feel a sense of purpose, and they are creative and nurturing. They experience a different sense of time. These individuals have a sense of higher order and oneness. Their state of mind is positive and open to new ideas, and a full sense of self is manifest.

Individuals with work spirit exhibit synergy; they discover common threads when there appears to be nothing but opposites and conflicts in situations. They work with self and others to produce greater results. These people exhibit *hardiness. They can make frequent shifts in thinking and can release old mindsets. They understand that patterns and processes in any project create the whole, rather than focusing on isolated parts. They value input from colleagues, seek meaningful relationships, and also praise co-workers' talents and resources. They focus on win–win situations.*

Individuals who have low levels of work spirit can create dysergy in the workplace. They focus on an isolated action that promotes one function, but impedes the progress of another person or the group working together. These individuals tend to work alone or evoke unnecessary competition among colleagues. They exhibit poor communication skills, aggressiveness, and insecurity, and they emphasize win–lose outcomes and reject meaningful interaction from co-workers.

Organizations can increase individual work spirit by having an identified purpose that workers can share and articulate. When this purpose is clearly communicated, supervisors or managers recognize individual strengths and talents and channel creative energy toward the organizational goals. Those organizations that offer praise and rewards that encourage risk taking and problem solving, while not imposing punishment for mistakes, also increase individual work spirit.

NOTES

1. S. Kobasa et al., Hardiness and Health: A Prospective Study, *Journal of Personality and Social Psychology* 42 (1982):168–177.

2. J.F. Wane (Issue Editor), Hardiness and Health, *Holistic Nursing Practice* 13, no. 3 (April) 1999. [This entire issue focuses on many aspects of hardiness and health.]

Chapter 3

The Art of Holistic Nursing and the Human Health Experience

H. Lea Barbato Gaydos

NURSE HEALER OBJECTIVES

Theoretical

- Explore the art of holistic nursing.
- Discuss the dynamic, dialectic relationship of health-wellness-disease-illness that comprises the human health experience.
- Discuss the facilitation of healing through the processes of engagement, values clarification, and change.

Clinical

- Describe the ways in which you are an artist in your practice.
- Identify the relationship of health-wellness-disease-illness in at least two clients.
- Identify the stages of change with a client and co-create a plan to implement appropriate strategies for motivation and sustained changed behaviors.
- Explore with a colleague the ways in which cultural variations in values affect the responses of clients.

Personal

- Reflect on the steps of personal integrity and their relationship to your values.

- Identify the dynamic, dialectic relationship of health-wellness-disease-illness in your life.
- Write down two action steps that will guide you in living your personal values.

DEFINITIONS

Art of Nursing: the manifestation of the nurse's fundamental self and source of being through the mastery of acts of caring.

Attitudes: feelings arising out of thoughts, emotions, and behaviors associated with a particular person, idea, or object.

Beliefs: a subset of attitudes that indicate faith in a particular person, idea, or object.

Dialectic: the art of discourse, implying a relationship in which there is a synthesis of objective and subjective perspectives.[1,2]

Disease: a discrete entity causing specific symptoms; more broadly, a phenomenon causing a deviation from normal.[3]

Engagement: the process of commitment, involvement, and performance of value-consistent health behaviors.[4]

Health: a state or process in which the individual experiences a sense of well-being, harmony, and unity; a process of becoming; expanding consciousness (Neuman).[5]

Human Health Experience: that totality of human experience that encompasses health-wellness-disease-illness.[6]

Illness: a subjective experience of symptoms and suffering to which the individual ascribes meaning and significance; not synonymous with disease.

Motivation: the internal spark or desire necessary for a person to be committed to change, set goals, and succeed.

Self-Responsibility: the ability to choose behaviors that are congruent with personal values.

Values: endowment of a particular person, idea, object, or behavior with worth, truth, or beauty.

Values Clarification: a process whereby one becomes more aware of how life values are established and how these values influence one's life.

Wellness: integrated, congruent functioning aimed toward reaching one's highest potential.

THE ART OF HOLISTIC NURSING

Nursing is a science, and it is also an art. Nursing has made many advances in describing the science of nursing. Exactly what constitutes the art of nursing is less clear. Interpreting the art of nursing as the "nursing arts" places the emphasis on the proper techniques employed in the tasks of nursing, such as bathing the patient, making the bed, and administering medication. In 1859, however, Florence Nightingale defined the art of nursing as a fine art having to do with the spirit. "Nursing is an art; and if it is to be made an art it requires as exclusive a devotion, as hard a preparation as any painter's or sculptor's work; for what is the having to do with dead canvas or cold marble, compared with having to do with the living body."[7]

Art is compelling and out of the ordinary. Art uses symbols and has meanings beyond those that are readily apparent. Art in nursing may be understood as a particular kind of asking (research) and knowing, learning, practice, and reflective experience.[8] The characteristics of art are apparent in the language of nursing, stories of nursing, nursing education, and nursing research. The art of nursing is a performance art. It happens in the moment, and it is full of dancelike movement. The quality of movement suggests that the art of nursing is fluid, flexible, and responsive.

The everyday arts, such as "the art of cooking" or "the art of bookbinding," involve doing a task creatively and well. The core behavioral tendency to "make special" in this way meets the universal human need to be artful.[9] "Making special" is a behavior as important to survival as other core behavioral tendencies, such as aggression and attachment.[10] Thinking of art as having survival value and as the effort to "make special" suggests the reason that nursing may be considered an art. In art-filled nursing, practitioners "make special" the relationship between nurse and client. Through this specialness, they co-create the circumstances for healing and sometimes for survival.

Art, like ritual, is a container for feelings.[11] When nurses are artful, they are able to receive another's feelings and to hold them. "The art of nursing is the capacity of a human being to receive another human being's expression of feelings and to experience those feelings for oneself."[12] Nurses and other health care professionals have appropriated the term *empathy* to mean that special kind of relating that allows them to feel the suffering of another without losing their professional bearings. Clients describing the art of nursing noted that artful nurses develop a deep connection characterized by empathy and intuition.[13]

Art arises out of the imagination, that realm of the mind that relies on intuitive judgment. Intuitive judgment has six aspects.[14] These aspects are not sequential, but are used in combination in artful nursing:

1. **Pattern recognition:** the ability to see a pattern without analyzing the separate components

2. **Similarity recognition:** the ability to relate one pattern to another, even if there are significant differences in the objective components
3. **Common sense understanding:** a deep understanding of culture and language that allows the nurse to understand the experience of the client and not just the disorder or the disease
4. **Skilled know-how:** the combination of knowledge, expertise, and experience that allows flexibility in actions and judgment
5. **A sense of salience:** the ability to discern what is significant in a situation
6. **Deliberate rationality:** the use of past experience and analysis to generate multiple interpretations of a clinical situation

Both science and art are creative and aesthetic. In truth, the best solutions to problems in both science and art are often the most aesthetic ones.[15] Because holistic nursing is both science and art, the holistic nurse is obligated to uncover or recover, support, and celebrate the creative self. Awakening and cultivating the imaginative mind requires uncovering the heart, opening the mind, letting loose the imagination, creating an environment conducive to creativity, working to master a form, and demonstrating the courage to take risks and be vulnerable.[16] Vulnerability is a key to authenticity,[17] which is requisite because the creative process is a manifestation of the spirit. In the creative process, artists touch their innermost selves and the source of their being through the mastery of a physical form.[18] The physical form of nursing is manifest in acts of caring.

Although the capacity for creativity is universal, there seem to be gender differences in the actualization of the creative impulse.[19] Firestone suggested that women tend to define creativity as a response to life, a way of living. In contrast, many studies on creativity that have been done with men emphasize the *products* of creativity, such as exceptional scientific or artistic innovations. It may be that creativity in the art of nursing (an essentially feminine art, whether it is performed by women or men) has something to do with a characteristic way of responding or living in which the nurse expresses creativity through the mastery of acts of caring.

Appleton found that a fundamental act of caring in nursing is the gift of self.[20] Clients described artful nurses as really being "there for them." Being there meant that the nurse saw the client as a whole person, unique, and worthy of respect, and the primary focus of attention. Being there was also characterized by truth telling and competent helping. In addition, clients described the artful nurse as someone who enabled them to be fully themselves, assisting them in preparing for personal well-being, helping them make responsible decisions, and guiding self-expression. The themes that emerged in this study, considered as a whole, established a unity of meaning; they created a "transcendent togetherness," an intimate union between the client and the nurse in which the client felt safe, secure, and bonded to the nurse. In transcendent togetherness, the client and the nurse are liberated from conventional responses and instead respond uniquely to each other. The client trusts the nurse to respect and safeguard the client's wholeness.[21] Artistic nursing brings into being a relationship between nurse and client that is "made special" as transcendent togetherness.

The increase of technology in nursing may at first appear to preclude an artistic approach, but it actually enables the nurse to be more present (and thus more artful) to the client. "Technology reduces the time spent in 'having to do things' and provides the means to carry out the care with less effort. . . . Technologies can shorten the time spent in completing a task and make procedures less invasive, more comfortable and more private."[22] In art of any sort, it is important to master the needed technology so that skill development is no longer the focus, but a means to the aesthetic end. When technology is used with beauty, grace, and the intent to "make special," it enhances rather than decreases an act of aesthetic caring.

Art as practice has a moral dimension. It reflects the moral consciousness of the artist and informs the moral consciousness of the spectator, observer, or participant.[23] In transcendent togetherness, the client relies on the integrity of the nurse, and the nurse supports the client's integrity. The nurse's moral sense lies in his or her awareness of the vulnerability of clients.[24] In other words, the morality demonstrated by the art of holistic nursing has integrity that is located in an acute sense of responsibility and an awareness of the vulnerability of clients. Because nursing occurs when people are at their most vulnerable, there is no art that has a greater need for moral awareness than the art of nursing. The ethic that supports this position is the ethic of care.[25] It is an ethic arising out of the moral development of women, and it is based in the feminine value of the primacy of relationship.

The art of holistic nursing is about the "making special" of the relationship between client and nurse, an effort that reveals the nurse's most fundamental self and source of being. This is a psychologic and spiritual penetration that is potentially healing for both nurse and client. Thus, artistic nursing is healing, and in this, the nurse is an artist healer who lives a life that is responsive to the call to service that is spiritual as well as practical.[26] Grounded in science and in aesthetics, holistic nursing is fluid, beautiful, creative, compelling, and moral. It has healing as its aim, and it is fundamentally a spiritual process that "manifests in the physical, mental and emotional realms."[27] As Stewart said, "The real essence of nursing, as of any fine art, lies not in the mechanical details of execution, nor yet in the dexterity of the performer, but in the creative imagination, the sensitive spirit and the intelligent understanding lying back of these techniques and skills."[28]

ASPECTS OF THE HUMAN HEALTH EXPERIENCE

Holistic nurses practice their art within the human health experience, the totality of the human condition that contains and reveals the dynamic relationships among health-wellness-disease-illness.[29] Wellness and illness, like health and disease, are often thought of as mutually exclusive and opposite outcomes. In holistic nursing, however, wellness-illness and health-disease are neither mutually exclusive, nor polar opposites, but are part of a process and part of the whole. Events of wellness-illness-health-disease within the human health experience unfold in a dynamic, dialectic relationship that makes it easier to understand that the individual is a changing person in a changing world.

All aspects of the human health experience have both cognitive and affective dimensions.[30] Cognitive dimensions of health-disease can be seen as comprehensible/incomprehensible, manageable/unmanageable, and meaningful/meaningless. Affective themes that appear are joy/despair, acceptance/resentment, power/fear, and anticipation/confusion. In the practice of artful nursing, the nurse acknowledges the meaning of the health experience for clients.[31] Therefore, developing a more artful practice requires exploration of the dynamics of health-wellness-disease-illness to gain a deeper understanding of the patterns, meanings, and client responses. Through greater understanding of the range of meanings in general and the meaning for an individual client in particular, nurses can facilitate the healing process.

Culture and the Human Health Experience

Cultural beliefs deeply influence the perceived meaning of health and illness for clients and family members, and a nurse's understanding of the cultural context of the human health experience can facilitate the development of the transcendent togetherness. The development of empathy, the artful use of intuitive judgment and creativity, truth telling, competent care, and the facilitation of the expression of the client's true self are more likely when the nurse understands the cultural context of the client's health experience. Furthermore, care that has integrity is culturally congruent. Therefore, clients need to receive care within the context of their cultural backgrounds, health beliefs, and values.

One way of gaining insight into a client's dominant cultural values is to answer the following five questions regarding the culture under consideration:

1. What is the inherent nature of human beings? Are humans good, evil, or a combination?
2. What is the relationship of human beings to nature? Does nature dominate human beings, do humans dominate nature, or do humans co-exist in harmony with nature?
3. What is the temporal focus of human experience? Is the perception of time predominantly focused on the past, present, or future?
4. What is the human mode of activity? Is human potential found in being (spontaneity is valued), growing (personal control and self-actualization are valued), or in doing (action is valued)?
5. What is the pattern of human relationships? Are significant relationships linear and hereditary, collateral and group-oriented, individual-oriented

with an emphasis on independence and autonomy?[32]

Nurses can gain cultural competency by reading and studying the literature of, or about, the culture under consideration.[33] Reading this literature provides a window through which a nurse can participate through imagination in the dramas, joys, values, and experiences unique to the culture. In addition, nurses who become familiar with the various studies that have been done on the healing beliefs and practices of other cultures can base culturally sensitive care on an assessment of the client's health-illness beliefs, attitudes, and values; the beliefs about causative agents of symptoms and illness; the way in which healers within the culture diagnose the symptoms or illness; and the treatments recommended by the healers. Knowledge of general patterns of responses for specific cultural and ethnic groups is necessary in order to provide a foundation for further assessment and individualized care (see Chapter 13, Table 13–2).[34] This information serves as a guideline for individualized care. *It should never be used as the basis for ethnocentric or stereotypic responses by health care providers.* The art of nursing depends on the recognition of the uniqueness of each person and the development of a unique relationship with a client.

Values Clarification and the Human Health Experience

The pioneering work of Raths and colleagues explores the complexity and differences in values, beliefs, and attitudes.[35] Values are affective dispositions about the worth, truth, or beauty of a thought, object, person, or behavior. Values influence decisions, behavior, and nursing practice. Attitudes and beliefs are closely related to values. Attitudes are feelings toward a person, object, or idea that include cognitive, affective, and behavioral elements. Beliefs are a subclass of attitudes. The cognitive factors involved in beliefs have less to do with facts and more with feelings; they represent a personal confidence or faith in the validity of some person, object, or idea.

Values are more dynamic than attitudes because, in addition to the cognitive, affective, and behavioral elements, values possess motivational characteristics. They provide direction and meaning to life and guide behavior. They provide a frame of reference by which to integrate, explain, and evaluate new thoughts, experiences, and relationships, both personally and professionally. Personal values are not always consistent with professional values. A direct conflict between a strong personal value and a professional value may lead to confusion, frustration, and dissatisfaction. Sometimes, the stories of nursing, a valuable source of understanding about the art of nursing, reveal confusion, doubt, and ambiguities regarding values.[36] A nurse has the right not to participate in any activity or experience that violates personal values. Usually, when confronted with a situation that requires action, individuals have a variety of alternatives. When choosing among alternative actions, it is important to focus on values in order to choose the best alternative.

Values are transmitted by moralizing, modeling, adopting a laissez-faire attitude, explaining, manipulating, and using a reward/punishment approach. Values clarification is a dynamic process that emphasizes an individual's capacity for intelligent, self-directed behavior. By taking the time to deliberate about values, individuals find their own answers to a variety of questions or concerns. There is no "correct" set of values, because no one set of values is appropriate for everyone. Rather, the process of values clarification establishes a closer fit between what a person does and what that person says.

The process of values clarification has three steps: choosing, prizing, and acting.[37]

In the first step, the person chooses the value freely and willingly, although only after evaluating each alternative and its consequences. The second step is to prize and cherish the decision and to affirm or communicate the choice publicly. The last step in the valuing process is to incorporate the choice into behavior. These steps translate a value into a consistent, repeated behavioral change that confirms the adoption of the particular value. A true value passes through all steps, but not necessarily in the order discussed. Many beliefs do not meet all the criteria of true values. Such beliefs, which tend to be more numerous than are actual values, are termed value indicators. If the individual is motivated to undergo the values clarification process, a value indicator may become a true value.

Values clarification is a critical component of successful client education.[38] Helping clients to achieve the full expression of their true selves involves teaching them about choices, supporting them in their decisions, and creating circumstances in which they feel free to change their decisions.[39] The art of nursing requires that the nurse and client co-create a common aim and work creatively together toward that aim. Nurses can help clients examine their values in terms of alternatives, evaluate the consequences of their choices, and choose an alternative behavior that is consistent with their values. Coaching and following through are two ways in which nurses provide guidance and support.[40] When the client has made the decision to change based on internally consistent values, positive outcomes are more likely. The following demonstrates values clarification in clinical practice.

> Mr. B.Z. is a 49-year-old man who was admitted to the coronary care unit with a diagnosis of acute myocardial infarction. He was executive vice-president of a large company. Following admission,

his condition was stable, and no major complications developed. On the second day of his hospital stay, he was found lying in the hospital bed with his briefcase open, surrounded by papers. He was writing a report and requested a telephone in his room. The nurse handled the situation as follows:

Nurse: It sure looks like you have a lot of work.

Client: Yes, I have so many deadlines this week, I cannot believe it. I really do not have time to be here. I sure hope my wife brings my fax machine soon.

Nurse: It seems that your work is very important to you. I certainly can understand deadline problems. Could we take just a minute to discuss some other things that are important to you right now?

Client: Sure. Getting better and getting out of here are important to me, and having the energy to deal with the demands of my job. This better not happen to me again.

Nurse: Tell me what you know about preventing another heart attack.

Client: Well, I know I am going to have to lose some weight and get some regular exercise. I'm not sure how I will fit that into my schedule though.

Nurse: Do you think that the heavy demands of work had anything to do with this illness?

Client: Well, I know a lot of stress can make people sick. I've got to admit that I have had a stressful couple of months at work. Yes, I suppose all of that didn't help.

Nurse: You've told me that your work is important to you. You've also told me that preventing another heart attack is important. You have said that it will be important to lose weight, exercise, and perhaps reduce some of your daily stress. If you could begin to work on one of these areas, which area would you choose?

Client: I guess learning to deal with stress.

Nurse: That is a great place to start. Many techniques can be used to reduce stress levels. They can have a profound impact on your mind, as well as a positive effect on your body. If you are willing, I'd like to take a few minutes now and guide you in a relaxation technique that can be of help to you right now and later after your discharge. Would you be willing to try this with me?

Client: Sounds good. I'm willing to try. I suppose I should have thought about this stuff a long time ago.

As nurses apply values clarification in their own lives, they become more aware of the best ways to help clients clarify their values. Clarification is important, because being clear about values helps nurses live and practice the art of nursing congruently and with integrity.

Health Behaviors and the Human Health Experience

Within the human health experience, people make choices that have significant effects on the relationships of health-wellness-disease-illness. Some choices are oriented toward changing behaviors in order to have healthier and longer lives.

People usually adopt preventive behaviors when they are asymptomatic, but wish to enhance their lifestyles. Changing may or may not be independent of the health care system. Illness behaviors often accompany symptoms and involve the health care system for evaluation and any necessary treatment. People who do not adhere to recommended health behaviors are often labeled *noncompliant,* a term that implies client failure in meeting professional expectations and is inconsistent with holistic nursing philosophy and ethics. Terms such as *engagement* and *lack of engagement* in recommended health behaviors are less paternalistic and judgmental.[41] Additionally, the term *engagement* underscores the fact that, in artful nursing, the client and the nurse work together toward common aims.

The Health Belief Model

Three factors that significantly influence a client's motivation to change are his or her health attitudes, beliefs, and social support. The health belief model identifies the specific attitudes and beliefs that influence people to choose preventive health care and to engage in recommended medical regimens. According to this model, the motivation to change behavior comes from the perception that the reward is greater than the perceived cost and the perceived barriers. The major factors in determining engagement include

- the health and willingness of the client to accept medical recommendations
- the client's subjective estimate of his or her susceptibility, vulnerability, and extent of bodily harm
- the extent to which engagement interferes with the client's social roles
- the client's perception of the efficacy and safety of the proposed regimen[42]

Criticisms of this model are that it focuses primarily on cognition and does not explicitly integrate affect. It also places the burden of action entirely on the client and does not address the larger issues impinging on clients, such as the range of choices available as a result of organizational and governmental policy and funding.[43] These criticisms demonstrate that this model is somewhat incongruent with the philosophical and ethical foundations of holistic nursing. The model does emphasize the personal context of decision making, however, and understanding personal context is essential to the practice of artful nursing. Furthermore, because the model is widely used in health care as the basis for research studies on client motivation,[44] it may serve as a starting point for understanding client choices.

Engagement

The Health Belief Model focuses on the perceptions of the client rather than those of the provider. It does not predict or screen persons who are at risk for nonengagement. It is possible, however, to identify four categories that describe individuals according to the relationship of health beliefs, attitudes, and social support to facilitate engagement. Categorization of client characteristics is inconsistent with the art of nursing, because that art demands unique responses within a unique relationship. Even so, if used judiciously as a starting place for understanding and potential intervention, and not as a model for labeling or otherwise objectifying people, categorization can be a helpful cognitive device. The four engagement categories are

1. positive health beliefs and attitudes, as well as adequate social support
2. negative health beliefs and attitudes, but adequate social support
3. positive health beliefs and attitudes, but little or inadequate social support
4. negative health beliefs and attitudes, and little or inadequate social support[45]

Exploration with the client of his or her values regarding the following facilitates the use of this cognitive device:

- general beliefs regarding health
- willingness to seek health care advice
- willingness to accept health care advice
- perception of the seriousness of the high-risk behavior and its consequences
- perception of susceptibility and vulnerability to the consequences of the behavior
- perception of the risks, benefits, and degree of interference that the new behavior will have on current roles[46]

The category that best describes the client's attitudes and circumstances determines the choice of strategies to facilitate engagement. When they become ill, individuals described by Category 1 believe that their illness is serious and that their therapy will be helpful. Nurses will be more effective with these individuals if their teaching efforts facilitate affective, cognitive, and psychomotor learning. Matching the information presented to the client's coping style and locus of control demonstrates caring. To accommodate different coping styles, those persons who use denial receive basic survival information, whereas those who cope by focusing on the problem receive detailed information. Those persons who are internally controlled (i.e., who believe that what they do will affect the outcome of the illness) receive specific instructions on ways to manage or control the situation. Those who are externally controlled (i.e., who believe that others or fate will determine the outcome of the illness) will benefit if an authority figure presents the information to them. For individuals with an external locus of control, a caring response is to discuss the most important points first and then repeat them.

In caring for individuals described by Category 2 (i.e., those who have negative health beliefs and attitudes, but adequate social support), focusing on consciousness-raising techniques can be effective. If the client desires, the nurse can arrange or facilitate the client's efforts to arrange self-help group meetings. In this way, the client can talk with other individuals who have similar problems and concerns. They can share effective strategies and perhaps resources. The social support network of the client can strengthen and facilitate healthy client choices. Values clarification is useful in exploring alternatives for healthy behaviors. Behavior modification techniques are also helpful with people who demonstrate the characteristics of this category. If the client desires, cues that stimulate healthy behavior are recommended. Small rewards can be suggested to support the healthy behaviors of the client's choice. The rewards should follow the behaviors and should be as small as possible, yet still be rewarding (e.g., taking 30 minutes off to read a good book following the daily exercise program). Clients may find that keeping a diary for several days to identify the cues and consequences of a particular behavior is helpful in identifying a list of rewards before attempting the behavior change.

Increased social support and cognitive strengthening are likely to benefit individuals described by Category 3. Providing family and friends with important information and encouraging their involvement with recommended therapy, discussion, or values clarification sessions increase and strengthen social support. Client involvement with community agencies and self-help groups may also be appropriate. Cognitive strengthening through training in assertiveness, relaxation, imagery, problem solving, and goal setting may enhance coping skills.

A "foot-in-the-door" strategy that requires minimal behavioral change may be effective with clients described by Category 4. Even small changes can produce positive outcomes. Mutually establishing basic goals and simple ways to meet these goals will support client choices and self-esteem. As with any behavior change, rewards and reinforcement may be effective. Breaking down complex behaviors into more easily accomplished steps will facilitate mastery and, thus, self-esteem. Written rather than verbal contracts may serve to remind clients of the nurse's support and concern, and of a mutual commitment.

Stages of Change in Addictive Behavior Patterns

Nurses frequently come into contact with clients because of the health or social consequences of addictive behaviors. Whether nurses are designing programs for population groups or co-creating individual care plans with clients, nurses must realize that the modification of addictive behavior is complex and involves a progression through five stages of change: (1) precontemplation, (2) contemplation, (3) preparation, (4) action, and (5) maintenance.[47]

In the precontemplation stage, individuals have no intention to change behavior in the near future. They are usually unaware of their problems, although their family, friends, employers, and neighbors are very aware of the problems. If people in this stage agree to therapy, it is usually under pressure from others. Most often, they feel coerced into changing and will demonstrate change only as long as the pressure continues.

At the contemplation stage, an individual is aware of the problem and is thinking seriously about overcoming it, but has not yet made a commitment to take action. Serious consideration of the problem solution is the central feature of contemplation. The individual knows what action to take, but weighs the pros and cons of the problem and its solution. The struggle to cope with the effort, energy, and loss required to overcome the addiction can last 2 years or longer.

The stage of preparation combines both intention and behavioral criteria. In this stage, individuals who have unsuccessfully taken action in the past year plan to take action again within the next month. Although some action may have reduced the addictive behavior, the criterion for effective action has not been reached.

During the action stage, individuals modify their behaviors, experiences, or environment in order to overcome their addictions. The hallmarks of this stage are significant overt efforts and modification of target behaviors to an acceptable criterion. It is in this stage that individuals receive the most external recognition from others. This stage requires an enormous amount of time, energy, and commitment. Individuals are in the action stage if they have successfully altered the addictive behaviors for a period of 1 day to 6 months.

The maintenance stage, in which individuals work to prevent relapse, represents a continuation of change rather than a stop and start of addictive behaviors. The criterion for this stage is that healthy behaviors replace addictive behaviors for longer than 6 months. In reality, this stage extends for 6 months to an indeterminate period past the initial action.

Each stage of change represents a period of time, as well as a set of tasks needed for movement to the next stage. Regardless of whether individuals try to change on their own or seek professional help in changing, they typically move through these stages several times before termination of the addiction. Figure 3–1 illustrates the spiral pattern in which most people actually move through the stages of change. Individuals may progress from contemplation to preparation to action to maintenance, but most will relapse. The spiral model suggests that most people who relapse do not revolve endlessly in circles, nor do they regress all the way back to where they began. Rather, they learn from their mistakes and try different behaviors the next time. The number of suc-

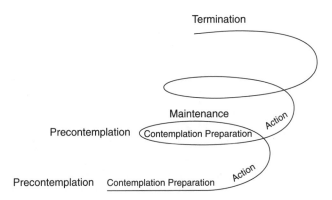

Figure 3–1 A Spiral Model of the Stages of Change. *Source:* Reprinted from Prochaska, J., et al., In Search of How People Change, *American Psychologist* Vol. 47, No. 9, pp. 1102–1114. Copyright © 1992 by the American Psychological Association. Reprinted with permission.

cesses continues to increase over time; thus, the more action taken, the better the prognosis and success.[48]

To assist individuals with changes in addictive behaviors, the nurse first helps them to identify clearly their stage of change. Each stage suggests treatment choices. For example, action-oriented therapies may be effective with individuals in the preparation or action stages, but very ineffective or even detrimental to those in the precontemplation or contemplation stages. The stages of change represent a temporal dimension that guides nurses in understanding when particular shifts in attitudes, intentions, and behaviors occur. Professionals who counsel individuals with addictions use a transtheoretical approach; they examine recommended change techniques across different theories and then integrate them.[49] Exhibit 3–1 presents ten processes with definitions and examples of interventions for each process. These processes are potent predictors of change both for clients who make changes on their own and for clients who change with professional therapy.

One of the most important findings to emerge from the self-change in addictive behaviors research of Prochaska and colleagues is the integration between the processes and stages of change.[50] Exhibit 3–2 represents this integration from cross-sectional research involving thousands of people who changed on their own at each of the stages of change for smoking cessation and weight loss.[51–56] This research indicates that people in the precontemplation stage process less information about the problem, devote less time and energy to it, and experience fewer negative reactions to it. People in the contemplation stage are more open to consciousness-raising techniques, such as confrontation, observation, and interpretations. As people in the precontemplation stage become more aware of the problem, they evaluate the effect of their behaviors on the people to whom they are the closest. Thus, moving from precontemplation to contemplation increases the use of cognitive, affective, and evaluative processes of change. The research also shows that, during the action stage, people begin to believe that they have the autonomy to change their lives. Like the maintenance stage, the action stage involves high degrees of preparation. In these stages, clients consider what leads to relapse, how to avoid relapse, and what alternative responses are available for effective coping. The important key here for change is the individual's conviction

Exhibit 3–1 Titles, Definitions, and Representative Interventions of the Processes of Change

Process	Definitions: Interventions
Consciousness raising	Increasing information about self and problem: observations, confrontations, interpretations, bibliotherapy
Self-reevaluation	Assessing how one feels and thinks about oneself with respect to a problem: value clarification, imagery, corrective emotional experience
Self-liberation	Choosing and making a commitment to act or belief in ability to change: decision-making therapy, New Year's resolutions, logotherapy techniques, commitment-enhancing techniques
Counterconditioning	Substituting alternatives for problem behaviors: relaxation, desensitization, assertion, positive self-statements
Stimulus control	Avoiding or countering stimuli that elicit problem behaviors: restructuring one's environment (e.g., removing alcohol or fattening foods), avoiding high-risk cues, fading techniques
Reinforcement management	Rewarding one's self or being rewarded by others for making changes: contingency contracts, overt and covert reinforcement, self-reward
Helping relationships	Being open and trusting about problems with someone who cares: therapeutic alliance, social support, self-help groups
Dramatic relief	Experiencing and expressing feelings about one's problems and solutions: psychodrama, grieving losses, role playing
Environmental reevaluation	Assessing how one's problem affects physical environment: empathy training, documentaries
Social liberation	Increasing alternatives for nonproblem behaviors available in society: advocating for rights of repressed, empowering, policy interventions

Source: Reprinted from Prochaska, J., et al., In Search of How People Change, *American Psychologist*, Vol. 47, No. 9, 1102–1114. Copyright © 1992 by the American Psychological Association. Reprinted with permission.

that to maintain change means to operate from a sense of self-value.

The underlying structure for change of addictive behaviors is neither technique-oriented nor problem-specific. It is a performance art that demands a perfect match between process and stage. In other words, efficient self-change or therapy change depends on doing the right things (processes) at the right time (stages). In artful caring practice, the nurse and client work together to co-create the circumstances that will facilitate successful change.

The Workplace and the Human Health Experience

Sometimes nurses encounter people who are seeking changes in their health experience in the context of their work environment. Many workplace wellness programs are now being developed throughout the United States because of the escalating health care costs of employees, cumulative research findings that document the rising health care costs associated with unhealthy employee behaviors, and em-

Exhibit 3–2 Stages of Change in Which Particular Processes of Change Are Emphasized

Precontemplation	Contemplation	Preparation	Action	Maintenance
Consciousness raising Dramatic relief Environmental reevaluation				
	Self- reevaluation			
		Self- liberation		
			Reinforcement management Helping relationships Counterconditioning Stimulus control	

Source: Reprinted from Prochaska, J., et al., In Search of How People Change, *American Psychologist*, Vol. 47, No. 9, 1102–1114. Copyright © 1992 by the American Psychological Association. Reprinted with permission.

ployer support of these programs. Generally, workplace wellness programs focus on stress management, nutritional education, weight control, exercise/physical fitness, smoking cessation, management of hypertension, alcohol and drug control, accident prevention, and early cancer detection. Because of their education and holistic focus, nurses are in an ideal position to develop wellness programs within businesses and all areas of the community.[57] Ideally, such nurses should have knowledge of current health care practices, existing workplace wellness programs, and marketing and health care reimbursement. They also need leadership skills. Community health nursing theory can provide specific guidance for nurses seeking to develop community wellness programs.

Effective wellness programs help individuals identify their motivation for change, that is, the spark or desire to improve their present situation. Imagination is a prerequisite of motivation, for it is necessary to answer the question, What do I really want? Discipline and determination must also be engaged. Some of the circumstances that may block motivated behavior are

- self-doubts and fears of unknown consequences that can override a person's desire to learn new health behaviors
- belief that prior commitments or high-priority projects leave little time for learning or implementing new behaviors
- perception of the person who is learning new skills that the new behaviors are distasteful
- previous failures in changing behavior
- lack of confidence in the ability to implement new strategies
- cultural beliefs that discourage the new behavior
- lack of support from family, co-workers, or other groups[58]

Whether in the workplace, the hospital, or other health care environment, the wise nurse recognizes that some people do not perceive the degree to which culture conditions their beliefs, attitudes, and values. Though wellness may be desired, people sometimes feel helpless under the burden of their role responsibilities and have a pervasive sense that they can do nothing to resolve existing problems. Artful caring can help people clarify their values and beliefs, identify obstacles to change, and rename these obstacles as challenges. Naturally, nurses will be more effective in motivating clients if they model wellness themselves. More than ever, nurses are placing an emphasis on wellness in their own lives. They are teaching self-care, self-responsibility, and choices that lead toward health and becoming powerful role models for the message of health that they bring.

CONCLUSION

Nursing is an art as well as a science. The artistry of nursing is embodied in the nurse's gift of self in a co-creative relationship with the client. The intent of artistic nursing is healing, which is an essentially spiritual process. Understanding the human health experience as a complex and dynamic dialectic relationship of health-wellness-disease-illness can facilitate the finding of meaning in the experience and, thus, the process of healing. Understanding the role of perceptions, values, beliefs, attitudes, the stages of change in addictive behavior patterns, and blocks to motivation helps to explain the complexities that people confront when making health choices. As nurses seek to provide the care, support, guidance, and commitment that facilitate healing, this understanding enhances the art of nursing.

DIRECTIONS FOR FUTURE RESEARCH

1. Describe the art of nursing with population groups.
2. Determine whether nurses who understand the health-disease-wellness-illness dialectic relationship and use this understanding with clients use holistic therapies more often than nurses who do not understand and use this model of the human health experience.
3. Evaluate to what degree matching nursing interventions to the client's stage of change enhances client outcomes.

NURSE HEALER REFLECTIONS

After reading this chapter, the nurse healer will be able to answer or begin a process of answering the following questions:

- How am I an artist in my nursing practice?
- How do my values influence my practice?
- How would I describe my experience of health-wellness, disease-illness?
- What motivates me to change?
- What is my self-image?
- What is my current quality of life?

NOTES

1. R. Barnhart, ed., *The Barnhart Concise Dictionary of Etymology* (New York: HarperCollins Publishers, 1995).

2. L. Jensen and M. Allen, Wellness: The Dialect of Illness, *Image* 25, no. 3 (1993): 220–224.

3. Jensen and Allen, Wellness: The Dialect of Illness.

4. S. Leddy and J.M. Pepper, *Conceptual Bases of Professional Nursing Practice*, 3rd ed. (Philadelphia: J.B. Lippincott, 1995).

5. Leddy and Pepper, *Conceptual Bases of Professional Nursing Practice*.

6. Jensen and Allen, Wellness: The Dialect of Illness.

7. J. Watson, Introduction: Art and Aesthetics as Passage between the Centuries, in *Art and Aesthetics in Nursing*, ed. J. Watson and P. Chinn (New York: National League for Nursing, 1994), xv.

8. J. Watson and P. Chinn, eds., *Art and Aesthetics in Nursing* (New York: National League for Nursing, 1994).

9. E. Dissanayake, *Homo Aestheticus: Where Art Comes From and Why* (Seattle: University of Washington Press, 1992).

10. Dissanayake, *Homo Aestheticus.*

11. Dissanayake, *Homo Aestheticus.*

12. Watson, Introduction: Art and Aesthetics as Passage between the Centuries, xvi.

13. C. Appleton, The Gift of Self: A Paradigm for Originating Art in Nursing, in *Art and Aesthetics in Nursing,* ed. J. Watson and P. Chinn (New York: National League for Nursing, 1994), 91–116.

14. P. Benner and C. Tanner, Clinical Judgement. How Expert Nurses Use Intuition, *American Journal of Nursing* 87 (1987): 23–31.

15. F. Barron et al., *Creators on Creating* (New York: Tarcher/Putnam, 1997).

16. Barron et al., *Creators on Creating.*

17. L.E. Daniel, Vulnerability as a Key to Authenticity, *Image* 30, no. 2 (1998): 191–192.

18. B. Willis, *The Tao of Art* (London: Century Paperbacks, 1987).

19. L.A. Firestone, *Awakening Minerva: The Power of Creativity in Women's Lives* (New York: Time Warner, 1997).

20. Appleton, The Gift of Self.

21. Appleton, The Gift of Self.

22. A. Bernado, Technology and True Presence in Nursing, *Journal of Holistic Nursing Practice* 12, no. 4 (1998): 42.

23. K. Maeve, Coming to Moral Consciousness through the Art of Nursing Narratives, in *Art and Aesthetics in Nursing,* ed. J. Watson and P. Chinn (New York: National League for Nursing, 1994), 67–90.

24. S. Gadow, Existential Advocacy: Philosophical Foundation of Nursing, in *Nursing Images and Ideals,* eds. S. Spicker and S. Gadow (New York: Springer, 1980), 79–101.

25. C. Gilligan, *In a Different Voice: Psychological Theory and Women's Development* (Cambridge, MA: Harvard University Press, 1982).

26. D.W. Wardell and J. Englebretson, Professional Evolution, *Journal of Holistic Nursing* 6, no. 1 (1998): 57–67.

27. M.A. Burkhardt, Reflections: Awakening Spirit and Purpose, *Journal of Holistic Nursing* 16, no. 2 (1998): 165.

28. P. Donahue, *Nursing: The Finest Art* (St. Louis, MO: Mosby, 1985), 467.

29. Jensen and Allen, Wellness: The Dialect of Illness.

30. Jensen and Allen, Wellness: The Dialect of Illness.

31. Appleton, The Gift of Self.

32. M.M. Andrews, Cultural Diversity and Community Health Nursing, in *Community Health Nursing: Promoting the Health of Aggregates,* eds. J.M. Swanson and M. Albrecht (Philadelphia: W.B. Saunders, 1993), 371–403.

33. G.M. Bartol and L. Richardson, Using Literature to Create Cultural Competency, *Image* 30, no. 1 (1998): 75–78.

34. K. Shadick, A Practice Model for Promoting Cultural Diversity (Paper presented at the American Nephrology Nurses Association Annual Conference, Dallas, TX, 1994).

35. L. Raths et al., *Values and Teaching: Working with Values in the Classroom* (Columbus, OH: Charles E. Merrill, 1978).

36. Maeve, Coming to Moral Consciousness.

37. Raths et al., *Values and Teaching: Working with Values in the Classroom.*

38. J. Havens, The Valuing Process, *Journal of Holistic Nursing* 11, no. 1 (1993): 56–63.

39. Appleton, The Gift of Self.

40. Appleton, The Gift of Self.

41. D. Lauver, A Theory of Care-Seeking Behavior, *Image* 24, no. 4 (1992): 281–287.

42. I. Rosenstock, The Health Belief Model: Explaining Health Behavior through Expectancies, in *Health Behavior and Health Education,* eds. K. Glanz and B. Rimer (San Francisco: Jossey-Bass Publishers, 1990), 39–62.

43. Lauver, A Theory of Care-Seeking Behavior.

44. J. Mirotznik et al., Using the Health Belief Model To Explain Clinic Appointment-Keeping for the Management of a Chronic Disease Condition, *Journal of Community Health* 23, no. 3 (1998): 195–210.

45. Rosenstock, The Health Belief Model.

46. J. Prochaska et al., In Search of How People Change, *American Psychologist* 47, no. 9 (1992): 1102–1114.

47. Prochaska et al., In Search of How People Change.

48. Prochaska et al., In Search of How People Change.

49. Prochaska et al., In Search of How People Change.

50. Prochaska et al., In Search of How People Change.

51. R. Kaplan and H. Simon, Compliance in Medical Care: Reconsideration of Self-Prediction, *Annals of Behavioral Medicine* 12 (1990): 66–71.

52. L. Beutler and J. Clarkin, *Systematic Treatment Selection* (New York: Brunner/Mazel, 1990).

53. C. DiClemente, Motivational Interviewing and the Stages of Change, in *Motivational Interviewing: Preparing People for Change,* eds. E. Miller and S. Rollnick (New York: Guilford Press, 1991), 191–202.

54. C. DiClemente and S. Hughes, Stages of Change Profiles in Alcoholism Treatment, *Journal of Substance Abuse* 2 (1990): 217–235.

55. C. DiClemente et al., The Process of Smoking Cessation: An Analysis of Precontemplation, Contemplation, and Preparation Stages of Change, *Journal of Consulting and Clinical Psychology* 59 (1991): 295–304.

56. T. Glynn et al., Essential Elements of Self-Help/ Minimal Intervention Strategies for Smoking Cessation, *Health Education Quarterly* 17 (1990): 329–345.

57. J. Dunham-Taylor, Nurses Cut Health Care Costs, *Journal of Holistic Nursing* 11, no. 4 (1993): 398–411.

58. J. Achterberg et al., *Rituals of Healing* (New York: Bantam Books, 1994).

VISION OF HEALING

The Web of Life

Human beings are embedded in the web of life.[1] We are part of a highly complex, integrative living system consisting of cyclic processes in which we participate and on which we depend. What we call objects are actually networks of relationships. What we call parts are, in fact, patterns in networks of relationships. All networks, with their patterns, contain or are nested in other networks and are inseparable. Human beings are engaged in an evolving process that affects and is affected by the patterns and rhythms that they support and in which they dwell. We are interconnected and interdependent with each other, as well as with the objects and parts that we try to view as other. We are engaged in an ongoing dance that proceeds through a subtle interaction of competition and cooperation, creation and mutual adaptation.[2]

As nurses, we need to de-emphasize the classification and categorization of objects and parts. We need to shift our thinking to take into account configurations, connections, and contexts rather than just attending to "affected" parts of wholes. Our thinking needs to expand to a holistic and ecologic perspective grounded in a natural and social environment. We need to shed the common notion of hierarchical structures, which are too often seen in terms of domination and control. Instead, we need to consider the multileveled order found in nature that comprises the web of life. Our models need to allow the creation of new structures and modes of behavior absorbed in the process of development, learning, and co-evolution. We need to recognize that we are engaged with open systems that operate far from equilibrium and to appreciate the nonlinear interconnectedness of all the components of the network(s).

It is especially important to remember that nurses are networks included in other network(s). Nurses are wounded healers. As nurses, we are often tempted to ignore our own woundedness. We must learn to acknowledge our wounds, as well as to recognize our strengths. When a nurse and a client who come together embrace their woundedness, healing occurs for both. Healing does not simply flow from the nurse to the client, for the potential to heal already exists within the client. The nurse simply encourages the client's process of inner healing. Healing occurs as the client and the nurse both acknowledge their life processes and cooperate to promote growth.

As the best of traditional practices continues to merge with the best of holistic practices, the art of healing will likewise progress. Creativity and spontaneity will be released as we admit our own weaknesses in order to open creatively to our clients. Only then will we know the powerful part of our being and fully realize our interconnections. The use of self, directed by intention and with presence, provides us with wondrous possibilities for healing.

NOTES

1. F. Capra, *The Web of Life* (New York: Doubleday, 1996), 46.

2. Capra, *The Web of Life,* 36.

Chapter 4

The Psychophysiology of Bodymind Healing

Genevieve M. Bartol and Nancy F. Courts

NURSE HEALER OBJECTIVES

Theoretical

- Articulate a comprehensive conceptual model of bodymind interactions.
- Interpret the application of selected models, theories, and research in the field of psychoneuroimmunology.
- Explain the interconnections of mind modulation and the autonomic, endocrine, immune, and neuropeptide systems.

Clinical

- Recognize the implications of bodymind interactions for clinical practice.
- Incorporate the knowledge of bodymind interactions in planning nursing interventions.

Personal

- Identify one's own patterns of bodymind interactions as expressed in attitudes, tensions, and images.
- Recognize the implications of one's own bodymind patterns for self-care and self-healing.

DEFINITIONS

Autopoiesis: the self-organizing force in living systems.

Bodymind: a state of integration that includes body, mind, and spirit.

Information Theory: a mathematical model that helps explain the connections between consciousness and bodymind healing.

Limbic–Hypothalamic System: the major anatomic modulating link connecting the brain/mind and the autonomic, endocrine, immune, and neuropeptide systems.

Mind Modulation: the bidirectional interrelationships of thoughts and feelings with neurohormonal messengers of the nervous, endocrine, immune, and neuropeptide systems that support bodymind connections.

Network: interconnected and interrelated system.

Neuropeptides: messenger molecules produced at various sites throughout the body to transmit bodymind patterns of communication.

Neurotransmitters: chemicals that facilitate the transmission of impulses through nerves in the body.

Psychoneuroimmunology: a branch of science that strives to show the connections among psychology, neuroendocrinology, and immunology.

Receptors: sites on cell surfaces that serve as points of attachment for various types of messenger molecules.

Self-Regulation Theory: a person's ability to learn cognitive processing of information to bring involuntary body responses under voluntary control.

Ultradian Performance Rhythm: rhythmic repetition of certain phenomena in living organisms that occur in less than 24 hours, such as varying patterns of activity and rejuvenation.

NEW SCIENTIFIC UNDERSTANDING OF LIVING SYSTEMS

New developments in science reveal human beings in a new light. The mechanistic view of the world of Descartes and Newton is giving way to a holistic and ecologic view. The habit of looking at persons from the perspective of the body, mind, or spirit is misleading and creates problems of its own. The body can no longer be considered a machine powered by the mind or spirit to which health care practitioners apply assorted therapies to effect healing. Rather, humans are complex, highly integrative systems embedded in and supporting other systems. The term bodymind can include the body, mind, and spirit as a unified whole.

Quantum Theory

In the 1920s, discoveries in quantum physics shocked the scientific community. The old ways of viewing phenomena no longer fit. Heisenberg described the changed world "as a complicated tissue of events, in which connections of different kinds alternate or overlap or combine and thereby determine the texture of the whole."[1] In the past, the properties and behavior of the parts were believed to determine those of the whole. These advances in quantum physics made it clear that the whole also defines the behavior of the parts.

The realization that systems are integrated wholes that cannot be understood simply by analysis shattered scientific certitude. No longer was it possible to believe that given enough time, effort, and money, all questions would have answers. Rather, all scientific concepts and theories have limitations. Scientific explanations do not provide complete and conclusive answers, but instead generate other questions.[2] The more we learn, the more we discover how much we do not know. Even one additional piece of data will change the whole configuration. It is important to remain open to all possibilities, because absolute certainty is an illusion.[3]

Increasingly, scientific findings demonstrate a changing world. Planck found radiant energy was emitted from light sources in discrete amounts or "quanta" and that changes in the amount of radiant energy occurred in leaps, not sequential steps.[4] Bohr extended Planck's discovery to the field of subatomic particles and argued that electrons could move from one orbit of energy to another. The behavior of light does not follow one set of rules. Light possesses the qualities of both waves and particles. One explanation is not correct and the other wrong; both interpretations are useful in explaining the behavior of light in different situations.

The world is complex and unified; parts complement one another and participate in the whole. Similarly, all parts of the body work together. Health and illness are indivisible; both are natural and necessary. Hyperpyrexia (fever) may be seen as a sign of illness, as well as a sign of the body's healthy response to a threat. Fever indicates that the hypothalamic set point of the body has changed.[5] Such an alteration occurs in the presence of pyrogens (e.g., bacteria, viruses). A mild temperature elevation up to 39°C (102.2°F) stimulates the body's immune system, increases white blood cell production, and reduces the concentration of iron in blood plasma, thereby suppressing the growth of bacteria. Fever also stimulates the production of interferon, which protects the body against viruses. Fever can be beneficial because it helps to defend the body against pyrogens. Using medications to lower the body temperature prematurely, particularly in the first 24 hours, may actually interfere with this important defense mechanism

Systems Theory

The major traits of systems thinking appeared concurrently in several disciplines during the first half of the twentieth century, but it was von Bertalanffy's concept of the open system and his general systems theory that established systems thinking as a predominant scientific movement.[6] The resultant theories and models of living systems initiated a radical shift in perceptions of human beings. It is now believed that persons and their environments make up an interconnected dynamic system in which a change at any point may effect changes at other points. The idea that the world is hierarchical, with each level organized separately, has been replaced with a new understanding of relatedness and context.

Human beings are living systems, organizationally closed and structurally open, embedded within the web of life.[7] They are "organizationally closed" because they are self-organizing; that is, they establish their own order and behavior rather than submitting to those imposed by the environment. They are "structurally open" because they engage in a continual exchange of energy and matter with their environment. Words like *feedback, integration, rhythm,* and *dynamic equilibrium* account for the continually changing components of living systems.[8] These components do not operate in isolation from each other. A dysfunction in any one system of the body reverberates in the other systems. For example, a dysfunction of the endocrine system referred to as hypothryroidism may manifest itself by thinning hair or clinical depression.[9] Hypothyroidism, in fact, may be secondary to a dysfunction in another organ system and not represent primary failure of the thyroid gland.[10] Thyroid deficiency may occur when the pituitary gland is malfunctioning or when there is damage to the hypothalamus. It is not possible to identify conclusively a single cause of what was formerly named a primary dysfunction. All body systems participate in the biodance; changes in one system result in changes in the other systems and, in circular fashion, changes itself, just as the pituitary gland will increase its secretion of thyroid-stimulating hormone (TSH) when the thyroid gland is underproducing thyroid hormone.

Theory of Relativity

Early in the twentieth century, Einstein developed a system of mechanics that acknowledges the relative character of motion, velocity, and mass, as well as the interdependence of matter, time, and space.[11] The theory is based on the principle that there is no absolute frame of reference independent of the observer. Each person views others from his or her own perspective, including his or her particular biases. Einstein characterized his feelings about this scientific revelation as having the ground pulled out from under him.[12]

Scientists can no longer describe their work as finding a piece to one gigantic puzzle or as adding a building stone to a firm foundation of knowledge. Rather, it has become increasingly apparent that scientific knowledge is a network of concepts and models, none of which is any more fundamental than the other. All things (objects) and events (happenings) in one's life are connected and relative within the whole. The mind and body are inseparably intertwined. Whatever happens in one's life is interconnected. Thoughts, feelings, and actions influence a person's state of health and illness.

Even religious beliefs have an impact, though it is not clear in what way. Koenig and associates reported that Christian persons who attend religious services at least once per week and who read the Bible or pray regularly have consistently lower diastolic blood pressure readings than those who do not.[13] A lower diastolic reading, which indicates the blood pressure when the heart relaxes, is associated with improved health. It is not known how these religious activities influence the blood pressure or if a specific spiritual orientation accompanies these activities and accounts for the difference. Other groups with different practices need to be studied.

Principles of Self-Organization

The key ideas of current models of self-organizing systems were refined and extended during the 1970s and 1980s, and a unified theory of living systems emerged.[14] These models encompassed the creation of structures and modes of behavior in the processes of development, learning, and co-evolution. In the past, living systems were viewed from two perspectives: in terms of physical matter (structure) and the configuration of relationships (pattern). Structure is concerned with quantities, things weighed and measured. Pattern is concerned with qualities and is expressed by a map of the configuration of relationships. Qualities, such as color or size, were considered accidental characteristics. For example, a bicycle may be red or green; may stand 24 or 26 inches high; may have a light or heavy frame, and remains a bicycle as long as it has the configuration of relationships consistent with a bicycle.

Systems, whether nonliving or living, are configurations of ordered relationships whose attributes are the properties of pattern. The bicycle, a nonliving system, consists of a number of components arranged to perform a particular function. The various kinds of bicycles (e.g., mountain bicycles, touring bicycles) embody the essential characteristics known as a bicycle. In brief, bicycles have a structure with specific components and operate as bicycles as long as the pattern of relationships that defines it as a bicycle remains.[15] Living systems, however, are fundamentally different from nonliving systems. Living systems do not function mechanically and are not explained just by physical principles. The components of living systems are interconnected by internal feedback loops in a nonlinear fashion and are capable of self-organization.

Not only is the activity of living systems purposeful, but also it appears to be under the direction of an overall design or purpose.[16] The pattern of organization of living systems includes a fundamental self-organizing force known as autopoiesis.[17] Yet, if the pattern of a living system is destroyed, the system dies even though all the components of the system remain intact. The living system cannot be restored simply by recreating the pattern, whereas a nonliving system, like a bicycle, will regain function if the parts are reassembled correctly. Living systems do not rest in a steady state of balance as do nonliving systems but rather operate far from equilibrium.[18] Stability in living systems embodies change. Relationships are not linear, but extend in all directions and generate feedback loops. Living systems regulate and recreate themselves.

Life process (cognition) is the link between pattern and structure in a living system.[19] Life process is "the activity involved in the continual embodiment of the system's pattern of organization."[20] It is related to autopoiesis, and they may be considered two distinct facets of the same phenomenon of life. All living systems are cognitive systems, and cognition indicates the existence of an autopoietic network.[21] Structure, pattern, and process are inextricably intertwined in a living system.

Organisms appear to be under the direction of an overall design or purpose and do not just function mechanically. For example, the symptoms experienced by humans represent attempts to gain health and, therefore, are signals of stability, not breakdown. The human immune system recognizes an invading organism as dangerous and quickly reacts to counter the threat. Symptoms are really signs of the inherent organization and adaptability of a living system. Even invading organisms, also living systems, learn and adapt. The ability of pathogens to modify themselves and develop resistance to antibiotics is another striking example of the ability of a living system to reorganize.

Bell's Theorem

Cause-and-effect thinking with its before, after, now, and later sequence is no longer acceptable. According to Bell's theorem, the whole determines the actions of the parts, and changes occur instantaneously.[22] Thus, even a fleeting thought or passing feeling can change the system. Changes do not happen in an orderly stepwise sequence. Furthermore, healing does not take time, but is dependent on hope and belief beyond time. Beliefs, thoughts, and feelings are all part of the configuration, and each affects the human states of wellness and illness.

Personality and Wellness

Researchers have unsuccessfully tried to link specific illnesses with particular personality constellations.[23] It has been found, for example, that individuals with peptic ulcers have as many personality configurations as does the general population. Several researchers, however, have uncovered particular personality traits associated with wellness.[24] Schwartz discovered that persons who attend to symptoms, sensations, and feelings; who connect those signals to events in their lives; and who express what is occurring have a stronger immune profile and healthier cardiovascular system than those who do not.[25] This capacity became known as the Attend, Connect, Express (ACE) Factor. Kabat-Zinn developed a training program in mindfulness (healthy attention) to help persons cope with a variety of chronic illness and intractable pain.[26]

Pennebaker found that persons who admit their feelings to themselves and others have healthier psychologic profiles and fewer illnesses than those who do not.[27] After observing that criminals seemed to relax and experience relief after confession, despite the fact that their confessions also brought certain punishment and loss, Pennebaker devised an experiment to test if disclosure of sexual and other traumas would bring similar relief. He asked 46 male and female students to go into a room and to write continuously for 20 minutes about the most upsetting or traumatic experience of their lives on 5 successive days. Many students wrote about experiences that they had never mentioned to others and had even tried to erase from their memory deliberately. Students reported that the first day was disturbing and painful, but by the fifth day, they experienced resolution and calm. Later, Pennebaker teamed up with Kiecolt-Glaser to study the effect of disclosure through writing on health.[28] Students who wrote about traumas had improved immune systems and fewer reports of illness, even though they had no other therapeutic intervention.

Ouellette discovered that individuals who have a sense of control over their quality of life, health, and social conditions; have a strong commitment to work (or creative activity) and relationships; and view stress as a challenge, not a threat, have stronger immune systems.[29] Ouellette collaborated with Maddi to show that this combination of qualities, known as the "hardiness factor," is not simply a reflection of well-being that comes from good health practices. Even after these researchers controlled for good health practices, including exercise, diet, relaxation regimens, and social support, hardiness emerged as the most powerful protector of health.

Solomon showed that persons who assert their needs and feelings have more balanced immune responses.[30] McClelland argued that persons who are strongly motivated to form relationships with others based on unconditional love and trust have more vigorous immune systems and fewer illnesses.[31] Luks discovered that altruistic persons suffer fewer illnesses than others.[32] Linville found that persons who explore many facets of their personalities can better withstand stressful life circumstances.[33] Although a direct cause-and-effect relationship between any personality factor and health or illness cannot be determined, this research indicates that developing personality strengths to protect one from the stresses of living seems also to bolster one's defense against illness.

Information Theory

Patterns of communication and patterns of organization in organisms can be viewed analogously.[34] Information theory, a mathematical model, was developed to define and measure amounts of information transmitted through telegraph and telephone lines. The theory was used to explain how to get a message coded as a signal in order to determine what to charge customers for messages. A coded message (signal) is essentially a pattern of organization. Information flow (i.e., pattern of communication and pattern of organization) in human beings is able to unify physiologic, psychologic, sociologic, and spiritual phenomena in a holistic framework. Information flow is the missing piece that makes it possible to transcend the bodymind split, because information resides in both the body and the mind.[35]

Santiago Theory of Congition

Derived from the study of neural networks, the Santiago theory of cognition is linked to the concept of autopoiesis (continual embodiment of the system's pattern of organization).[36] Cognition is generally defined as the process of knowing or perceiving; it is associated with the mind, implicitly with the brain and nervous system. Yet, the Santiago theory offers a radical expansion of the traditional concept of cognition. In this new view, cognition involves the whole process of life, including perception, emotion, and behavior. Even the cells that make up the immune system perceive the characteristics of their environment and will, for example, move to the site of a wound and increase in numbers to deal with an invading organism. Despite the absence of a brain, cognition is present; in this event, it can be described as "embodied action."[37] Perception and action in these cells are inseparable.

A living organism is an interconnected network (system) that undergoes structural change while preserving its pattern of organization as it interacts with other systems.[38] Actually, changes in both autopoietic networks take place. In other words, one living system may trigger an autopoietic network response in the other, but does not direct or control the response. A living organism chooses which stimuli from the environment will trigger structural changes. Moreover, not all changes in an organism are acts of cognition. A person who is injured in an accident does not specify and direct those structural changes, for example. Other structural changes (e.g., perception and response of the circulatory system) that accompany the imposed changes are acts of cognition, however.

The Santiago theory helps explain how humans receive, generate, and transduce information. New ideas and events evoke bodymind changes; that is, neural pathways and consciousness couple to enable information transduction.[39] For example, a client with severe episodes of asthma that increasingly interfere with her activities may remember that her mother's asthma also became more severe as she aged, and she may begin to become despondent at what she views as an inevitable decline in her health. After a nurse teaches her how to monitor her asthma with the help of a flow meter, the client begins to see a pattern to her attacks and identifies potential triggers. She gains a new understanding of body-mind connections and uses both traditional and holistic interventions to interrupt the triggers. These interventions not only lead to or result in change in the pattern of her attacks, but also provide her with a greater sense of control over her asthma. The asthma attacks decrease in severity and frequency. The client had a personal experience of information transduction and acquired a new understanding of the interconnectedness of body-mind-spirit.

The extent of the interactions that a living system can have with its environment outlines its "cognitive domain."[40] Emotions are not just an accompaniment of perception and behavior, but are an inherent part of this domain. For example, a fear response to a situation initiates an entire pattern of physiologic processes. Blood goes to the large skeletal muscles, making it easier to run, while the face blanches. Freezing for a moment allows time to assess the situation and determine if hiding may be a wiser choice. Circuits in the brain's emotional centers trigger a flood of hormones that sounds a general alert. Although experience and culture modify responses, emotions occur simultaneously with and are part of every cognitive act.

EMOTIONS AND THE NEURAL TRIPWIRE

The traditional view in neuroscience has been that the sensory organs transmit signals to the thalamus and from there to the sensory process areas of the neocortex,[41] which translates the signals into perceptions and attaches meanings. The signals then move to the limbic system, which sends the appropriate response to the body. This has all changed, however, with the discovery of a smaller bundle of neurons that leads directly from the thalamus to the amygdala—in addition to those that connect with the neocortex (Figure 4–1). Sensory impulses go directly from the sensory organs to the amygdala, allowing for a faster response. The amygdala triggers an emotional response even before the person fully understands what is happening. Taking immediate action, the amygdala sends impulses through the brain to the body. If the stimulus is traumatic, the amygdala responds with extra strength. Key changes take place in the locus ceruleus, which regulates catecholamines; adrenaline and noradrenaline are released. Other limbic structures, such as the hippocampus and the hypothalamus respond, and the main stress hormones bring about the typical body responses labeled fight or flight, faint or freeze. Changes in the brain opioid system that secretes endorphins prepare the person to meet the danger. Meanwhile, the neocortex processes the impulse, and a more considered response follows. Emotions are not dispensable, but rather an integral part of the whole.

State-Dependent Memory and Recall

What people learn depends on their mood or feelings at the time of the experience.[42] Feelings are integral to human living; not just an extravagance or an annoyance. The emotion-carrying molecules or ligands, which accompany all human activity, bind to cellular receptors and send an informational message to the cell where they can be stored as memories.

Feelings and actions are intertwined. People are more likely to help others when

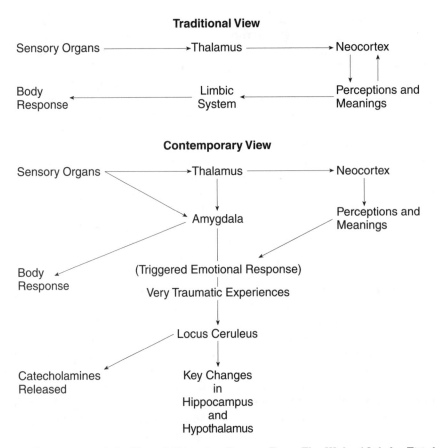

Figure 4-1 Emotions and the Neural Tripwire. *Source:* From *The Web of Life* by Fitjof Capra. Copyright © 1996 by Fitjof Capra. Used by permission of Doubleday, a division of Bantam Doubleday Dell Publishing Group, Inc.

they are in a good mood and more likely to hurt others when they are in a bad mood. Likewise, feelings and memories are intertwined. Thoughts that occur throughout daily routines are repeated patterns of memories and their associative emotional connections. Memories are accompanied by emotions that, in turn, are influenced and affected by the context in which they were acquired. A particularly traumatic experience is stamped in the memory with special strength. Subsequent stimuli in new situations and emotional experiences can attach to and reactivate past memories. These thoughts and emotions direct and shape people.

Feelings or mood also play a major role in bodymind healing. Recent work with persons suffering from post-traumatic stress disorder (PTSD) has revealed that relearning is the route to healing. Writing therapy, bibliotherapy, art therapy, and even the traditional talk therapies are all ways of unfreezing a picture frozen in the amygdala that is capable of triggering the fight or flight, freeze or faint response provoked by seemingly benign stimuli. At the same time, body work is often used to release these pockets of energy that are frozen in the body. Because people have network responses with the systems that they contain and those with which they nest, healing can occur from multiple directions.

Location of the Brain Centers

Old models for brain functioning were the telegraph or telephone by which messages were sent from one point to another.[43] Another model compared brain functioning to that of a computer. A more accurate way of understanding brain function, however, is to use the model of a hologram. A specially processed photographic record, a hologram provides a three-dimensional image when a light from a laser is beamed through it. If any part of the hologram should be destroyed, any one of the remaining parts is capable of reconstructing the whole image. The brain operates like a hologram. This later model does not negate the earlier models, but is congruent with the new understanding of the way in which information is transmitted, received, and stored (learned). Current data on brain functioning modify the following elements of the traditional model:

- Memories are not stored in any specific part of the brain, but rather in multiple overlapping areas. They can be retrieved in their entirety by a stimulus to more than one area of the brain. Loss of specific memory is related more to the amount of brain damage than to the site of the injury.
- The ability to recall what was lost when the brain was first injured by gunshot wounds or cardiovascular accident (stroke) often returns, even though regeneration of neurons is not generally believed to be possible.
- Paranormal events, including the transpersonal healing associated with shamanism and other approaches to metaphysical healing, involve communicating information in ways that do not conform to the current understanding of receiving, processing, and sending energy.

- Phenomena such as phantom limb sensations and auras that extend beyond the corpus challenge traditional perceptions of body image, as well as the understanding of the physical boundaries of the body.
- Mechanisms of consciousness, such as the ability of the person to reflect on the self or create and retrieve images, cannot be explained simply in terms of the structure and function of current anatomic models.

Viewing the brain in a holographic manner reveals its influence on psychophysiologic functioning. People who believe that they do not have the conscious ability to effect a physical change with their imagination do not try to do so. They will not explore memories and patterns formed of past experience and will continue to respond unconsciously as they always have in the past.

ULTRADIAN RHYTHMS

Humans have various natural, biologic rhythms that mirror those found in nature.[44] Infradian rhythms are those that recur in a period longer than a day, such as a woman's menstrual cycle. Circadian rhythms are those that rise and fall, usually within a 24-hour period, such as sleep and wake patterns. Ultradian rhythms refer to the cyclic patterns of rhythmic repetition that occur in cycles of less than 24 hours, such as varying levels of energy associated with activity and rest. These rhythmic patterns vary for each person, and individuals can shift them with changing demands and daily circumstances.

The body periodically offers important physiologic and psychologic information about keeping healthy, energetic, creative, and productive. This information comes from the circadian and ultradian rhythms experienced throughout the day. For example, the general pattern of the ultradian rhythm is 90 to 120 minutes of activity, followed by a 20-minute recovery period (Figure 4–2). Periods of high energy regularly alternate with signals suggesting a need for rest. Ignoring those signals and continuing to work disturbs the ultradian rhythms and leads to stress. Responding appropriately to these signals with a rest period allows the ultradian rhythms to regain their normal pattern and relieves the stress. Thus, heeding this natural call promotes rejuvenation and recovery. Nurses can use their knowledge of natural cycles to help themselves and their clients optimize their level of wellness.

MIND MODULATION

Indirect and direct anatomic and biochemical pathways connect the nervous, endocrine, and immune regulatory systems. Communication among these systems is multidirectional with signal molecules and their receptors regulating the cellular outcomes.[45]

Stress Response

The biochemical functions of the major organ systems are modulated by the mind.[46]

Thoughts and feelings are transduced into chemicals (i.e., neurotransmitters, neurohormones, and peptides) that circulate throughout the body and convey messages via cells to various systems within the body. The stress response is a good example of the way in which systems cooperate to protect an individual from harm.

A young man is walking to his car alone late at night when a stranger grabs his arm and attempts to rob him. His immediate response is one of fear, and his body prepares him to manage the danger by preparing him physically. The locus ceruleus with nerve endings in the forebrain instantaneously secretes norepinephrine directly into the cortex. Not only does the sympathetic nervous system (SNS) secrete norepinephrine, but the SNS fibers also extend into the adrenal medulla, stimulating medulla secretion of norepinephrine. The young man's body is now full of norepinephrine, and he feels the effects. In addition, muscular ten-

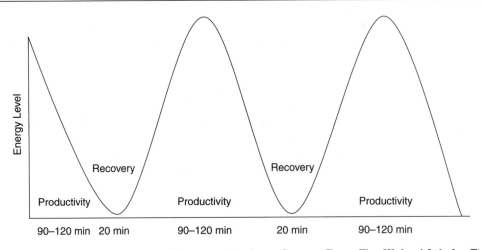

Figure 4–2 General Pattern of Ultradian Rhythms. *Source:* From *The Web of Life* by Fitjof Capra. Copyright © 1996 by Fritjof Capra. Used by permission of Doubleday, a division of Bantam Doubleday Dell Publishing Group, Inc.

sion occurs from neural messages and stimulation of the SNS to prepare him for physical challenges.[47] All of this happens even before he is fully aware of the danger.

Quickly, the young man registers what is happening. The hypothalamus secretes corticotropin-releasing factor (CRF) into the hypothalamic–pituitary circulation in the brain. Within approximately 15 seconds, CRF triggers the release of the pituitary hormone adrenocorticotropic hormone (ACTH). In a matter of minutes, the adrenal cortex releases glucocorticoids.[48] Hypothalamic, pituitary, and adrenal neuropeptides and other substances interact with the immune response, completing the multidirectional circle of communication among the nervous, endocrine, and immune systems. The young man has now experienced a full-blown psychophysiologic stress reaction to the fear of being robbed and possibly hurt.

Physiologically, the cascade of changes associated with the stress response appears as increased heart and respiratory rates, tightened muscles, increased metabolic rate, and a general sense of foreboding, fear, nervousness, irritability, and negative mood. Other physiologic responses include elevated blood pressure, dilated pupils, stronger cardiac contractions, and increased levels of blood glucose, serum cholesterol, circulating free fatty acids, and triglycerides. Although these responses prepare a person for short-term stress, the effects on the body of long-term stress responses can include structure damage and chronic illness. The memory of this experience, stored in the brain and other body cells, has psychologic and spiritual out-

comes. The individual may experience the same reaction in future similar events with less intense stress, such as having a friend touch his arm as they walk toward the car. Indeed, just thinking about this experience can initiate a stress response. Table 4–1 contains a review of the effects of sympathetic and parasympathetic stimulation.

The stress response is designed to meet the demands of stressful stimuli, including experiences such as surgery, burns, and infections. Long-term and unremitting stress can exacerbate angina, tension headaches, cardiac arrhythmias, and pain.[49] The long-term presence of high levels of cortisol over an extended period of time promotes lipolysis in the extremities and lipogenesis in the face and back, suppresses the inflammatory process, increases the risk of osteoporosis and ulcers, and leads to atrophy of immune system organs. Levels of various reproductive hormones (e.g., progesterone, estrogen, testosterone), growth and thyroid hormones, and insulin decline during stress, probably to conserve energy.[50] For example, Hippocrates recognized the stress–spontaneous abortion link when he recommended that pregnant women avoid emotional disturbances.[51] The stress of compulsive marathon running can lead to amenorrhea in women.

Nervous System

The interconnectedness of the central nervous system (CNS) means that frontal cortex thoughts and images are in intimate communication with the emotion-related limbic center. As the biochemicals transduced from thoughts and ideas circulate through the limbic–hypothalamic system, memory cells from past experiences affect their structure. The hypothalamus, the central control center, coordinates the biochemical cascade, integrating neuroendocrine functions by secreting releasing and inhibiting hormones, and stimulating the autonomic nervous system (ANS). The sympathetic branch of the ANS is connected to the limbic system, has

Table 4–1 Effects of Sympathetic and Parasympathetic Stimulation

Structure	Sympathetic Stimulation	Parasympathetic Stimulation
Pupil of eye	Dilates	Contracts
Ciliary muscle	Relaxes, accommodates for distance vision	Contracts, accommodates for close-up vision
Bronchial tubes	Dilates	Constricts
Heart	Accelerates and strengthens actions	Depresses and slows actions
Stomach muscles	Depresses activity	Increases activity
Glands	Alters secretion	Increases secretion
Liver	Stimulates glycogenolysis	
Visceral muscle of intestine	Depresses peristalsis	Increases peristalsis
Adrenal medulla	Causes secretion of epinephrine	
Sweat glands	Increases activity	Decreases activity
Coronary arteries	Dilates	Constricts
Abdominal and pelvic viscera	Constricts	
Peripheral blood vessels	Constricts	
External genitalia	Constricts blood vessels	Dilates blood vessels, causes erection

fibers extending into the adrenal medulla, and a pathway of nerves to the thymus, lymph nodes, spleen, and bone marrow. Hence, the connections are not only biochemical, but also anatomic.

Understanding the psychophysiologic stress response as it affects the nervous system helps to clarify how the different holistic therapies work. It is possible to interrupt feelings of anxiety by using a relaxation technique to calm oneself or a cognitive restructuring technique to change thought patterns. When patients learn to use relaxation, imagery, music therapy, or certain types of meditation training, their sympathetic response to stress decreases, and the calming effect of the parasympathetic system takes over, leading to bodymind healing. Benson described two phases to the relaxation response.[52] The first phase includes the physiologic responses of the relaxation response, that is, decreased sympathetic nervous system activity. Encouraging patients to breathe deeply and slowly, breathing with patients, or instructing patients to synchronize their breathing with the nurse's own can help them to become calmer. In the second phase, when they are relaxed and calm, patients are more recep-

tive and open to new information, and able to solve problems and make decisions. This is a good time to use visual imagery to heal from stress. In addition, the body is protected, since the regular practice of relaxation exercises serves to block the potency of stress hormones.[53]

Often used in conjunction with relaxation techniques, biofeedback can also reduce arousal and tension.[54] It is so effective that it has become a common intervention for a number of conditions induced or exacerbated by uncontrolled stimulation of the stress response. To illustrate, warming the fingers decreases the discomfort that accompanies Raynaud's disease.[55] Connecting the patients' images, emotions, feelings, and spirit with their physiology is the basis for these major changes.[56] Physiologic changes flow in a circular pattern with feedback loops to the frontal cortex and limbic system affecting thoughts and feelings. Conversely, physiologic changes affect the frontal cortex and limbic system, in turn modifying thoughts and feelings, as well as the ability to make decisions and learn.

Medications are used to treat conditions, such as panic attack, that consist of a hyperreaction of the SNS. Beta blockers, for example, block the alpha adrenergic receptors, producing lower heart rate and blood pressure. Patients who are taking beta blockers may not exhibit the normal reactions to threat. Also, older people often have decreased psychophysiologic stress responses, as their reactions to SNS stimulation are blunted.

Endocrine System

Hormones are the specialized chemical messengers that act to modulate both cellular and systemic responses.[57] They are always present in body fluids, but their concentrations vary. They produce both localized and generalized effects. Furthermore, one hormone can stimulate a variety of effects in different tissues, and a single function may be subject to regulation by more than one hormone. Hormones include amines and amino acids (e.g., norepinephrine, epinephrine, dopamine), peptides, polypeptides, proteins, and steroids.[58]

Each cell has a multitude of receptor molecules that can be modified or altered, and hormones act by binding to their specific receptor on target cell surfaces. Treatment with methadone is effective for heroin addicts, for example, because the methadone binds to the opioid receptor sites. A decrease in hormone levels can increase the number of receptor sites available. This is up-regulation. Conversely, an elevated hormone level leads to a decrease in receptors, or down-regulation.[59] In addition, many of the hormones have a negative feedback loop that maintains the balance in serum hormonal levels.

Stimuli such as circadian rhythms, the environment, and emotional and physical stressors influence the secretion of hypothalamic hormones. The opioids (i.e., endorphins, enkephalins, dynorphin) are synthesized in the pituitary and other parts of the CNS. They have a morphinelike effect with receptors throughout the body. These naturally occurring hormones produce the "runner's high," increase a person's pain threshold, and explain how people can "ig-nore" their own serious injury to save a loved one.

Immune System

The immune system shares anatomic connections and signal molecules with the nervous and endocrine systems.[60] Anatomically, the nervous system has direct connections to immune system organs (thymus, bone marrow, lymph nodes, and spleen).[61] There are receptors on the immune system cells for the neurotransmitters such as the opioid peptides, dopamine, and the catecholamines.[62] All the neuropeptide receptors found in the brain are also found on monocytes.[63] The SNS pathways of norepinephrine and epinephrine secretion and the hypothalamus–pituitary–adrenal axis with glucocorticoid secretion have direct effects on immune system cells. It has long been known that the glucocorticoids suppress the immune system. Cortisol, for example, suppresses white blood cells, and it is even administered to suppress the immune system in people with autoimmune diseases.

Recent findings indicate that CNS and ANS neuropeptides and endocrine hormones stimulated by the nervous system directly affect immune system cells. Receptor sites located on the surface of the T and B lymphocytes have the ability to activate, direct, and modify immune function. For example, CRF suppresses monocytic macrophages and T helper lymphocytes. Lymphocytes produce the stress hormone ACTH and the brain peptide endorphin.[64] Endorphins have both enhancing and suppressing effects on immune system cells, depending on their concentration. Immune system cells also have receptors for ACTH and other endocrine hormones.[65]

In turn, cytokines, secretions of immune system cells, affect the nervous and endocrine systems. Cytokines such as the interleukins can stimulate the hypothalamus–pituitary–adrenal axis, thus increasing the levels of glucocorticoids.[66] Cytokines stimulate white blood cell proliferation, phagocytosis, and antibody production. They also induce fever, initiate the inflammatory process, and repair tissue as a healing influence. New evidence suggests that interleukin-2 or cell growth factor is able to up-regulate ACTH from the pituitary.[67] In other words, no system functions in isolation, but all are interconnected, thus demonstrating a vital, bidirectional communication among the systems.

Interventions to reduce the stress response can have a positive effect on the immune system. Some of the direct effects of stress and holistic interventions on immunity include the following:

- Wound healing takes significantly longer in women caregivers of relatives with dementia.[68]
- The response of T lymphocytes improves following writing about traumatic experiences.[69]
- Significant increases of natural killer (NK) cells and NK cell cytotoxic activity occur following a structured psychiatric intervention with cancer patients.[70]
- Significant immunologic changes are evident in students during examination periods; NK cell cytotoxicity decreases significantly, and there are increases in polymorphonuclear superoxide release and lymphocyte proliferative responses.[71]

Interventions that induce the parasympathetic response have healing effects on the body. Because all systems are interconnected, holistic interventions contribute to health and healing.

Neuropeptides

With their receptors, neuropeptides help explain bodymind interconnections and the way that emotions are experienced in the body.[72] Circulating throughout the body, neuropeptides are considered the messengers that connect body and mind. The first neuropeptides were discovered in the intestine, which has many receptors; this explains those "gut feelings." Neuropeptides are secreted in the cortex, hypothalamus, limbic system, and pituitary,[73,74] with the limbic brain containing most of the 88 neuropeptides identified to date.[75] The frontal lobes of the cerebral cortex have the greatest number of opiate receptors.[76] High concentrations of neuropeptides are also found in the spinal cord, accounting for the connection of body sensations and emotions.[77] This open network of neuropeptides with their receptors allows messages to enter and/or be changed at any point.

The limbic system and hippocampus are rich with neuropeptide receptors, containing almost all of them and connecting emotions and learning. The concept of emotions as neuropeptides explains why people have trouble remembering and learning when they are experiencing psychophysiologic stress. Performance, too, is affected. Those who experience severe anxiety and panic before speaking in public or performing a violin concert benefit from relaxation techniques and cognitive restructuring. This ability to alter biochemicals and the consequent effects on memory and learning occur when the unconscious mind is brought into consciousness with hypnosis.[78] Pert wrote that "peptides serve to weave the body's organs and systems into a single web that reacts to both internal and external environmental changes with complex, subtly orchestrated responses."[79]

Emotions cannot be separated from the body. Nurses who attend to the body without also attending to emotions are not providing holistic care. Furthermore, because the immune system cells produce the biochemicals that affect mood, emotional expressions may be the first sign of physiologic changes.[80] Holistic interventions prepare the physiologic environment that promotes healing and has great potential for healing and wholeness.

Pain Response

Pain and suffering are universal and multidimensional experiences. Pain has physical interconnections and physiologic outcomes. As a stressor, pain stimulates the same physiologic responses as other stressors that affect the nervous, endocrine, and immune systems, and pain memories produce the same psychologic and spiritual outcomes. As stress is designed to meet demands, so pain is designed to alert people to problems. The significance of the pain shapes the experience. The more threatening the diagnosis, the more intense the suffering. For example, a woman who suspects that she may have cancer when she discovers a lump in her breast reacts with the psychophysiologic stress response. Throughout diagnosis and treatment, she must face uncertainty, fear, and pain. Any new pains are forever after interpreted as a return of the cancer, thus stimulating psychophysiologic responses.

Somatic pain or cutaneous pain results from the stimulation of nociceptors in superficial structures such as skin and mucosa. Superficial somatic pain is sharp and prickly, such as that associated with a superficial paper cut on the finger. Deep somatic pain begins in the deep body tissues and is more diffuse than superficial somatic pain. Visceral pain results from damage to visceral organs. It is mediated by the SNS. The pain is diffuse, not easily localized, and is often referred.

Acute and chronic pain differ in several ways. First, acute pain is time-limited, because it occurs with an identifiable problem that generally responds to diagnosis and treatment. Surgery, injury, and trauma result in acute pain. Healing of tissue damage usually eliminates the pain. If untreated for 24 hours or longer, however, severe, acute pain can cause neuroplastic changes that lead to "incurable chronic pain syndromes."[81] Neuroplasticity refers to alterations in neuron structure and function resulting from stimulation. Learning and memory produce both chemical and physical neuroplastic changes.

Chronic pain is prolonged, lasting longer than anticipated based on the etiology of the pain. It may be ongoing or may be cyclic, with remissions and exacerbations (such as pain associated with sickle cell anemia, lupus, arthritis, or migraines). Prolonged chronic pain may progress to the point that it becomes the disease or condition. If this occurs, lifestyle changes affecting the person and the family and/or the system of support are common. As coping resources and sympathoadrenal responses are depleted, patients become depressed and irritable. Well established chronic pain patterns can be changed with nonpharmacologic holistic interventions such as cognitive restructuring, biofeedback, and mental imagery.

Neuroanatomic Pain Pathways

Pain perception is shaped by afferent pathways, the CNS, and efferent pathways. Nociceptors, pain receptors located in tissues, carry signals to the dorsal horn of the spinal cord. Large, myelinated A-delta fibers transmit pain quickly and localize it precisely. The smaller, unmyelinated or lightly myelinated C fibers not only transmit pain impulses slower, but also localize it only poorly. In addition, there are millions of sensory nerve endings in tissues and organs that, when injured, release pain-producing substances such as serotonin, histamine, bradykinin, prostaglandins, and substance P.[82] Painful stimuli can stimulate post-traumatic stress in the spinal cord, leading to a hypersensitive state that persists after cessation of the stimuli. Interruption of the afferent pain pathways before surgery is preemptive analgesia.[83]

From the dorsal horn, pain messages travel to the CNS, where they pass to the reticular formation, limbic system, thalamus, hypothalamus, medulla, and cortex. Awareness of the pain occurs in the thalamus. Pain discrimination is dependent on the interconnections between the thalamus and the somatosensory cortex. The meaning of the pain, based on past experiences, is identified in the cortex. If only the thalamus is functional, an individual can experience pain in the leg; however, an intact sensory cortex is necessary for the individual to identify that it is the lower part of the anterior leg that is hurting.[84] Other CNS cortical interconnections of the thalamus and limbic cortex determine hurtfulness, mood, and attention abilities.

Efferent fibers in the periaqueductal gray (PAG) area in the midbrain can stimulate or block pain. This area receives information from the spinal cord, reticular formation, hypothalamus, and cortex, and it is associated with the limbic system. Moreover, descending fibers connect this area with the dorsal horn of the spinal cord. Stimulation of the periaqueductal gray region produces analgesia. In addition, this area is rich with the opioids, so naturally occurring endorphins serve to mediate pain.

Pharmacologic approaches to pain management include anti-inflammatory medications, analgesics such as nonsteroidal anti-inflammatory drugs (NSAIDs), acetaminophen, and aspirin. The NSAIDs and aspirin block pain transmission centrally and peripherally. They also inhibit prostaglandins, making tissues less sensitive to the tissue damage chemicals such as bradykinin. The opioid analgesics work by binding to the same receptor sites as the endogenous opioids. Morphine and endorphins act at the receptor level to produce analgesia. Adjuvant analgesics include antidepressants and antiseizure medications, which can produce analgesia in some patients and some pain conditions. These medications are especially effective after nerve damage, as they suppress neuronal firing.[85]

Psychosocial Pain Pathways

Past experiences with pain, emotional state at the time of the pain, and interpretation of the meaning of the pain affect the degree to which the pain is experienced. Both pain recollection and pain anticipation elicit the pain response, just as the recollection of a stressful experience can elicit the stress response (i.e., state-dependent learning). The patient with leukemia who has experienced a number of bone marrow aspirations may begin to cry when the physician orders yet another bone marrow aspiration—even before being prepared for the procedure. Thus, both cognitive and affective factors influence pain perception.

Cognitive factors affect pain interpretation. Changes in the way that a person thinks about the pain, reframing self-talk, thinking about other things (distraction), or anything that takes the focus off the pain tends to increase the person's tolerance for the pain. Increased tolerance, in turn, increases the person's sense of control over the pain by diminishing feelings of helplessness. Opportunities to make decisions about care and to solve problems lead to a greater sense of control, increasing pain tolerance and decreasing pain perception (i.e., mind modulation). Remember the man who was robbed.

Affective factors such as emotional state, beliefs, values, and goals affect the meaning of the pain and influence the pain experience. When the pain experience leads to loss of hope or interferes with goals, the intensity of the pain is worse. For example, a sprained ankle may be uncomfortable and a nuisance to someone who tends to be sedentary, but it can be viewed as a disaster for someone who planned to run a 5-mile marathon. Fear of the unknown, anxiety resulting from psychophysiologic reactions to stress, and pain are circuitous, as each intensifies the others.

Psychologic coping factors, too, modulate pain.[86] The depletion of coping resources leads to feelings of helplessness, loss of control, and pain anticipation that worsen pain perception. In addition, the inability to cope leads to counterproductive behaviors that worsen the pain. It is necessary to design individualized, supportive nursing interventions to reduce the sense of helplessness and increase the sense of control, thus strengthening coping abilities. It is important to identify the needs of patients who get secondary gains from the attention for their pain so that they can learn more effective ways to get their needs met. Pain modulation, then, becomes increasingly challenging.

Pain can reactivate repressed or unresolved past, painful physical and emotional experiences, such as physical or sexual abuse.[87] For example, adults expressing multiple complaints of pain and seeking medical care from a variety of physicians without a definitive diagnosis may be victims of childhood abuse. When issues associated with such abuse remain repressed and unresolved, they tend to aggravate other problems, psychologic and/or physical, often leading to "acting out" behaviors. Unresolved grief experiences can also affect the pain experience, as individuals may be coping well until they have an experience with pain. When sensitive, caring nurses tolerate uncomfortable emotions and allow patients to grieve and express their pain, pain medication requests often decrease. The nurse's ability to model acceptance of grief and pain in appropriate ways encourages patients to decrease behaviors that intensify pain.[88]

Pain and suffering are different phenomena. Each can occur without the other, but they can also occur simultaneously. Suffering results when self-image is threatened. Suffering includes spiritual and/or psychosocial anguish,[89] which may be identified through sensitive assessment or by the fact that the pain reaction is greater than expected from the injury. Pain and suffering may appear indistinguishable.[90] A distraught, weeping cancer patient may be complaining of pain, for example, but assessment reveals that her physician has just told her about new metastatic lesions.

As she talks, she begins to calm down, and her complaints of pain diminish. Suffering, then, can intensify pain. Patients who experience high levels of suffering have low levels of pain tolerance and often "act out" behaviorally.

The pain response is also shaped by gender, culture, current health states, coping strategies, support, and other issues such as feelings of control and helplessness. Both men and women are taught to be stoic about their pain in some cultures. These people tend to deny pain when questioned about hurting and to refuse pain medication. In our culture, little boys learn at an early age that "big boys don't cry." Even though there is some evidence that this is changing, many men find it difficult to admit to pain.

CONCLUSION

New scientific understandings of living systems, such as principles of self-organization and mind modulation of the bodymind systems, provide a theoretical base for holistic healing interventions. Understanding the physiologic principles that are involved in nursing interventions helps nurses to design individualized and appropriate holistic care for clients. Nurses, aware of their own wounds and sensitive to the wounds of clients, are strategically placed to lead clients in facilitating health and healing.

Holistic interventions are science-based.[91] Clients often know more about these interventions than those who care for them. It is essential, therefore, to educate nurses to empower themselves as well as clients. For, if truth be known, nurses who do not care for themselves are unable to provide holistic care for their patients. Knowledge of the communication of the nervous, endocrine, and immune systems is necessary, but not sufficient for holistic nursing—nor does it explain all aspects of illness.

The new scientific information invalidates the idea of the dualism of mind and body. Thoughts, emotions, and consciousness do not reside solely in the brain, but are projected to various body parts—the brain, the glands, and the immune, enteric, and sexual systems. The research data have overwhelmingly documented the bodymind interrelationships. There are still many unanswered questions, however. Does the mind exist after the physical death? Does the soul survive death of the body? Why do some people experience phantom pain after an amputation? Nurses must continue to incorporate wholeness into their own lives while exploring effective ways to integrate care and document the effectiveness of holistic interventions. The meaning of the illness, the method of giving the diagnosis, the tone of voice and the touch of the nurse, the relationships to family and friends must all be investigated. The goal is to integrate the human spirit with physiologic interventions. As L. Dossey wrote,

> We will never achieve the validation of our spiritual intuitions by scrutinizing monocytes, neuropeptides, and receptor sites. What we will achieve is an expanded view of what it means to be human. The point that we will continue to emphasize is that the physiological and the spiritual are not equivalent, and if we ignore the difference between these two domains it will be at the risk of our spiritual impoverishment. These scientific insights are im-

portant signposts pointing to the nonlocal nature of consciousness. They get the mind out of the brain and into the body at large. Any science that helps us toward this understanding that is contained in the sublimest of the most acute seers of our race deserves, I would submit, our deepest respects.[92]

DIRECTIONS FOR FUTURE RESEARCH

1. Develop instruments that accurately measure psychophysiologic responses to particular holistic nursing interventions.
2. Explore the effectiveness of holistic interventions in preventing illness and promoting health.
3. Investigate the effects of holistic nursing practice on nurses.
4. Carry out longitudinal studies to examine the effects of the regular use of holistic nursing interventions.

NURSE HEALER REFLECTIONS

After reading this chapter, the nurse healer will be able to answer or begin a process of answering the following questions:

- Do I attend to my own bodymind communication?
- Do I provide time for self-reflection?
- How do I heighten my awareness of who I am?

NOTES

1. F. Capra, *The Web of Life* (New York: Doubleday, 1996), 30.
2. Capra, *The Web of Life*, 41.
3. G.M. Bartol and N.F. Courts, Psychophysiology of Bodymind Healing, in *Core Curriculum for Holistic Nursing*, ed. B.M. Dossey (Gaithersburg, MD: Aspen Publishers, 1997), 35.
4. A. Bullock and S. Trombley, *The Harper Dictionary of Modern Thought* (New York: Harper & Row, 1988), 652.

5. M.A. Boyd and M.A. Nihart, *Psychiatric Nursing* (Philadelphia: Lippincott-Raven Publishers, 1998), 197–198.

6. L. von Bertalanffy, *General Systems Theory* (New York: George Braziller, 1968).

7. Capra, *The Web of Life*, 167.

8. G.M. Bartol and N.F. Courts, Psychoneuro-immunological Aspects of Nursing, *Journal of Holistic Nursing* 11, no. 4 (1993):332–340.

9. Boyd and Nihart, *Psychiatric Nursing*, 197–198.

10. B.J.F. Clark et al., *Pharmacological Basis of Nursing Practice*, 5th ed. (St. Louis: Mosby, 1997), 738.

11. Bullock and Trombley, *The Harper Dictionary of Modern Thought*, 735.

12. Capra, *The Web of Life*, 39.

13. H.G. Koenig et al., The Relationship between Religious Activity and Blood Pressure in Older Adults, *International Journal of Psychiatry in Medicine* 28, no. 2 (1998):189–213.

14. I. Prigogine, *The End of Certainty* (New York: The Free Press, 1997), 9–56.

15. Capra, *The Web of Life*, 85.

16. Bartol and Courts, Psychophysiology of Bodymind Healing, 35.

17. Capra, *The Web of Life*, 158–159.

18. Bartol and Courts, Psychophysiology of Bodymind Healing, 35.

19. Capra, *The Web of Life*, 150–161.

20. Capra, *The Web of Life*, 162.

21. Capra, *The Web of Life*, 160.

22. Bartol and Courts, Psychophysiology of Bodymind Healing, 35.

23. G.M. Bartol and G.G. Eakes, A Study of the Meanings Assigned to the Term Psychosomatic among Health Professionals, *Perspectives in Psychiatric Care* 31, no. 1 (1995):24–29.

24. H. Dreher, *The Immune Power Personality* (New York: Plume, 1996), 2–4.

25. Dreher, *The Immune Power Personality*, 48–74.

26. J. Kabat-Zinn, *Wherever You Go, There You Are* (New York: Hyperion, 1994), xiii–xxiv.

27. J.W. Pennebaker, *Opening Up: The Healing Power of Confiding in Others* (New York: William Morrow, 1990), 46–48, 202–206.

28. Dreher, *The Immune Power Personality*, 104.

29. Dreher, *The Immune Power Personality*, 125–146.

30. Dreher, *The Immune Power Personality*, 137–138.

31. Dreher, *The Immune Power Personality*, 230–239.

32. A. Luks, *The Healing Power of Doing Good* (New York: Fawcett Columbine, 1991), 16–18, 27–34, 80–130.

33. Capra, *The Web of Life*, 267.

34. Capra, *The Web of Life*, 64–65.

35. C.B. Pert, *Molecules of Emotion: Why You Feel the Way You Feel* (New York: Charles Scribner's Sons, 1997), 261.

36. Capra, *The Web of Life*, 266–267.

37. Capra, *The Web of Life*, 268.

38. Capra, *The Web of Life*, 160–161.

39. Capra, *The Web of Life*, 269.

40. Capra, *The Web of Life*, 175.

41. Pert, *Molecules of Emotion*, 350.

42. D. Goleman, *Emotional Intelligence* (New York: Bantam Books, 1995), 6–7, 206–206.

43. B.M. Dossey et al., eds., *Holistic Nursing: A Handbook for Practice*, 2d ed. (Gaithersburg, MD: Aspen Publishers, 1995), 92–93.

44. Goleman, *Emotional Intelligence*, 205–206.

45. J. Shelby and K.L. McCance, Stress and Disease, in *Pathophysiology: The Biologic Basis for Disease in Adults and Children*, ed. K.L. McCance and S.E. Heuther (St. Louis: Mosby, 1998), 298.

46. Dossey et al., *Holistic Nursing: A Handbook for Practice*, 95.

47. C.L. Wells-Federman et al., The Mind-Body Connection: The Psychophysiology of Many Traditional Nursing Interventions, *Clinical Nurse Specialist* 9 (1995):59–66.

48. R.M. Sapolsky, *Why Zebras Don't Get Ulcers* (New York: W.H. Freeman, 1998), 33.

49. Wells-Federman et al., The Mind-Body Connection, 61.

50. Shelby and McCance, Stress and Disease, 290.

51. Sapolsky, *Why Zebras Don't Get Ulcers*, 120.

52. H. Benson, The Relaxation Response, in *Mind Body Medicine: How to Use Your Mind for Better Health*, ed. K Boleman and J. Gurin (Yonkers, NY: Consumer Reports Books, 1993), 253.

53. Benson, The Relaxation Response, 255.

54. M.S. Schwartz and M.A. Schwartz, Biofeedback: Using the Body's Signals, in *Mind Body Medicine: How to Use Your Mind for Better Health*, ed. K. Boleman and J. Gurin (Yonkers, NY: Consumer Reports Books, 1993), 306.

55. Schwartz and Schwartz, Biofeedback: Using the Body's Signals, 307–308.

56. Dossey et al., *Holistic Nursing: A Handbook for Practice*, 99.

57. C.M. Porth, *Pathophysiology Concepts of Altered Health Status* (Philadelphia: Lippincott-Raven, 1998), 775.

58. Porth, *Pathophysiology Concepts of Altered Health Status*, 776.

59. Porth, *Pathophysiology Concepts of Altered Health Status*, 778.

60. Porth, *Pathophysiology Concepts of Altered Health Status*, 1239.

61. K.L. McCance and S.E. Heuther, eds., *Pathophysiology: The Biologic Basis for Disease in Adults and Children* (St. Louis: Mosby, 1998), 297.

62. M. Jenny, Psychoneuroimmunology, in *Comprehensive Human Physiology from Cellular Mechanism to Integration*, ed. R. Greger and U. Windharst (New York: Springer, 1996), 1735.

63. Pert, *Molecules of Emotion*, 182.

64. Pert, *Molecules of Emotion*, 161.

65. Shelby and McCance, Stress and Disease, 297.

66. Post-White, The Immune System, *Seminars in Oncology Nursing* 12 (1996):89.

67. McCance and Heuther, *Pathophysiology*, 297.

68. J.K. Kiecolt-Glasser et al., Slowing of Wound Healing by Psychological Stress, *Lancet* 346 (1995):1194–1196.

69. J.W. Pennebaker et al., Disclosure of Traumas and Immune Function: Health Implications for Psychotherapy, *Journal of Consulting and Clinical Psychology* 56 (1998):239–245.

70. F.I. Fawzy et al., A Structured Psychiatric Intervention for Cancer Patients: 2. Changes over Time in Immunological Measures, *Archives of General Psychiatry* 47, no. 8 (1990):729–735.

71. D.H. Kang et al., Immune Responses to Final Exams in Healthy and Asthmatic Adolescents, *Nursing Research* 46 (1997):12–19.

72. Dossey et al., *Holistic Nursing: A Handbook for Practice*, 104–105.

73. Dossey et al., *Holistic Nursing: A Handbook for Practice*, 105.

74. Pert, *Molecules of Emotion*, 133.

75. Pert, *Molecules of Emotion*, 67.

76. Pert, *Molecules of Emotion*, 134.

77. Pert, *Molecules of Emotion*, 141.

78. Pert, *Molecules of Emotion*, 147.

79. Pert, *Molecules of Emotion*, 148.

80. Pert, *Molecules of Emotion*, 183.

81. P. Arnstein, The Neuroplastic Phenomenon: A Physiologic Link between Chronic Pain and Learning, *Journal of Neuroscience Nursing* 29, no. 2 (1997):179–186.

82. L. Jonathan and S. Heuther, Pain, Temperature Regulation, Sleep, and Sensory Function, in *Pathophysiology: The Biologic Basis for Disease in Adults and Children*, ed. K.L. McCance and S.E. Heuther (St. Louis: Mosby, 1998), 428.

83. D. Carr, Preempting the Memory of Pain, *Journal of the American Medical Association* 279, no. 14 (1998):1114–1115.

84. S. Curtis et al., Somatosensory Function and Pain, in *Pathophysiology Concepts of Altered Health Status*, ed. C.M. Porth (Philadelphia: Lippincott-Raven, 1998), 970.

85. Porth, *Pathophysiology Concepts of Altered Health Status*, 980.

86. N. Frisch and L. Frisch, *Psychiatric Mental Health Nursing: Understanding the Client as Well as the Condition* (New York: Delmar Publishers, 1998), 452.

87. Frisch and Frisch, *Psychiatric Mental Health Nursing*, 593.

88. N.F. Courts, Nonpharmacologic Approaches to Pain, in *Pain Management Handbook*, ed. E. Salerno and J. Willens (New York: Mosby, 1996), 143.

89. E.J. Cassell, Recognizing Suffering, *Hastings Center Report* 21, no. 3 (1991):24–31.

90. P.H. Coluzzi, A Model for Pain Management in Terminal Illness and Cancer Care, *Journal of Care Management*, no. 4 (1996):45–46, 64, 68, 70, 72, 74–76.

91. B.M. Dossey et al., *Holistic Nursing: A Handbook for Practice*, 107.

92. L. Dossey, *Medicine and Meaning* (New York: Bantam Books, 1991), 108.

VISION OF HEALING

The Evolving Process of Life's Dance

The dance of human life is an evolving process that can be compared to the rhythms in nature of day and night, and the shades of light and darkness between. This analogy of light and darkness applies to our own lives, with the shades between seen only as contrasts. Without the light, we have no concept of the darkness. Contrast is essential in every aspect of our life. The familiar contrasts of daily experience include happiness and sadness, strengths and weaknesses, and wellness and illness. The only way that we have a concept of personal wellness is to have at some point in our life a firsthand experience with illness or major life stressors. Particularly in Western culture, the high peaks in life are emphasized, while the low points are ignored. In order to understand our wholeness, however, it is essential to recognize these differences. The human psyche does not cope well with these differences, for the ego loves clarity. Yet, it is when we repress these differences that ambiguity is taken into our unconscious and leads to disharmony and psychophysiologic disturbances.

When major stressors such as disaster or illness occur, the tendency is to repress the meaning of these events. When we repeatedly fail to recognize these life situations, we move away from our internal healing resources of hope, strengths, and new insights. At some point, we must address these life processes be-cause they are always present. There is a part of us that always needs healing—the wounded healer—yet we are tempted to ignore this woundedness. We must learn to embrace our limitations, as well as to recognize our strengths. All great healers acknowledge their inherent weaknesses and fallibilities.

When a client and nurse come together with both denying their woundedness, the outcome of care is mechanical at best. Neither the client nor the nurse is able to use his or her inner wisdom to activate self-healing. Both have devalued this innate potential. Inner healing does not flow from the nurse to the client. The nurse cannot give inner healing to the client, for it already exists within the client. Rather, the nurse acts as a facilitator to evoke the client's process of inner healing. Healing occurs when the client and the nurse both acknowledge their life processes and use them to move toward balance and harmony.

As the best of traditional and holistic practices merge, much of the work that remains to be learned is the art of healing. When we recognize personal traits, attitudes, and stressors that are in need of healing, this time of reflection can also be a source of creativity and spontaneity. Hence, we need to acknowledge our own stressors in order to open creatively to our clients. Being a healer requires work on the self, our imperfect, fallible self. We must affirm our weaknesses and strengths, and acknowledge our inadequacies. Only then can we know a powerful part of our being and allow new strengths to be born. The use of self, in a loving and compassionate way, provides us with our most powerful instrument for healing.

Chapter 5

Spirituality and Health

Margaret A. Burkhardt and Mary Gail Nagai Jacobson

NURSE HEALER OBJECTIVES

Theoretical

- Describe spirituality.
- Compare and contrast spirituality and religion.
- Discuss common elements of spirituality and their varying manifestations in different people.
- Recognize mystery, suffering, love, forgiveness, hope, and grace as spiritual issues.
- Discuss the interplay of spirituality and psychology.

Clinical

- Explore the efficacy and place of prayer in healing.
- Discuss listening as intentional presence.
- Incorporate different approaches to spirituality assessment into holistic care.
- Discuss the use of story in spirituality assessment and care.
- Describe approaches for responding to spiritual concerns.

Personal

- Explore the need for nurses to nurture their own spirits and ways to do so.

- Discuss ways in which ritual, rest and leisure, play, and creativity relate to spirituality.
- Explore ways of naming and nurturing important connections.

DEFINITION

Spirituality: the essence of our being, which permeates our living and infuses our unfolding awareness of who and what we are, our purpose in being, and our inner resources; and shapes our life journey.

THEORY AND RESEARCH

We join spokes together in a wheel
but it is the center hole that makes the
wagon move.
We shape clay into a pot,
but it is the emptiness inside that holds
whatever we want.
We hammer wood for a house,
but it is the inner space that makes it
livable.
We work with being,
but non-being is what we use.[1]

Spirituality is perhaps the most basic, yet least understood aspect of holistic nursing. Spirituality often eludes the cognitive mind because it is intangible in many ways and defies quantification. The term *spirituality* derives from the Latin *spiritus*, meaning breath, and relates to the Greek *pneuma* or breath, which refers to the vital spirit or soul. Spirituality is the essence of who we are and how we are in the world and, like breathing, is essential to our human existence.

All people are spiritual. By virtue of being human, all persons, at all ages, are bio-psycho-social-spiritual beings. Attending to spirituality across the life span implies an understanding of the developmental aspects of spirituality, particularly an awareness that expressions of spirituality may vary with age. Some people describe themselves or others as not spiritual because they do not attend religious services or believe in God. This reflects the common practice of describing spirituality in terms of religious beliefs and practices. For years, nurses and other health care providers have linked spiritual caregiving with determining a patient's religious affiliation and understanding the health-related beliefs, norms, and taboos of that religion. Although such knowledge is important for holistic nursing, spiritual caregiving requires an understanding that spirituality is broader than religion and a recognition that, although some people may not be religious, everyone is spiritual.

Relationship between Spirituality and Religion

The nursing and health care literature makes it clear that spirituality and religion are not synonymous.[2–11] Spirituality, as noted, is an integral dimension of all persons. As the essence of who we are, spirituality is a manifestation of each person's wholeness and being that is not subject to choice, but simply is. Religion per se is not essential to existence. Religion is chosen. Spirituality is expressed and experienced in many ways, often, but not always, within the context of religion.

Religion refers to an organized system of beliefs shared by a group of people and the practices, including worship, related to that system. Because culture influences a person's values and beliefs, religious, as well as other spiritual expressions, often relate to personal culture. Religions reflect particular understandings of spirituality, but are only one of many ways of understanding or accessing spirituality. Religious precepts and practices often assist persons in attending to their spiritual selves; at times, however, these actions do little to nurture a person's true spirituality. Life issues that are spiritual in nature may, or may not, relate to religion. Knowledge of the histories, symbols, beliefs, practices, and languages of various religious traditions increases the nurse's ability to hear, recognize, and address religious needs of patients, but information about religious affiliation and practices alone offers only a glimpse into a person's spiritual self.

The literature suggests that nurses may be more comfortable discussing spiritual concerns when they arise within an identifiable religious context than when they occur within a broader perspective of spirituality. Mansen cautioned that when it is assumed that satisfying the rites and rituals of a particular religion meets a patient's spiritual needs, interventions may become standardized rather than individualized to the patient's needs.[12] This is of concern, especially when a patient's spirituality is not expressed through an affiliation or alignment with the practices of a particular religion.

Understanding Spirituality

One of the barriers to incorporating spirituality into holistic nursing care is the paucity of language within Western societies for discussing and expressing matters of the spirit or soul. This difficulty with the language of spirituality is evident in the nursing literature.[13–18] Hall noted that, in Western cultures, the choice of a language for expressing spirit has generally been limited to that of science or that of religion derived from the Judeo-Christian tradition.[19] Indeed, much of the discussion of spirituality within nursing and other health care literature reflects Judeo-Christian values and perspectives regarding the Divine, relationships with others and the world, experience of suffering, prayer, and the like. Because spirituality is the essence of every person and is not limited to a particular religious perspective, nurses need to strive to find or create a language that allows room for each person's unique expression of spirituality.

According to Engebretson,[20] the Western cultural bias can lead to misinterpretation of spiritual expression and concerns. She noted that not all assumptions of Western Judeo-Christian-Islamic traditions (e.g., monotheism, transcendence, dualism) are shared with Eastern and nature religious traditions. Monotheism is a belief in one god that is above and beyond nature, contrasted with a belief in the existence of many gods (polytheism) or the existence of the sacred in all living things (pantheism) found in Eastern and nature religions. Transcendence, which means to exist above material existence, is implied in the Western view of God as separate from humanity. People from such Western traditions often seek connection with the Divine by focusing outward through ritual and prayer. Eastern and nature traditions focus on immanence, the experience of the Divine within each person. Looking inward through meditation and spiritual exercises are ways of connecting with the Divine in these traditions. Dualism, the separation of spirit and matter, is a basic concept in Western traditions, while reality is conceived as a unified whole in Eastern metaphysical traditions of monism. Engebretson noted that the polarization of science and religion found in the West reflects the institutionalization of dualism. She stressed the importance of recognizing the impact of these assumptions on percep-

tions, definitions, and expectations of the spiritual experience within health care. She was especially concerned about labeling spiritual issues as pathology or not recognizing them at all because they do not fit a familiar paradigm.

Many people experience a blurring of boundaries and a blending of various religious traditions in relation to their own spirituality. Some people express and experience their spirituality best in the distinctiveness of a particular religious tradition; others address their spirituality through blending different religious and philosophical traditions; and still others experience their spirituality outside organized religious systems. Holistic nursing practice recognizes that religion and spirituality are different and honors the unique ways in which people express, experience, and nurture their spiritual selves.

Elements of Spirituality

The resurgence of interest in spirituality and health that has occurred in the past decade has generated many definitions and descriptions of spirituality within the health care literature. In many ways, however, trying to define spirituality is like trying to lasso the wind. The wind can be felt and its affect on things seen, but it cannot be contained within imposed boundaries, conceptual or otherwise. The similar nature of spirituality poses a particular challenge for minds that feel more at home with phenomena that can be categorized, quantified, and measured. Rather than being hostile to scientific debate, spiritual discourse actually complements it.[21] Understanding spirituality requires both cognitive and intuitive knowing.

Although the health care literature provides no single agreed upon understanding of spirituality, many authors note that spirituality reflects the essence of being, unifying and animating force, and life principle of each person.[22-28] Spirituality can be considered the eternal form of the body-mind, a state of being that does not go away. Our deepest core is spirit, and it is this spirit that animates all that we are and do. No words can truly describe the experience of this essence.

Spirituality permeates life; shapes our life journey; and is vital to the process of discovering purpose, meaning, and inner strength. Although matters of spirit transcend all cultures, a person's cultural perspective influences that person's expressions of spirituality. Personal values are rooted in and flow from spirituality, which may or may not be aligned with a particular religious tradition, and are reflected in a cultural perspective. Spirituality helps to ground one's sense of place and fit in the world. Because it is practical and relevant to daily life, people experience spirituality in the mundane as well as in the profound, the secular as well as the sacred.

A sense of peace, often described as inner peace, is among the positive qualities attributed to an awareness of spirit or spirituality. Peace in this context implies a deep confidence and an ability to remain calm in the midst of the storm, to know somehow that all is well. In the Judeo-Christian tradition, references to "a peace which passeth understanding" flow from an awareness of life beyond immediate circumstances and unbounded by the past. Peace is a product of living that acknowledges and nurtures the soul. For some, peace is inseparable from justice. Inner peace reflects a way of being, a space from which one is able to live and be in ways that nurture and heal.

A sense of trust that people have or are given the resources needed for dealing with whatever comes their way—expected or not—is a manifestation of spirituality. These resources include both strength and guidance from within and support from sources beyond themselves. Through encountering obstacles along their life path, learning through experiences, and developing new awarenesses, people gain appreciation for the ways that spirituality

shapes and gives meaning to their unfolding life journey. To reach this point, people may find it necessary to reconcile new experiences with previously held values, resulting in new values and understandings. Often, the pattern of the journey and the meaning of life events become clear only in retrospect.

Research and other writings on spirituality reflect a strong element of interconnectedness between individuals and all that is within and around them. Nolan and Crawford summarized this in saying "the spirit is that which enlivens, empowers, and motivates, and spirituality has to do with what takes place within, between, and beyond people."[29] This is borne out in research findings indicating that spirituality is expressed and experienced in and through connectedness, which includes relationships with the Absolute, nature, others, and the self.[30-34]

Connectedness with the Absolute

The Absolute may be experienced as a person, a presence, or as mystery, that which is beyond words. The Absolute is called by many names, including Life Force, Source, God, Allah, Lord, Goddess, Higher Power, Spirit, Inner Light, Tao, The Way, Universal Love, and the One with no name. The Absolute is often experienced within one's inner being as a power greater than the self, yet wholly the self, both within and beyond the self. Connecting with the Absolute may involve such things as prayer, ritual, reconciliation, stillness. Teachings of different religious traditions offer their own perspectives and guidance on how to be in a relationship with the Absolute. Discovering how persons seek and experience connection with the Absolute and what might be perceived as blocks to such a connection is an important part of spirituality assessment.

Connectedness with Nature

Spirituality is frequently expressed and experienced in and through a sense of connectedness with nature, the earth, the cosmos, the environment, and the universe. Animals, birds, fish, and other creatures of the earth are often important in providing meaning and joy for people of all ages. An awareness of all the life forms of the earth and their place within the natural order is a source of connection with and appreciation of the spiritual. Beavers at work on a dam, birds in flight, or bees among the flowers all illustrate the wonder of various life forms that may provide deeply spiritual experiences.

Awareness of a connectedness with the earth and, indeed, the entire cosmos is particularly evident within indigenous spiritual traditions. A speech attributed to Chief Seattle emphasizes that all things are connected.[35] Individuals are not the weavers of the web of life; rather they are each but a strand in the web. What they do to the web they do to themselves. Thus, what happens to the earth and environment affects them, and conversely, their choices and actions in all levels of their being affect the earth. Such an understanding of the interconnectedness of spirit and matter is basic to some religious traditions and known at some level in all spiritual traditions.

Many people, particularly those who live close to the land, experience a sense of connection with the Absolute through nature, regardless of their religious background. As Lamb noted, there is something extraordinarily alive among members of long established Southwestern cultures that comes "from paying close attention to matters of the spirit and living so intimately with the land that its seasons are felt in the heart."[36] People often express a particular feeling of closeness to their spiritual selves while walking a beach, sitting by their favorite tree, viewing a sunset, listening to flowing water, watching a fire, caring for plants, and otherwise experiencing the natural order. Being in nature can be a source of strength, inspiration, and comfort, all of which are attributes of spirituality. A sense of awe at the wonder of life and a feeling of connectedness with all things, with or without a belief in a Divine being, is an experience of spirituality. Connection with nature for some flows from a sense of finding God in all things, and many people experience a relationship with the earth and all its creatures at an energetic level. Appreciating, respecting, and caring for the earth and all its inhabitants are elements of spirituality.

Connectedness with Others

Spirituality is known and experienced in relationships. People express and experience spirituality through an appreciation of a common bond with all humanity and in their particular relationships with others. People often speak of their spirituality in terms of their relationships, both harmonious and discordant. Being with others in loving and supportive ways is an expression of spirituality, as is struggling with painful and difficult relationships with family, friends, and acquaintances. Relationships that need healing are as important to spirituality as those that provide support and comfort. Spirituality embraces both the joys and sorrows of relationships, and it prompts reconciliation where the connection has been frayed. A lack of connections produces a dispiriting sense of aloneness and isolation and often leads to spiritual crisis.

Spiritual connectedness with others involves both giving and receiving. Receptive openness to Love, Light, Life, and the Absolute is a spiritual stance. Although it is common to think of spirituality in terms of doing for another, being able to receive from others, both the gift of themselves and the things that they do or say, is also an expression of spirituality. Indeed, the genuine presence that people share with another, with its implicit loving honesty and intimacy, is a manifestation of spirituality.[37,38] Spirituality is evident in both common experiences of daily living and special times shared with others, times of joy, sorrow, ritual, loving sexuality, prayer, play, encouragement, anger, reconciliation, and concern. The recognition that relationships are a source of growth and change reflects spirituality. Social structures that provide a context for relationships with others are often instrumental in the development of spiritual aspirations. Such structures include health care, educational, and other institutions; religious and social organizations; and informal affiliations with others, and are often places that mediate spiritual aspirations.

Connectedness with Self

Being, knowing, and doing reflect connectedness with self. Spirituality infuses the ever-unfolding awareness of who one is, of self-becoming. The ability to be in the place of awareness that flows from the spirit or soul is a pivotal element of connectedness with self. Awareness opens people to the experience of living in the moment, present to their own body-mind-spirit, and allows them to receive all aspects of themselves without judgment. They experience awareness through being, the art of stillness and presence with self, others, the Absolute, and nature. Being asks for nothing and expects nothing. Being simply is. Being includes experiencing the present moment more deeply, aware from the physical experience of all levels of one's body-mind-spirit-energetic self in interaction with all in the environment. It is bringing one's whole self—alert, quiet, aware—to an experience. Within being it is possible to pay attention to the quiet place inside and come to experience inner peace, synchrony, harmony, and openness. Attentiveness to being allows a person to attune to sources of inner strength and tap into the deepest knowing.

Spirituality manifests itself through knowing, in one's awareness of self and one's place in the cosmos. Knowing has both cognitive and intuitive dimensions of awareness about physical, mental, emotional, energetic, and spiritual natures; connections; and surroundings. Knowing flows from a stance of openness and attuning to an inner source. It may involve actively seeking knowledge and insights or maintaining a posture of open receptivity to a deeper understanding of life matters. Spirituality reflected in one's knowing includes a gratitude for all experiences of living, both those of joy and those of struggle, and an appreciation that each moment is a gift.

From being and knowing flows doing, the outward, visible expression of spirituality. Because doing is more tangible and measurable, it is the manifestation of spirituality that is most often addressed in health care literature. Generally, the concept of doing brings to mind activities such as attendance at religious services or ceremony, scripture study, prayer or meditation, participation as student or teacher in religious education, and spiritual reading. Spirituality can be demonstrated as well, however, through actions such as assisting others, gardening, becoming involved in environmental concerns, attending to the sick, caring for family, spending time with friends, taking a walk, taking time to nurture one's own spirit, and creating sacred space for self and others.

The concept of sacred space applies both to one's inner being and to places in one's environment. Although to "create" sacred space suggests doing something, inner sacred space is often the result of being in awareness and stillness. Many people acknowledge that buildings such as religious edifices or monuments represent sacred space. Special places in nature are often experienced as sacred. Any place can become sacred space if someone intentionally brings awareness of the spirit into the setting. Words, actions, sounds, scents, colors, and objects may shape such spaces. Sacred spaces are home for the spirit, providing rest, stillness, nurture, and opportunities for opening to various connections. A special plant in a sunlit space, the garden or workshop, a room for prayer or meditation, the corner of a porch with a rocking chair, family surrounding a loved one in a hospital bed, each space touched by the intention of those who arrange it, are examples of sacred spaces.

SPIRITUALITY AND THE HEALING PROCESS

In a holistic paradigm, body-mind-spirit is an intertwined and interpenetrating unity; thus, every human experience has body-mind-spirit components. In considering spirituality and healing, it is useful to remember that the words *healing, whole,* and *holy* derive from the same root: Old Saxon *hal,* meaning *whole.* This suggests that, by its nature, healing is a spiritual process that attends to the wholeness of a person. The work of healing requires recognition of the spiritual dimension of each person, including the healer, and an awareness that spirituality permeates every encounter. The shared relationship acknowledging the common humanity and connectedness between the caregiver and the receiver, which is basic to healing, is a manifestation of spirituality.

Spiritual View of Life Issues

Spiritual issues are core "life issues" that often draw people to look into the deepest places in their beings. These issues are not quantifiable and are more authentically expressed as questions, tentative definitions, or as mysteries that cannot be fully explained. They challenge the individual to experience life at its highest heights and deepest depths. Considerations of mystery, love, suffering, hope, forgiveness, grace, and prayer are all inherent in the spiritual domain.[39,40]

Mystery

Because it is an inherent part of life, mystery is inherent to spirituality as well. Mystery may be described as a truth that is beyond understanding and explanation. Many life experiences prompt questions of why and wonderings about what if. Appreciation of the mystery inherent in life events often sustains people in the unknowing. As people encounter that which is troubling and unexplainable, spirit recognizes mystery and helps them survive the unknowing. Spirituality supports and encourages them in the questioning and seeking that often emerges when they are faced with such mystery. The spiritual self calls them ever further into the darkness in order that they may come to know and appreciate the light. Accepting and finding a comfort level with mystery is part of the spiritual journey.

Love

The source of all life, love fuels spirituality, prompting each person to live from the heart, the center where the ego is detached from outcomes. Love, like the spirit, is nonlocal, transcending place and time, and enabling its energy to be shared for healing at many levels.[41] The relationship of love to healing is a continuing source of exploration and wonder.[42-44] In its truest sense, love is a mystery that involves both choice and emotion, and it often underlies acts of courage and compassion that defy explanation. It is in both giving and receiving care that love is experienced and expressed. Love is both personal and universal. Flowing from and prompting interconnectedness, love includes dimensions of self-love, divine love, love for others, and love for all of life. Loving presence is a key component of spiritual care.

Suffering

In both its presence and its meaning, suffering is one of the core issues and mysteries of life. It occurs on physical, mental, emotional, and spiritual levels. People throughout the ages have struggled to understand the nature and meaning of suffering. Their attempts to make sense of suffering have helped to shape cultural and religious traditions. Suffering may be a transformative experience, the nature of the transformation varying with each individual. For some, suffering enhances spiritual awareness; for others, suffering appears meaningless and engenders feelings of anger and frustration. One interpretation of burnout among health care professionals is that it represents the inability to find ways to tend the spirit as one suffers the suffering of another.

Depending on one's perspective, certain forms of suffering may be seen as a blessing, something to be endured, or evidence of a curse. Not all people seek to alleviate suffering immediately. Sociocultural, religious, familial, and environmental factors influence an individual's response to suffering. Thus, having knowledge of personality, culture, religious traditions, and family background may assist the nurse in understanding the nature and meaning of suffering for a particular person. In the same vein, nurses need to be aware of their own responses to and understanding of suffering so as not to confuse their perceptions with those of the patient. This awareness enables nurses to be more fully present in an intentional, healing way with those who are suffering. Such presence allows nurses to discern whether honoring another's suffering requires action, presence, absence, or a combination of these. The ability to be with another who is suffering is crucial, particularly when nurses confront suffering that cannot be alleviated and must simply be borne. Listening with one's whole being as another wonders aloud and expresses deep feelings regarding some of life's unanswered questions is a very important part of being with those who suffer.

Hope

Because it is a desire accompanied by an expectation of fulfillment, hope goes beyond believing or wishing. Hope is future-oriented. The saying "hope springs eternal" reflects this energy of the spirit and prompts the anticipation that tomorrow things will be better, or at least different!

There are two levels of hope. Specific hope implies a goal or desire for a particular event or outcome. Hope can also include a more general sense that the future is somehow in safekeeping. Hope is a significant factor in overcoming illness and in living through difficult situations.[45] It helps people deal with fear and uncertainty, and enables them to envision positive outcomes. It is not surprising that there is a positive correlation among hope, spiritual well-being, intrinsic religiosity, and other positive mood states.[46]

Forgiveness

Ultimately a matter of self-healing, forgiveness is a deep need and hunger of the human experience. Religious beliefs, cultural traditions, family upbringing, and personal experience all help to shape an individual's attitudes about forgiveness, both given and received. The understanding of the nature of God or the Absolute influences one's ability to offer and receive forgiveness. Difficulties with forgiving others, forgiving oneself, and accepting forgiveness from others often relate to a misunderstanding of the nature of forgiveness. Simon and Simon suggested that forgiveness is not forgetting, condoning, absolving, or sacrificing; nor is forgiveness a clear-cut one-time decision.[47] Rather, they noted that, as a byproduct of an ongoing healing process, forgiveness is an internal letting-go of intense emotions attached to incidents from the past, recognizing that there is no longer any need for grudges, resentments, hatred, and self-pity; releasing the desire to punish people who have done hurtful acts; and accepting that no punishment of others will promote internal healing. Forgiveness, a sign of positive self-esteem, allows a person to put the past in proper perspective; free up energy once consumed by grudges, resentments, and nursing unhealed wounds; and use this energy for opening to healing and moving on with life. Releasing the desire or need to berate or punish oneself for past actions is an important part of this process.

Kollmar addressed the importance of self-forgiveness for spiritual growth and healing, noting that self-forgiveness is not about regret or guilt, but rather concerns acknowledgment of responsibility for one's actions.[48] Self-forgiveness is a gift to oneself that provides an opportunity to remove the energetic consequences from past actions and thoughts so that the cumulative energy of one's past actions will not adversely affect the self. The notion of free will, that the actual or energetic result of one's actions and thoughts cannot be bypassed by God or the universe, is basic to self-forgiveness. The process of self-forgiveness removes the barriers to receiving help from God or the universe through acknowledgment of personal responsibility for past thoughts and actions, and the willingness to let go of any energetic attachment to these thoughts and actions. Kollmar used the following analogy to illustrate the self-forgiveness process. If someone goes for a walk and along the way steps on a thorn, every step from that point is painful. The more the person walks, the more it hurts. The body cannot heal as long as the thorn is in the foot; however, once the thorn is removed, the body can begin the healing process. Self-forgiveness, like pulling out the thorn, enables the natural self-healing energy that is a part of the universe to begin and gives all of God's grace room to provide comfort.

Grace

- And he just showed up at the door right when I needed him.
- I didn't know how I was going to pay for everything; then this check arrived.
- I don't know why my spirits lifted that morning; perhaps it was the rain after such a long drought.
- I didn't think I could stand another bout of chemotherapy, but my friend said she will go with me and we'll take one day at a time.
- My CT scan was clear for the third time, something that the doctors didn't expect and that I didn't dare hope for.

The experiences expressed in these remarks may be described as grace by some and as coincidence or circumstances by others. Grace is a blessing that comes into one's life unearned. It is often spoken of as a gift from the Absolute, or from life itself, that enables, assists, and empowers a person in the midst of difficult and sometimes seemingly overwhelming circumstances. Indeed, grace provides a framework for understanding those gifts of life that are frequently attributed to providence or coincidence. Grace may offer a measure of peace and acceptance or courage and endurance.

Prayer

An expression of the spirit, prayer is a deep human instinct that flows from the core of one's being where the longing for and awareness of one's connectedness with the source of life are blended. Prayer represents a longing for communion or communication with God or the Absolute. The most fundamental, primordial, and important language that humans speak, prayer is an endeavor that starts and ends without words. In this understanding, prayer flows from yearnings of the soul that arise from a place too deep for words and move to a space beyond words.

The forms and expressions of prayer are as varied as the people who pray. Prayer, which is intrinsic to many religious traditions and rituals, may be public or private, individual or communal. It is not always a fully conscious activity. Speaking (sometimes silently), singing, chanting, listening, waiting, moaning, being with what is going on in the present moment, and being silent may all be elements of prayer. Prayer includes petition, intercession, confession, lamentation, adoration, invocation, thanksgiving, being, and showing care and concern for others. Some people incorporate processes and techniques such as relaxation, quieting, breath awareness, attention training, focusing, imagery, and visualization into their prayer. Movement such as walking, dancing, or drumming may be expressions of prayer. A reminder of our nonlocal, unbounded nature, prayer is infinite in space and time. It is divine, the universe's affirmation that we are not alone.[49,50]

That prayer is an appropriate consideration for nursing is grounded in the writings of Florence Nightingale.[51] Research is now affirming the truth that people have known for ages: prayer can affect healing.[52,53] Both directed prayer, which focuses on a specific outcome, and nondirected prayer, which focuses on the greatest good of the organism, can affect healing and other outcomes, although nondirected prayer may be more effective. Even at a distance, prayer alters processes in a variety of organisms, including plants and people. Furthermore, the observed effects of prayer do not depend on what the one prayed for thinks. In his book, *Be Careful What You Pray For*, Larry Dossey reminds us that prayer is a potent force that is best used thoughtfully, with care and discernment.[54]

Spiritual and Psychologic Dimensions

The term *psyche* means soul or spirit, reflecting the relationship between the spiritual and the psychologic that is evident even in the spoken language. Before the time of Freud, phenomena of the sentient realm that could not be explained physically were often considered matters of the spirit and viewed in religious terms. With the advent and ongoing development of psychology, matters of the soul have often been subsumed into psychologic theory, and frequently interpreted as pathology. Within a holistic paradigm, spiritual and psychologic elements are interconnected because the body-mind-spirit is an integrated whole. Failing to differentiate the spiritual and psychologic dimensions, however, can lead nurses to miss cues regarding spiritual concerns and inappropriately label spiritual issues as psychopa-

thology.[55-57] Although spiritual awakenings and deepenings may be accompanied by elements of psychologic distress, the "dark night of the soul" may be a very important part of the process of moving to greater awareness and enlightenment. Fortunately, more contemporary psychologic models such as psychosynthesis; logotherapy; and transpersonal, humanistic, and Jungian psychology address the spiritual dimension.

Unlike Eastern and indigenous traditions around the world, Western traditions have only a limited familiarity and comfort with the spiritual nature of different levels of awareness. The misinterpretation of behaviors, emotions, and reactions associated with individual experiences and expressions of the spiritual is keenly evident in the life of Florence Nightingale, and the many interpretations of her life.[58-61] Some have interpreted the behaviors and health concerns evident throughout her life after her return from the Crimea as psychologic pathology, such as anxiety neurosis, malingering, depression, and stress burnout. Approaching Nightingale's life from a spiritual as well as psychologic perspective, however, allowed Dossey to recognize Nightingale for the mystic that she was.[62,63] In a similar vein, appreciating the difference between spiritual and psychologic domains enables nurses to assess spiritual cues and spiritual crises more effectively, as well as to recognize opportunities to foster spiritual growth.

SPIRITUALITY IN HOLISTIC NURSING

Nurturing the Spirit

The way that nurses care for and nurture themselves influences their ability to function effectively in a healing role with another. The spiritual path is a life path. Attentiveness to one's own spirit is a key component of living in a healing way and is foundational to integrating spirituality into clinical practice. Care of their spirit or soul requires nurses to pause for reflecting and taking in what is happening within and around them; to take time for themselves, for relationships, and for other things that animate them; and to be mindful about nourishing their spirits.[64] The many ways to nurture their spirits and respond to their spiritual concerns are the same as those that they suggest to their patients.

Care of the spirit is a professional nursing responsibility and an intrinsic part of holistic nursing. Wright argued that within a holistic perspective, providing spiritual care is an ethical obligation as well.[65] Nurses must become competent and confident with spiritual caregiving, expanding their skills in assessing the spiritual domain and in developing and implementing appropriate interventions. A persistent barrier to the incorporation of spirituality into clinical practice is the fear of imposing particular religious values and beliefs on others. Nurses who integrate spirituality into their care of others need to recognize that, although each person acts out of and is informed by her or his own spiritual perspective, acting from this foundation is not the same as imposing these beliefs and values on another. In fact, many practitioners believe that the more grounded they are in their own spiritual understandings, the less likely they are to impose their values and beliefs on others.

Assessing and Investigating Spirituality in Practice and Research

The renewed appreciation of the role of spirituality in health and healing that has emerged in the past decade is evident in the literature, in the number of professional conferences that include spirituality as a major theme, and in efforts to incorporate courses on spirituality into education programs for health care professionals.[66–68]

The literature reflects attempts to make some sense of spirituality within a scientific frame of reference, and clinicians and researchers continue to struggle with difficulties surrounding how to assess and measure a phenomenon that defies definition. Many researchers have attempted to measure the expression of spirituality primarily through religious beliefs and practices.[69–72] This approach can be problematic, however, in that many people do not express their spirituality within a religious tradition; conversely, religious practices do not necessarily indicate a person's true spirituality. Some assessment scales that have been used in research on spirituality reflect a strong bias toward Judeo-Christian beliefs, suggesting that those who do not ascribe to these traditions may not be spiritual.

Attempts to quantify spirituality, even with more broadly applicable scales, must be viewed with some caution regarding the results and the effect of such instruments on care. Hatch and colleagues suggested that credible, objective, quantitative instruments for spiritual inquiry will facilitate the integration of spirituality into health care by providing a mode of assessment similar to that of the mental status examination.[73] Hall, on the other hand, asserted that "allusive spiritual phenomena have been operationalized into constructs that have been developed as scales that measure such concepts as spiritual dimension, spiritual well-being, and spiritual needs that are supposed to stand for spirituality and are taken by researchers to be spirituality."[74] She noted that, when this occurs, both the concepts and their measurements may obscure rather than reveal the individual meanings associated with the spiritual journey and are poor substitutes for a holistic understanding of the person.

The difference in these two perspectives represents an ongoing question about how best to approach spirituality assessment in clinical practice and research. A goal of holistic nursing is to know a person in the fullness and complexity of her or his wholeness. Knowledge obtained about a person through any process of assessment is not an end in itself; rather, it is useful inasmuch as it contributes to understanding and knowing more of the essence of the person. Knowledge about a person enables nurses to come to know more of who the person is when it is enhanced by the person's perspective of the meaning of such knowledge. Although quantification may more readily capture the attention of the scientific and medical community,[75] reliance on quantitative measurements may indeed promote the use of diagnostic reasoning and structured interview formats as a substitute for listening.[76]

Listening and Being Present Intentionally

Attentive listening and focused presence are at the heart of caring for the spirit, and they are essential in any approach to spirituality assessment. Like many others related to matters of the spirit, this concept is simple in many ways, but not easy. Good therapeutic communication skills facilitate the exploration of spiritual issues, and broad, open-ended questions are often useful. Questions and statements such as "Tell me more about . . . ," "What was that like for you?" "Help me to understand what you need," and "I feel that I didn't understand what you were trying to say" are useful as nurses seek a deeper understanding of their patients. Creating a sacred space in which spirituality can be expressed and having clarity about their own spiritual perspective enhance nurses' ability to conduct spirituality assessments. The practice of various spiritual disciplines such as prayer, centering, awareness, and meditation make it easier for nurses to be fully present, available to be with and listen to another. In the face of distractions from within and without, the nurse's ability to

focus on the relationship with a particular person in a particular moment is an important aspect of being a healing presence that greatly enhances spiritual care.

One of the gifts of intentional, active listening is that the client, in sharing with an open-hearted and fully present listener, often hears herself or himself with greater clarity and understanding. Such a listener provides a safe space for expression of negative as well as positive feelings and experiences. The contradictions, pains, questions, and struggles can be heard without judgment or advice. The person is able to express and, thereby, often to hear and better understand her or his situation in all of its richness and complexity and move toward the future with more awareness.

Holistic nurses assess their own abilities as listeners, considering barriers to intentional listening that are part of their personal journeys. There may be topics that make one uncomfortable. Although discomfort alone need not make one an unsuitable listener to another, being aware of one's discomfort, its source and manifestations, is an important part of a self-evaluation. Nurses should consider how external distractions such as the environment or the pressure of time affect their ability to listen, and they should be attentive to how body posture conveys presence and attention. A hospice patient illustrated an experience of intentional listening and presence in describing his relationship with one of the hospice workers on his team. "It just makes me feel good to see him come in. One day he and I both fell asleep, kind of took a nap for a bit. He probably knows as much about me as anyone—because he's the kind of guy who's interested in everything I talk about, my family, my worries, my sickness. Sometimes he asks a question, but mostly he just listens—but I mean really listens, like he wants to know about whatever is on my mind."

Intentional listening and presence foster authenticity in the nursing process. Such listening and presence demand a recognition of both verbal and nonverbal cues in communication and the validation by the patient of any interpretations that the nurse may make. Nurses should ask themselves the following questions: When have I been intentionally present for another, listening with my whole being and with an open heart? What factors, internal and external, make that difficult for me? When have I been in the presence of one who was fully present for me? How did I recognize that full presence? How did that affect me? The core of active listening and healing presence lies in the intention and spirit of the nurse who recognizes all persons as spiritual beings. Exhibit 5–1 lists important considerations for nurses as they strive to listen in healing ways to their clients. According to Bruchac,[77] "It all begins with listening. There are stories all around us, but many people don't notice those stories because they don't take the time to listen."

Exhibit 5–1 Listening in Healing Ways

- Be intentionally present.
- Maintain focus on the patient/client as a whole person.
- Set aside the need to "fix," "answer," or "correct."
- Learn to be with another in silence.
- Interrupt as little as possible, recognizing that even what is not said at a particular time has meaning and that the way and sequence in which a story is told are part of the story.
- View the other as embodied spirit, ongoing and unfinished story.
- Hear the journey, the relationships, the meanings in the story.
- Listen with all your senses.
- Do not prematurely diagnose.
- Let the conversation flow, being with silence as well as words.
- Breathe!

Source: M.G. Nagai Jacobson and M. Burkhardt, © 1997.

Using Story and Metaphor in Spiritual Care

Recognizing all persons, including themselves, as ongoing and unfolding stories offers nurses a valuable perspective from which to approach spiritual caregiving.[78,79] Spirituality is multidimensional, reflecting the depth and complexity of a person's being, and embracing that person's connections with the Absolute, the earth, other persons, and the self. Story and metaphor often provide a language and form for conveying the richness of one's spirituality when factual statements of experience fail to do so. Stories bring people enjoyment, teach them to solve problems, help them form identity, and are wonderful teachers. Few things help a person to understand the world better than a good story.[80] Through the vehicle of story, people learn to know another from many perspectives, as one who experiences relationships, emotions, conflicts, and struggles, and one whose responses are at once personal and universal. Nurses become, however briefly, a part of the life stories of those for whom they care. Nurses own life stories inform and form them, and an understanding of those stories deepens the awareness with which they hear another's story.

Listening and encouraging people to share their stories can be both assessment and intervention in spiritual care. Stories make it possible to move beyond physical symptoms, diagnoses, and theoretical constructs, which may be similar for any number of patients, to an appreciation of the wholeness and uniqueness of each person and the particular way in which he or she fits into the family and community. As an assessment approach, story and metaphor provide insight into spiritual concerns such as supportive and disruptive relationships, questions of meaning, values and purpose, issues of forgiveness, hope and hopelessness, and experiences of grace. Listening is a reminder that life stories are ongoing and unfinished.

The sharing of story and metaphor can also be a nursing intervention. In sharing with a fully present listener, patients hear their own stories with new insights and appreciation for their own lives—affirmations and validations, conflicts and struggles, questions of meaning and dark times—life in its variety and fullness. In a safe space, patients can express fears and perceived failures, hopes and wonderings, disappointments and achievements, as they consider pages of their life stories. Through such a process, patients may come to see themselves more clearly and, in an atmosphere of acceptance, accept themselves in their full humanity. From such a stance, patients are able to participate more consciously in the present situation.

The case of Mr. M. is an example of the power of the story:

Mr. M. has been diagnosed with probable cancer of the lungs and is scheduled for exploratory surgery in a few days. Several times, he has asked the nurse, "How serious do you think this is?" After he asks once again, the nurse says, "Mr. M., you seem to be asking me more than how serious this is. Can you tell me more about what is concerning you?" He responds, "Well, to be honest, I've been thinking about telling the kids, . . . especially my son in Chicago. You see, we haven't been on very good terms." And so begins an important story for Mr. M. to tell, and for the nurse to hear. The medical information about Mr. M.'s illness is but one piece of the greater fabric of his life as a family man and father. The nurse now hears Mr. M. talk about his concerns for his family and the relationships within the family as his upcoming surgery and uncertain future affect them. In telling his story, Mr.

M. participates in both the assessment and intervention related to his spiritual care. The nurse learns about his relationships and his concerns surrounding them, and Mr. M. begins to understand what the most important aspects of his situation are, from his unique perspective. With that understanding, he can begin to plan what he will do and what help he needs to seek. The nurse becomes a partner in his plan, which will be revised and updated as his story continues to be told.

Sharing a story brings the listener face to face with quandaries, insights, struggles, joy, suffering, pain, and healing moments. Stories may make the listener feel helpless in the face of perceived hopeless situations, but they may also help the listener recognize the hope that lies in such a situation. Stories challenge nurses to understand the wholeness of a person, to listen for the meaning of a life. One nurse commented that "I used to think that people who told me stories about their lives were just wasting my time and theirs, but now I realize that they are telling me about what is really important. I've learned to listen and to use what they say to help them see who they really are, what they can really do. Even when they tell me things that are really hard to hear, or even to understand, it seems like they just want me to know that it is part of their life, too." Perhaps stories are a way of helping the nursing process fit the patient rather than requiring the patient to fit the process.

Some shared wonderings and questions that may help others share their stories include the following:

- If you were writing your life story, what would be the title?
- What is the title of the current chapter?
- Who are some of the heroines and heroes of your story?

- How would you like this chapter to turn out?
- Tell me more about how you handled your child's accident.
- I wonder where you get your spunk.
- I wonder what it's like to live with your physical limitations.
- You've mentioned several times that your sister is ill, and you seem worried.

Nurses can affirm the sharing of stories through statements such as "your sharing has helped me see this in a different light." As nurses encourage clients to share their stories, it is helpful to encourage the significant people in the clients' lives to participate in the process. The exercises presented in Exhibit 5–2 may increase attentiveness to story, both among nurses themselves and with clients.

Using Guides and Instruments To Facilitate Spirituality Assessment

Different approaches to assessing spirituality are available to facilitate the integration of spirituality into holistic care.[81,82] Although many assessment instruments are based primarily on conceptualizations of spirituality in the literature, the JAREL Spiritual Well-Being Scale, which was developed as an assessment tool for nurses, is grounded in qualitative research on spiritual well-being in older adults.[83] When incorporated into a clinical setting, these spirituality assessment guides are a means of gaining a deeper understanding of a person from a holistic perspective. Rather than considering the completion of an instrument to be an end point, nurses can use the questions of an assessment guide as openings or referent points for discussing spirituality with patients and ultimately coming to know and understand them better as unique persons. Furthermore, they can adapt the various guides to the specific situation and person. Assessing a person's understanding of and ways

Exhibit 5–2 Exercises To Facilitate Awareness of Story

1. Take a few moments to become quiet, perhaps using some breath awareness. In this quiet space, allow yourself to remember, in as much detail as possible, something about yourself, some event or incident that comes to mind. How has this experience or event become a part of who you are? What meaning does it have for your life at this moment?
2. Keep a journal in which you record events, feelings, experiences, insights, questions in your life. Periodically review your writings, noting themes flowing through your story. Reflect on your story as it is evolving.
3. Think about books, stories, songs, fairy tales, movies, plays, or works of art that have special meaning for you. Take time to consider why and how they hold that meaning for you. Think about the images, characters, colors, and sounds that are found in each of these and how they are reflective of your own story. What meanings do you find that provide insight into your own unfolding journey?
4. Write an autobiography for your eyes only. Take your time. Re-read and reflect on it. Are there parts you want to share? With whom would you share? What new awarenesses and learnings have come to you?
5. Look at some old family photos or photos of friends. What story do they tell? What memories and feelings come with these pictures? Do you want to tell someone else about them? What do you want to say? Would you like to hear someone else's story about these same photos?

Source: M. Burkhardt and M.G. Nagai Jacobson, © 1997.

of expressing spirituality includes exploration of important connections and their role and influence in the present circumstances, issues related to meaning and purpose, important beliefs, values and practices, prayer or meditation styles, and desire for connection with religious groups or rituals.

The Spiritual Assessment Tool (Exhibit 5–3) is based on a conceptual analysis of spirituality derived from Burkhardt's critical review of the literature.[84] This instrument poses open-ended, reflective questions that can assist nurses in developing more awareness of spirituality for themselves and others. These questions are meant to be prompts that the nurse can use in focusing on pertinent spiritual concerns. Other, simi-

---

Exhibit 5-3 Spiritual Assessment Tool

To facilitate the healing process in clients/patients, families, significant others, and yourself, the following reflective questions assist in assessing, evaluating, and increasing awareness of the spiritual process in yourself and others.

MEANING AND PURPOSE These questions assess a person's ability to seek meaning and fulfillment in life, manifest hope, and accept ambiguity and uncertainty.

- What gives your life meaning?
- Do you have a sense of purpose in life?
- Does your illness interfere with your life goals?
- Why do you want to get well?
- How hopeful are you about obtaining a better degree of health?
- Do you feel that you have a responsibility in maintaining your health?
- Will you be able to make changes in your life to maintain your health?
- Are you motivated to get well?
- What is the most important or powerful thing in your life?

INNER STRENGTHS These questions assess a person's ability to manifest joy and recognize strengths, choices, goals, and faith.

- What brings you joy and peace in your life?
- What can you do to feel alive and full of spirit?
- What traits do you like about yourself?
- What are your personal strengths?
- What choices are available to you to enhance your healing?
- What life goals have you set for yourself?
- Do you think that stress in any way caused your illness?
- How aware were you of your body before you became sick?
- What do you believe in?
- Is faith important in your life?
- How has your illness influenced your faith?
- Does faith play a role in regaining your health?

INTERCONNECTIONS These questions assess a person's positive self-concept, self-esteem, and sense of self; sense of belonging in the world with others; capacity to pursue personal interests; and ability to demonstrate love of self and self-forgiveness.

- How do you feel about yourself right now?
- How do you feel when you have a true sense of yourself?
- Do you pursue things of personal interest?
- What do you do to show love for yourself?
- Can you forgive yourself?
- What do you do to heal your spirit?

These questions assess a person's ability to connect in life-giving ways with family, friends, and social groups and to engage in the forgiveness of others.

- Who are the significant people in your life?
- Do you have friends or family in town who are available to help you?
- Who are the people to whom you are closest?
- Do you belong to any groups?
- Can you ask people for help when you need it?
- Can you share your feelings with others?
- What are some of the most loving things that others have done for you?
- What are the loving things that you do for other people?
- Are you able to forgive others?

These questions assess a person's capacity for finding meaning in worship or religious activities and a connectedness with a divinity or universe.

- Is worship important to you?
- What do you consider the most significant act of worship in your life?
- Do you participate in any religious activities?
- Do you believe in God or a higher power?
- Do you think that prayer is powerful?
- Have you ever tried to empty your mind of all thoughts to see what the experience might be like?

continues

Exhibit 5–3 continued

- Do you use relaxation or imagery skills?
- Do you meditate?
- Do you pray?
- What is your prayer?
- How are your prayers answered?
- Do you have a sense of belonging in this world?

These questions assess a person's ability to experience a sense of connection with all of life and nature, an awareness of the effects of the environment on life and well-being, and a capacity or concern for the health of the environment.

- Do you ever feel at some level a connection with the world or universe?
- How does your environment have an impact on your state of well-being?
- What are your environmental stressors at work and at home?
- Do you incorporate strategies to reduce your environmental stressors?
- Do you have any concerns for the state of your immediate environment?
- Are you involved with environmental issues such as recycling environmental resources at home, work, or in your community?
- Are you concerned about the survival of the planet?

Source: Based on Margaret Burkhardt: Spirituality: An Analysis of the Concept, *Holistic Nursing Practice*, Vol. 3, No. 3, p. 69. 1989. Reprinted from B.M. Dossey, *AHNA Core Curriculum for Holistic Nursing*, pp. 46–47, © 1997, Aspen Publishers, Inc.

lar types of questions can be equally as appropriate. Some areas may be addressed more fully than others, depending on particular client needs. This instrument is meant to be a guide for nurses, to support and enhance their comfort and skills with spirituality assessment, and is not designed as a self-administered survey.

Howden's Spirituality Assessment Scale (SAS; Exhibit 5–4) is a 28-item instrument based on a conceptualization of spirituality as a phenomenon represented by four critical attributes.[85] These attributes and the corresponding items on the scale are

1. *purpose and meaning in life*—the process of searching for or discovering events or relationships that provide a sense of worth, hope, or reason for existence (Items 18, 20, 22, 28)
2. *innerness or inner resources*—the process of striving for or discovering wholeness, identity, and a sense of empowerment, manifested in feelings of strength in times of crisis and calmness or serenity in dealing with uncertainty in life, a sense of being guided in living and being at peace with oneself and the world, and feelings of ability (Items 8, 10, 12, 14, 16, 17, 23, 24, 27)
3. *unifying interconnectedness*—the feeling of relatedness or attachment to others, a sense of relationship to all of life, a feeling of harmony with self and others, and a feeling of oneness with the universe or Universal Being (Items 1, 2, 4, 6, 7, 9, 19, 25, 26)
4. *transcendence*—the ability to reach or go beyond the limits of usual experience; the capacity, willingness, or experience of rising above or overcoming body or psychic conditions; or the capacity for achieving wellness or self-healing (Items 3, 5, 11, 13, 15, 21)

Exhibit 5–4 Spirituality Assessment Scale

DIRECTIONS: Please indicate your response by circling the appropriate letters indicating how you respond to the statements.

MARK:
  SA if you STRONGLY AGREE
  A if you AGREE
  AM if you AGREE MORE than DISAGREE
  DM if you DISAGREE MORE than AGREE
  D if you DISAGREE
  SD if you STRONGLY DISAGREE

There is no "right" or "wrong" answer. Please respond to what you think or how you feel at this point in time.

1.	I have a general sense of belonging	SA A AM DM S SD
2.	I am able to forgive people who have done me wrong.	SA A AM DM S SD
3.	I have the ability to rise above or go beyond a physical or psychological condition.	SA A AM DM S SD
4.	I am concerned about destruction of the environment.	SA A AM DM S SD
5.	I have experienced moments of peace in a devastating event.	SA A AM DM S SD
6.	I feel a kinship to other people.	SA A AM DM S SD
7.	I feel a connection to all of life.	SA A AM DM S SD
8.	I rely on an inner strength in hard times.	SA A AM DM S SD
9.	I enjoy being of service to others.	SA A AM DM S SD
10.	I can go to a spiritual dimension within myself for guidance.	SA A AM DM S SD
11.	I have the ability to rise above or go beyond a body change or body loss.	SA A AM DM S SD
12.	I have a sense of harmony or inner peace.	SA A AM DM S SD
13.	I have the ability for self healing.	SA A AM DM S SD
14.	I have an inner strength.	SA A AM DM S SD
15.	The boundaries of my universe extend beyond usual ideas of what space and time are thought to be.	SA A AM DM S SD
16.	I feel good about myself.	SA A AM DM S SD
17.	I have a sense of balance in my life.	SA A AM DM S SD
18.	There is fulfillment in my life.	SA A AM DM S SD
19.	I feel a responsibility to preserve the planet.	SA A AM DM S SD
20.	The meaning I have found for my life provides a sense of peace.	SA A AM DM S SD
21.	Even when I feel discouraged, I trust that life is good.	SA A AM DM S SD
22.	My life has meaning and purpose.	SA A AM DM S SD
23.	My innerness or an inner resource helps me deal with uncertainty in life.	SA A AM DM S SD
24.	I have discovered my own strength in times of struggle.	SA A AM DM S SD
25.	Reconciling relationships is important to me.	SA A AM DM S SD
26.	I feel a part of the community in which I live.	SA A AM DM S SD
27.	My inner strength is related to belief in a Higher Power or Supreme Being.	SA A AM DM S SD
28.	I have goals and aims for my life.	SA A AM DM S SD

Source: Copyright © 1992, Judy W. Howden.

The SAS is a 6-point response-rating scale using the following numerical rating: strongly disagree (SD) = 1; disagree (D) = 2; disagree more than agree (DM) = 3; agree more than disagree (AM) = 4; agree (A) = 5; strongly agree (SA) = 6. There is no neutral option. It is scored by summing the responses to all 28 items; subscale scores may also be obtained by summing the responses to subscale items. Psychometric evaluation resulted in a high internal consistency (alpha = 0.9164) for the SAS, indicating that the instrument appears to be a valid and reliable measure of spirituality.

The usefulness of numerical scores derived from quantitative spirituality assessment instruments may be more apparent within the context of a research study. In a clinical setting, however, a scale such as the SAS can enable a nurse to gain an overall sense of a person's spirituality, either when administering the instrument or when discussing it with a client who has already completed it. It is the pattern of responses to individual items, more than a numerical score, that provides nurses with insights into areas of spiritual strengths and concerns, enabling them to support the strengths and address the concerns. For example, discovering that a person may be experiencing a lack of kinship with others and a lack of connection to life provides an opportunity for the nurse to explore these concerns further and plan appropriate interventions. In the clinical arena, nurses need to remember that a quantitative measure should be an adjunct to, not a replacement for, listening presence.

Barker offered yet another approach to spirituality assessment in her Personal Spiritual Well-Being Assessment (PSWBA) and Spiritual Well-Being Assessment (SWBA), presented in Exhibit 5–5.[86,87] These instruments, which originate in her clinical experiences and research,[88] were developed initially as a short process for assessing spiritual well-being among cancer patients. The SWBA is intended for use by clinicians as they elicit information about the patient's place in the spiritual walk. The PSWBA was originally intended for use by clinicians in determining and clarifying their own spiritual well-being prior to addressing the spiritual well-being of others, but it may be useful with patients as well. Key guide questions are provided, and the respondent is asked to verbalize thoughts in the area. Each instrument uses four broad facets of spiritual well-being: relationship to self, relationship to God/Creative Source, relationship to others, and relationship to nature. Although this type of assessment format can be self-administered, a greater depth of information and insight can be gained by using an interactive process that allows for an exploration of responses.

Barker cautioned nurses to be aware of certain barriers related to spiritual well-being assessment. These barriers include believing that there is not enough time to do the assessment, being embarrassed about asking the questions, thinking that doing the assessment means that the nurse has to solve all the patient's problems (rescue fantasy), doubting that the nurse can make a difference in the patient's life, feeling responsible for the patient's place in the cosmos, and accepting responsibility for the patient's choices. When experiencing such reactions, nurses can utilize the PSWBA or other processes to explore their own understanding of spirituality, to develop the necessary skills, and to become comfortable with this area of holistic nursing care.

Each of the assessment guides that have been discussed provides a process for exploring the elements of spirituality. For example, spirituality involves relationships, and each instrument offers a different way in which a nurse may enhance the patient's awareness of significant relationships. The Spiritual Assessment Tool addresses the area of harmonious interconnectedness; Howden's work asks the patient to consider questions related to unifying interconnectedness; and Barker clearly

Exhibit 5–5 Spiritual Assessment Instruments

Personal Spiritual Well-Being Assessment

Relationship to Self

Overall, in the last month, I feel _____ about myself.

Overall, this feeling is _____ .

Overall, my "well" feels _____ .

Relationship to God/Creative Source

Overall, in the last month, my sense of connection to God/my Creative Source is _____

_____ .

Overall, I feel a purpose to being where I am today _____ .

Overall, I feel _____ about my place in the world.

Relationship to Others

I feel most connected to _____ .

This connection feels _____ .

Overall, my relationships are _____ .

I have one intimate relationship _____ .

This relationship brings me _____ .

Relationship to Nature

My favorite part of creation is _____ .

The last time I was able to experience this part of creation was _____ .

When I experienced this part of creation, I felt _____ .

Spiritual Well-Being Assessment

What is *(the illness or other concern)* _____ like for you?

What do you do to cope with *(the illness or other concern)* _____ ?

What makes you smile? _____

If you could be anywhere, where would you be? _____

What relationships are most important to you? _____

How can I help?

Source: Copyright © 1996, Elizabeth R. Barker.

---

asks what relationships are most important to the patient. As nurses become more at home with the concept of spirituality and its language, they will form their own questions and make their own observations in understanding another person as a whole being whose essence is spirit.

HOLISTIC CARING PROCESS CONSIDERATIONS

Spiritual caregiving requires an understanding of the holistic caring process that is integrative, in which assessment and intervention may well be the same process, and where description may be more useful than labeling. Identification of needs in the area of spirituality does not necessarily indicate pathology or impairment. Hall clearly stated the importance of exploring and describing the human spirit in the language of those who are living with particular health care needs and concerns, and exploring individual meaning according to the particular person's values.[89] Holistic nurses recognize that spirituality is an important consideration with any health concern, and they use the evolving nursing diagnoses regarding spirituality appropriately. Nurses need to collaborate with clients and their families in determining appropriate outcomes, developing a plan, and organizing overall care to ensure the incorporation of each person's selfhood, values, and world view. Nurses facilitate this process when they promote an atmosphere that is accepting and encouraging of spiritual expression in its many and varied forms. Understanding and awareness of their personal spiritual perspective improve nurses' ability to be alert to its influence on their relationships and work. Nurses are thereby able to recognize their own discomfort with a client's spiritual perspective and involve others in order to provide the needed care for the client.

Tending to the Spirit

Care of the spirit, a fundamental aspect of holistic nursing care, takes place in the context of the significant connections in a person's life. The nurse, for a time, enters the client's world and, through intentional presence in this relationship, may facilitate healing. Assessment, diagnosis, planning, and intervening are all experienced within a unique and particular relationship. Recognizing that all persons are spiritual beings provides the basis for being alert to the many and varied ways in which persons express their spirituality. Often, simply hearing and validating questions and concerns of the spirit are not only part of the assessment, but a part of the intervention as well. Simply opening the opportunity for clients to discuss and reflect on spiritual concerns enables them to become more aware of their spirituality and personal spiritual journeys.

Awareness of and care for self as a spiritual being is an important aspect of holistic nursing care. Spiritual "co-counseling" among colleagues who also deal with spiritual issues and consciously pursue a spiritual path can nurture a nurse's spirit. Forming spiritual companionship, mentoring, or support groups within the work environment, even with one or two colleagues, can help nurses maintain their spirits in the midst of the daily demands on their energies.

Regular practices of prayer, centering, mindfulness, or meditation enable nurses to access more readily the space of their own wholeness and be intentionally present in each client encounter. With intentionality and consciousness, busy nurses can use common activities as processes or rituals for leaving past client encounters behind to be more fully present in a current client encounter. For example, when washing hands between patients, nurses can release the concerns of the previous patient and, thus, be more open to those of the next patient. Similarly, by consciously taking a breath before entering an examination room, nurses can clear their beings of other distractions so as to focus on the person to be seen. Simply pausing to center and focus, "stepping back" from a confusing, distressing situation in order to reenter from a point of calmness and being silent as one listens deeply are skills that develop as nurses attend to spirit. With awareness and creativity, nurses can use most any activity as a way to foster spiritual presence.

Touching

Physical contact through touch in its myriad forms may foster connection. Sensitivity to the meaning of touch for each person is essential in using touch therapeutically. When appropriate, a hand on the shoulder can provide support, a handclasp can convey understanding and presence, an arm around the waist can literally and figuratively give a lift! One patient described a nurse's support in saying, "When the doctor came in to give me the news, she was standing beside me, and I could feel her hand on my arm the whole time he was talking. . . . I was so glad that she was just there with me."

Families and friends may need encouragement to share physical expressions of care and concern in the sometimes intimidating hospital environment. Nurses may encourage them with statements such as "It's OK to hold her hand; you won't interfere with the tubes." "He mentioned that you give a wonderful back rub; would you like to give him one today?" "She seems to know when you are here and holding her hand." "I can show you how to massage her feet." "Would you like to brush her hair?" Persons vary in their degree of comfort with touch and the conditions in which they may want to share touch. The nurse's own personal feelings about and comfort with touch help in assessing the place and potential use of touch in the patient's situation. At times when words cannot be found, or in circumstances where persons are more comfortable with physical expression than with words, touch is a powerful expression of spirit and instrument of healing.

Fostering Connectedness

Relationships are a major aspect of spirituality. An awareness and an appreciation of important relationships in the client's life enable the nurse to help strengthen meaningful and supportive bonds. Some family members may need encouragement and guidance in visiting and calling. Clients may need assistance in sharing some aspects of their situation with others—even when they very much want to explain what

is happening to them and express their feelings about it. Nurses can remind clients of their network of care and support by recognizing and affirming the support of significant others. Statements such as "You seem especially close to Marta" may provide an opportunity for sharing about a special relationship. Having photographs, artwork, and other memorabilia of loved ones provides reminders of connections beyond the confines of illness or injury. Pictures or discussions of special places or pets are evidence of other special connections. Visits from pets may be as spiritually uplifting for some people as those from human companions! Using imagery, pictures, and stories can help persons connect with important places, people, and experiences.

Contact with persons from religious, social, business, neighborhood, school, hobby, or interest groups may provide reminders of connections with and participation in the larger community and world. In some health care settings, such as intensive care or long-term care facilities, bonds of mutual caring develop among various patients, families, and caregivers. These networks of support can become very significant in the lives of all those involved. Holistic care implies a recognition of the healing potential in such relationships and impels nurses to foster their development actively.

The client's sense of connection with the environment may be an important source of comfort and strength. For persons to be able to feel the wind, see the stars, smell the flowers, touch the trees, and simply to experience the world may be a significant aspect of healing. Is there a window with a view of nature? Can the patient spend some time outside? Is there a photograph of a scene from nature on the wall, or one of a special place that can be placed at the bedside? Would the patient enjoy a plant, a bouquet of flowers, or a single rose? Some people enjoy audiotapes of music or of nature sounds. Spiritual uplifting can occur when visitors share the progress of the vegetable garden, the news of a recent fishing trip, or reflect on the weather conditions.

Spirituality may call to mind one's relationship with the sacred. People have different, unique, and personal understandings and experiences of the sacred, and language may pose a problem when talking about this aspect of spirituality. Those who are comfortable with the Judeo-Christian tradition of God or Lord, or the Islamic Allah, may find themselves less comfortable with understandings expressed as Higher Power, Tao, Universal Light, or Absolute. The reverse may also be true. For some people, "new age" is a relevant term that connotes spiritual growth and expansion; for others, however, anything "new age" is suspect and can be spiritually distressing. Listening beyond specific words to hear what is most sacred for this person and how his or her relationship with the sacred may be nurtured is important in addressing spiritual concerns. Are particular words of importance to this person? What is the place of formal religion and a person's own rabbi, priest, shaman, minister, or spiritual leader? What is the place of music, prayer, sacred texts, books, particular objects, foods, or rituals in nurturing spirit for this person?

Sensitivity to and appreciation of persons who profess atheism (i.e., disbelief in the existence of a supreme being) or agnosticism (i.e., doubt surrounding the existence of God or ultimate knowledge) involve moving beyond what is not believed. Instead, the nurse must listen for that which gives meaning and purpose to the patient's life, including that which brings joy and satisfaction, the nature of hopes and fears, and the recognition of important relationships. How does this particular health crisis fit into the patient's understanding of her or his life, and how is she or he dealing with it? For example, an astronomer who noted that she was not religious and did not believe in God described her understanding and awe in regard to the evolution of the universe as a cause of deep won-

der to her that all that had gone before led to this particular time. This sense gave her a feeling "that I belong." The words voiced were not traditionally religious language, but her expressions of appreciation, awe, wonder, and meaning spoke of spirituality.

A nurse who is attending to spiritual concerns needs a willingness to be present with mystery, uncertainty, pain, or suffering, seeking not to "fix" or to "answer," but to be in the mystery with another. Learning to let the client know that the nurses are willing, with their whole being and intention, to stay the course through times of difficulty, pain, and mystery provides encouragement when they can only say, "I don't understand this either." This willingness on the part of the nurses may help family and friends to understand that, when they feel that there is nothing they can do, their presence and expressions of love and care are important and valuable components of their healing support.

As the nurses learn to understand the relationships and connections that frame a client's life, they begin to be more aware of recurring themes and concerns. When such themes are noted, the nurse can reflect on and validate them with the client. Statements such as "It seems I have often heard you speak of . . . with great concern" gives the client the opportunity to know the nurse's perceptions and to validate or correct them. In general, it is reassuring to the client to know that the nurse is indeed listening and responding to deep concerns.

Using Rituals To Nurture the Spirit

Rituals serve as reminders to allow sacred time and space in our lives. Both the ritual behavior and the mindfulness that accompanies it are important aspects of ritual. Achterberg and colleagues described three phases of ritual.[90] The first phase is the symbolic breaking away from everyday busyness. The second phase is the transition phase, which calls for the identification and focus on areas of life that need attention. The third and final phase, referred to as the return phase, is the reentry into everyday life. In essence, ritual gives a person time apart so that he or she may return to the world in a clearer, more centered way. Ritual then can enable nurses to be more intentionally present in healing ways with another. Exhibit 5–6 provides an example of a ritual that can enhance the healing process.

Either shared with others or highly personalized, rituals are significant aspects of various religious traditions and cultures. Rituals come in many shapes and forms. Routine morning walks, daily prayer time, sharing of the day's experiences with family over dinner, or a soothing bath can all be rituals. Anything done with awareness may serve as a ritual. Rituals provide a rich resource in caring for the spirit, and consid-

---

Exhibit 5–6 The First Ritual Guide to Getting Well

This ritual helps you decide what to do if you are diagnosed with the unknowable, the unthinkable, the awful, or the so-called incurable. By doing this, you can better determine how to survive treatment, yourself, your friends and family, and life in general.

1. Find a quiet place, a healing place, and go there. This might be a corner of your favorite room where you have placed gifts, pictures, a candle, or other symbols that signal peace and inner reflection to you. Or it might be in a park, under an old tree, or in a special place known for its spirit, such as high on a sacred mountain or on the cliffs overlooking a coastline or in the quiet magnificence of a forest.
2. Ask questions of your inner self about what your diagnosis or treatment means in your life. How will life change? What are your resources, your strengths, your reasons for staying alive? These deeply philosophical or spiritual issues often come to mind when problems are diagnosed. Listen with as quiet a mind as possible for any answers or messages that come from within, or from your higher source of guidance.
3. Take this time, knowing that very few problems advance so quickly that you must rush into making decisions about them immediately, without first gaining some perspective.
4. Find at least one friend or advocate who can be level-headed when you think you are going crazy; who can be positive for you when you are absolutely certain you are doomed; who can listen when your head is buzzing with uncertainty.
5. Love yourself. Ask yourself moment by moment whether what surrounds you is nurturing and life-giving. If the answer is no, back off from it. Kindly tell all negative-thinking people that you will not be seeing them while you are going through this. You may need never to see them again, and this is your right and obligation to yourself.
6. Assess your belief system. What do you believe? How did you get to believe it in the first place? What is really happening inside you and outside you? How serious is it? What will it take to get you well?
7. Gather information, keeping an open mind. Everyone who offers to treat you or give you advice has their lives invested in what they tell you. Stand back and listen thoughtfully.
8. Now go and hire your healing team. Remember, you hired them—you can fire them. They are in the business of performing a service for you, and you are paying their salaries. Sometimes this relationship gets confused. Make sure they all talk to each other. You are in command. You are the captain of the healing team.
9. Don't let anyone talk you into treatment you don't believe in or don't understand. Keep asking questions. Replace anyone who acts too busy to answer your questions. Chances are, they're also too busy to do their best work for you.
10. Don't agree on any diagnostic or lab tests unless someone you trust can give you good reasons why they are being ordered. If the tests are not going to change your treatment, they are an expensive and dangerous waste of your time.

continues

Exhibit 5-6 continued

11. Sing your own song, write your own story, take your own spiritual journey through a journal or diary. A threat to health and well-being can be a trigger to becoming and doing all those things you've been putting off for the "right" time.

12. Consider these maxims in your journey:
    - Everything cures somebody, and nothing cures everybody.
    - There are no simple answers to complex issues, like why people get sick in the first place.

- Sometimes disease is inexplicable to mortal minds.

13. You will not be intimidated by the overbearing world of medicine or alternative health know-it-alls but can thoughtfully take the best from several worlds.

14. You can teach gentleness and compassion to the most arrogant doctor and the crankiest nurse. Tell them that you need your mind and soul nurtured, as well as the best medical treatment possible in order to get well. If they are not up to it, you'll find someone someplace who is.

Source: From *RITUALS OF HEALING: Using Imagery for Health and Wellness,* by J. Achterberg, B. Dossey, and L. Kolkmeier. Copyright © 1994 by Jeanne Achterberg, Barbara Dossey, and Leslie Kolkmeier. Used by permission of Bantam Books, a division of Bantam Doubleday Dell Publishing Group, Inc.

ering the place of rituals in one's life is an important aspect of self-care.

Developing an awareness of the place of ritual in their own lives establishes a basis from which nurses can facilitate and provide opportunities for patients to consider and experience the place of ritual in their lives. What rituals are significant for a particular patient? Are there rituals that might support the patient's healing process? Nurses need to consider what constitutes sacred space for various patients and to explore with patients resources that might help them better understand and include supportive rituals in their lives.

Developing Centering, Mindfulness, Awareness

Spiritual disciplines are those practices that cause people to pause in the midst of their activities and busyness to attend to matters of the spirit or soul. The practice of spiritual disciplines requires intention and attention. Eastern and many indigenous traditions around the world emphasize the importance of mindfulness and awareness as disciplines that permeate all of life. Like the practice of centering prayer in Judeo-Christian traditions, the mystical path of

many traditions calls one to quietness. Making the intentional decision to pause and be mindful of the present moment and all that it holds nurtures the ability to be centered and aware. Taking the time to observe what is going on within oneself, without judgment or elaboration, and to note thoughts, feelings, physical sensations, and distractions provides valuable experiences in the practice of awareness. Observing what is going on in the environment, attending to all senses, and experiencing all sensations enhance a person's full presence in the moment.

Processes of relaxation and imagery facilitate awareness and centering. The practice of spiritual disciplines provides access to a centered space from which the nurse and client can work together, confronting significant life experiences in an environment that is often busy and complex. Some clients may be experienced practitioners of such disciplines, while others may be almost unaware that they have already incorporated spiritual disciplines into their lives that can assist them in times of health crises. Many clients may be ready to learn about such practices when they are presented in clear language that is appropriate to their cultural and spiritual perspectives. Questions such as "Have you ever tried any particular methods of relaxing?" or "What kinds of activities help you find calm in the middle of a busy day?"may facilitate a person's practice of spiritual disciplines in a more intentional way.

Praying and Meditating

Prayer and meditation are spiritual disciplines practiced in many traditions, both cultural and religious. Appreciating the personal nature of these disciplines, the nurse, with respect and sensitivity, can help patients remember or explore ways in which they reach out to and listen for God or the Absolute. Recalling the place and meaning of prayer and the ways in which they experience the presence of and communion with God or the Absolute provides patients with a rich resource. In the clinical setting, both the nurse's and the patient's understanding of prayer will determine the role of prayer. Clarifying the patient's understanding of and need for prayer is a part of holistic care. Some patients want others to pray with or for them, while others do not believe in prayer. Nurses should support each patient's requests and needs for prayer, which may mean inviting others to take part in various forms of prayer with and for the patient, or simply praying with the patient themselves. The nurse can encourage expression of the patient's desire for shared prayer, for participation in religious worship, or for quiet, uninterrupted periods of time for personal spiritual practices. Facilitating the appreciation and practice of prayer in a patient's life is an important aspect of caring for the spirit.

When a person is physically confined to a hospital room, the practice of imagery may enable him or her to experience another space. Imagery can take a person to a temple, an ocean, a place of religious worship, a breakfast nook, or any "sacred space," that is, a life-giving and healing place for the patient. In this other space, the patient may feel more comfortable in spirit and more able to engage in prayer. Family and friends, as well as other patients and staff, may be resources in the practice of imagery.

Exploring as many aspects of the prayer experience as possible enriches both the nurse's and the patient's understanding of the nature and place of prayer for a particular individual. Sacred or inspirational readings, music, drumming, movement, light or darkness, aromas, and time of day are among the many factors that may be important considerations in one's prayer life. The patient's prayer life, in all of its fullness and meaning, nurtures the spirit, and the nurse may be able to support the patient's prayer needs by facilitating changes in the environment or schedule. It is wise to remember that merely the process of listening to and appreciating the prayer life of another nurtures the spirit and acknowledges the spiritual dimension of that person.

Ensuring Opportunities for Rest and Leisure

Integral aspects of holistic living and care of the spirit, rest and leisure enhance growth, creativity, and renewal.[91] Assisting persons to consider the place of rest and leisure in their lives is part of holistic nursing. Taking stock of the way that they integrate rest and leisure into their own lives is a necessary part of self-care for nurses as well. In an increasingly busy society, where filling each moment is viewed in terms of increasing productivity and where even leisure happens according to a schedule, the notion of rest and leisure deserves thoughtful consideration.

Holistic nurses try to enhance the patient's conscious awareness of how rest and leisure are, or are not, part of their lives. Such awareness makes those areas available for intentional evaluation, and, if desired, change. Observations and question that may be helpful in the exploration of this aspect of spirituality include the following:

- I notice that you read a lot. What does reading do for you?
- You say you just can't rest. When have you been able to rest? Are there things that usually help you to rest?
- What is a real vacation like for you?
- What time of the day (year, season, week) is most restful or peaceful for you?
- How do you relax?
- Some people just help us to relax . . . who does that for you?
- Is there something I can do to help you to relax?

Regular exercise, music, imagery, a specific time for rest and quiet, and the commitment to incorporating these experiences into daily life encourage rest and leisure. Validating the importance of rest and leisure, and encouraging a commitment to making time for renewal a part of one's life are important aspects of holistic care.

ARTS AND SPIRITUALITY

The arts have a role in the life of the spirit. Many persons find that various forms of artistic endeavor are doors to and expressions of the spirit. The term *artist* can include anyone who creates—the homemaker who cooks and sews and the carpenter who designs and builds, as well as the more often recognized persons whose works are heard in symphonies or seen in galleries. As an expression of her or his wholeness, an artist's work is also a reflection of spirituality. L'Engle expressed this well:

> As I listen in the silence, I learn that my feelings about art and my feelings about the Creator of the Universe are inseparable. To try to talk about art and about Chris-

tianity is for me one and the same thing, and it means attempting to share the meaning of my life, what gives it, for me, its tragedy and its glory. It is what makes me respond to the death of an apple tree, the birth of a puppy, northern lights shaking the sky, by writing stories.[92]

Literature contains life stories, both real and fictional, to which people relate and from which they learn, gain comfort, and garner encouragement. Poetry contains deep truths, often in a few well chosen words, a rhythm, and spaces for silence. Music expresses feelings that are beyond words. Songs bring back memories or capture what people would like to say. Pottery awakens the senses of touch and sight as one forms a vessel or holds a favorite mug. Dance moves people, literally and figuratively, in space and time. Photography connects individuals, and sometimes moves their hearts for those known only through the images seen all over the world. Drumming awakens deep, basic yearnings, and calls some to worship. Gardens nourish not only the body, but also the senses of sight, touch, and smell. Cave drawings are reminders of civilizations past and awaken a sense of wonder.

Creativity nourishes both observers and participants. People are in awe of ancient castles and of children building sand castles, reveling in the sea, wind, and treasures of the ocean. They marvel at monuments and buildings that have stood the test of time, while joining with friends and neighbors to build a playground for today's children can enliven them. The passing down of skills joins the generations over time and space. How many gifts of the spirit came as one learned to bake cookies with a special grandparent or to play the fiddle under the guidance of a beloved mentor?

An awareness of the breadth of the possibilities of using the arts to enrich the life of the spirit increases the nurse's ability to help the patient use the world of the arts for his or her own journey. The nurse and patient may recognize in books or movies struggles and questions that the patient now confronts, or they may share an appreciation for a special painting, musical piece, or homemade dessert. Providing an atmosphere that, as much as possible, is pleasing to the sensibilities of the patient may promote rest and relaxation. It may also facilitate the use of other interventions, such as imagery. Encouraging and facilitating opportunities for people to engage in or share stories of their creative endeavors is one of the many ways that nurses include spirituality in care.

CONCLUSION

Because all persons, nurses as well as patients, are spiritual beings, care of the spirit is an integral component of holistic nursing care. Care of the spirit requires the evolution of language to express this dimension of ourselves better, and an approach to nursing process that is integrative rather than linear. Spirituality assessment and intervention, which are often the same process, require intentional listening, presence, and a willingness to hear another's story. Spiritual care is based on a recognition that people express and experience their spirituality in and through relationships with the Absolute, others, nature, and self.

Spiritual care may incorporate "experts" such as representatives of particular religious traditions or other spiritual support people, but nurses need to do more than merely refer matters of the spirit to these persons. Although spiritual matters are both deep and personal, they often come to the forefront of life when health crises cause a person to stop, to take stock, to experience anxieties and fear, and to seek that which is at the heart of his or her life. Nurses offer spiritual support as they are able to be present with mystery and the life questions of others. Tending to matters of

the spirit may include incorporating ritual, prayer, meditation, rest, art, and any activity that enhances awareness of oneself and one's place in the world.

DIRECTIONS FOR FUTURE RESEARCH

1. Further explore understandings of spirituality in health and illness across cultures and in different age groups, using qualitative methodologies.
2. Explore the influence of spirituality on staying healthy and on healing related to specific health concerns.
3. Investigate how attentiveness to spirituality in clinical practice may influence health outcomes, including economic considerations.

NURSE HEALER REFLECTIONS

After reading this chapter, the nurse healer will be able to answer or begin a process of answering the following questions:

- In recognizing my wholeness, how would I describe my physical being, my psychologic–emotional being, and my spiritual being?
- What signals spiritual distress in my own life?
- How do I nurture my spirit?
- How would I describe the most significant connections in my life—the giving, receiving, and interplay in relationship with family, colleagues or peers, God or the Absolute, friends, and nature/environment/cosmos?
- What areas of the spirit need intentional care in my own life, perhaps because of pain or distress, or because there are areas in which I want to focus and grow?
- As I reflect on my own story, how is the growth and development of my spirit reflected in the events of my life?
- How have I experienced intentional presence?

NOTES

1. L. Tzu, *Tao Te Ching* (London: Penguin Books, 1988).

2. M.A. Burkhardt, Spirituality: An Analysis of the Concept, *Holistic Nursing Practice* 3 (1989):69–77.

3. M.G. Nagai-Jacobson and M.A. Burkhardt, Spirituality: Cornerstone of Holistic Nursing Practice, *Holistic Nursing Practice* 3 (1989):18–26.

4. J.D. Emblen, Religion and Spirituality Defined According to Current Use in Nursing Literature, *Journal of Professional Nursing* 8 (1992):41–47.

5. T.J. Mansen, The Spiritual Dimension of Individuals: Concept Development, *Nursing Diagnosis* 4 (1993):140–147.

6. N.C. Goddard, Spirituality as Integrative Energy: A Philosophical Analysis as Requisite Precursor to Holistic Nursing Practice, *Journal of Advanced Nursing* 22 (1995):808–815.

7. J. Engebretson, Considerations in Diagnosing the Spiritual Domain, *Nursing Diagnosis* 7 (1996):100–107.

8. R.J. Fehring et al., Spiritual Well-Being, Religiosity, Hope, Depression, and Other Mood States in Elderly People Coping with Cancer, *Oncology Nursing Forum* 4 (1997):663–671.

9. B.A. Hall, Spirituality in Terminal Illness, *Journal of Holistic Nursing* 15 (1997):82–96.

10. P. Nolan and P. Crawford, Towards a Rhetoric of Spirituality in Mental Health, *Journal of Advanced Nursing* 26 (1997): 289–294.

11. S. Sussman et al., On Operationalizing Spiritual Experience for Health Promotion Research and Practice, *Alternative Therapies in Clinical Practice* 4 (1997):120–124.

12. Mansen, The Spiritual Dimension of Individuals.

13. Burkhardt, Spirituality: An Analysis of the Concept.

14. Emblen, Religion and Spirituality Defined.

15. Fehring et al., Spiritual Well-Being, Religiosity, Hope, Depression, and Other Mood States.

16. Nolan and Crawford, Towards a Rhetoric of Spirituality.

17. Sussman et al., On Operationalizing Spiritual Experience.

18. P.G. Reed, An Emerging Paradigm for the Investigation of Spirituality in Nursing, *Research in Nursing and Health* 15 (1992):349–357.

19. Hall, Spirituality in Terminal Illness.

20. Engebretson, Considerations in Diagnosing the Spiritual Domain.

21. Nolan and Crawford, Towards a Rhetoric of Spirituality.

22. Burkhardt, Spirituality: An Analysis of the Concept.

23. M.A. Burkhardt, Becoming and Connecting: Elements of Spirituality for Women, *Holistic Nursing Practice* 8 (1994):12–21.

24. Emblen, Religion and Spirituality Defined.

25. Mansen, The Spiritual Dimension of Individuals.

26. M.G. Nagai-Jacobson and M.A. Burkhardt, Awareness and Relatedness: Elements of Spirituality for Men (Unpublished data).

27. Reed, An Emerging Paradigm.

28. J. Walton, Spiritual Relationships: A Concept Analysis, *Journal of Holistic Nursing* 14 (1996): 237–250.

29. Nolan and Crawford, Towards a Rhetoric of Spirituality, 291.

30. Burkhardt, Becoming and Connecting: Elements of Spirituality for Women.

31. Nagai-Jacobson and Burkhardt, Awareness and Relatedness: Elements of Spirituality for Men.

32. E.R.D. Barker, Being Whole: Spiritual Well-Being in Appalachian Women: A Phenomenological Study (Unpublished doctoral dissertation, University of Texas, Austin, 1989).

33. J. Walton, Spirituality of the Patient Recovering from an Acute Myocardial Infarction: A Grounded Theory Study (Unpublished doctoral dissertation, University of Missouri, Kansas City, 1997).

34. Reed, An Emerging Paradigm.

35. S. Jeffers, *Brother Eagle, Sister Sky* (New York: Dial Books, 1991).

36. S. Lamb, *Pueblo and Mission* (Flagstaff, AZ: Northland Publishing, 1997), 2.

37. M.J. McKivergin and M.J. Daubenmire, The Healing Process of Presence, *Journal of Holistic Nursing* 12 (1994):65–81.

38. J. Walton, Spirituality of the Patient Recovering from an Acute Myocardial Infarction.

39. Nagai-Jacobson and Burkhardt, Spirituality: Cornerstone of Holistic Nursing Practice.

40. M.A. Burkhardt and M.G. Nagai-Jacobson, Reawakening Spirit in Clinical Practice, *Journal of Holistic Nursing* 12 (1994):9–21.

41. L. Dossey, What's Love Got To Do with It? *Alternative Therapies in Health and Medicine* 2 (1996):8–15.

42. B. Siegel, *Love , Medicine, and Miracles* (New York: Harper & Row, 1986).

43. L. Dossey, What's Love Got To Do with It?

44. J. Green and R. Shellenberger, The Healing Energy of Love, *Alternative Therapies in Health and Medicine* 2 (1996):46–56.

45. V. Frankl, *Man's Search for Meaning* (New York: Washington Square Press, 1984).

46. Fehring et al., Spiritual Well-Being, Religiosity, Hope, Depression, and Other Mood States.

47. S.B. Simon and S. Simon, *Forgiveness: How To Make Peace with Your Past and Get on with Your Life* (New York: Warner Books, 1990).

48. D. Kollmar, *Manifestation* (Workshop sponsored by The Complete Self-Attunement Associates, Charleston, WV, August 30, 1998).

49. L. Dossey, *Healing Words: The Power of Prayer and the Practice of Medicine* (San Francisco: Harper, 1993).

50. L. Dossey, *Prayer Is Good Medicine* (San Francisco: Harper, 1996).

51. M.D. Calabria and J.A. Macrae, eds., *Suggestions for Thought by Florence Nightingale: Selections and Commentaries* (Philadelphia: University of Pennsylvania Press, 1994).

52. L. Dossey, *Healing Words*.

53. L. Dossey, *Prayer Is Good Medicine*.

54. L. Dossey, *Be Careful What You Pray For* (San Francisco: HarperCollins, 1997).

55. Engebretson, Considerations in Diagnosing the Spiritual Domain.

56. Mansen, The Spiritual Dimension of Individuals.

57. Nolan and Crawford, Towards a Rhetoric of Spirituality.

58. B.M. Dossey, Florence Nightingale: A 19th-Century Mystic, *Journal of Holistic Nursing* 16 (1998):111–164.

59. B.M. Dossey, *Florence Nightingale: Mystic, Visionary, Healer* (Springhouse, PA: Springhouse Corporation, 1999).

60. B.M. Dossey, Florence Nightingale: Her Crimean Fever Chronic Illness, *Journal of Holistic Nursing* 16 (1998):168–196.

61. B.M. Dossey, Florence Nightingale: Her Personality Type, *Journal of Holistic Nursing* 16 (1998):202–222.

62. B.M. Dossey, *Florence Nightingale: Mystic, Visionary, and Healer.*

63. B.M. Dossey, Florence Nightingale: A 19th-Century Mystic.

64. T. Moore, *Care of the Soul* (New York: HarperCollins, 1992).

65. K.B. Wright, Professional, Ethical, and Legal Implications for Spiritual Care in Nursing, *Image* 30 (1998):81–83.

66. D. Barnard et al., Toward a Person-Centered Medicine: Religious Studies in the Medical Curriculum, *Academic Medicine* 70 (1995):806–813.

67. D.B. Larson et al., *Model Curriculum for Psychiatry Residency Training Programs: Religion and Spirituality in Clinical Practice* (Rockville, MD: National Institute for Healthcare Research, 1996).

68. H.D. Silverman, Creating a Spirituality Curriculum for Family Practice Residents, *Alternative Therapies in Health and Medicine* 3 (1997):54–61.

69. Fehring et al., Spiritual Well-Being, Religiosity, Hope, Depression, and Other Mood States.

70. D.B. Larson et al., Systematic Analysis of Research on Religious Variables in Four Major Psychiatric Journals 1978–1982, *American Journal of Psychiatry* 143 (1986):329–334.

71. D.B. Larson, Health: What Does God Have To Do With It? (Paper presented at the Third Annual Alternative Therapies Symposium: Creating Integrated Healthcare, San Diego, CA, April 3, 1998).

72. J.S. Levin et al., Religion and Spirituality in Medicine: Research and Education, *Journal of the American Medical Association* 278 (1997):792–793.

73. R.L. Hatch et al., The Spiritual Involvement and Beliefs Scale: Development and Testing of a New Instrument, *Journal of Family Practice* 46 (1998):476–486.

74. Hall, Spirituality in Terminal Illness, 86.

75. Larson, Health: What Does God Have To Do With It?

76. Hall, Spirituality in Terminal Illness.

77. J. Bruchac, *Tell Me a Tale* (New York: Harcourt, Brace, 1997), 1.

78. M.G. Nagai-Jacobson and M.A. Burkhardt, Viewing Persons as Stories: A Perspective for Holistic Care, *Alternative Therapies in Health and Medicine* 2 (1996):54–58.

79. M.A. Burkhardt and M.G. Nagai-Jacobson, Psychospiritual Care: A Shared Journey Embracing Wholeness, *Bioethics Forum* 13 (1997):34–41.

80. J. Bruchac, *Tell Me a Tale*.

81. Hatch et al., The Spiritual Involvement and Beliefs Scale.

82. J. Hunglemann et al., Focus on Spiritual Well-Being: Harmonious Interconnectedness of

Mind-Body-Spirit—Use of the JAREL Spiritual Well-Being Scale, *Geriatric Nursing* 17 (1997): 262–266.

83. J. Hunglemann et al., Use of the JAREL Spiritual Well-Being Scale.

84. Burkhardt, Spirituality: An Analysis of the Concept.

85. J.W. Howden, Development and Psychometric Characteristics of the Spirituality Assessment Scale (Unpublished doctoral dissertation, Texas Woman's University, Denton, 1992).

86. E.R. Barker, Patient Spirituality Assessment: A Tool That Works (Paper presented at the Uniformed Nurse Practitioners Association Meeting, November, 1996).

87. E.R. Barker, How To Do Research, Get Finished, and Not Lose Your Balance (Presentation at the Nursing Research Symposium, San Diego, 1998).

88. Barker, Being Whole: Spiritual Well-Being in Appalachian Women.

89. Hall, Spirituality in Terminal Illness.

90. J. Achterberg et al., *Rituals of Healing: Using Imagery for Health and Wellness* (New York: Bantam Books, 1994).

91. L. Doohan, *Leisure: A Spiritual Need* (Notre Dame, IN: Ave Maria Press, 1990).

92. M. L'Engle, *Walking on Water: Reflecting on Faith and Art* (Wheaton, IL: Harold Shaw Publishers, 1980), 16.

VISION OF HEALING

Toward Wholeness

Within the philosophy underpinning energetic healing is the view that the soul/mind/psyche precedes energy and energy precedes biology. Radical? Yes, it changes everything. If the soul/mind/psyche somehow determines the form that energy will take, it is ultimately the builder of biology, chemistry, emotions, relationships, and all experience. The holistic view that the body, mind, emotions, and spirit are integrated can be rephrased as the idea that the body, mind, emotions, and spirit are different reflections of the same energy. Thus, healing requires us to turn from individual biologic, psychologic, emotional, and spiritual healing paths and to begin a journey toward the energy and to the soul/mind/psyche that precedes the energy. Healing is returning to one's wholeness as a soul.

One way to begin such a journey is to become acquainted with our own energy. As we do, we will explore the body, mind, emotions, and spirit differently. We will discover areas that are darker than we want to believe—and lighter. Eventually, we will discover someone that we like and respect very much, someone whose wholeness surprises us and whose wisdom is breathtaking. It is a hero's or heroine's journey, one that begins with the wound of believing that we are separate within ourselves and from each other. It progresses through dark and seemingly perilous experiences until we begin to understand the meaning of the journey in its wholeness. We gradually enter more and more of the light and discover that it is not blinding, but filled with joy, wonder, and love.

The journey to the wholeness is the journey of a lifetime, everyone's lifetime. It can involve any path that will help the individual learn of his or her own history and its meaning and purpose. Some people will find that exploring their own energy and the information it contains is a useful path. Traveling this path can be an extraordinarily rich experience. The journey is an adventure, one that must be taken with intention and deliberateness; it must be entered through choice. When the journey to wholeness begins in earnest, everything changes. As we embark or continue our journey to wholeness, we must explore and enjoy all of the avenues open to us. In one way or another, each will reveal more information, and with each new piece, we step closer to our own wholeness.

Chapter 6

Energetic Healing

Victoria E. Slater

NURSE HEALER OBJECTIVES

Theoretical

- Name and describe three major energetic structures.
- Apply electromagnetic characteristics to the human.
- Discuss a structural and a process view of chakras.
- Compare chakras to a Fourier analyzer or a spectrometer.
- Compare meridians to a direct electric current.
- Discuss the quantum theories of holography and consciousness-created reality.
- Apply Battista's information process model and Assagioli's model of the dimensions of the psyche to holistic healing.

Clinical

- Identify and use the most appropriate energetic healing modalities for each client/patient.
- Recognize the information level and the dimensions of psyche used by clients/patients.

Personal

- Explore a variety of forms of energy to access information from the dimensions of the psyche.
- Discover how to deliberately use chakras, meridians, and aura to further one's own health.
- Explore energetic healing modalities.

DEFINITIONS

Aura: an atmosphere; a vague, luminous glow surrounding something.

Centering: the act of focusing one's attention on the heart, resulting in an increase in measurable extra low frequency magnetic pulses 0.3 to 3.0 cycles per second (Hertz) emitted by the hands.

Chakra: an energy center in the subtle, or energetic, body that is described as a whirling vortex of light.

Consciousness-Created Reality: the quantum theory that proposes that reality (matter) emerges from the potentialities (wave functions) of the universe because a consciousness observed all possible potentialities and selected one. Until a consciousness makes such an observation, there is no reality.

Energetic: having a capacity for work; active, showing great physical or mental energy.

Energetic Healing: the process of healing one's energetic structures (meridians and chakras) and the information carried within the electromagnetic field (aura).

Hologram: a three-dimensional image produced by an interference pattern of light (as laser light). Each individual part of the interference pattern contains the entire image. The entire image is revealed when the interference pattern is exposed to coherent light of the proper frequency.

Intention: the establishment of a healing activity that results in "intensity of feelings, heart-felt motivation, lowered heart rate variability, and brain wave synchronization."[1]

Meridian: parallel pathways that are low-voltage electrical conduits. In Eastern philosophies, the meridians are said to conduct chi, qi, prana, or ki, or universal energy.

Psychosynthesis: Assagioli's psychologic theory that proposes a multidimensional human psyche.

Self-Referencing Biofeedback: biofeedback in which the internal responses are the feedback reference. Centering with intention is a self-referencing biofeedback state.

Three sources contribute to the definition of energetic healing: (1) traditional understandings of energetic structures and functions, (2) physics, (3) and the personal experiences of energetic healers. To physicists, physics is defined by experimental results and mathematical formulas. Until a theory is confirmed experimentally, it is a metaphor. Thus, physics concepts operate as metaphors because there are limited experimental data and no mathematical support for the energetic structures and processes described by energetic healers. Because there are no machines that measure all that energetic healers experience, the healer becomes the tool of measurement. Because each person experiences energy slightly differently and everyone is unique, people should use descriptions of energetic processes given by others as guidelines. Ultimately, the experience that matters is each individual's personal relationship with his or her own chakras, meridians, aura, and the information contained within.

More important than the theory of energetic anatomy and processes is the use of the meridians, chakras, the aura, and the information that they contain. The goal of holistic nursing is to assist each other's growth as integrated body-mind-emotion-spirit people. Such growth is a deliberate process; it does not just happen.

NATURE'S LOVE OF REDUNDANCY AND ENERGETIC HEALING

The International Society for the Study of Subtle Energies and Energy Medicine (ISSSEEM) has identified and defined two concepts associated with energetic healing:

> *Energy medicine* includes all energetic and informational interactions resulting from self-regulation or brought about through other energy couplings to mind and body. In addition to various therapeutic energies which we may use, there are also energy pulses from the environment which influence humans and animals in a variety of ways. For instance, low level changes in magnetic, electric, electromagnetic, acoustic, and gravitational fields often have profound effects on both biology and psychology.

> *Subtle energy* is more difficult to discuss in a scientific paradigm. The traditional subtle energies re-

ferred to as chi (or ki), prana, etheric energy, fohat, orgone, odit force, mana, homeopathic resonance, etc., are said to move in the so-called etheric body (subtle body), and seem to be difficult to measure at present. A number of therapeutic methods prevalent today, however, appear to be concerned with facilitating the flow of these subtle energies through the dense physical body.

In addition, it is traditionally accepted that expansions of consciousness often are related to changes in subtle energies that cannot be quantified. These latter "energies," which are said to be associated with interactions and with transcendence, may not, in fact, actually be involved with known physical fields.[2]

Green, the president of ISSSEEM, refined the definition of subtle energies as

detected only by the work associated with its use, that is detected by its effects, [and] hypothesized to be the carrier of informational and interactive processes in both mind-over-matter, inside-the-skin (INS) processes, as in psychophysiologic self-regulation, and mind-over-matter outside-the-skin (OUTS) processes, as in parapsychology, psychokinesis, and traditional healing.[3]

The ISSSEEM definitions of energy medicine and subtle energy are useful, but they do not satisfy the needs of a holistic nurse trying to understand how energetic approaches to health care may assist someone in working with and integrating body, mind, emotion, and spirit. Energetic healing is defined here as integrating the information that is stored, carried, and processed by the subtle energy system of aura, meridians, and chakras. Such healing includes releasing information that no longer enhances life and bringing it into the person's conscious awareness. Integration of that information contributes to one's conscious wholeness and results in healing. An energetic healer uses energy in any form, including energy medicine and subtle energies, to enable clients to access and process the information stored within their personal energetic field so it can be used for healing.

The energetic and informational interactions and the energy pulses from the environment defined by ISSSEEM as energy medicine do not, in and of themselves, lead to energetic healing, nor does merely "facilitating the flow of . . . subtle energies through the dense physical body." Dossey and White postulated that it is not energy that is healing, but one's consciousness.[4,5] White emphasized this point:

Some spiritual seekers, failing to understand [the] distinction, become "energy junkies." They learn with fine detail how to manipulate energy inside themselves or attract energy to themselves from outside. . . . Yet when the experience is over, their consciousness has not changed a whit. . . . After the internal pyrotechnics have subsided, it is consciousness alone that can bring understanding to the person.[6]

As practitioners of energetic healing have experienced, physical, emotional, mental, and spiritual changes accompany subtle energy treatments. The more profound changes are not immediately noticeable, even though the treatments result in relaxation followed by relief of pain and stress, increased rates of wound healing, and more. The changes that are healing (i.e., enabling one to become more whole) take time—often weeks, months, and years of participating with energetic modalities.

Energetic healers talk about dealing with their own painful emotional issues as a prerequisite to being an effective healer, rather than just a technician of energetic modalities. There seem to be two levels of energy work: the technical level, which is concerned with proper form of the auric, chakra, and meridian techniques, and the healing level, which is aimed toward emotional, mental, spiritual, and physical interpretation and integration. Benner's novice-to-expert model illuminates this distinction.[7] One begins by learning the steps of various techniques and practicing them hundreds of times until becoming the expert who works through the techniques, rather than merely performing them. Slater's study found that after receiving a single treatment from a novice energetic practitioner, clients reported transient physical changes, such as relaxation and pain relief.[8] After receiving the identical treatment from an expert practitioner, some clients experienced permanent physical changes, such as relief of pain that had continued for many years. The difference was not the technique; it was the practitioner.

Merely practicing techniques hundreds of times does not inevitably make one an expert healer. Practicing techniques is only one aspect of becoming an expert energetic healer; actively pursuing a personal healing is more important. This pursuit opens the energetic healer to a greater understanding of the possibilities within him or her as an instrument of healing and of the energetic medium through which to express that healing for others. Thus, the expert healer has done the same techniques differently hundreds of times and is familiar with their possibilities.

An expert healer has learned that there are levels of wounding and healing, but, ultimately, all healing is spiritual. For example, chakras may be damaged physically and unable to process energy adequately. Chakras also process informa-

tion and the damage may result in destructive emotional and mental habits. A novice healer will notice and work with the changes in the ability of the chakra to process energy physically, while the expert will work with both the physical changes and the information's energy pattern (energy information) to relieve its constriction and to assist healing the information that led to the problem. All energetic healing treatments work with the physical and informational energetic patterns, but the expert who is aware of the pattern of information and the physical distortions is likely to help a client move toward wholeness more easily. The art of energetic healing is learning that the same form, chakras, serves several functions and it is necessary to adjust one's treatment to work with the several functions at the same time.

Nature uses successful forms repeatedly for similar, but seemingly different functions. Several examples of successful forms are trees, orifices, and spirals. The branching form of trees and bushes is seen in the neurologic and vascular system, organizations, and in spiritual symbols. In the neurologic system, the roots are the neurons from the extremities and trunk that carry electrochemical information to the spinal cord, and then to the branches within the brain and back again. The roots of the vascular system are the interosseous origins of blood cells, which are carried to and through the heart and branching vessels to supply oxygen and nutrients to the cells, carry waste products away, and defend and help heal the physical body. Similarly, organizations gather their nutrients from the environment (e.g., information, money, employees, ideas, markets), circulate those through the organizational tree, and send them back into the branching environment. The Tree of Life, an ancient spiritual symbol, is portrayed as a tree with a wide and bushy canopy of leaves connected through a broad trunk to a plethora of roots branching deep into the ground. In each case, a similar form is used to accomplish the same function, that of spreading nutrients, power, and information throughout the organism, whether physical, social, or spiritual.

Another example of a repetitive form is illustrated by the eye, uterine cervix, and crown chakra (as described by Leadbeater[9]). All three have the same structure—several concentric circles of cell-like structures with an orifice in the middle that opens and closes. Each is involved with the transfer of information: the eye is the doorway for information carried on electromagnetic waves of light; the uterine cervix is the doorway for information carried by menstrual blood, sperm, and, later, the delivery of a baby; and the spiritual chakra is believed to be the doorway for information about one's spiritual relationships with the divine and with one's own soul/spirit. The form has been repeated, and the function of carrying information is the same. Only the type of information changes—electromagnetic, physical, spiritual.

The spiral is another form that nature uses widely, as in the electron circling a nucleus, the solar system and galaxies, tornados, water going down a drain, and ice skaters spinning. In each case, the spiral form maintains or increases energy. Nature seems to decide what function is required and then adapts an existing form that may serve the purpose.

Meridians, chakras, and the aura are also repetitive forms while serving different functions. On the physical level, each serves the same function as a common electrical device; at the more abstract level, they address perceptions and their emotional accompaniment. Meridians are described as the conductors of a very low frequency direct electric current;[10] they also act as messengers. Chakras act like modulators and processors of energy,[11] and as a data-processing program. The aura, which resembles an electromagnetic field, serves as the site of information storage. The me-

ridians, chakras, and aura do more than just transmit, process, and store physical energy; they collect, process, prioritize, and store information about one's environment and experiences. They do not, however, interpret that information. A conscious aspect of oneself that is external to and co-extensive with the physical and emotional–mental nature of the human seems to determine the meaning of information. The interpreter may be one's soul/spirit, but is defined here as one's eternal consciousness.

MERIDIANS

Tradition and Data

Traditionally, meridians are portrayed as 12 pairs of superficial and deep pathways that carry throughout the body the human energy called *chi* by the Chinese and *qi* by the Japanese. The superficial meridian pathways are associated with a series of acupuncture points that are stimulated by pressure, heat, and needles to reduce pain and illness, and improve or maintain health. Weil pointed out that, although the meridians have names like the organs (e.g., liver meridian), they do not absolutely equate with the organ of their name.[12] Because the Chinese tradition prohibits autopsies, the Chinese had to rely on their observations of the meridians' functions. The liver meridian refers to the sphere of influence of that meridian, not the organ by the same name.

In 1988, Gerber reviewed the literature about meridians and found radiographic, histologic, and Kirlian photographic studies of their locations and possible function.[13] In the 1960s, for example, a Korean research team headed by Kim Bong Han had injected radioactive phosphorus into the acupoints and veins of rabbits.[14] The phosphorus injected into the acupoint was taken up by a ductlike tubule approximately 0.5 to 1.5 microns in diameter. When injected in the nearby vein, little or none of the phosphorus could be detected in the meridian. A French researcher, De Vernejoul, found that radioactive technetium 99m injected into acupoints moved along the meridian associated with that acupoint for a distance of 30 centimeters in 4 to 6 minutes.[15] Random injection of the same isotope in the skin, veins, and lymphatic system did not produce similar results. These two radiographic studies suggest that the meridian system is separate from the vascular and lymphatic networks.

Kim's histologic studies suggested that there are four layers of meridians and they are associated with the vascular and lymphatic systems, the organs, the skin, and the nervous systems. From deepest to most superficial, he named these layers (1) the internal duct system, (2) the intra-external duct system, (3) the external duct system or superficial duct system, and (4) the neural duct system. The internal duct system wove in, out, and through the vascular and lymphatic vessels, and its fluids traveled independently of the blood and lymph flow. The meridian fluid might travel in the same direction or in a different direction of the surrounding vessel, as if there were a channel within a larger river. The ducts of the intra-external duct system were found along the surface of the internal organs, and the external duct system ran along the outer walls of the blood and lymphatic vessels and in the layers of the skin. The latter system is the one used for acupuncture and acupressure. The fourth system, the neural duct system, is spread throughout the central and peripheral nervous system. In 1985, Becker and Selden reported that meridians conduct an electric current that flows into the central nervous system and that perineural cells appear to conduct the current physically.[16] Perineural cells surround every nerve cell, such as in the Schwann cell sheath, and compose 90 percent of the brain. The cytoplasm of all Schwann cells is linked through holes in their adjacent membranes, forming an uninterrupted pathway for the electric current. Broken bones begin to heal normally only after the perineural sleeve mends, indicating that the electric current conducted by the Schwann cells is required for healing to begin.

In other studies, Kim found that the meridian ducts were formed within 15 hours of an embryonic chick's conception, which is prior to the formation of even the most rudimentary organs. His data suggested that the arteries, veins, and lymphatic vessels grow around a preexisting meridian system as the organism develops, and the meridians may act as the spatial guide for the vascular and lymphatic system. Kim also discovered that the four meridian duct systems are interconnected in much the same manner that veins and arteries are linked at the capillary level.[17] The capillary-type structures are called terminal ductules, and they have branches that feed into the nuclei of tissue cells. Thus, the meridian-to-cell nucleus chain is an unbroken pathway. Meridian fluid contains DNA, RNA, amino acids, hyaluronic acid, free nucleotides, adrenaline, corticosteroids, estrogen, and other hormonal substances in different concentrations and levels than usually found in the bloodstream.

When Kim severed the meridian going to a frog's liver, microscopic changes showed enlarged hepatocytes with turbid cytoplasm. Within 3 days, vascular degeneration took place throughout the entire liver. When perineural meridian ducts were cut, neural reflexes were prolonged by more the 500 percent within 30 minutes, and the effects lasted longer than 48 hours with only minor changes. The Schwann cell sheath that lines every neuron is made of perineural cells; multiple sclerosis is characterized by destruction of these cells and subsequent diminishing of neural reflexes.

Kim and Becker both studied the meridian acupoints. Kim found small corpuscles beneath the acupoints that contained 10 times the level of adrenaline in the blood. Becker, who was interested in the electrical nature of the meridians, found that the electric current carried by meridians was a low-voltage, low-amplitude direct current somewhere between a trillionth (a picoamp) and a billionth (a nanoamp) of an ampere.[18] All direct currents lose strength with distance and must be boosted at regular intervals. Becker calculated that a microvolt, nanoamp current would need boosters every few inches and that about half of the traditional acupoints have electrical characteristics consistent with a microvolt direct electric current amplifying booster. He also found that the current strength at the acupoints had a 15-minute rhythm, which may relate to De Vernejoul's discovery that meridian fluid travels 30 centimeters in 4 to 6 minutes, or 90 centimeters in 15 minutes. The wrist and elbow are about 30 centimeters apart, which suggests that meridian fluid and, thus, information could flow throughout most of the human body in 15 minutes.

Gerber proposed that the "presence of hormones and adrenaline within ductal fluids would certainly suggest some link between the meridian system and the endocrine glands of the body."[19] Pert's[20] discovery that the neuroendocrine cells, peptides, act like a mobile neurologic system carrying emotional information throughout the body may support Gerber's conclusion.

Kirlian photographs of acupoints demonstrate that they have distinct electrographic characteristics and that the brightness of the acupoints changes prior to the onset of physical illness, sometimes even weeks before the advent of symptoms.[21] This evidence supports the traditional teaching that illnesses are reflected in the energy field before the individual experiences them physically.

Intuition

The meridian system seems to act like part of the body's defense system. It appears to have an alertness to the environment,

though not an awareness, and acts like an ever vigilant sentry or searchlight scanning for danger. Meridians can be hyperalert or sluggish, as if their flow were partially dammed and/or traveled a tortuous path, rather than an easy course downstream.

> Pause for a moment and sense your own meridians. The Chinese teach that the meridian flow is from foot and hand to head, so it might be easiest to sense your flow if you begin by focusing your attention on your feet or your hands. Notice a flow that may feel like an underground river or may suggest a sense of movement. Relax into this experience, letting yourself become aware of a new and more subtle aspect of yourself. Keep trying.

A glance at the evolution of life may help explain meridians. The first life form was likely only one cell, such as a paramecium. As it floated in its aquatic environment, it had to gather and transmit information throughout its one cell effectively and efficiently enough to survive.

> Imagine yourself as a one-cell organism gathering information from your environment. How does the information about your environment come to you? Is it in the form of pressure waves as another organism moves or floats by, or does it come in another form? What would the wave feel like if it came from something you could eat? How about one that came from something that could eat you? How do those waves differ? Do they differ only in their strength and direction, or do they have different frequencies? What additional information can the frequency of a wave give you?

A one-cell organism may not have awareness, but it undoubtedly gathers enough information to survive. The paramecium has primitive motility, digestion, respiration, circulation, and elimination. Perhaps the movement of its cell wall in response to pressure waves of various frequencies is a primitive information-gathering, information-processing, defense system. Perhaps the meridian system is a series of one cells that transmit pressure and frequency information from cell to cell as rapidly as they can handle the flow.

> Return to your experience as a one-cell organism. How might that primitive defense system work in a higher organism such as a human? Imagine your skin and superficial duct meridian system receiving the pressure and frequency waves in the room, giving you more information than you can gather by your five senses. Imagine data moving through your meridians at cell speed and into each cell nucleus. What subtle nuances are you aware of that you did not cognitively notice before?

Meridian techniques such as the Scudder, which is taught in the Healing Touch program, Jin Shin Jyutsu,[22] and Touch for Health act quickly. Recipients experience rapid relaxation of tissues and mood. Acupuncture, which works directly with meridians, is reputed to bring a body into balance. The same technique given to a hyperthyroid and a hypothyroid patient brings both closer to normal thyroid functioning. Perhaps the effect of acupuncture, the Scudder, or any meridian technique is to calm down a hyperalert meridian system and stimulate a sluggish one.

The relaxing, balancing effect of meridian techniques is temporary if the internal and external environment remain the same. If the meridian system is a defense mechanism, then it will return to its hyperalert state if the environment continues to appear threatening. Threats may be physical, emotional, mental, spiritual or, more accurately, a combination of all four.

CHAKRAS

Tradition and Data

The word *chakra* means wheel, vortex, or wheel (vortex) of light in Sanskrit. Chakra lore is vast and varied, but there are two commonalities: chakras exist, and they are ports for energy exchange with the universe. Their locations, colors, tones, and functions have been identified intuitively and differently. Five representative views of chakra functioning are listed in Table 6–1.[23–27] In each, the first chakra is believed to function on the most concrete level, the seventh, at the most abstract. Most views have the first chakra relating to survival and its requirements, the fourth to love, the fifth to expression, the sixth to insight, and the seventh to spirituality. Views of the second and third chakras vary widely. Nurses are familiar with a chakra sequence in Maslow's hierarchy of needs (Figure 6–1).[28] Maslow described seven levels of needs, although most people are familiar only with the first five, physiologic survival needs to self-actualization. He also listed a sixth level of needs, the need to know and understand, and a seventh level, aesthetic needs.

Although some traditions identify as many as 12 chakras, most recognize 7 major chakras, all associated with the nervous system structure or a neuroendocrine gland (Table 6–2). Some authors list a splenic chakra and/or a gonadal chakra;[29] others list a chakra at the manubriosternal joint (the Angle of Louis), below the collar bone at the junction of the manubrium and sternum.[30] The spinal joints have been described as five octaves of chakras.[31] Some sources talk about 9 to 12 chakras, 7 on the physical body and up to 5 off-body chakras.

Table 6-1 Five Perspectives of Chakras*

Chakra	Bruyere	Brennan	Judith	Lansdowne	Sharamon and Baginski
7th	Release, surrender	Integration of total personality, spiritual aspects	Wisdom	Spiritual will, dynamic	Perfection, enlightenment through inner contemplation, universal consciousness
6th	Inspiration, insight	Visualization, implementation of ideas	Clairvoyance	Vision, intuition, soul force	Realization, intuition, inner senses
5th	Expression	Sense of self, taking in and assimilating	Communication	Creative energy, sound	Communication, creative self-expression, independence
4th	Secondary feeling (usually contrary to first feeling)	Love, openness to life, ego will	Love	Life force, group consciousness	Unfolding qualities of heart, love, sharing, selflessness, devotion, compassion, healing
3rd	Opinion	Healing, position in the Universe	Power	Emotion, desire	Unfolding one's personality, assimilating feelings and experience
2nd	Feeling	Pleasure, sexual energy	Sex	Life force, vital energy	Primordial feelings, enthusiasm, sensuality, creativity, awe
1st	Concept, original idea	Physical energy, will to live	Survival	Will energy, universal life	Primordial life energy, stability, power to achieve trust

*Data taken from R.L. Bruyere, *Wheels of Light: A Study of the Chakras,* Vol. 1 (Sierra Madra, CA: Bon Productions, 1989); B.A. Brennan, *Hands of Light: A Guide to Healing through the Human Energy Field* (New York: Bantam Books, 1987); A. Judith, *Wheels of Life: A User's Guide to the Chakra System* (St. Paul, MN: Llewellyn Publications, 1990); A.F. Lansdowne, *The Chakras and Esoteric Healing* (York Beach, ME: Samuel Weiser, 1986); and S. Sharamon and B.J. Baginski, *The Chakra Handbook* (Wilmot, WI: Lotus Light Publications, 1991).

These are considered additional spiritual chakras. A number of authors discuss the seven major chakras and a number of minor ones. Minor chakras include the palm, sole of the foot, the base of the skull, and all joints in the body. In this scheme, there are more than 360 chakras in the human body.[32] The following oral tradition format is generally acceptable, however:

Root chakra: survival and security
Second chakra: sexuality, pleasure, primal creativity, sensuality, what arouses passion
Third chakra: emotions, "feel it in my gut"
Fourth (heart) chakra: love, heart-felt love, self-esteem
Fifth (throat) chakra: expression of the state of the first four chakras; expression of security, creativity, emotions, what stirs love
Sixth chakra: third eye; intuition insight, gestalts of awareness, perception; ability to provide insight into the first four chakras and modify the fifth chakra's expression
Seventh chakra: Gateway to the spiritual realm and to the higher chakras

Chakras can be detected in the same areas as major nerve plexi and with two neuroendocrine glands, the pituitary and pineal. They can be stimulated with specific colors and tones. They have been assigned

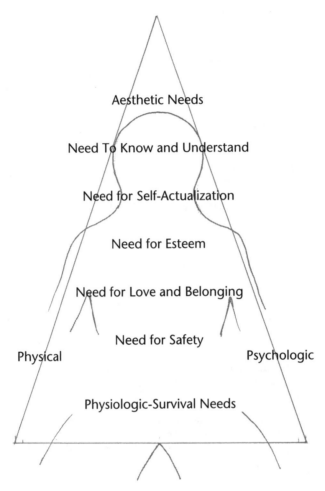

Figure 6-1 Maslow's Hierarchy of Needs. *Source:* Data from A.H. Maslow, *Motivation and Personality,* © 1954, Harper & Bros., and A.H. Maslow, *Psychological Review,* No. 50, pp. 370–396, © 1943.

the colors of the rainbow and the tones of an octave (see Table 6–2). The root chakra is associated with the gonads, is seen as red, and is heard as the note middle C, for example. The following exercise will help individuals become aware of their own chakra energy.

Place one hand lightly over your perineum or coccyx (first or root chakra), and place the thumb of your other hand at your umbilicus. Rest your upper hand lightly on your lower abdomen (second chakra). Just notice whatever you notice. Now, ask the chakra under

your upper hand to close. What do you feel? Then ask it to open. What do you feel? Do this several times. Move your hands so that the thumb of one hand and the little finger of the other are at your umbilicus so one hand is resting on your lower abdomen (second chakra or sacral plexus chakra) and the other on your upper abdomen over your stomach (third chakra or solar plexus chakra). Notice any subtle movement under your hands. Now, ask the chakra beneath your lower hand

Table 6–2 Chakra Locations, Associated Organs and Nervous Structures, and Attributes

Chakra Location	Nervous System Structure	Function	Gland	Color	Tone
7 Crown of head	Pineal gland	Spiritual	Pineal or pituitary	Violet/white	B
6 Brow	Pituitary gland Carotid plexus	Intuition insight	Pituitary or pineal	Indigo (red–blue)	A
5 Throat and shoulders	Pharyngeal plexus	Expression Speak own truth	Thyroid	Blue	G
4 Heart and knees	Carotid plexus	Heart, love	Thymus	Green	F
3 Stomach	Solar plexus	Emotions	Adrenals	Yellow	E
2 Lower abdomen Wrists and ankles	Pelvic plexus	Reproduction, Creativity Passion	Lymphatic tissue	Orange	D
1 Groin Palms and soles	Coccygeal plexus	Survival, Security	Gonads	Red	C

Source: Data from B.A. Brennan, *Hands of Light: A Guide to Healing Through the Human Energy Field,* p. 48, © 1987, Bantam Books, R.L. Bruyere, *Wheels of Light: A Study of the Chakras,* Vol. 1, p. 42, © 1989, Bon Productions, R. Gerber, *Vibrational Medicine: New Choices for Healing Ourselves,* p. 130, © 1988, Bear & Company, A. Judith, *Wheels of Life: A User's Guide to the Chakra System,* p. 23, © 1990, Llewellyn Publications, Z.F. Lansdowne, *The Chakras & Esoteric Healing,* p. 56, © 1978, Samuel Weiser, Inc., A.E. Powell, *The Etheric Double,* p. 56, © 1978, Theosophical Publishing House, C.W. Leadbeater, *The Chakras,* pp. 40–41, © 1927, Theosophical Publishing House.

to close. And open. And close. And open. And quicken. And radiate. And blend with the chakra under your upper hand. What do you feel? Do this several times. When you ask a chakra to close, what physical sensation do you have under your hands, and what happens with the rest of your body? What emotional response do you have? What are your thoughts?

Move your hands to the middle of your chest, right over the sternum, about where you would do closed chest cardiac massage. That is the fourth or heart chakra. Ask it to open and close several times. What happens to your breathing? Are there changes in the tension in your back? Your fifth chakra is at your throat in the area of the Adam's apple and suprasternal notch. It is the smallest of the seven major chakras, about the size of a 50-cent piece. Put your hands over the front of it, and ask it to close and open. What happens? Now put one hand in front and one in back of it, and ask it to open and close. By this time, you may have noticed that each time you ask a chakra to open and close, you feel a slight sensation or change of pressure or temperature under your hands. You may feel a movement like a flower opening.

Your sixth chakra is in the center of your forehead. Place one or both hands lightly over your sixth chakra, also called the third eye. Move your hands so that your fingers are over your third eye; then move your hand so that your palm is over your third eye. Is there a different sensation? Remember, the palms of your hands have chakras, and so do each of the joints in your fingers. Your seventh chakra is at the top, or crown, of your head where your soft spot was. Sense your body and your emotions as you ask it to close and open. What do you experience?

Give yourself a chakra treatment. Place one hand over your first chakra at your perineum or coccyx and the other hand over the second chakra. For 1 minute, visualize that universal energy is flowing through your hands into your chakras as if you were intravenous tubing. Then, move your hands to cover your second and third chakra, above and below the umbilicus. For 1 minute imagine universal energy flowing into these chakras. Do the same for the third and fourth chakras, fourth and fifth, fifth and sixth, sixth and seventh. How do you feel?

Hiroshi Motoyama of Japan recorded the electrical state and changes over chakra areas of control subjects, advanced meditators, and people with histories of psychic experiences.[33] Chakras that the meditators believed were "awakened" showed electrical readings of increased frequency and amplitude compared to chakras of control subjects. Motoyama also found that subjects who could consciously project energy through their chakras displayed significant electrical field disturbances over the activated chakras. When Valerie Hunt, professor of physical therapy at the University of California at Los Angeles (UCLA) placed electromyographic (EMG) electrodes on the skin of chakra areas, she found regular, high-frequency, wavelike electrical signals from 100 to 1600 cycles per second, which is higher than any previously recorded human body frequency.[34] The frequency band of brain waves is between 1 and 100 cycles per second; muscle frequency reaches 225 cycles per second; and the heart frequency is as high as 250 cycles per second.

Physics Metaphors

Like meridians, chakras receive and process data carried on electromagnetic frequencies. Unlike meridians, each chakra perceives and processes only a small range of frequencies, and each alters the data on the frequency before sending it to the next higher chakra. The chakra tree, from root to the highest chakra, refines the data so that the individual, the consciousness who will act on the data, is not overwhelmed by all of the information. The chakra system provides an efficient means of data management.

Individual chakras and the chakra tree have analogs in physics. Chakras act like inductance–capacitance (L–C) circuits. An L–C circuit is constructed to amplify only one frequency from the many it receives. Radios are collections of L–C circuits, each one amplifying only its specific frequency.

While it may be a natural chakra function, Motoyama's finding that advanced meditators could consciously project energy through their chakras suggests that people can deliberately enhance this natural ability and control their own energy. Gerber suggested that the "ability to activate and transmit energy through one's chakras is a reflection of a rather advanced level of consciousness development and concentration by the individual."[35]

Like a Fourier analyzer, the chakra tree acts as if it analyzes the strength and distribution of frequencies in its environment. Chakras also act like transformers, devices that efficiently change voltage and currents. Any change in a primary coil's current will induce a voltage change in the adjacent coil.[36] The energy of the first chakra radiates to the second, inducing a voltage surge. Each chakra stimulates the one above it, changing its power. Chakras act like both step-up and step-down transformers; step-up transformers increase the power in the second coil, and step-down transformers modify the energy so that the lower coil can handle it. Hindu tradition teaches that the soul/spirit enters the body through the crown, or seventh chakra. It steps down through each chakra until it reaches the root chakra, where its energy can be used for life and survival. The root chakra, then, steps up the current so it can be used constructively by each chakra in turn. Chakras are examples of redundant structures. The same form acts like a step-down transformer to bring in and modify universal energy so the body can handle it. It also acts like a step-up transformer to fuel each chakra in its moment-to-moment task. Perhaps the step-down process reflects the spiritual function of chakras; the step-up process, the physical, emotional, and mental functions.

Intuition

For a one-cell organism, all information came in pressure waves of particular frequencies. When the first animal walked out of the primordial swamp, however, it needed more detailed information to cope with its more diverse environment. The bundle of information carried in a pressure wave needed to be separated into its various components so that the animal could perceive and interpret gradations, rather than bursts, of information. What was needed were devices that were able to take in the entire environment, separate the waves into their component parts (a Fourier analyzer function), and analyze and amplify the information within each frequency (L–C circuit function); what was needed were chakras.

The feet and palms, or paws for four-legged animals, act like root chakras. Land-based animals are rooted to the earth, not only through their first chakras, but also through the chakras in their paws. The survival, security function of the root chakra is the first requirement for life, and animals have paw chakras to gather and analyze the pulses coming from the earth. The animal's body may be designed to gather information from the subtle and not so subtle pulsings of the earth beneath it. The trunk and legs contain five ports for each of the first five chakras. A glance at the dog and cat drawings in Figure 6–2 suggests that the legs act as streams collecting data that flow into the larger river of the trunk. The standing animal has paws and metatarsal joints firmly planted to absorb data; the sitting animal is resting on its root. Both are gathering the pulses from within the environment. Very little crucial data is likely to escape detection by such a finely crafted system.

> Take a moment to sense your hand–feet–spine chakras as if you were an animal needing information about your environment. You may want to place your hands and feet on the earth itself. Allow each palm, sole, toe, and finger to come alive to information. Open your

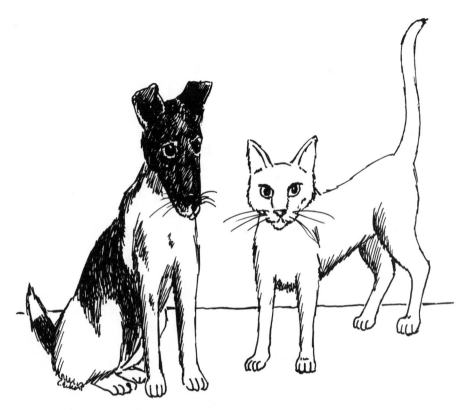

Figure 6-2 Dog Sitting and Cat Standing on Chakras. *Source:* Copyright © 1999, Carol Eckert.

spinal chakras. What do you feel? How do you feel? Is there a barely perceptible flow in your hands and feet that you did not distinguish before? What about your spine? Do you sense your environment as safe and secure, or is there danger present? What are your emotional and mental responses to what you sense?

When *Homo erectus* stood up and took two chakras off the ground, it needed an adjustment to its L–C circuit chain. With only two-fifths of its input sites in constant contact with the ground, it had to use the available information more efficiently and effectively. Like the one-cell organism that evolved to walk on land, it needed to refine the data available. Chakras that could do more than receive, process, and transmit

information were needed; *Homo erectus* needed perception, insight, intuition, and gestalts of awareness, all of which are provided by the sixth chakra in the brow. Over time, *Homo erectus* evolved into *Homo sapiens*, the Wise Human. As it processed more and more data with insight, gestalts of awareness, and intuition, at some point the Wise Human realized that it was more than body, that it had a spiritual nature. It was beginning to awaken the seventh chakra.

Imagine yourself as a newly upright *Homo erectus*. Feel the energy flow stop at the fifth chakra in your throat. How does that feel, and what do you know about your environment? Allow the energy to move into the sixth chakra. What happens? What do you sense differently? How does the sixth chakra receive and process information differently from the ones below it? Sense the information flow into the seventh chakra at the top of your head. What do you experience? Some may get the impression of an entirely different realm of energy, one that is 360 degrees, lighter, softer, flowing up and around you like a fountain of mist or soft air. This energy is different from that of the first five chakras, which is more rugged with a lower frequency and higher amplitude (bigger, slower waves). The energy of the seventh chakra acts more like fine ripples than waves. Tradition calls the seventh chakra the spiritual chakra. What do you intuit?

The imagined evolution of chakras suggests that they have evolved with the species; they also may develop with age. Bruyere stated that each chakra develops at a particular time of life (Table 6–3).[37] Another developmental pattern is suggested by the Fibonacci number sequence, a particular pattern in the growth of plants and other organisms. When a plant begins to put out leaves in the spring, it will put out one leaf. Then one more leaf. Then two leaves and three leaves. Then five leaves. The pattern of 0-1-1-2-3-5-8-13-21-34-55-89... is consistent throughout nature. In addition to plant growth, this sequence is seen in DNA, RNA, and the branching of the dendrites throughout the nervous system.[38] Each number after the first is the sum of the two preceding numbers. If the Fibonacci number sequence is a pattern that nature finds useful, perhaps chakras develop along the same pattern.

If there are 12 chakras, the pattern suggested by the evolution of the species and the Fibonacci number sequence would indicate that *Homo sapiens* is only one stage in the development of the human species. Perhaps the eighth chakra can be expected to mature at age 89, the ninth at age 144, tenth at age 233, and so forth. Of course, if the evolution of the species is tied to the evolution of the chakras, there is no way to know what additional information humans will be able to process or what life will be like with matured eighth and ninth chakras. Perhaps before the advent of Rogers's hypothesized *Homo spatialis,*[39] *Homo sapiens* will evolve into *Homo spiritualis,* representing the dominance of the seventh chakra and the opening of the eighth.

Table 6–3 Theoretical Ages of Chakra Development

Chakra	Chakra Function	Fibonacci Number	Bruyere Teaching*
1, Root, sacrum	Survival	1 (conception ?)	Birth to 3 or 4
2, Pelvic plexus	Reproduction, creativity	1, 2 (first cell division)	4 to 7
3, Solar plexus	Emotion	3, 5 (years?)	8 to 12
4, Heart	Love	8 (years?)	13 to 19
5, Throat	Expression	13 (years?)	19 to 25
6, Brow	Insight	21, 35 (years?)	25 to 35
7, Crown	Spiritual	55 (years?)	35+
8, ?	?	89 (years?)	
9, ?	?	144 (years?)	
10, ?	?	233 (years?)	
11, ?	?	377 (years?)	
12, ?	?	610 (years?)	

*The information in column four is data from R.L. Bruyere's oral teachings.

Not all 35-year-old people are insightful, and not all 55-year-old adults are wise. Some people, it has been said, grow wise and some just grow older. What makes the difference? Transformers and L–C circuits are designed to function optimally, but time, overuse, or abuse will damage the coils and diminish the functional capacity. The structures may still be present, but their functioning is compromised. Chakras, likewise, will still be present, but their functioning may be diminished or damaged. The most basic function of chakras is to receive, process, and transform energy, but they also have been given the more abstract function of processing, transforming, and transmitting data.

Battista's informational processing model may apply to chakras.[40] He identified seven states of consciousness and the level of information they handle:

1. Sensation
2. Sensation + perception about the sensation (e.g., good, bad; pleasant, perilous)
3. Sensation + perception + emotion
4. Awareness: cognition (reflective knowing about levels 2, 3, 5, 6, and 7) and intuition (nonreflective knowing about levels 2, 3, 5, and 6)
5. Self-awareness (knowing the nature of one's own awareness): awareness (level 4) + unition (level 6)
6. Unition (the experience of the process of awareness): self-awareness (level 5) + pure awareness (level 7)
7. Absolute (pure awareness, an integrated awareness of all the levels)

Each level adds more information to the information it receives. According to this model, people experience a sensation and have a perception about it. They add emotion and then become cognitively and intuitively aware of their emotional response to their perception of the sensation (emotion + perception + sensation). At the fourth level, awareness, they have access to the (initially) limited information in levels 5 through 7. As they become self-aware, they are able to know that they are aware, as well as knowing what they are aware of. This is a radical departure from just adding data to data. Battista depicted this fifth stage, which equates with the fifth chakra of insight, as looking in two directions. It processes information coming from the levels both below and above it, as if it were a data manager. Unition, Battista's sixth level, blends information about self-awareness (level 5) and the actual experience of pure awareness (level 7), which is an integration of all the levels of awareness.

Many views of chakra functions list a mental chakra, a function that is not included in the chakra format used here. The ultimate decision about what to do with the data seems to be external to the chakras, as if the individual were the overseer of the responses, rather than the responses being merely instinctual or habitual. This is the individual who decides when it is time to seek a new approach to life and leads to the most appropriate one. This may be the individual's eternal consciousness, the soul/spirit/mind.

Traditions have given the chakras various tasks as shown in Table 6–1 and Maslow's hierarchy of needs triangle (see Figure 6–1). Chakras are more complex than these models suggest. Chakras receive and process information according to preestablished data-processing programs, which are culminations of prior experiences. When a person has the same or a similar experience frequently, a depth or weight of data develops, and chakras process any event containing familiar elements according to the established response for those elements. During a new experience, chakras will seek an established response (a similar form) to deal with the new data. For example, a "stimulus" that has elicited fear, anger, or love in the past will do so again, even if many of the details within the new situation are different. The continuity provided by repeatedly using established responses is efficient and contributes to a person's self-image and identity.

People may repeat the same painful or self-destructive behaviors because they are operating with programs that have not been transformed since they were created, perhaps even in utero. It is important to heal both the physical trauma that chakras may experience and the programs created to process experiences. While any energetic experience will influence chakras physically and has the potential to provide insight into habitual responses, energetic healing at the hands of an expert can do both with relative ease. Early data can lose their grip on perceptions and interpretations of current life events. The deciding factor, however, is not the energetic experience or the expertise of the energetic healer, but the individual's decision to heal.

Energetic healing involves using either subtle or more easily noticed energy, such as sound, to assist a person to uncover his or her established programs and change them. The information management function of an energetic healer is not just to apply energy or, as the ISSSEEM stated, "to facilitate the flow of . . . subtle energies through the dense body."[41] The goal of facilitating the flow of subtle energies is to assist the energetic river to clear out the informational boulders and dams that block the flow, one twig, one byte at a time. As the programs begin to emerge from obscurity and reveal their contents, the person can deliberately modify a childhood or any other response to situations. With fewer obstacles, the energetic and information flow from chakra to chakra can move up the chakra chain from survival and emotional issues, to loving responses, to insight, and to wisdom. The reverse flow can bring additional insight to the existing data of the sensation–perception–emotion pattern. It is as if the higher level chakras tell the lower ones, "Pay more attention, give more weight to the experiences of love, abun-dance, and fulfillment. Pay less attention to experiences that outrage the ego. They're not so important." As Yomata noted, "you can only solve a problem from a higher chakra," for only a higher chakra can give old data the new perspectives and insights that allow healing.[42] Not only must the chakras mature in the species and the individual, but also the statistical programs that process the information must do so.

THE AURA

Tradition and Data

Complementing the meridians and chakras is the aura, traditionally described as a multilayer field of energy surrounding the physical body. Brennan's seven-layer system is a well-known auric description among Western nurses (Table 6–4).[43] It includes the physical, astral, and spiritual planes. The physical plane is composed of three layers: the etheric body, which is closest to the physical body; the emotional body; and the mental body, which is involved with linear thinking. Etheric is "the state between energy and matter."[44] Between the physical and spiritual planes lies the astral plane, which comprises only one body and one function—the astral body that moderates the love of others and humanity. The spiritual plane, like the physical plane, includes three layers: the etheric template, which connects higher will more to divine will; the celestial body, which involves love that extends beyond human love; and the ketheric body, the higher mind, which integrates the spiritual and physical. Brennan described every other layer (1, 3, 5, 7) as highly structured as if they serve as boundaries for the other, more fluid layers. The structured layers appear to be standing waves of scintillating light patterns with tiny electrical charges moving along them. The three fluid layers appear as constantly moving colored fluids. According to Brennan, the aura is not like an onion, with separable layers.

Rather, each layer interpenetrates all the other layers, including the physical body, which is considered the most dense layer. Brennan's seven-layer model also reflects chakra functions, and each auric level is associated with a chakra. Brennan's aura scheme reflects the ancient and holistic awareness of the human body, mind, emo-

Table 6-4 Chakra, Aura, Information, and Dimensions of the Psyche Models*

Chakra Levels and Function	Brennan's Aura Levels	Kunz's Aura Levels	Battista's Information Stages	Assagioli's Dimensions of the Psyche
7: Spiritual	Ketheric body Higher mind, knowing and integration of spiritual and physical makeup		Absolute (pure awareness)	The higher unconscious or superconscious Higher knowings and feelings
6: Intuition, insight	Celestial template Love that encompasses all life	Innate qualities or character potentials	Unition (the experience of the process of awareness)	The conscious or personal self or *I* Individuality and identity
5: Expression	Etheric template Higher will connected with divine will		Self-awareness (knowing the nature of one's own awareness)	The field of consciousness Direct awareness
4: Heart, Love	Astral body lover of other and humanity	Green band	Awareness: cognition (reflective knowing) and intuition (nonreflective knowing)	
3: Emotions	Mental body Linear thinking	Qualities and emotions active in the moment	Emotion: information about the meaning of perception + sensation	The middle unconscious Skills and states of mind
2: Reproduction Creativity Passion	Emotional body	Influences of early experiences and past events	Perception: information about information, the meaning of sensation	The lower unconscious Repressed complexes Long-forgotten memories
1: Survival, Security	Etheric body Automatic and autonomic functioning		Sensation: information level 1	

*Data taken from B.A. Brennan, *Hands of Light: A Guide to Healing through the Human Energy Field* (New York: Bantam Books, 1987); D.v.G. Kunz, *The Personal Aura* (Wheaton, IL: Quest Books, 1991); J.R. Battista, The Holographic Model, Holistic Paradigm, Information Theory and Consciousness, in *The Holographic Paradigm and Other Paradoxes: Exploring the Leading Edge of Science*, ed. K. Wilbur (Boston: Shambhala, 1985); and R. Assagioli, *Psychosynthesis: A Collection of Basic Writings* (New York: Penguin Books, 1965).

tion, and spiritual natures, with the body, mind, and emotions reflected in both physical and spiritual planes.

Kunz defined the aura as dense light and as "the personal emotional field."[45] She described it as a 12- to 18-inch multicolored elastic oval light interpenetrating and surrounding the physical body. Two colorful hemispheres are linked by a green band encircling the middle of the physical body (Table 6–4). The upper hemisphere embodies "the innate qualities or character of a person: one's potential, which may or may not be fully realized in life. In one way these colors represent what a person essentially is, or can be."[46] It is more stable than the lower band, but does change over a lifetime. The lower hemisphere reflects past experience and action, and is influenced by one's emotions. The auric colors from the waist to the knees reflect the person's usual emotions, and colors below the knees to beneath the feet carry memories of his or her past experiences. The green band encircling the middle of the physical body begins to appear in children. "It indicates our ability to put our ideas, feelings and interests into action, or, to state it differently, to actualize our potentialities."[47] The width and intensity of the band reflects the person's level of maturity and ability to express himself or herself intellectually, artistically, and physically. The width relates to one's capacity and the color to one's work. For example, Kunz saw yellow-green bands in people engaged in intellectual activities, blue-green in artists, and darker green bands in physical laborers. She added that chakras are an integral part of the anatomy of the aura.

When Benor studied multiple healers making simultaneous intuitive diagnoses of the same person, Benor and the healers were surprised that the differences in impressions far exceeded the similarities.[48] According to Benor, each healer "had the impression that he or she was perceiving THE true picture of each patient's condition, rather than one

out of many possible pictures of this reality."[49] The patients found most of the healers' information relevant and helpful, even though substantially different. Benor proposed that intuitive diagnosticians obtain their impressions through a "window of observation" and that individual healers may have "blind spots." He recommended that intuitive diagnoses and healing treatments given by multiple healers may be more useful than those given by one healer only.

Just as Benor's healers saw different truths in the same aura, perhaps Brennan and Kunz have each seen different accurate auric structures and colors. Brennan's seven-layer model contains two planes, the physical and spiritual, bridged by the astral plane. Kunz's model identifies an upper hemisphere of potential linked by a green band to the lower hemisphere of the present moment. (See Table 6–4.) Both believe that chakras are integral to the aura. Bruyere perceived the heart chakra as green, suggesting that Kunz's green band and Brennan's astral body may be the same phenomenon seen through different eyes. Both Brennan and Kunz described the astral plane and green band as if it were acting like a transformer.

Physics Metaphors

Brennan's description of the aura as layers of magnetic density that surround a physical body and diminish in intensity as one moves further away from the body resembles physics descriptions of an electromagnetic field (Figure 6–3). An electromagnetic field results any time electrical charges change locations, such as in the flow of electrons in the meridians, neurons, blood, and lymphatic fluid. Many electromagnets have iron cores; red blood cells contain hemoglobin, or iron. Furthermore, every atom involves moving electric charges (electrons) that create a magnetic field. Collections of atoms in cells and or-

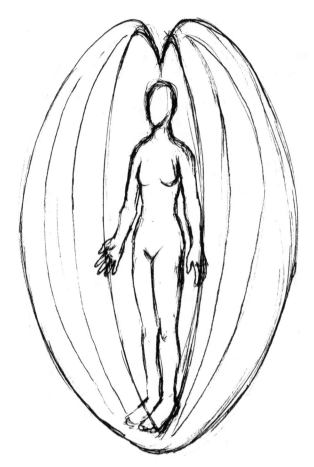

Figure 6–3 The Electromagnetic Human. *Source:* Copyright © 1999, Carol Eckert.

gans produce magnetic fields that can be used to image body structures. Thus, the human body has all the requirements of an electromagnet: an iron core and moving electrical charges that produce magnetic fields. Human magnetic fields can be calculated, such as the heart's field measured with a magnetocardiogram and the head's weak magnetic field assessed with a magnetoencephalogram. Nuclear magnetic resonance (NMR) produces pictures of the body at the cellular level.[50]

Electromagnetic fields decrease in density in continuous fashion from the core out, varying in strength with the square of the distance from the source. The electromagnetic field layer closest to the core is the most dense, the next one is one-fourth as dense, the third one is one-ninth as dense. Field strength decreases rapidly at first, but never reaches zero; hence, physicists say that a field becomes undetectable, but not that it disappears.

Take a moment to sense your own electromagnetic field. Begin by stirring up the electrons in your hands. Rub your hands vigorously until you feel heat. Separate your hands slightly, and notice the amount of pressure, heat, or other sensations between them. Slowly, move your hands further apart. Do you feel changes in the density, heat, or sensations as your hands separate? Change directions, and move your hands closer to each other. Do you sense any changes in pressure, density, temperature, tingling, movement, or anything else? Move your hands in and out several times, varying the speed and distance. Sometimes, it is easier to feel other people's electromagnetic field levels than your own, so try this exercise by sensing the electromagnetic layers surrounding several people. Notice the differences in the fields of an athletic person versus a sedentary one, a man and a woman, a child and an adult. Sense your pet's field. Sense your own field again. What have you discovered about the electromagnetic nature of your family, friends, pets, and yourself?

Intuition

A person's electromagnetic field, including a strong heart magnetic field, may have the electrical and magnetic potentials to influence another's energetic field. Each heart beat begins with an electrical pulse that flows through the heart muscle. Like all moving electrical fields, the beating heart produces a strong magnetic pulse that spreads out in front and behind the body and can be detected up to 15 feet away.[51] The electrical pulse that begins each beat is responsible for the heart's rhythm and variation. Its variability is due to the interaction between the sympathetic nervous system, which causes the heart rate to increase, and the parasympathetic system, which causes the heart rate to decrease. The autonomic nervous system, which responds to a person's mental and emotional responses of the moment, further modulates the heart rate.

Studies by the Institute of HeartMath have shown that, when subjects were asked to shift their attention to their heart intentionally and feel specific emotions or think specific thoughts, their heart rate variability changed.[52] When they were asked to feel frustration, there was a great deal of variability; when they were asked to feel appreciation, heart rate variability decreased. It decreased even more when they were asked to feel love. The reduction of heart rate variability to near zero (i.e., the heart firing at regular intervals), along with a decrease of random thoughts and feelings, is defined as internal coherence. The subjects in these studies had practiced a centering technique for 6 to 36 months and were able to increase internal coherence by increasing their degree of mental and emotional self-management. "It appears that when a person is in a state of deep peace and inner harmony the heart shifts to a very regular and coherent rhythm."[53] Pathologic heart conditions, however, do not respond to this level of conscious control.

Energetic healers are taught to center, to enter a heart-centered state of awareness before providing energetic healing. As the HeartMath data illustrate, the act of centering leads to a state of deep peace, inner harmony, and a coherent heart rate. Thus, the healer's heart emits a coherent magnetic pulse that may influence the electromagnetic field of a client, just as one magnet influences another. The energetic healer's centered state and coherent heart rate also may assist the client's heart to adopt a similar coherent heart rate, contributing to the deep peace and inner harmony that is common among clients during energetic healing treatments. An expert healer will be able to maintain a more deeply centered state longer and more consistently than will a novice.

Healers also identify a healing intention, often that a treatment will be for the highest good of the client, with harm to none, and aligned with Divine will. Gough and Shacklett defined intention as focused choice and listed four physiologic consequences of intention: "intensity of feelings, heart-felt motivation, lowered heart rate variability, and brain hemisphere synchronization."[54] Brain waves have been measured in a variety of situations. Practicing meditators routinely increase their alpha during meditation healing sessions with the client present, and long-distance healing sessions without the client's presence were accompanied by high-frequency high-amplitude beta and gamma rhythms and low-amplitude theta rhythms. Of greater interest than the actual rhythm were the findings that the within-healer alpha, beta, theta, and gamma rhythm synchrony was higher and less variable than the client's in all conditions and that there was synchrony between the electroencephalogram (EEG) patterns of client and healer even when they were not together.[55] In one study, two subjects casually interacted and then separated. When one was shown a flashing light, EEG patterns in the subject who was not stimulated by the flashing light changed synchronously with the one who was.[56] Other studies have shown similar synchrony between people, such as an EEG synchronicity between psychoanalyst and patient in proportion to the amount of empathy between them. Intention may add to the effect of an energetic healing treatment by increasing the intensity of heart-felt caring, the sense of peace due to decreased heart rate variability, and increased brain wave synchronicity between client and healer. Synchrony between the weak magnetic fields of a healer's head and a client's head may account for the common experience of each person seeing the same scene during a treatment or having the same gestalt at the same time.

Electroencephalograms of energetic healers have shown high-amplitude alpha, beta, and gamma rhythms during relaxation and meditation. Theta EEG activity is electrical energy between 4 and 8 cycles per second; alpha activity occurs between 8 and 13 cycles per second. While a great deal of effort has gone into studying the brain wave patterns of meditators, energetic healers, and others, no one knows precisely what alpha or theta mean, just that they are present during meditative, healing, and other contemplative states.[57]

In the 1980s, Zimmerman studied the magnetic fields of therapeutic touch practitioners' hands with the superconducting quantum interferometric (interference) device (SQUID).[58] Superconductors are materials that conduct electric current perfectly; that is, they offer no resistance to the electrical flow. Superconductors may one day be used in supersensitive electronic devices, powerful miniature motors, and other very tiny electrical and mechanical devices. Researchers have already used the SQUID to detect some of the weakest human biomagnetic fields, such as in the brain. During Zimmerman's study of therapeutic touch practitioners, the client and practitioner were in a magnetically shielded chamber. To get a baseline reading, the practitioner first touched the client before entering a centered-intention state. Immediately upon centering, the SQUID detected a huge biomagnetic field emerging from her hand. The field was so strong that the equipment had to be readjusted in order to record the response. The therapeutic touch signal pulsed from 0.3 to 30 cycles per second, mostly in the 7 to 8 cycles per second range, meaning that the biomagnetic field coming from the healer's hands swept or scanned through a range of electromagnetic frequencies concentrating in the theta to alpha range. Zimmerman was unable to detect such pulses from nonhealers.

Similar results have been found with practitioners of a variety of energetic healing modalities, martial arts, yoga, meditation, and others. Their overall fields measured 10^{-3} gauss (the unit of measurement of magnetic fields), which is 1,000 times stronger than that of the heart (10^{-6} gauss), which is the strongest human biomagnetic field, and 1,000,000 times stronger than that produced by the brain. Medical science uses the same extra low frequencies (ELF) produced by energetic healers to accelerate healing of bones and wounds. These ELF magnetic fields that energetic healers' hands emit may account for research results showing that energetic healing accelerates the rate of wound healing in mice and humans.[59,60]

The human body readily conducts electricity. The main flow is through the circulatory system, which is filled with a saline plasma solution. Muscles conduct electricity, especially along their longitudinal axis, such as the long muscles in the arms. The body also produces heat, and Qi Gong masters have been shown to project and absorb measurable infrared energy, or heat, from their hands. Like the heart rate, skin temperature is under the control of the autonomic nervous system,[61] the system shown in the HeartMath studies to be responsible for lowering heart rate variability. It appears that the human body is designed to conduct, produce, absorb, and emit electromagnetic energy and that practice enables one to do so in a manner that not only alters one's own heart rate, skin temperature, and brain waves, but also can influence brain waves in others.

A centered and intended state may be a type of self-referencing biofeedback, as described by Green and Green.[62] Self-referencing biofeedback does not involve machines to provide feedback for biologic control, but uses the self as the reference. Healers learn to use their own internal clues, such as heart rate, sense of peace, and inner calm, to enter a deeper meditative theta brain wave state that is associated with brain wave synchronization. Centering with intention may be a self-referencing biofeedback state.

TWO QUANTUM THEORIES

Two quantum theories, holography and consciousness-created reality, offer tentative assistance in determining the role of energetic healing in helping people extract the data packages that they laid down in childhood and eliminate perceptions now interfering with their lives. Holographic theory is a theory of how information may be stored, and consciousness-created reality is the theory that purports that consciousness is the force that selects which potentiality (what information) will become an actuality.

Holographic Theory

Herbert described the holographic quantum theory of the universe as a universe of undivided wholeness, "a seamless and inseparable whole."[63] Holograms are ways of storing information in a network of interference patterns or the interaction of energy waves of various frequencies (e.g., light waves). The holographic characteristics useful for a discussion of data storage within an energy field come from the discovery that 10 billion bits of information have been stored holographically in a cubic centimeter. A similar amount of data stored by conventional means would fill a shoe box. Holography stores data by distributing it over the entire surface of a photographic film in diffuse patterns of light and particles. Like ripples on a pond after several rocks are thrown into it, the ripples of light interfere with each other. According to Pribram,[64] those ripples contain surprising order hidden within them. When needed, data contained within those ripples can be extracted by coherent light of the right wave length.

All data received by the human body—including that carried on light, sound, taste, smell, touch, and pressure waves—is transferred into an electrical signal that is sent to the brain for interpretation. Data from intuitions and insights may be included. If such data were stored holographically, then the experiences of a lifetime could be stored within the human body and field. Energetic healers and recipients seem to experience such holographic images when, suddenly, an entire picture of a client's past may appear in either or both the healer's and recipient's minds. The event, the place, emotions, and thoughts of the person at that time are revealed. The recipient can be asked to step back from the situation to see the larger picture, which provides additional insight and allows modification of the data pattern.

Information that emerges during an energetic healing session often arrives in a whole package of sensation–perception–emotion that the client and energetic healer can dissect into its components. Once perception and emotion are separated from the situation and from each other, a client can learn more about her or his own history and process it through more mature eyes and chakras. One result is greater insight into that history. For example, the knee jerk reaction of a childhood program is mitigated and the automatic response replaced by cognitive/intuitive awareness and insights. The client now has the ability to choose a response, rather than react automatically, and heal the wounds of the past.

If data are stored holographically in the human energy field, the physical body may be a storage medium as well. Snippets of data may be revealed during a lymphatic drainage massage in which the skin is gently moved to stimulate the lymphatic channels, suggesting that data may be stored holographically in the lymph and blood in the same manner that information is stored in homeopathic solutions. Because meridians reach through the cytoplasm to the cell's nucleus, all of one's physical, emotional, mental, and spiritual experiences may be stored within the cell's cytoplasm and nucleus. As the sperm merges with the egg during conception, each brings the record of the parent's experiences down through the ages. This may explain the collective unconscious, tribal memories, and past life memories. If one's consciousness is eternal and experiences more than one physical lifetime, those memories may be holographically stored in the pattern of the information that reincarnates life after life.

Holographic storage of data may explain why some data are revealed in snippets and some in gestalts. Clients who have been sexually abused tend to reveal data in snippets, for example. Sexual abuse begins physically, and the experience may be stored in tissues. Other types of energetic abuse, such as hatred, anger, witnessing abuse, and other less directly physical situations, may be stored primarily in the hologram of the energy field, rather than body tissues. More distantly experienced data may be able to be revealed in a gestalt, while physical assaults are remembered in bits and bytes.

As noted earlier, holographic images are revealed when coherent light of the right frequency shines on the hologram. The system is incoherent when each quantum particle interacts with other particles separately by colliding and exchanging energy in various ways. Coherence occurs when individual particles begin to work together, as if in a ballet, and an electromagnetic field arising from the same dance keeps them in phase.[65] Because each particle moves with the others, very strong forces are generated. The ELF pulses that a healer's hands emit when she or he is centered with intention may be the right coherent frequency to elicit a client's data stored holographically within lymph, blood, cells, tissues, and the energy field.

Consciousness-Created Reality

Quantum theory is concerned with the particles and their activity that are at and below the level of the atom. Relative to the size of the bodies involved, the distance between the nucleus of an atom and its electrons is even greater than the distance between the moon and the earth. Between atoms and between the nucleus of an atom and its electrons is an immense space filled with electromagnetic energy.

> Imagine that you are constructed of many atoms. How much space exists in you? There isn't much that is solid in the atoms that make up molecules, cells, organs, and you. Sense the space that you

are and sense the power that fills that space. Now sense you. Are you just your body, or are you more? Take a moment to consider the more that you are.

The matter that quantum physics deals with is the minuscule particles moving within quantum space. As they move, they create waves, like a motor boat on a river. Those waves are called radiation, electromagnetic waves, or light. The tangible world that people sense emerges, somehow, from those waves of visible and invisible light. How? One theory is that all possibilities reside within those quantum waves (which really have no substance, they are inferred, mathematical, and called a quantum wave function). Perhaps all possibilities are stored holographically in quantum waves; perhaps not. When something measures (a physics word) or observes the quantum activity, some actuality "collapses" out of all possibilities. One quantum theory is that the act of observing the quantum potentialities is what forces the actual to appear. But what does the observing? The theory of consciousness-created reality suggests that the observer is consciousness,[66] perhaps yours, mine, and the Divine's.

As people sense something, they add perception and then emotion to it. The act of adding perception and emotion changes the sensation. No other person has exactly the same perceptual and emotional response to the same sensation. As data move up the chakras, more information based on past experience refines the original data. Everyone will interpret an event differently; some will sense the event as loving, others as neutral or threatening. In that light, each person creates his or her own reality.

If the theories of consciousness-created reality and Battista's informational theory are correct, then what type of consciousness has the potential to grow from merely sensing to awareness to insights to spiri-

tual reflection? Assagioli's seven dimensions of the psyche offer a useful model.[67] As can be seen in Table 6–4, he portrays the psyche as containing three levels of the unconscious and two *I*s. The three levels of the unconscious—the lower, middle, and higher—contain the past, present, and future. Like Kunz's aura model, the lowest level, the lower unconscious, contains fundamental drives, emotionally charged complexes, phobias, delusions, and the elementary psychologic activities that enable the organism to survive. The middle unconscious is like the waking consciousness, the place where experiences are assimilated and gestate before the person becomes aware of them. The higher unconscious or superconscious is the realm of higher intuitions, inspirations, and feelings. It is much like Kunz's upper hemisphere and Maslow's seventh level of aesthetic needs (see Figure 6–1). The two selves are the conscious self, the "I" that is the center of consciousness, and the higher, or transpersonal self. The conscious self is directly aware of the sensations, images, thoughts, feelings within the field of consciousness of direct awareness, which may contain data that the meridians and chakras process. Assagioli added two layers of consciousness that are not shown on Table 6–4 and that have no corresponding structure in Kunz's, Brennan's, or Battista's models. He proposed a Transpersonal Self that sees the data more globally and the collective unconscious, which is the sea of unconscious in which our psyches are bathed. We are separated from and united with collective unconsciousness by a semipermeable consciousness boundary. His depiction of the three levels of the unconscious surrounded by a semipermeable membrane resembles Kunz's and Brennan's portrayals of the aura. The Field of Consciousness and the Conscious self and Transpersonal Self remind one of the chakras' information-processing function and the You who interprets with insight all data and experiences.

The quantum theory of consciousness-created reality holds that consciousness is the observer that selects one actuality from the quantum collective of all possibilities. Assagioli's dimensions of the psyche suggest that the conscious self, "I," may prioritize the various sensations and perceptions gestating within the pre-waking middle unconscious. It may be the consciousness that, based on preestablished programs, selects the possibility that will become actual. The conscious self may not be able to separate the emotions and perceptions given to sensations until the sensation–perception–emotion package reaches the higher chakras and, in time, the higher self with their wider viewpoints. The higher self is the consciousness that is present when a person is asleep, unconscious, or in meditation and contemplation. It may be the aspect of consciousness that is instrumental in healing the primitive sensation–perception–emotion programs by enabling a return to the sensation–perception–emotion packages of childhood. This self returns the original material with its new insights to the conscious self and to the field of consciousness to be examined and restructured.

USE OF OTHER FORMS OF ENERGY

Any form of energy has the potential to elicit information from that stored within a person's field. All of the senses receive data. In fact, it appears that nature designed the senses to receive data from a wide variety of media. Eyes receive electromagnetic light, which moves in a shearing, back-and-forth motion. Ears process data carried on sound waves that move in a pulsing, forward motion. The tongue and structures of the nose interpret taste and smell. Touch, from a quantum perspective, is an electromagnetic interaction. People can use their senses deliberately to create any energetic state they desire, such as a calm environment, an anxiety state, or a memory-filled experience.

In addition to the laying-on-of-hands approach to energetic healing of meridian, chakra, and auras, the senses offer other physics-based approaches to healing. Aromatherapy uses scents with and without massages to calm, excite, heal wounds, clear lungs, and loosen tight chests, among other goals. The body responds to the frequencies of odors in fairly predictable ways; the mind and emotion responses are more personal. One may remember a long-forgotten person or event when smelling an aroma associated with an earlier time. Sound and music therapies use both the pressure of the sound waves and musical tones to calm, excite, or stimulate people in comas, and to assist the dying. Sound at a soccer game or rock concert can stimulate root chakras; perhaps one reason for violence during and after games and concerts is that the energy stimulated in the root chakra is not dissipated. Symphonies are written to stimulate the root chakra and then resolve the energy through each of the chakras. Another sound energy experience is to listen to a tape of Himalayan bells. As the pressure of the bells' sounds stimulates their chakras, people notice physical and emotional responses. The effects of colors on mood is widely recognized and used by such diverse organizations as hospital emergency departments and prisons to calm the waiting patients or prisoners. Each of the senses can be stimulated energetically. Thus, any stimulus that involves application of energy can become a means of energetic healing.

CONCLUSION

All of the models presented indicate that as individuals, people evolve from primitive animal-like functioning to a higher spiritual nature. Several models of chakras and the aura describe slightly different anatomies of the energetic field, but they are similar in visualizing movement from the most basic survival to a higher spiritual development. Energetic healing techniques can mend chakras and help mobilize information, such as Joy's chakra connection and therapeutic touch.[68,69] Meridians, chakras, and the aura can be differentiated by function and form, but cannot be separated. It is impossible to do an aura technique without working with chakras and meridians, to do chakra techniques without influencing the aura and meridians, or to work with meridians without affecting the aura and chakras. Each is integral to the others. Therapeutic touch and Reiki are probably among the best examples of techniques that work with the entire field, without concern for the particular structure. Other techniques, such as Mentgen's pyramid technique,[70] concentrate on the chakras, but assist the aura and meridians to process and reveal the data held within the holographic energy field. The goal of energetic healing is to assist individuals to heal their energetic structures and help reveal the information carried within. The individual, ultimately, must choose how to handle what is revealed.

Energetic healing is more than a technique or a deliberate exposure to overt or subtle energy; it is the art of helping oneself or someone else extract and heal personal history and its legacy. The key to energetic healing is the intention, not the source of the energy, subtle or otherwise. The key to energetic healing is consciousness and a deliberate intention coupled with the action and technique. The goal of holistic nursing and energetic healing is the same: an integration of body, mind, emotion, and spirit, which can only lead to healing, peace, love, and joy within the self. As people change, so must the energy that they emit, and it will change their world.

Ultimately, the person each of us needs to heal the most is ourselves. Both novice and expert healer usually can take most clients only as far as the healer has gone in her or his own healing. A few people are on such an active healing path that they use the skills of even the most novice healer

optimally; an expert healer can assist more clients more rapidly. Most people who begin working as energetic healers soon realize that, if they do not do their own healing work, the energy they are working with will make them. They will either move deliberately into counseling, meditating, journaling, and receiving healing treatments regularly, for example, or they will go into crisis and be forced to do so.

The holistic philosophy recognizes that the body, mind, emotions, and spirit are not separate aspects of a person, as if they were cubicles in an office. A more accurate image is a carnival of mirrors in which each mirror reflects a different image. The essential person stands within the center of a circle of mirrors. One mirror is the physical reflection, another is the emotional reflection, a third is the mental, and the last is the spiritual. Each reflects part of the same truth of who the person is. In a holistic understanding, the essential spirit/soul/consciousness who is seeking to understand more of itself uses the physical, emotional, mental, and spiritual mirrors to experience and gather information. Sometimes it seems to misunderstand and creates responses that become painful, hurting, grief-filled, fearful, and/or angry and more. Healing is the act of looking at the mirrors and piece by piece reconstructing the past to understand the present and change the future. The wise energetic healer will deliberately begin a conscious healing journey.

Take a moment to assess your journey. Is it deliberate? If so, what means do you use to help you extract and heal your own data, resolve your hurts and pains and the things that separate you from yourself and others? If your journey is not deliberate, review what has happened to you since your first encounter with energetic healing and holistic nursing. What, if anything, has changed?

What would you like to change and to heal?

Look through the *AHNA Holistic Nursing: A Handbook for Practice* or another source and select one modality that you have not used before. Consciously use it every day for 1 month. After you decide what to use, establish your healing intention: the intensity of feeling and heart-felt motivation that synchronizes your brain waves and lowers your heart rate variability. Write down your goal for this modality. What is your state now that you want this modality to change? In 30 days, review your goal and your state. What is today's date? On what date will you review your progress? Put it in your calendar.

Understanding how meridians, chakras, the aura, and the senses bring you data and process it can be interesting, but it is useless if you do not use it for your personal benefit. If meridians gather data and act as a part of your defense system, what data are yours giving you? Close your eyes and sense your environment. Go into another room and do the same. When you are with your family, do the same. When you are with friends or at work, do the same. What have you learned about your response to your family, friends, home, and work environments that you need to change? How will you approach that aspect of your healing journey?

Remember one thing that makes you angry, fearful, hurt, or any other painful emotion. When was the last time you experienced this emotion? What was the situation? Analyze your perception. Now that you have looked at it again, notice what age you felt like during the interaction. Remember that time in your life. Are you responding now with the same response you used then? What healing modality can you use to move this painful emotion toward healing and joy? When do you intend to start?

DIRECTIONS FOR FUTURE RESEARCH

Professional

1. Examine the life changes that occur after individuals receive any type of energetic modality, including subtle energies, sensory energy, or any other energetic intervention.
2. Determine whether meridians participate in the immune function and if meridian techniques are followed by psychoneuroimmunologic responses.
3. Investigate the possibility that meridian techniques consistently relieve pathologic conditions such as hypertension, multiple sclerosis, and stress-related conditions.
4. Explore whether routine chakra/meridian techniques retard symptoms of diseases of the perineural cells, such as multiple sclerosis.
5. Determine how chakra techniques influence recovery from addictions.
6. Study the effect of energetic interventions on the process and results of counseling.
7. Examine the emotional responses that occur and the information that emerges when someone is exposed to the pressure waves of sound.

Personal

1. Study the short-term effects of each energetic modality you use (1) when you engage it with an intention and (2) when you passively receive it.

2. Determine when it is best for you to be active and when you should passively receive an energetic healing modality.

3. Study the long-term effects of your energetic healing journey.

NURSE HEALER REFLECTIONS

After reading this chapter, the nurse healer will be able to answer or begin a process of answering the following questions:

- How do my meridians contribute to my awareness?

- How do my chakras participate in processing information in my life?

- What data about me do I want to interpret differently?

- When I feel anger (other emotion), what other emotions are present? What situation elicits them? What perception do I have about the situation that calls for those emotions? Is my response rational, or does it come from a latent internal program?

- Which energetic modalities best help me extract my own information?

- What does my healing journey look like? How could I improve it?

NOTES

1. W.C. Gough and R.L Shacklett, The Science of Connectiveness, Part III: The Human Experience, *Subtle Energies* 4, no. 3 (1993): 187–214.

2. International Society for the Study of Subtle Energies and Energy Medicine, Founding Statement, 6th Annual ISSSEEM Conference Proceedings, 1997, p. 2.

3. E.E. Green, Mind over Matter: Volition and the Cosmic Connection in Yogic Theory, *Subtle Energies* 4, no. 2 (1993): 152.

4. L. Dossey, Healing, Energy, and Consciousness: Into the Future or a Retreat to the Past? *Subtle Energies* 5, no. 1 (1994): 1–33.

5. J. White, Consciousness and Substance: The Primal Forms of God, *Journal of Near Death Studies* 5, no. 2 (1987): 73–78.

6. White, Consciousness and Substance, 75.

7. P. Benner, *From Novice to Expert* (Menlo Park, CA: Addison-Wesley, 1984).

8. V.E. Slater, Safety, Elements, and Effects of Healing Touch on Chronic Non-Malignant Abdominal Pain (Unpublished doctoral dissertation, University of Tennessee, Knoxville, 1996).

9. C.W. Leadbeater, *The Chakras* (Wheaton, IL: Quest Books, 1927).

10. R. Becker and G. Selden, *The Body Electric: Electromagnetism and the Foundation of Life* (New York: William Morrow/Quill, 1985).

11. V.E. Slater, Toward an Understanding of Energetic Healing, Part I: Energetic Structures, *Journal of Holistic Nursing* 20, no. 10 (1995): 209–224.

12. A. Weil, *Health and Healing* (Boston: Houghton Mifflin, 1983).

13. R. Gerber, *Vibrational Medicine: New Choices for Healing Ourselves* (Santa Fe, NM: Bear & Company, 1988), 122–127.

14. S. Rose-Neil, The Work of Professor Kim Bong Han, *The Acupuncturist* 1 (1987): 15.

15. P. De Vernejoul et al., Étude des Meridiens D'Acupuncture par les Traceurs Radioactifs, *Bulletin de L'Academie Nationale Medecine* 169 (1985): 1071–1075.

16. Becker and Selden, *The Body Electric*, 236–239.

17. Rose-Neil, The Work of Professor Kim Bong Han, 15.

18. Becker and Selden, *The Body Electric*, 142, 234.

19. Gerber, *Vibrational Medicine*, 124.

20. C.B. Pert, *Molecules of Emotion: Why You Feel the Way You Feel* (New York: Charles Scribner's Sons, 1997).

21. Gerber, *Vibrational Medicine*, 127.

22. M. Burmeister, *Jin Shin Jyutsu Is* (Scottsdale, AZ: Jin Shin Jyutsu, 1985).

23. R.L. Bruyere, *Wheels of Light: A Study of the Chakras*, Vol. 1 (Sierra Madra, CA: Bon Productions, 1989).

24. B.A. Brennan, *Hands of Light: A Guide to Healing through the Human Energy Field* (New York: Bantam Books, 1987).

25. A. Judith, *Wheels of Life: A User's Guide to the Chakra System* (St. Paul, MN: Llewellyn Publications, 1990).

26. Z.F. Lansdowne, *The Chakras and Esoteric Healing* (York Beach, ME: Samuel Weiser, 1986).

27. S. Sharamon and B.J. Baginski, *The Chakra-Handbook* (Wilmot, WI: Lotus Light Publications, 1991).

28. A.H. Maslow, *Motivation and Personality* (New York: Harper, 1954).

29. Gerber, *Vibrational Medicine*.

30. B. Joy, *Joy's Way* (Los Angeles: J.P. Tarcher, 1987).

31. T. Gimbel, *Form, Sound, Colour and Healing* (Essex, UK: Daniel Company, 1987), 65.

32. Gerber, *Vibrational Medicine*.

33. Gerber, *Vibrational Medicine*, 128–130.

34. Electronic Evidence of Auras, Chakras in UCLA Study, *Brain/Mind Bulletin* 3, no. 9 (1978).

35. Gerber, *Vibrational Medicine*, 132.

36. I.M. Freeman, *Physics Made Simple* (New York: Doubleday, 1990), 164.

37. R.L. Bruyere, oral teachings.

38. E.S. Wilson, The Transits of Consciousness, *Subtle Energies* 4, no. 2 (1993): 177.

39. V.M. Malinski, The Rogerian Science of Unitary Human Beings as a Knowledge Base for Nursing in Space, in *Visions of Rogers' Science-Based Nursing*, ed. E.A.M. Barrett (New York: National League for Nursing, 1990), 375–386.

40. J.R. Battista, The Holographic Model, Holistic Paradigm, Information Theory and Consciousness, in *The Holographic Paradigm and Other Paradoxes: Exploring the Leading Edge of Science*, ed. K. Wilber (Boston: Shambhala, 1985), 143–150.

41. International Society for the Study of Subtle Energies and Energy Medicine, p. 2.

42. H. Yomata, oral teachings.

43. B.A. Brennan, *Hands of Light*.

44. Brennan, *Hands of Light*, 49.

45. D.v.G. Kunz, *The Personal Aura* (Wheaton, IL: Quest Books, 1991), 11.

46. Kunz, *The Personal Aura*, 39.

47. Kunz, *The Personal Aura*.

48. D.J. Benor, Intuitive Diagnosis, *Subtle Energies* 3, no. 2 (1992): 41–64.

49. Benor, Intuitive Diagnosis, 49.

50. F.A. Wolf, *The Body Quantum: The New Physics of Body, Mind, and Health* (New York: Macmillan, 1986).

51. J.L. Oschman, What Is "Healing Energy"? Part 2: Measuring the Fields of Life, *Journal of Bodywork and Movement Therapies* 1, no. 2 (1997): 117–122.

52. R. McCraty et al., New Electrophysiological Correlates Associated with Intentional Heart Focus, *Subtle Energies* 4, no. 3 (1993): 251–268.

53. McCraty et al., New Electrophysiological Correlates, 262.

54. Gough and Shacklett, The Science of Connectiveness, Part III: The Human Experience, 198.

55. S.L. Fahrion et al., EEG Amplitude, Brain Mapping, and Synchrony in and between a Bioenergy Practitioner and Client during Healing, *Subtle Energies* 3, no. 1 (1992): 19–52.

56. J. Grinberg-Zylberbaum et al., Human Communication and the Electrophysiological Activity of the Brain, *Subtle Energies* 3, no. 3 (1992): 25–43.

57. M.A. Tansey, Boundary Conditions: The Surrounds of a State of Mind, *Subtle Energies* 5, no. 2 (1994): 180–194.

58. J. Zimmerman, Laying-on-of-Hands Healing and Therapeutic Touch: A Testable Theory, *BEMI Currents: Journal of the Bio-Electro-Magnetics Institute* 2 (1990): 8–17.

59. D.J. Benor, Survey of Spiritual Healing Research, *Contemporary Medical Research* 4, no. 3 (1990): 9–32.

60. D. Radin, Beyond Belief: Exploring Interactions among Mind, Body and Environment, *Subtle Energies* 2, no. 3 (1991): 1–42.

61. J.L. Oschman, What Is "Healing Energy"? Part 2B: Polarity, Therapeutic Touch, Magnet Therapy and Related Methods, *Journal of Bodywork and Movement Therapies* 1, no. 2 (1997): 123–128.

62. E. Green and A Green, *Beyond Biofeedback* (Ft. Wayne, IN: Knoll, 1977).

63. N. Herbert, *Quantum Reality—Beyond the New Physics: An Excursion into Metaphysics and the Meaning of Reality* (New York: Doubleday, 1985), 18.

64. K.H. Pribram. What the Fuss Is All About, in *The Holographic Paradigm and Other Paradoxes: Exploring the Leading Edge of Science*, ed. K. Wilber (Boston: Shambhala, 1985), 27–43.

65. T.M. Srinivasan, Coherence and Pattern: Scientific and Aesthetic, *Subtle Energies* 3, no. 3 (1992), i–v.

66. Herbert, *Quantum Reality*.

67. R. Assagioli, *Psychosynthesis: A Collection of Basic Writings* (New York: Penguin, 1965).

68. Joy, *Joy's Way*.

69. D. Krieger, *The Therapeutic Touch: How To Use Your Hands To Help or To Heal* (New York: Prentice Hall, 1979).

70. D. Hover-Kramer, *Healing Touch: A Resource for Health Care Professionals* (New York: Delmar Publishers, 1996), 135–136.

CORE VALUE II

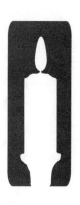

Holistic Ethics, Theories, and Research

VISION OF HEALING

Ethics in Our Changing World

Albert Einstein believed that the most important human endeavor is striving for morality in our actions. Our inner balance and even our very existence depend on it. Only morality in our actions can give beauty and dignity to life. Ralph Waldo Emerson relayed a similar message when he said that character is a natural power—light and heat and all nature cooperate with it.

For healing modalities to operate in a natural environment, the disposition of the intellect, will, emotions, and spirit of the healer must be balanced and centered. Such balancing and centering effects are enhanced by knowledge of self. Belief structures and the reasoning behind such belief structures place the individual healer's spirit in a dynamic equilibrium or cybernetic relationship with the powers in the cosmos. It is in this way that conscious evolution proceeds. It is a give and take—a continuous ongoing dialogue between the healer and the cosmic environment that empowers the healer to heal. Healing is a psychophysiologic psychospiritual experience that enables the healer to cooperate with nature and, indeed, exigently coerce nature to cooperate with the healer.

Holistic ethics provides guidelines for the development of this spirit in the healer and spells out the steps needed to develop the healing attitude. Ethics thus serves as a guide to tap into the wisdom of the cosmos, teaching the individual strategies to release the self to become more participatory in the Greater Self. The participation in the Greater Self forms the linkages between the powers of the cosmos, the healer, and the one to be healed.

Nursing and ethics have been intertwined since the inception of modern nursing. The ethics of nursing encompasses both a bedside ethic and a social ethic, as nurses have always concerned themselves in such matters of public policy as urban slums and tenements, war and disaster, and special needs of the underserved. Recently, the ethics of public policy has also addressed environmental concerns, population issues, human rights, health care delivery, and health promotion. Nurses, both individually and collectively, are directly in the forefront not only of ethical decision making, but also of public policy formation. Many aspects of future health care delivery will be based on the ethical decisions that we make now. Thus, nurses must examine current and future healing activities from ethical perspectives. All of us must strive to understand the concept and application of ethics.

Chapter 7

Holistic Ethics

Lynn Keegan

NURSE HEALER OBJECTIVES

Theoretical

- Review the classic principles of ethics.
- Synthesize the basic tenets from the work of traditional ethical theorists.
- Explore the new concept of holistic ethics.

Clinical

- Relate ethical theory to clinical situations.
- Gain the knowledge necessary to serve on institutional ethics committees.

Personal

- Begin to see daily choices as opportunities to make a positive impact on the world.
- Clarify your own values and ideas.

DEFINITIONS

Being: the state of existing or living.

Consciousness: a state of knowing or awareness.

Ethical Code: a written list of a profession's values and standards of conduct.

Ethics: the study or discipline concerned with judgments of approval or disapproval, rightness or wrongness, goodness or badness, virtue or vice, and desirability or wisdom of actions, dispositions, ends, objects, or states of affairs; disciplined reflection on the moral choices that people make.

Holistic: concerned with the interrelationship of body, mind, and spirit in an ever-changing environment.

Holistic Ethics: the basic underlying concept of the unity and integral wholeness of all people and of all nature that is identified and pursued by finding unity and wholeness within the self and within humanity. In this framework, acts are not performed for the sake of law, precedent, or social norms, but rather from a desire to do good freely in order to witness, identify, and contribute to unity.

Morals: standards of right and wrong that are learned through socialization.

Nursing Ethics: a code of behavior that influences the way nurses work with those in their care, with one another, and with society.

Personal Ethics: an individual code of thought and behavior that governs each person's actions.

Planetary Ethics: a code of behavior that influences the way in which we individually and collectively interact with the environment and other peoples and animals of the earth.

Values: concepts or ideals that give meaning to life and provide a framework for decisions and actions.

THE NATURE OF ETHICAL PROBLEMS

Because ethical issues consist of diverse values and perspectives, they are extremely complex. Ethical questions arise from all areas of life. The ramifications of the population explosion, euthanasia, genetic engineering, and allocation of resources, for example, are only a few of a whole host of controversial ethical issues. Furthermore, four specific recent developments in our society have dramatically increased ethical awareness: (1) advances in medical technology, (2) greater recognition of patients' rights, (3) malpractice cases and court-ordered treatment, and (4) scarcity of resources.[1] Jonsen noted the element of mystery intertwined with ethics when he stated that no matter how much is revealed about antibodies, osmolality, immunoglobulins, or any of the other mysteries of the body, mystery remains at the heart of the science of medicine. The patient also participates in the mystery, for the patient knows himself or herself intimately.[2] Naturally then, mystery adds to the element of complexity.

Unfortunately, ethical dilemmas are usually characterized by the fact that there is no right answer. There are often two or more unsatisfactory answers or conflicting responses. In addition, nurses often find that the expectations of employers, physicians, patients, or other nurses themselves are sources of conflict.[3]

Changes in the knowledge that forms the basis of our values are changing the sources of some of our ethical dilemmas. For example, technologies related to computers and communication have affected patient confidentiality. Improved life support technology has been used to keep patients alive against their wishes. Sophisticated technology has the clear disadvantage of being able to reduce persons to objects.[4] Thus, advances in procedures (e.g., organ transplantation, amniocentesis) and equipment (e.g., respirators, dialysis machines) have opened the doors to new possibilities for extending or prolonging life, but they also prompt the critical ethical question, Does the fact that it can be done mean that it should be done?[5]

MORALS AND PRINCIPLES

Over the past two decades, biomedical ethicists have identified several moral principles. Three primary principles are (1) respect for persons, (2) beneficence, and (3) justice. Sometimes these principles are stated as obligations; sometimes, as rules. Whether primary or secondary, these principles represent obligations to respect the wishes of competent persons, obligations not to harm others, obligations to benefit others, obligations to produce a net balance of benefits over harm, obligations to distribute benefits and harms fairly, obligations to keep promises and contracts, obligations to be truthful, obligations to disclose information, and obligations to respect privacy and to protect confidential information.[6]

Within natural law ethics, the principle of double effect has special importance for nurses. Oftentimes, nurses are involved in actions that have untoward consequences. For example, administering a drug to relieve a cancer patient's pain may shorten that patient's life. In double effect situations, four conditions must be met before an act can be justified:

1. The act itself must be morally good or at least indifferent.
2. The good effect must not be achieved by means of the bad effect.
3. Only the good effect must be intended, although the bad effect is foreseen and known.
4. The good effect intended must be equal to or greater than the bad effect.[7]

Ethics addresses three types of moral problems: moral uncertainty (unsureness about moral principles or rules that may apply, or the nature of the ethical problem itself); moral dilemma (conflict of moral principles that support different courses of action); and moral distress (inability to take the action known to be right because of external constraints). Ethical debate helps to relieve moral uncertainty by clarifying questions and illuminating the ethical features of the situation. Discussion helps to clarify moral dilemmas by revealing general and specific obligations and values.[8] Milner urged nurses to use principles and theory to deal with issues of relationships as well as health care concerns, as following principles rather than emotions or feelings in conflicting situations may reduce moral distress. Basic ethics that involves how we treat each other as human beings is a necessary first step before we can appropriately deal with broader issues.[9]

TRADITIONAL ETHICAL THEORIES

Many nurse clinicians turn away in frustration when confronted with the details of ethical theories. Perhaps this is because it has been difficult in the past to see how these historical philosophical theories relate to contemporary clinical situations. In order to make these theories meaningful to the work setting, it is helpful to think of situations in which they may apply to current clinical practice.

A number of ethical theories have played a role in Western civilization and have laid the foundation for the development of modern ethics. Aristotelian theory is based on the individual's manifesting specific virtues and developing his or her own character. Aristotle (384–322 B.C.) believed that an individual who practices the virtues of courage, temperance, integrity, justice, honesty, and truthfulness will know almost intuitively what to do in a particular situation or conflict.[10] The system of Emmanuel Kant (1724–1804) formulated the historical Christian idea of the Golden Rule. "So act

in such a way as your act becomes a universal for all mankind."[11] Kant was very much concerned with the "personhood" of human beings and "persons" as moral agents.

Other theories that are helpful in understanding a holistic approach to ethics include the consequentialism theory of Jeremy Bentham (1748–1832) and John Stuart Mill (1806–1873), the natural rights theory of John Locke (1632–1714), and the contractarian theory of Thomas Hobbes (1588–1679). Briefly stated, the consequentialist or utilitarian view of Bentham and Mill is that the consequences of our actions are the primary concern, the means justify the ends, and every human being has a personal concept of good and bad. The natural rights theory of Locke was the forerunner of the U.S. Declaration of Independence, as it included the tenet that individuals have inalienable rights and that other individuals have an obligation to respect those rights. The contractarian theory of Hobbes contends that all morality involves a social contract indicating what individuals can and cannot do.[12]

Another way of viewing ethics is in terms of the two traditional forms: the deontologic (from a Greek root meaning knowledge of that which is binding and proper) style and the teleologic (from a Greek root meaning knowledge of the ends) style. The former assigns duty or obligation based on the intrinsic aspects of an act rather than its outcome; action is morally defensible on the basis of its intrinsic nature. The latter assigns duty or obligation based on the consequences of the act; action is morally defensible on the basis of its extrinsic value or outcome.

DEVELOPMENT OF HOLISTIC ETHICS

The holistic view of reality reopens vistas of thought that were dominant in the pretechnologic era, times when people were generally closer to their environment and the earth. The allure of new science and technology sidetracked many of us into primarily linear, rational, unidirectional thought. Furthermore, while technology has provided conveniences and easy solutions, it has also contributed to a tendency to objectify the universe.

Holistic ethics is a philosophy that couples both reemerging and rapidly evolving concepts of holism and ethics. It involves a basic underlying concept of the unity and integral wholeness of all people and of all nature that is identified and pursued by finding unity and wholeness within the self and within humanity. Within the framework of holistic ethics, acts are not performed for the sake of law, precedent, or social norms, but rather from a desire to do good freely in order to witness, identify, and contribute to unity of the self and of the universe of which the individual is a part. Encompassing traditional ethical views, the holistic view is characterized by the Eastern monad in the yin–yang mode and the Western concept of masculine and feminine. Holistic ethics is not grounded or judged in the act performed or in the distant consequences of the act, but rather in the conscious evolution of an enlightened individual of raised consciousness who performs the act. The primary concern is the effect of the act on the involved individual and his or her larger self.[13]

Presuppositions

Ethics is the study of the paths of practical wisdom. It is concerned with judgments of goodness and badness, rightness and wrongness based on a philosophic view of the nature of the universe. All ethical theories have presuppositions. The following are some of the presuppositions of holistic ethics:

- There is a Being or Spirit who is actively involved with humanity and with the universe and in whose image we are created.
- There is a divine plan. Although modeled on it, the material universe is but an infinitesimal part of the overall plan.
- The Spirit is active in the inner life of individuals.
- Persons (personalities) have a dual existence. One existence is on a material plane (body, mind, and spirit), and another is on the divine plane (soul).
- Humankind has a purpose or task—the evolution of itself and the universe into a more perfect image of its Creator.
- The concept of unity is the key to the path of critical wisdom.
- The matter of which our entire universe (body, mind, and spirit) is comprised is subject to dynamic development under the influence of dialectic laws. These principles operate on a psychologic, as well as a physical, plane.
- The Spirit is operative in the universe. This cosmic view embraces two paths. The first is the scientific or phenomenologic path, which has as its byproduct holistic ethics, and the other approach is the theologic path. The two paths intersect at a point called Omega, the apex both of the scientific and of the religious view of nature. According to this concept of time and space, Omega is not only present in the universe, but also represents a different, much larger reality. The symbol of Omega transcends matter.
- There is purposefulness in the universe. All occurrences—the entire range from good to bad, from complex to simple—are in some way part of the divine plan. There is purpose and reason, although oftentimes consciously

incomprehensible, for things that happen.[14]

Holistic ethics originates in the individual's own character and in the individual's relationship to the universe. In some way, the universe is present totally in each individual; paradoxically, the person is just a small part of that same universe. Gregorios believed that wisdom is a condition in which the self and the world are in communion with each other within the larger communion with Being in its integrity.[15] A holistic view takes into account the relationship of unity of all being. Albert Einstein, in the course of a serious illness, was asked if he feared death. He replied, "I feel such a sense of solidarity with all living things that it does not matter to me where the individual begins and ends."[16]

An a priori belief for a holistic person is probably, I believe in being, or even more simply, I am. In this belief system, no act, principle, or person is independent, but all are interrelated; all are "I." Each and every action is a moral action, either contributing to the unity of being or diminishing it. It is the enlightened and totally expanded "I" that creates a holistic view of ethics.

Moral acts may be judged not solely in terms of their intrinsic nature nor solely in terms of their ends, but in both ways. The act may affect the nature of the person performing the act (the "I") and his or her relationships, as well as the object of the act and the object's relationships. In addition, it can be helpful to explore the relationship of the act to the present and future of humanity. Through use of this construct, holistic ethics is both deontologic and teleologic. Holistic ethics is specifically teleologic in questioning the meaning and quality of life.

As a philosophic design for living, holistic ethics is a system for the individual. It appeals to the emotions, senses, aesthetic appreciation, and the inner self as revealed by meditative techniques. Such techniques may be active (e.g., the body movements of Tai Chi or jogging), passive (e.g., sitting meditative posture), or traditional prayer.

The educative process of holistic ethics is not a matter of memorizing facts or historical perspectives, but is instead a process of developing an attitude of awareness of the sacredness of ourselves and all of nature. It is a process in which there is an expanded view that, for both internal and external transformation, our inner self and the collective greater self have stewardship not only over our bodies, minds, and spirits, but also over our planet and the total universe.[17]

Based on this emergent ethical theory, the American Holistic Nurses' Association has developed a position statement on holistic nursing ethics (Exhibit 7–1).

Holistic Ethics and Consciousness

The underlying principle in a holistic ethical view is being, and its corollary is consciousness. Being and consciousness can be further defined as having their origin in the spirit.[18] Not only is consciousness accepted in the holistic system as the product of an evolutionary process, but also it is believed to become operative through the effect of the spirit. Our personal will becomes the motivator for continued evolution. In the holistic concept of ethics, moral decisions affect both the spirit of humankind as a whole and our own individual spirits.[19] As each of us evolves our own individual consciousness, we assess and direct the evolution of the consciousness of our species and contemplatively examine our relationship with the universal being.

Holistic ethics is not grounded or judged either in the act performed or in the distant consequences of the act, but rather in the

Exhibit 7-1 American Holistic Nurses' Association Position Statement on Holistic Nursing Ethics

Code of Ethics for Holistic Nurses

We believe that the fundamental responsibilities of the nurse are to promote health, facilitate healing and alleviate suffering. The need for nursing is universal. Inherent in nursing is the respect for life, dignity and right of all persons. Nursing care is given in a context mindful of the holistic nature of humans, understanding the body-mind-spirit. Nursing care is unrestricted by considerations of nationality, race, creed, color, age, sex, sexual preference, politics or social status. Given that nurses practice in culturally diverse settings, professional nurses must have an understanding of the cultural background of clients in order to provide culturally appropriate interventions.

Nurses render services to clients who can be individuals, families, groups or communities. The client is an active participant in health care and should be included in all nursing care planning decisions.

In order to provide services to others, each nurse has a responsibility toward him/herself. In addition, nurses have defined responsibilities towards the client, co-workers, nursing practice, the profession of nursing, society and the environment.

Nurses and Self

The nurse has a responsibility to model health behaviors. Holistic nurses strive to achieve harmony in their own lives and assist others striving to do the same.

Nurses and the Client

The nurse's primary responsibility is to the client needing nursing care. The nurse strives to see the client as a whole, and provides care that is professionally appropriate and culturally consonant. The nurse holds in confidence all information obtained in professional practice, and uses professional judgment in disclosing such information. The nurse enters into a relationship with the client that is guided by mutual respect and a desire for growth and development.

Nurses and Co-Workers

The nurse maintains cooperative relationships with co-workers in nursing and other fields. Nurses have a responsibility to nurture each other, and to assist nurses to work as a team in the interest of client care. If a client's care is endangered by a co-worker, the nurse must take appropriate action on behalf of the client.

Nurses and Nursing Practice

The nurse carries personal responsibility for practice and for maintaining continued competence. Nurses have the right to utilize all appropriate nursing interventions, and have the obligation to determine the efficacy and safety of all nursing actions. Wherever applicable, nurses utilize research findings in directing practice.

Nurses and the Profession

The nurse plays a role in determining and implementing desirable standards of nursing practice and education. Holistic nurses may assume a leadership position to guide the profession toward holism. Nurses support nursing research and the development of holistically oriented nursing theories. The nurse participates in establishing and maintaining equitable social and economic working conditions in nursing.

Nurses and Society

The nurse, along with other citizens, has responsibility for initiating and supporting actions to meet the health and social needs of the public.

Nurses and the Environment

The nurse strives to manipulate the client's environment to become one of peace, harmony, and nurturance so that healing may take place. The nurse considers the health of the ecosystem in relation to the need for health, safety and peace of all persons.

Source: Courtesy of the American Holistic Nurses' Association, Flagstaff, Arizona.

conscious evolution of an enlightened individual who performs the act. The primary concern is the effect of the act on the individual and his or her larger self (that unity of which the individual is a part). Unethical acts are those that degrade or brutalize the individual who performs the act and detract from his or her conscious evolution. The effect of an unethical act is to make us aware of the deprivation of divinity within humanity and of humanity itself. The unethical act dissolves the unity of matter and takes away wholeness. Acts must be judged in this setting to determine whether they promote wholeness and integration of either an individual or the collective whole.[20]

Clearly, it is within the emergence of consciousness that the evolution of ethical action begins. Anthropologist Richard Leakey suggested that consciousness supplied primitive human beings with their first capacity for empathy. For example, when the early human recognized that a particular action would injure the self, that human inferred that a particular action would cause injury to another person (another self). Leakey contended that the mechanism of consciousness (i.e., recognition of self) provided the rudiments of a kind of Golden Rule: "Do not do unto others what you would not have done unto you."[21]

Seshachar described three levels of consciousness:

1. Knowledge and awareness of the external world by exoceptors (e.g., organs of sight, hearing).
2. Inner sensing, not directly derived from sensory data, but triggered by them (e.g., emotions, intentions, memories, dreams, imagination).
3. Knowledge of one's self (other than body) characterized by the ability to recognize the present from the infor-

mation of the past and to project the future, establishing a continuity in one's lifetime. The belief that there is an "I," a self who does the perceiving, makes possible the creation of aesthetic, ethical, and spiritual values that are unique to persons.[22]

Of these three levels, it is possible that only the first is present in lower animals. In some higher mammals, there may be an element of the second. The absence of language, however, makes it difficult for them to express, to compare, and to evaluate these experiences and for humans to make a valid assessment of the extent to which this inner sensing has been developed in animals. There is little doubt that the third level of consciousness is exclusive to human beings. Seshachar continued to explain that a fusion of the totality of impressions and experiences makes the consciousness an attribute unique to humans.

Holistic ethics embraces and strives for the fusion between self and others. In the process, it becomes a cosmic ecology, a flowing with the universal tide of events and a co-creator of celestial harmony. All events and ethical decisions become part of the unfolding of a harmonious order and a realization of potentialities. Even tragic events can be analyzed within this harmonious spectrum with full realization of the fusion of relationships. One's own actions can become courageous, truth-full, being-full, beauty-full, assured, detached, and virtuous.[23]

DEVELOPMENT OF PRINCIPLED BEHAVIOR

Health care providers with a holistic ethics perspective and high standards of principled behavior are best prepared to analyze clinical dilemmas. Burkhardt and

Nathaniel asserted that principled behavior flows from personal values that guide and inform one's responses, behaviors, and decisions in all areas of one's life.[24]

Values Clarification

Values develop over time and have cultural, familial, environmental, and educational components. Values clarification is a never ending process in which an individual becomes increasingly aware of what is important and just—and why. Understanding the truth of a situation is usually more accurate, however, if people appreciate different views and openly share these perspectives.[25]

Sometimes organizations must clarify their values. They may begin by determining what staff, board members, management, and workers value about the elements of the organization's philosophy and identifying specific expectations for each group. In selected groups under the direction of a guide, the members can do focus exercises on self-awareness, clinical priorities, and opinions about value-laden issues.[26]

Oftentimes, patients must clarify their values in order to participate fully in the ethical decision making. One such approach involves asking individuals to identify 10 health-related behaviors that they do and to explain why they do those behaviors. Doyle noted that the reasons given for practicing a behavior provide insight into the values surrounding the behavior, such as choosing not to exercise in order to have more time, or choosing to exercise because it helps in weight control.[27]

Legal Aspects

Health care providers must adhere to the law. All nurses are responsible and accountable to comply with the Nursing Practice Act and Rules and Regulations of the Board of Nurse Examiners in the state where they are licensed and work. Standards of professional nursing practice require that each nurse practice to the level of his or her knowledge and skills. This means that, whatever an individual nurse's personal ethic, he or she must still adhere to the standards of practice and to the law.

ANALYSIS OF ETHICAL DILEMMAS

We are all confronted daily with the need to make personal and professional ethical decisions. Some decisions are minor, but others are fraught with long-term multifaceted ramifications. In order to make these decisions appropriately, it is necessary, first, to operate from a set of principles and, second, to have some sort of analytical method to help sort out and classify the elements of the problem. When the cases are institutional and patient care–oriented, there are well established guidelines for analyzing individual cases in ethics that may be helpful.[28,29] Jonsen and colleagues divided the case analysis process into four components: (1) medical indications, (2) patient preferences, (3) quality of life, and (4) contextual issues. Present in every clinical ethical case, these four topics are necessary for a thorough analysis. The holistic approach adds questions of relationships: Who am I? What is my relationship to others? What other factors are contributing to my decisions? Am I wise and courageous enough to perceive and respect others' differences and honor them as I would honor my own beliefs?

Medical Indications

The underlying ethical principle in considering medical indications is beneficence: Be of benefit and do no harm. Discussion should focus on discerning the relationship between the pathophysiology and the diagnostic and therapeutic interventions available to remedy the patient's pathologic condition. Questions to be considered in this component are, What is the overall goal in this case? and What should be the goal in cases such as this one?[30] For the patient who is terminally ill, for example, there may be discussions about the futility of further treatment.

Patient Preferences

In all interventions, the preferences of the patient are relevant. The questions to be asked are, What does the patient want? Does the patient comprehend? Is the patient being coerced? In some cases, there is no certainty because the patient is incapable of self-expression. Whenever possible, it is essential to ensure the patient's right to self-determination, based on his or her personal values and evaluation of risks and benefits. It is necessary, however, to be clear about what is realistically feasible before considering the patient's wishes.

In the case of a child, nurses must ask the questions, Do the parents understand the situation? Do the parents appear to have the best interests of the child at heart? Are the parents in agreement or discord?

Quality of Life

A patient enters a health crisis situation with an actual or potential reduction in quality of life, manifested by the signs and symptoms of the illness. The objective of health care interventions is to improve quality of life. In each case, multiple questions surround quality-of-life issues. What does quality of life mean, in general? In particular? How are others responding to their perceptions of it? What levels of quality impose what obligations on providers? This component may be a difficult component of the analysis of clinical problems, but it is indispensable.

Contextual Issues

Every case has a patient at its center. The patient exists in a social, psychologic, economic, and relational environment. To be relevant, all decisions must be considered in the light of this expanded conceptual and holistic view of personhood and personality. The major impacts are psychologic, emotional, financial, legal, scientific, educational, and religious.

ADVANCE MEDICAL DIRECTIVES

The Patient Self-Determination Act, effective December 1, 1991, requires that all individuals receiving medical care also receive written information about their right to accept or refuse medical or surgical treatment and their right to initiate advance directives, such as living wills and durable power of attorney. Advance medical directives are of two types: treatment directives, often referred to as living wills, and appointment directives, often referred to as power of attorney or health proxies. A living will specifies the medical treatment that a patient wishes to refuse in the event that he or she is terminally ill and cannot make those decisions. A durable power of attorney for health care appoints a proxy, usually a relative or trusted friend, to make medical decisions on behalf of the patient if he or she can no longer make such decisions. It has broader applications than a living will and can apply to any illness or injury that could leave the patient incapacitated.

An advance directive applies only if a patient is incapacitated. It may not apply if, in the opinion of two physicians, the patient can make decisions. Individuals can cancel advance directives at any time. An advance directive may be as simple or as complex as necessary. Individuals should give a copy of the advance directive to family members and the physician, and should carry a copy if and when hospital admission is necessary.

As part of patient assessment, a nurse may consider asking the following questions:

- Have you discussed your end-of-life choices with your family and/or designated surrogate and health care team workers?
- Do you have basic information about advance medical directives, including living wills and durable power of attorney?
- Do you wish to initiate an advance medical directive?
- If you have already prepared an advance medical directive, can you provide it now?

CONCLUSION

Holistic ethics embraces both the traditional and the masculine–feminine historical perspectives, but transcends both by taking into account the unity of being. The holistic view of human beings is one of self-actualization, as it places the highest value on the development of the individual to attain higher levels of human awareness and, thus, advances the whole of humanity. Within this framework, a unique moral viewpoint takes its origin. The cybernetic relationship of an act to the universal "I" becomes the new categorical imperative of the holistic person. Evolution and consciousness should be directed toward positive ends. They should be directed toward the "good" of people perceived by a contemplation of the reality of being. The process begins with the individual and his or her own self-realization within a universal context. It is the development of total personality where consciousness shines through with self-luminosity.[31] The best utilization of this theory is to internalize these principles and begin to apply them practically within our own settings.

Many hospitals are developing ethics committees, and soon there may be legisla-tion requiring the participation of these committees in decision-making processes. Ethically knowledgeable nurses are poised to become active participants in ethics committees and decision-making discussions. When those opportunities arise, nurses can begin to articulate a holistic approach that supports the very essence of a comprehensive world ethical view.

DIRECTIONS FOR FUTURE RESEARCH

1. Determine how and where the new theory of holistic ethics fits into the continuum of emerging ethical theories.
2. Develop a process of clinical case analysis based on the process of holistic ethics.
3. Examine specific clinical situations through a process of holistic ethics.
4. Analyze the application of holistic ethics to planetary ethical issues.

NURSE HEALER REFLECTIONS

After reading this chapter, the nurse healer will be able to answer or begin a process of answering the following questions:

- What new insights do I have about the process of ethics?
- How does ethics fit into my clinical practice?
- Do I have the interest and beginning ability to become involved in an institutional ethics committee?
- What role does ethics play in my day-to-day personal life?
- Am I ready to look at planetary issues from a holistic ethical perspective?

NOTES

1. F. Hendrickson and G.L. Deloughery, Ethical Influences on Nursing, in *Issues and Trends in Nursing*, ed. G.L. Deloughery (St. Louis: C.V. Mosby, 1991), 180.

2. A. Jonsen, *The New Medicine and the Old Ethics* (Cambridge, MA: Harvard University Press, 1990), 138.

3. M. Corley and D. Raines, An Ethical Practice Environment as a Caring Environment, *Nursing Administration Quarterly* 17, no. 2 (1993):68–74.

4. Corley and Raines, An Ethical Practice Environment.

5. Hendrickson and Deloughery, Ethical Influences on Nursing.

6. R.M. Veatch, ed., *Medical Ethics* (Boston: Jones & Bartlett, 1989).

7. Hendrickson and Deloughery, Ethical Influences on Nursing, 187.

8. M. Fowler, Ethical Decision Making in Clinical Practice, *Nursing Clinics of North America* 24, no. 4 (1989):955–965.

9. S. Milner, An Ethical Practice Model, *Journal of Nursing Administration* 23, no. 3 (1993):22–25.

10. H. Sidgwick, *Ethics* (Boston: Beacon Press, 1960), 59–63.

11. Sidgwick, *Ethics*, 273.

12. Sidgwick, *Ethics*, 163–169.

13. L. Keegan and G. Keegan, A Concept of Holistic Ethics for the Health Professional, *Journal of Holistic Nursing* 10, no. 3 (1992):205–217.

14. L. Keegan and G. Keegan, Holistic Ethics, unpublished manuscript, 1994.

15. P.M. Gregorios, *Science for Sane Societies* (New York: Paragon House, 1987).

16. M. Born, *Born–Einstein Letters* (New York: Walker, 1971).

17. Keegan and Keegan, A Concept of Holistic Ethics.

18. L. Keegan and G. Keegan, Spirituality and the Technological Crisis, *Healing Currents* 11, no. 2 (1987):26–28.

19. D. Singh, The Psychology of Consciousness, in *The Evolution of Consciousness*, ed. K. Gandi (New York: Paragon House, 1983), 68–86.

20. Keegan and Keegan, A Concept of Holistic Ethics.

21. Singh, The Psychology of Consciousness.

22. B.R. Seshachar, Biological Foundations of Human Evolution and Consciousness, in *The Evolution of Consciousness*, ed. K. Gandi (New York: Paragon House, 1983), 28.

23. Keegan and Keegan, A Concept of Holistic Ethics.

24. M.A. Burkhardt and A.K. Nathaniel, *Ethics and Issues in Contemporary Nursing* (Albany, NY: Delmar Publishers, 1998).

25. B.C. Banois, Principled Behavior Applied to Everyday Life, unpublished manuscript, 1997.

26. B.S. Gingerich and D.A. Ondeck, Values Incorporated throughout the Organization, *Caring* 12 (1993):18–23.

27. E.I. Doyle, Recognizing the Value–Health Behavior Connection: "What I do and why I do it," *Journal of Health Education* 25 (1994):116–118.

28. A.R. Jonsen, Case Analysis in Clinical Ethics, *Journal of Clinical Ethics* 1, no. 1 (1990):63–65.

29. A.R. Jonsen et al., *Clinical Ethics*, 4th ed. (New York: Macmillan, 1998).

30. S.E. Shannon, Living Your Ethics, in *Critical Care: Body-Mind-Spirit*, ed. B.M. Dossey et al. (Philadelphia: J.B. Lippincott, 1992), 135–141.

31. Seshachar, Biological Foundations.

VISION OF HEALING

Active Listening

To achieve good listening, it is necessary to quiet the inner dialogue. Good listening has an enormous quality of nowness, the ability to throw away intellectualizations when a client goes off in an unexpected direction. Sometimes, because of a personal inner dialogue of analysis and intellectualization, a nurse will stop the flow of a client's story and bring the client back to a certain point, which then may block the client's insight. As nurses increase the process of nowness, clients also will move to a state of nowness that allows a place of inner wisdom to emerge. Questioning, and listening, that structures the answers only minimally is a great art.

Any communication process has three components. These are (1) a sender of the message, (2) a receiver of the message, and (3) the content of the material. In order to understand others, it is essential to listen actively. Being quiet while someone else is talking is not equivalent to real listening. The key to real listening is intention, which occurs when we focus with someone in order to move with purpose in our responses and interventions. This can lead others or ourselves toward effective actions or forward in personal growth. Real listening occurs when we have the intention to understand someone, enjoy someone, learn something, or want to give help to someone.

At times, we all lapse into pseudolistening when we try to meet the needs of others. Some signs of pseudolistening are

- silence to buy time preparing your next remark
- listening to others so that they will listen to you
- listening only to specific information while deleting the rest
- acting interested when you are not
- partially listening because you do not want to disappoint another person
- listening in order not to be rejected
- searching for a person's weaknesses in order to take advantage of them
- identifying weak points in dialogue so that you can be stronger in your response

We must continue to learn how to be with others. Active listening skills promote effective communication in several ways. They clarify the message. The receiver of the message can verify nonverbal messages communicated through body language or by silences. The receiver is also able to gather additional information that can help with interventions. Active listening facilitates a greater acceptance of the sender's thoughts and emotions. Thus, the receiver of the message may be in a better situation to choose the most effective behaviors that lead toward health and wholeness.

Chapter 8

Nursing Theory in Holistic Nursing Practice

Noreen Cavan Frisch

NURSE HEALER OBJECTIVES

Theoretical

- Describe the elements of holistic nursing and explain why the use of theory is one of the elements.
- Compare and contrast the nursing theories: Nightingale's Environmental Adaptation Model; the Roy Adaptation Model; the Modeling and Role-Modeling Theory, Watson's Theory of Humancare; Rogers' Theory of Unitary Human Beings; Newman's Theory of Health and Expanding Consciousness; and Parse's Theory of Human Becoming.

Clinical

- Apply the nursing theories discussed in the clinical setting.
- Determine how the perspective of the theory influences the nursing care and the evaluation of that care.

Personal

- Select a nursing theory(ies) that provides a framework and philosophy consistent with your own view.
- Use the theory(ies) and evaluate its effect on your personal world view.

DEFINITIONS

Concept: an abstract idea or notion.

Conceptual Model: a group of interrelated concepts described to suggest relationships among them.

Framework: a basic structure; the context in which theory is developed; the structure that permits theory to be understood.

Model: a representation of interactions between and among concepts.

Nursing Theory: a framework; a set of interrelated concepts that are testable; a way of seeing the factors that contribute to nursing practice and nursing thought.

World View: a perspective; a way of viewing, perceiving, and interpreting one's experience.

THEORY AND RESEARCH

By definition and by history, nursing is a holistic practice. Nursing's work is concerned with the restoration and promotion of health, the prevention of disease, and the supports necessary to help the client gain a subjective sense of peace and harmony. As a profession, nursing has never been focused solely on the physical body or the disease entity. Rather, taking into account the holistic nature of all persons, nursing is concerned with the client's experience of the condition. In addition, nurses attend to the environmental influences that promote recovery as well as the social and spiritual supports that promote a sense of well-being for clients. Nurses have found that nursing theories help to articulate the nature of nursing practice and guide nursing interventions to meet client needs.

Nursing Theory Defined

Simply defined, a nursing theory is a framework from which professional nurses can think about their work. Theory is a means of interpreting one's observations of the world. For example, most nurses have studied developmental theory, which provides a framework for viewing childhood behaviors expected with various ages and phases of child growth. Thus, when nurses observe a toddler crying when his mother must leave him alone with nurses in the hospital, nurses interpret the child's crying as separation anxiety—an expected and predicted toddler behavior according to the theory. The theory provides a means of understanding behavior that otherwise might seem random and, thus, is a framework from which to understand the child's actions.

Theory has also been defined as an abstraction of reality,[1] or "a creative and rigorous structuring of ideas that project a tentative, purposeful, and systematic view of phenomena."[2] There are ideas or concepts common to all nursing theories—the concepts of nursing, person, health, and environment. Different theories present differing definitions of these concepts and suggest different ways in which these concepts are linked to one another. For example, one theory may define the environment in direct, concrete terms, referring to the physical environment; another theory may define the environment as an energy field. Each of these theories would have a different perspective on the effect of the environment on a client's health. The way that a nurse defines concepts related to

nursing care and the way that nurse thinks about the relationship of these concepts affects the practice and, presumably, the outcome of nursing care.

Since the writings of Florence Nightingale,[3] considered the first nursing theorist and the founder of "modern secular nursing," nurses have had theories about how to practice nursing. Most nursing theories, however, were developed from the time period of the 1960s to the present. Several nurses have put forth their ideas of what nursing is and how nursing care can be delivered to assist clients in achieving health. Many practicing nurses are using theory without being aware that their care is based on a specific theory. They have learned what nursing is by going to nursing school and working with a set of beliefs or assumptions about nursing and the effects of nursing care. Nursing curricula are based on nursing theories—in some schools, theory is taught as an assumption; in others, it is more explicitly taught as a theory. Nonetheless, all nurses have learned what nursing is from a viewpoint that included definitions of the major concepts of nursing theory and have learned to practice nursing in a manner consistent with that viewpoint. When nurses study nursing theory, they have an opportunity to consider carefully the assumptions on which they base their practice. Knowledge of several theories gives nurses more choices in thinking about the situations in which they find themselves and their clients. Theory gives nurses tools to guide practice, and, because nursing theory is grounded in research, theory provides a scientific basis for nursing care.

The Need for Theory

Whenever the topic of nursing theory comes up, some nurses ask, "Why do I need a theory? Isn't being holistic enough?" These are very important questions. Nurses committed to holism are kind and compassionate nurses who share a philosophy that emphasizes a "sensitive balance between art and science, analytic and intuitive skills, self-care skills, and the ability and interconnectedness of body, mind, and spirit."[4] Theory suggests, in fact *demands*, that nurses reflect on this philosophy and consider how their practice is working (or not working) to achieve holistic ideals.

The Description of Holistic Nursing developed by the American Holistic Nurses' Association (AHNA) states that "holistic nursing practice draws on knowledge, theories, expertise, intuition, and creativity."[5] All five elements are necessary for the nurse to function in an ideal way. Nursing knowledge is essential for the understanding of health and disease states and the various regimens required to achieve health. Theories are needed for the ability to reflect on practice and to consider carefully all alternatives of care. Expertise is needed for the performance of nursing skills and for the ability to make accurate assessments and decisions about care. Intuition is needed to understand the client and to appreciate the subjective experiences of others. Creativity is helpful in solving problems in providing care that can seem insurmountable; it provides the nurse with novel ideas and ways of being with clients. Each one of these elements is as important as the others. Knowledge and theory are cognitive tools that help the nurse to know and to reflect about practice. Expertise is an experiential tool that comes from practice and a significant number of encounters in nurse–client situations. Intuition and creativity are affective tools that lead the nurse to feel, experience, and follow inner guidance in work with clients.

Professional practice requires that nurses use these different ways of being to bring the best possible results. A holistic nurse can move back and forth between intuitive knowing and logical reasoning; between a creative approach to care and a standard care protocol; between a hunch of what to do and a considered direction grounded in the predictions of a theory. All of the elements of practice come only by learning how to use them. Table 8–1 presents a summary of the five elements of holistic nursing practice.

Theory Development

Theories develop over time as a theorist defines concepts, suggests relationships between concepts, tests and evaluates the relationships, and modifies the theory based on research findings. In the first stage of theory development, when the theorist is providing definitions of the concepts and suggesting possible relationships, the theory is called a "conceptual model." The framework is being presented without strong research findings that the relationships exist as proposed in the theory. There is a research basis for all of the nursing theories presented in this chapter; however, many nurses believe that all nursing theories are more correctly called conceptual models because theory

Table 8–1 Five Elements of Holistic Nursing Practice

Element	Domain	Use in Practice
Knowledge	Cognitive	Understanding health and disease states; interpreting regimens of care
Theory	Cognitive	Reflection; considered judgments
Expertise	Experiential	Skilled performance
Intuition	Affective	Subjective knowing
Creativity	Affective	Spontaneity; solving problems or challenges

development in nursing is still relatively new. As theories develop and mature, they pass through various stages and serve increasingly complex purposes:

1. *Description.* The theory provides definitions of concepts, suggests a way of looking at the world, and provides a framework for describing the phenomena of nursing.
2. *Explanation.* The theory suggests relationships between and among various concepts and gives the nurse a means of explaining observed events.
3. *Prediction.* The theory has research findings that establish clear relationships between aspects of nursing, and the nurse is able to predict outcomes.
4. *Prescription.* The theory is well developed and permits a nurse to prescribe nurse or client actions with confidence in the outcomes.

Most nursing theories are developed to the stage of description and explanation, and theorists and researchers are currently developing nursing theories to the stages of prediction and prescription. Any aspect of a theory can be validated through research. For example, if a theory states that a person is a human energy field and suggests that there is an exchange of energy between two persons, research that evaluates such an exchange serves to validate the theory.

SELECTED NURSING THEORIES

There are several recognized nursing theories; a standard text on nursing theory covers more than 20 theories.[6] The following are those most commonly used by holistic nurses.

Florence Nightingale: Theory of Environmental Adaptation[7]

Nightingale gave nursing the first published theory by which to reflect on nursing. She presented views on the major concepts important to nursing and directed nurses in the provision of care. To Nightingale, *Nursing* is putting the patients in the best condition for nature to act upon them; *Nursing,* as a profession, is a calling. *Person* is described in relation to the environment; the person is the recipient of nursing care. *Health* is the "positive of which pathology is the negative."[8] *Environment* is stressed in relation to healing properties of the physical environment, such as fresh air, light, warmth, and cleanliness. In relation to healing, Nightingale wrote, "Nature alone cures."[9]

For Nightingale, the focus of nursing care is to create an environmental space so that natural healing may take place. Cleanliness, fresh air, and order are emphasized, as are the patient's needs for nutrition. While not stated as such in her writings, Nightingale and her nurses regularly provided emotional and interpersonal supports. The images of Nightingale with her lamp attending to patient's needs at night, writing letters for them, and being present as a caring nurse are as much a part of her theory of practice as preparing food and cleaning the sick room. Although Nightingale's theory has not been developed in the same sophisticated manner as more modern theories, her work stands as a remarkable writing on reflective and thoughtful practice. Nurses today are often surprised by the accuracy of her directions in guiding current practice. The theory has been studied and "modernized" by nurse scholars who have described the theory in terms of theory development used today. Selanders noted that "the principle of environmental alteration has served as a framework for research studies."[10] Nightingale's theory is clearly a wonderful heritage for holistic nurses.

The Roy Adaptation Model

Roy began work on her theory in 1964 and has continued its development over the years.[11,12] The theory is based on the idea that it is necessary to adapt to stressors and to achieve health as a state of balance or homeostasis. *Nursing* is defined in terms of the roles and activities of nurses to promote adaptive responses in support of a client's health. *Person* is defined as a holistic, adaptive system; individual aspects or parts of an individual act together to form a unified being. *Health* is a state or process of being and becoming an integrated, whole person; it is a state of balance. *Environment* includes any condition, circumstance, and/or influence that affects the development and behavior of persons or groups. Stimuli in the environment can be focal (the immediate situation), contextual (other current stimuli in the person's environment that provide the context for adapting to the current situation), or residual (all other internal factors).

Because the theory is based on the idea of adaptation, the nurse is directed to evaluate the stressors in the client's environment and determine the client's ability to adapt or cope with current stressors. Health is achieved when the client is able to adapt or cope to create a sense of balance and a physiologic state of homeostasis. Nursing care involves taking actions to promote healthy adaptation. This theory has been strongly influenced by systems theory—changes in one or any part of the system affect other parts of the system. For example, emotional stress produces stress for the physical body and requires adaptation. One current study using Roy's theory is an evaluation of stressors, adaptation, and coping of family members caring for chronically ill relatives.[13]

Modeling and Role Modeling

In 1983, Erickson and colleagues published a theory and paradigm for nursing called the Modeling and Role-Modeling theory.[14] The theory draws on work from many theoretical perspectives, including Maslow's Basic Needs, Erikson's Stages of Development, Piaget's Theory of Cognitive Development, and Selye's Stress Theory. The work of the psychiatrist Milton Erickson (the father-in-law of the theory's senior author), who provided a perspective of the mind-body connection in health, healing, and disease, and a belief that the most important thing a professional can do is understand the world from the client's perspective are also important to the theory. According to this theory, *Nursing* is a process that demands an interpersonal and interactive relationship with the client. Facilitation, nurturance, and unconditional acceptance should characterize the nurse's caregiving. *Person* is seen as a holistic being with interacting subsystems (biologic, psychologic, social, and cognitive) and with inherent genetic bases and spiritual drives; the whole is greater than the sum of its parts. *Health* is a dynamic equilibrium between subsystems. *Environment* is seen as both internal and external; environment includes stressors as well as resources for adapting to stressors.

The client is seen as an individual with strengths that can and should be used to mobilize resources to adapt to stress. Adaptation potential is a theory-specific term used to describe conditions of adaptation—equilibrium (which can be adaptive or maladaptive), arousal, or impoverishment. The theory presents five aims of all nursing interventions: (1) to build trust, (2) to promote positive orientation, (3) to promote perceived control, (4) to promote strengths, and (5) to set mutual goals that are health-directed. The nurse uses this theory by creating a model of the client's world (Modeling) and using that model to plan interventions and to demonstrate and support health-producing behaviors from within the client's world view (Role Modeling). An excellent case study applying the theory to a client with diabetes mellitus illustrates how the perspective can help the client develop strengths.[15] Some of the current research on the theory has focused on understanding the concepts of stress, well-being, and self-care.[16–19]

Watson's Theory of Humancare

First presented as a philosophy and science of caring in 1979,[20] Watson's theory of Humancare emphasizes the humanistic aspects of nursing, combined with scientific knowledge. Within this framework, *Nursing* is mediated by "professional, personal, scientific, esthetic, and ethical human care transactions."[21] *Person* is seen holistically with the knowledge that the whole is greater than, and different from, the sum of the parts; every person is a valued individual to be cared for, cared about, and understood. *Health* is a subjective state that has to do with unity and harmony; illness can be understood as disharmony. Caring is achieved through the *environment*. Although environment is not defined explicitly, Watson stated that the environment provides social, cultural, and spiritual influences that may be perceived as caring.

In using the theory of Humancare, the foremost role of the nurse is to establish an intimate, caring relationship with the client. The nurse must be able to understand the client's subjective experiences and interact with the client in a meaningful relationship. The nurse–client encounter may change both the nurse and the client. Watson drew significant attention to the fact that the nurse must never "objectify" another human being (treat the client as an object), as every human being must be approached with unconditional acceptance and positive regard. The strength of the theory relies on the nurse's ability to provide quality, caring interactions with the client while simultaneously promoting health through nursing knowledge and interventions. Watson's theory gave rise to numerous qualitative research studies that documented the lived experiences of clients as they received care in our health care system. Current research on the theory

has emphasized basic patterns of care across cultures, suggesting applicability of the concept in varied settings.[22,23] Other writers have emphasized the caring aspects of nursing as appropriate and imperative for the advanced practice nurse or nurse practitioner.[24]

Theories Based on Energy Fields

Martha Rogers was the first theorist to describe nursing in relation to the view that the person is an energy field. In addition, she believed that nursing is a "humanistic science dedicated to compassionate concern for maintaining and promoting health, preventing illness, and caring for and rehabilitating the sick and disabled."[25] Rogers' theory, an abstract system, is the basis for the Science of Unitary Human Beings. Within this theory, *Nursing* is the scientific study of human and environmental energy fields. *Person* is a unified whole, defined as a human energy field; human beings evolve irreversibly and unidirectionally in space and time. *Health* is understood in terms of culture and, according to Rogers, individually defined by the subjective values of each person. *Environment* is the environmental energy field that is in constant interaction with the human energy field. There are no boundaries to the environmental or the human energy field.

Margaret Newman included Rogers' concepts of energy patterns and unitary human beings in developing her own theory.[26] Newman viewed *Nursing* as a profession that is moving to an integrated role; nursing is caring, and caring is a moral imperative for nursing. *Person* is a dynamic energy field; humans are identified by their field patterns. *Health* is expanding consciousness that includes an individual's total pattern; pathologic conditions are manifestations of the individual's total pattern. *Environment* is the wholeness of the universe; there are no boundaries. Newman's theory is called the Theory of Health As Expanding Consciousness.

Rosemarie Rizzo Parse further developed the idea of the person as a unitary whole and suggested that the person can only be viewed as a unity.[27] *Nursing* is seen as a scientific discipline, but the practice of nursing is an art in which nurses serve as guides to assist others in making choices affecting health. *Person* is a unified, whole being. *Health* is a process of becoming; it is a personal commitment, an unfolding, a process related to lived experiences. *Environment* is the universe. The human–universe is inseparable and evolving together. This theory is called the Theory of Human Becoming.

Energy field theories have provided nurses with an entirely new view of the world and of themselves. The energy field is a powerful concept that prompted many to study it further. The theories suggest much about the interaction between the human energy field and the environmental energy field, as well as the interactions between the healer and client energy fields. Each of the theories that have been described has a different focus, but each demands that the nurse enter into a new way of thinking. Each has prompted research on the various concepts in the theories and their relationships with one another. Recent research on the Theory of Human Becoming has documented the importance of intersubjective dialogue in assisting clients to move toward different meanings and choices in their lives[28] for example, and has described the sense of caring that clients perceive from nurses guided by the theory.[29] Research on the use of therapeutic touch and other energy-based modalities in nursing practice continue at a rapid rate.[30–34]

A WORD ABOUT DEFINITIONS OF *PERSON*

Since the emergence of Rogers' theory, the definition of person as a unitary whole has challenged nurses to reflect on the meaning of *whole*. Parse has suggested that there are two world views in nursing: a summative paradigm in which the person is viewed as a combination of component parts (with the belief that the whole or the essence of the person is greater than the sum of the parts) and the simultaneity paradigm in which a person can be viewed only as a unity, that is, the person is a holistic energy field and cannot be broken into parts.[35] For Rogers, Newman, and Parse, the only appropriate definition of the person is in terms of the unitary whole. Adherents of their theories insist that it is impossible to think of persons as having component parts (e.g., bio-psycho-social-spiritual components) and that any discussion of a "part" is improper. Other theorists (e.g., Roy, Erickson, Watson) have concluded that discussion of the "part" is helpful in considering the various ways in which a person functions, feels, and reacts to the environment.

Over the years of this debate, the AHNA has been asked to take a stand on the meaning of *whole* in holistic nursing practice. The official AHNA Description of Holistic Nursing states that holistic nursing is defined primarily as all nursing practice that has the enhancement of healing of the whole person as its goal.[36] The AHNA recognizes that there are two views of holism and has publicly stated that "holistic nursing responds to both views, believing that the goals of nursing can be achieved within either framework."[37] The important aspect of nursing practice is that the nurse and the client believe that the care received is assisting the client to enhance healing and achieve a state of health. Any nurse who believes that a particular theory is helping to reach the goals mutually set between nurse and client should use the theory and reflect on how the theory's world view changed and assisted nursing practice.

THEORY INTO PRACTICE

The theories discussed are not the only theories in use today, and most certainly other theories will be suggested in the future. Nurses use these and others in making assessments and in interpreting assessment data. The interpretation of data based on the theory's world view leads the nurse to establish goals for care and to design interventions to achieve the best outcome. To illustrate the use of theory in a clinical situation, Exhibit 8–1 outlines the view of the following client situation according to each of the theories.

> Mr. S. is a 50-year-old man who comes to the emergency department with his wife. He is suffering from severe chest pain and is short of breath. He has never experienced this before, and he tells his nurse that he is very much afraid of having a heart attack, as his partner at work had a myocardial infarction just last year. His wife is supportive and, under the circumstances, appears relatively calm. She asks the nurse to help provide assurance and treatment, if needed.

Reflection on the use of nursing theory demands that the nurse think about practice in new and critical ways. For practice to be consistent, nursing interventions

---

Exhibit 8–1 Interpretation of Case, Mr. S., According to Selected Theories

Nightingale/Theory of Environmental Adaptation

The environment of care for Mr. S. should include order, light, air. Activities and actions must be carried out efficiently with minimal disturbance to others. Nursing actions should be professional and unobtrusive.

Roy Adaptation Model

Stressors for Mr. S. are to be assessed. The immediate (focal) stimuli are the experience of chest pain and Mr. S.'s fear of having a myocardial infarction; the contextual stimuli are the choice to come to the hospital for care and the fact that Mr. S. has a partner who experienced a myocardial infarction a few months ago. Residual stimuli are other factors unknown to the nurse at present that may affect Mr. S.'s feelings and ability to cope. Interventions are directed to reestablish physiological homeostasis and equilibrium.

Modeling and Role-Modeling

Mr. S. is currently in a state of arousal related to his pain and call for help. He needs to feel safe and secure in the hospital environment. His wife is one of the resources that he is using to help him to cope and adapt to his immediate condition. Care should be directed toward supporting Mr. S. to receive the treatments or care he wishes and to help him reestablish equilibrium. To promote perceived control, Mr. S. should be given choices about his care whenever possible.

Watson's Theory of Humancare

Both Mr. S. and his wife require the presence of a compassionate and caring human being to offer them unconditional acceptance and support throughout the evaluation and treatment in the hospital.

Energy Field Theories

The emergency department is part of the environmental energy field, in interaction with the client's energy field. Assessment of balance of the client's field is to be done; actions to reestablish balance are needed while other treatments and evaluations are being carried out. The pain and fear that brought Mr. S. to the hospital are part of the energy pattern. The art of nursing permits the nurse to guide Mr. S. in making choices about care; however, the nurse recognizes that by coming to the emergency department, Mr. S. has chosen to receive evaluation and treatment.

should be derived from the theory; that is, there should be a congruence between the "thinking" about the nurse–client interactions and the "doing" of the nursing care. For example, the Modeling and Role-Modeling theory requires that the nurse create a model of the client's world and step into that world before planning interventions. It is important for the nurse to consider the timing and pacing of his or her actions so that they are consistent with the client's. Thus, nurses acquainted with this theory frequently use the modalities of guided imagery and hypnosis because these techniques require the nurse's pacing interactions, breathing, and speech to be like the client's. One of the benefits of theory-based practice is that nurses are challenged to make their practice consistent. Further, the focus of the nurse's thought is on the theory, the world view, and the client rather than on the modality or the nursing activities and tasks. Table 8–2 presents common complementary modalities that are consistent with the nursing theories described in this chapter.

CONCLUSION

A theory provides a means of interpreting and organizing information. Nursing theories give nurses a tool to ensure that nursing assessments are comprehensive and systematic, and that care is meaningful. Holistic nurses use several theories, and each nurse must decide which theory to use, and when to use an alternative perspective. In selecting a theory, a nurse may ask two questions: What theory is most comfortable for me? and What theory is most comfortable for my client? The perspective selected must

Table 8–2 Nursing Interventions Most Consistent with Specific Nursing Theories

Theory	*Interventions*	*Rationale*
Nightingale: Theory of Environmental Adaptation	Care of the environment to promote order, fresh air, and light	Nursing care to the environment puts the patient in the best condition for nature to act upon him/her and promotes healing.
Roy Adaptation Model	Progressive relaxation Coping enhancement	The nurse evaluates stressors, assists the client to eliminate immediate stress (when possible), and enhances coping strategies in order to adapt to stressors.
Modeling and Role Modeling	Guided imagery Hypnotherapy	To "model the client's world," the nurse must focus on timing and pacing of nursing actions. To assist the client to mobilize resources to cope with stress, the modalities of imagery and hypnosis help the client to uncover inherent strengths.
Watson's Theory of Humancare	Therapeutic presence Healing presence	To establish a meaningful nurse–client relationship based on caring and the demand for authentic person-to-person exchange, presence is the most important and basic nursing action.
Energy Field Theories	Therapeutic touch (TT) Healing touch modalities	Interventions based on the concepts of the human and environmental energy field are clearly consistent with theories that describe this as their world view.

be comfortable for both. Many clients, as well as nurses, have strong feelings and opinions about what nursing is and what type of care they wish to receive. If the theory's perspective is not comfortable for the client, the nurse is ethically obligated to change her or his perspective and adopt a framework that is compatible with the client's needs.

DIRECTIONS FOR FUTURE RESEARCH

1. Holistic nurses should consider what is known and not known about any theory being applied to practice and evaluate the next steps needed to develop the theory in their own area of practice.
2. Evaluate theories related to the identification of specific outcomes of care.

NURSE HEALER REFLECTIONS

After reading this chapter, the holistic nurse will be able to answer or to begin a process of answering the following questions:

- What definition of the concept of *person* is a good fit with my own view of myself and others?
- Which of the nursing theories described can I use in my practice?
- Which of the nursing theories would be uncomfortable for me to use? Can I openly explore why a particular theory(ies) would be uncomfortable to use?
- How will I determine if the theory I am using is acceptable to my clients?
- In what ways am I able and willing to make a contribution to the use and development of nursing theory?

NOTES

1. J. Fawcett, *Analysis and Evaluation of Conceptual Models of Nursing*, 3d ed. (Philadelphia: F.A. Davis, 1995).
2. P.L. Chinn and M.K. Kramer, *Theory and Nursing: A Systematic Approach*, 3d ed. (St. Louis: C.V. Mosby, 1991), 123.
3. F. Nightingale, *Notes on Nursing* (London: Harrison, 1860).
4. B.M. Dossey, ed., *Core Curriculum for Holistic Nursing* (Gaithersburg, MD: Aspen Publishers, 1997), 5–6.
5. American Holistic Nurses' Association, *Description of Holistic Nursing* (Flagstaff, AZ: AHNA, 1998).
6. J. George, *Nursing Theories: The Base for Professional Practice*, 4th ed. (Stamford, CT: Appleton & Lange, 1995).
7. L.C. Selanders, The Power of Environmental Adaptation: Florence Nightingale's Original Theory for Nursing Practice, *Journal of Holistic Nursing* 16 (1998): 247–263.
8. Selanders, The Power of Environmental Adaptation, 260.
9. Nightingale, *Notes on Nursing*, 74.
10. Nightingale, *Notes on Nursing*, 74.
11. C. Roy and H.A. Andrews, *The Roy Adaptation Model: The Definitive Statement* (Stamford, CT: Appleton & Lange, 1991).
12. C. Roy, Future of the Roy Model: Challenge to Redefine Adaptation, *Nursing Science Quarterly* 10 (1997): 42–48.
13. D. Newman, Responses to Caregiving: A Reconceptualization Using the Roy Adaptation Model, *Holistic Nursing Practice* 12 (1997): 80–88.
14. H. Erickson et al., *Modeling and Role-Modeling: A Theory and Paradigm for Nursing* (Lexington, KY: Pine Press, 1983).
15. J. Sappington and J. Kelley, Modeling and Role-Modeling: A Case Study of Holistic Care, *Journal of Holistic Nursing* 14 (1996): 130–141.
16. B. Irvin and G. Acton, Stress Mediation in Caregivers of Cognitively Impaired Adults: Theoretical Model Testing, *Nursing Research* 45 (1996): 160–166.
17. G. Acton, Affiliated-individuation as a Mediator of Stress and Burden in Caregivers of Adults with Dementia, *Journal of Holistic Nursing* 15 (1997): 336–357.
18. G. Acton and E. Miller, Affiliated-individuation in Caregivers of Adults with Dementia, *Issues in Mental Health Nursing* 17 (1996): 245–260.

19. S. Bowman, *Self-care Activities of Adults Experiencing Acute Illness* (Unpublished doctoral dissertation, University of Texas at Austin, School of Nursing, 1998).

20. J. Watson, *Human Science and Human Care* (New York: National League for Nursing, 1988).

21. Watson, *Human Science and Human Care*, 54.

22. K. Eriksson, Understanding the World of the Patient, the Suffering Human Being: The New Clinical Paradigm from Nursing to Caring, *Advanced Practice Nursing Quarterly* 3 (1997): 8–13.

23. M. Ray, Consciousness and the Moral Ideal: A Transcultural Analysis of Watson's Theory of Transpersonal Caring, *Advanced Practice Nursing Quarterly* 3 (1997): 25–31.

24. C. Green-Hernandez, Application of Caring Theory in Primary Care: A Challenge for Advanced Practice, *Nursing Administration Quarterly* 21 (1997): 77–82.

25. M. Rogers, *The Theoretical Basis for Nursing* (Philadelphia: F.A. Davis, 1970), vii.

26. M. Newman, *Health as Expanding Consciousness*, 2d ed. (New York: National League for Nursing, 1994).

27. R.R. Parse, Human Becoming: Parse's Theory of Nursing, *Nursing Science Quarterly* 5 (1992): 35–42.

28. S. Baumann, Contrasting Two Approaches in a Community-Based Nursing Practice with Older Adults: The Medical Model and Parse's Nursing Theory, *Nursing Science Quarterly* 10 (1997): 124–130.

29. N. Janes and D. Wells, Elderly Patients' Experiences with Nurses Guided by Parse's Theory of Human Becoming, *Clinical Nursing Research* 6 (1997): 205–222.

30. T. Meehan, Therapeutic Touch as a Nursing Intervention, *Journal of Advanced Nursing* 28 (1998): 117–125.

31. J. Turner et al., The Effect of Therapeutic Touch on Pain and Anxiety in Burn Patients, *Journal of Advanced Nursing* 28 (1998): 10–20.

32. B. Daley, Therapeutic Touch, Nursing Practice and Contemporary Cutaneous Wound Healing Research, *Journal of Advanced Nursing* 25 (1997): 1123–1132.

33. D. Wirth et al., Multisite Electrolyographic Analysis of Therapeutic Touch and Qigong Therapy, *Journal of Alternative and Complementary Medicine* 3 (1997): 109–118.

34. K. Olson and J. Hanson, Using Reiki To Manage Pain: A Preliminary Report, *Cancer Prevention and Control* 1 (1997): 108–113.

35. Olson and Hanson, Using Reiki To Manage Pain.

36. AHNA, Description of Holistic Nursing.

37. AHNA, Description of Holistic Nursing.

VISION OF HEALING
Questioning the Rules of Science

Nothing is more important about the quantum physics principle than this, that it destroys the concepts of the world as "sitting out there," with the observer safely separated from it. . . . To describe what has happened, one has to cross out that old word "observer," and put in its place the new word "participator." In some strange sense the Universe is a participatory universe.[1]

*   *   *

Nurses traditionally have relied on accumulated practice experience as though it were synonymous with knowledge. Nothing is more effective in shaking this belief system loose than a confrontation with the fact that not everyone's experience leads to the same conclusion.[2]

*   *   *

We are a peculiar people, we European/North Americans. We often demand to know why and how something works before we ask if it does. It isn't enough for us to experience something and to accept it. We can't accept something of value until we are convinced that it is logical, that the system fits within some preconceived mechanism or that it has been "proven" (by someone else) to work. We have even developed a unique system, the scientific method, to prove things. Science has become one of the special religions of our culture: it both regulates and comforts us.[3]

*   *   *

Great discoveries have been made by means of experiments devised with complete disregard for well-accepted beliefs.[4]

NOTES

1. J.A. Wheeler, Not Consciousness but Distinction between the Probe and the Probed as Central to the Elemental Quantum Level of Observations, in *Role of Consciousness in the Physical World*, ed. R. Jahn (Boulder, CO: Westview Press, 1981), 87–111.

2. F.S. Downs, Relationship of Findings of Clinical Research and Development of Criteria: A Researcher's Perspective, *Nursing Research* 29(1980):94–97.

3. S. Eabry, *Massage* 47(1994):36.

4. W.I.B. Beveridge, *The Art of Scientific Investigation* (New York: Vintage Books, 1957).

Chapter 9

Holistic Nursing Research

Cathie E. Guzzetta

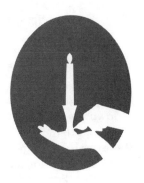

NURSE HEALER OBJECTIVES

Theoretical

- Discuss ways in which the wellness model has redirected priorities in nursing research.
- Compare and contrast qualitative and quantitative research methods.
- Read a qualitative research study (e.g., references 24 and 30 at the end of this chapter) and identify the holistic implications.

Clinical

- Collect data from various clients who are participating in some form of complementary and alternative therapies to determine their subjective evaluation of their outcomes.
- Discuss ways to enhance holistic research with a nurse researcher.
- Explore ways to establish a research-based practice in your clinical setting.
- Design a holistic research study based on one of the questions found in the section, "Directions for Future Research," at the end of this chapter.

Personal

- Read a research study on the effects of an alternative therapy (e.g., references 38 and 48 at the end of this chapter).

- Set aside some time to learn more about research methods.
- Attend a research conference.

DEFINITIONS

Heisenberg's Uncertainty Principle: the idea that one cannot look at a physical object without changing it.

Meta-analysis: a statistical technique that combines the results of many studies related to a topic to establish an overall estimate of the therapeutic effectiveness of an intervention.

Placebo: a medically inert medication, preparation, treatment, technique, or ritual that has no specific effects on the body and is intended to have no therapeutic value.

Qualitative Research: a systematic, subjective form of research that is used to describe life experiences and give them meaning. Qualitative research focuses on understanding the whole, which is consistent with the philosophy of holistic nursing.

Quantitative Research: a systematic, formal, objective form of research in which numerical data are used to obtain information about the world. Quantitative research embodies the principles of the scientific method and is used to describe variables, examine relationships among variables, and determine cause-

and-effect interactions between variables.

Reductionism: the approach of breaking down phenomena to their smallest possible parts.

Research: a diligent, systematic inquiry or investigation to validate and refine existing knowledge and generate new knowledge.

Triangulation: the use of multiple research techniques to collect and evaluate data on a specific topic in order to converge on a complete representation of reality and confirm the credibility of the research findings.

WELLNESS MODEL

The framework of client/patient nursing research is shifting from an illness to a wellness model of health care. The wellness model views individuals holistically as bio-psycho-social-spiritual units who assume responsibility for their own health. This model emphasizes the enormous potential that each individual has in healing his or her own body-mind-spirit. A significant body of research provides evidence of the enormous effects of consciousness on both health and illness. Investigations have shown that complementary and alternative therapies have the exciting potential to prevent illness and maintain high-level wellness. In addition, such research has been instrumental in guiding the development of humanistic and holistic approaches to health care. The challenge for nursing is to apply these findings in nursing practice.[1]

HOLISTIC RESEARCH METHODS

Quantitative Research

Research can be defined as a diligent, systematic inquiry or investigation to validate and refine existing knowledge as well as to generate new knowledge.[2] Descartes'

teachings in the seventeenth century did much to advance the use of the scientific method in medical research as we know it today.[3] His notion of reductionism in research—the idea of breaking down every question to its smallest possible parts—has been immensely beneficial in isolating those factors responsible for disease. For example, the physiologic part of a human being can be divided into organs, cells, and biochemical substances, then into molecular, atomic, and subatomic levels. Such an approach is useful for identifying the cause of disease (e.g., the finding that a virus causes acquired immune deficiency syndrome [AIDS]) and offers direction for studying the cure of disease (e.g., the use of antibodies to kill the bacteria associated with endocarditis).

Quantitative research is a systematic, formal, objective process in which numerical data are used to obtain information about the world. Embodying the principles of the scientific method, quantitative research involves (1) descriptive research, used to describe phenomena; (2) correlational research, used to examine relationships between and among variables; (3) quasi-experimental research, used to explain relationships, examine causal relationships, and clarify the reasons for events; and (4) experimental research, used to examine cause-and-effect relationships between variables.[4] It is the most commonly used method of scientific inquiry.

The gold standard in biomedical research is the randomized clinical trial (RCT), which includes elements of randomization, an experimental intervention, a control or placebo group, and blinding (often in the case of drug trials) in which neither the patient nor the investigator knows whether the patient is receiving the experimental treatment or placebo.[5] Randomized clinical trials are used in biomedical research because the design is believed to control threats to the internal and external validity of the study and, thus, to allow inferences about cause-and-effect relationships.[6] The internal validity of a study refers to the extent that it is possible to infer that the experimental treatment, rather than uncontrolled factors, is responsible for the outcome in a study. External validity refers to the generalizability of the findings to other samples and settings.[7] Thus, if a study has been properly designed and controlled, the quantitative method makes it possible to generalize the results obtained in one study to other, similar client populations and to replicate the results in similar studies. The key issue of the quantitative method is its ability to predict and control outcomes.

It has been argued that the RCT may not be the preferred strategy for evaluating holistic and complementary therapies because many of the therapies are not testable under blinded conditions, the choice of an appropriate control condition is not always clear, and eliminating threats to internal and external validity may not be ethically possible.[8] Thus, in holistic nursing, various quasi-experimental approaches, which may actually have greater internal or external validity than some RCTs, can also be used to produce important scientific findings characterizing cause-and-effect relationships.[9]

Biomedical research using quantitative methods abounds as scientists seek to identify unknown causes and cures for physiologic (and sometimes psychologic) illnesses. Efforts to find answers at the molecular level to such problems as the common cold, heart disease, cancer, AIDS, and essential hypertension, to name only a few, have consumed enormous numbers of personnel hours and dollars. Statistical analyses of isolated parts and group comparisons have indeed validated cause and effect in many cases. The quantitative method, however, does not take into account (1) the responses of the whole human being to variables, (2) the characteristics of one individual's pathway to a particular

problem, and (3) the unique patterns and interacting variables of one individual.[10] Thus, the distinctive features of unique individuals are lost in aggregate means, standard deviations, and various statistical analyses.[11] Historically, such distinctions have been deemed irrelevant in the biomedical paradigm.[12]

Qualitative Research

Current holistic and bodymind researchers have challenged the very roots of the biomedical paradigm. In his general systems theory (see Chapter 1), von Bertalanffy proposed that the study of systems requires an understanding of the whole rather than investigation of its separate parts. The field of psychoneuroimmunology has generated astounding research findings to support the interactive nature of psychophysiologic variables. There is conclusive evidence that thoughts and emotions affect the neurologic, endocrine, and immune systems at the cellular and subcellular levels. As a result, nurses have come to realize that the fit between quantitative methods and holistic nursing research is not always an ideal one.

Because quantitative methods seek to find answers only to parts of the whole, nurses have looked to alternative philosophies of science and research methods that are compatible with investigating humanistic and holistic phenomena.[13,14] Termed qualitative research, this approach is a systematic, subjective form of research that is used to describe and promote an understanding of human experiences such as health, caring, loneliness, pain, and comfort.[15] It is used to investigate the context and meaning of observed patterns, producing a richly articulate, in-depth, and coherent understanding of the phenomenon. Qualitative methods are used when little information is known about a phenomenon or in areas that are difficult to measure.[16] Qualitative research focuses on understanding the whole, which is consistent with the philosophy of holistic nursing.[17-20]

Five major types of qualitative research frequently used by nurses are (1) phenomenology, which is used to describe an experience as the whole person lives it; (2) hermeneutics, which focuses on meaning and is used to access the sociocultural experiences of individuals; (3) ethnography, which is used to study a culture and the people within the culture; (4) grounded theory research, which is used to uncover the problems in a social situation and the way in which the persons involved handle them; and (5) historical research, which is used to describe or analyze events that occurred in the past in order to understand the present better.[21,22] For example, Parse and associates used the phenomenologic research approach to describe the experience of health. They conducted a study to discover a definition of health as people live and experience it in everyday life. They asked the question, What are the common elements in a feeling of health among several different age groups?[23] One hundred subjects between 20 and 45 years old wrote a description of their feelings, thoughts, and perceptions of the experience during an episode in which they felt healthy. The researchers used the subjects' actual words when reporting the findings. From the data collected, they identified 30 descriptive expressions of health (Table 9–1). Three central themes emerged from these 30 descriptors: spirited intensity, fulfilling inventiveness, and symphonic integrity. Based on these central themes, the researchers then formulated the following definition: "health is symphonic integrity manifested in the spirited intensity of fulfilling inventiveness."[24] The descriptors in the table are so rich that they provide a clear understanding of the lived experience of health and make it possible to develop a definition of health that is fuller and much more holistic than the traditional biomedical view of health defined as the "absence of disease."

Table 9–1 The Experience of Health—Descriptive Expressions from Participants in a Phenomenological Study

Spirited Intensity	Fulfilling Inventiveness	Symphonic Integrity
1. Being enthusiastic	1. Finishing a project that takes up time	1. Being at ease
2. Catching a second wind	2. Accomplishment	2. Feeling of worth
3. Exercising and walking	3. Winning the game of life	3. Enjoying own space at that moment
4. Feel in peak condition	4. Trying some new endeavor	4. Peaceful feeling inside while bicycling
5. Positive outlook on life	5. Feeling something enriching my life	5. A "just right" feeling about everything
6. Feeling of refreshment	6. Doing what I struggled for	6. Drinking in the beauty of the day
7. Feeling full of energy	7. Pushing a little extra	7. Peaceful attitude
8. A glowing light of energy burning brightly in my eyes	8. Feel successful as a person	8. Rhythmical, easy, warm
9. A whip the world feeling	9. Ability to extend to limits of endurance	9. Glowing and good inside
10. A surge of energy	10. Accomplishing something	10. Feeling loved

Source: Reprinted with permission from R.R. Parse, A.B. Coyne, and M.J. Smith, *Nursing Research: Qualitative Methods,* p. 32, © 1985, Appleton and Lange.

It has taken centuries to generate convincing data that refute the idea of a separation between the body and the mind. Many health care professionals remain tied to the biomedical model, however, and perceive holistic principles and their corresponding research approaches as unscientific. They have doubted the psychophysiologic link between mind and body because the primary evidence supporting the link has been provided in the form of anecdotes or personal testimonials. "Hard core" researchers who embrace the quantitative method have not placed much value on the "softer" data obtained from qualitative studies. Even when quantitative studies support the link, questions arise about their retrospective designs, methodologic problems, or lack of measurement tools with psychometric properties.[25]

It is clear that, before the bodymind link is universally accepted, additional research is necessary. By virtue of their day-to-day care of clients, nurses are in a unique position to observe, document, quantify, and analyze the interactive relationship of variables in health and illness. The value of qualitative research methods will undoubtedly increase as important bodymind variables are discovered. The respectability of qualitative research findings will also increase as the authors of nursing research texts dedicate more attention to this content area, as research journal editors accept more qualitative studies for publication, and as more qualitative studies attract federal funding.[26] Moreover, the results of qualitative studies are supplying quantitative researchers with a plethora of potential research hypotheses that can be used as the focus for future investigations.

Qualitative and quantitative methods, however, should not be viewed from an either/or perspective. Both methodologies are needed in holistic research.[27] Both are important in scientific investigation (Exhibits 9–1 and 9–2). Often, qualitative findings augment the significance of quantitative results to enhance a real-world understanding of the results even when findings are statistically insignificant.[28] For example, Curtis and Wessberg found no physiologic changes when they evaluated various forms of self-regulation therapies, but their subjects reported positive

Exhibit 9–1 Quantitative and Qualitative Research Characteristics

Quantitative Research	*Qualitative Research*
Hard science	Soft science
Focus: concise and narrow	Focus: complex and broad
Reductionistic	Holistic
Objective	Subjective
Reasoning: logistic, deductive	Reasoning: dialectic, inductive
Basis of knowing: cause-and-effect relationships	Basis of knowing: meaning, discovery
Tests theory	Develops theory
Control	Shared interpretation
Instruments	Communication and observation
Basic element of analysis: numbers	Basic element of analysis: words
Statistical analysis	Individual interpretation
Generalization	Uniqueness

Source: Reprinted with permission from N. Burns and S.K. Grove, *The Practice of Nursing Research: Conduct, Critique and Utilization,* p. 27, © 1993, W.B. Saunders.

Exhibit 9–2 Investigating an Apple: A Quantitative vs. a Qualitative Approach

Quantitative Approach

A **quantitative** researcher might examine an apple by
    Inspecting the apple closely
    Carefully weighing it
    Cutting into it
    Separating the skin from the meat and
        Weighing each
        Analyzing each for sugar, salt, water, fiber, calories, vitamins, and then statistically analyzing
            the differences between the skin and the meat
    Counting the seeds and examining the inside of the seeds

Qualitative Approach

A **qualitative** researcher might examine an apple by
    Looking at the apple from all sides, top, and bottom
    Feeling it
    Smelling it
    Shining it
    Rolling it
    Appreciating its wholeness
    Biting into it, eating it, and enjoying it, describing its
        Sound
        Taste
        Texture
        Temperature
    Planting its seeds to determine what they might produce

Note: The author wishes to thank Elizabeth H. Winslow, PhD, RN, FAAN, for sharing this example.

evaluations of these therapies.[29] Thus, a rich, promising, and holistic source of data lies within the subjects' own estimates of their behavior and outcomes. Meaning and quality of life are essential tenets of the holistic model, and qualitative methods are well suited to tapping this subjective source of data.[30]

ENHANCING HOLISTIC RESEARCH

Triangulation

Researchers can use several strategies in planning studies to enhance the completeness and holistic nature of their investigations. For example, triangulation methodologies involve both holistic and multidimensional approaches to collect and evaluate data on a specific topic in a way that ensures a complete representation of reality and strengthens the credibility of the research results.[31] These methodologies, which are compatible with good science and holistic research, include data source triangulation, methodologic triangulation, investigator triangulation, interdisciplinary triangulation, theory triangulation, and analyses triangulation.[32]

Data source triangulation strengthens the rigor of the research by using several sources of data to assess a single clinical phenomenon. For example, in a study evaluating the effects of family presence at the bedside during cardiopulmonary resuscitation (CPR),[33] researchers conducted interviews with family members, nurses, and physicians present during the event to determine the benefits and problems of the experience from the perspective of all those involved. In addition to the interviews conducted in this study, questionnaires, attitude scales, and observations of family behavior during bedside visitation were also used. In this example of methodologic triangulation, the qualitative findings (identification of themes emerging from the interviews) confirmed and validated the quantitative findings (scores on the attitude scale, yes/no responses tallied from the questionnaire, and observations of family behavior). The understanding of the family presence experience, therefore, was more complete than if only one of the strategies had been used alone.[34] Likewise in this study, investigator triangulation played a role, because there were several clinical nurse co-investigators, a nurse research consultant, and a qualitative nurse researcher, who all independently evaluated the data and then collaboratively interpreted the findings on the families' and health care providers' perception of the experience. Interdisciplinary triangulation, collaboration between two or more investigators from different disciplines to examine a phenomenon, was also a factor, as a nurse–physician team developed the family presence study. The nurse and the physician later evaluated the results of the data collection independently and then collaborated in interpreting the findings based on their professional orientation to yield a more comprehensive perspective of the benefits and problems of family presence.[35]

Theory triangulation uses two or more conceptual frameworks to examine the phenomenon under study. For example, in a recent study examining the reasons that individuals use complementary and alternative therapies, researchers used health belief, motivational, and holistic theories to interpret predictors of complementary and alternative therapy use.[36] Data analysis triangulation involves the use of two or more methods of data analysis to evaluate a phenomenon. For example, regression analyses could be used to predict the effects of three kinds of distraction on pain, and analysis of variance could be used to determine any differences among the three types of distraction.[37]

Psychophysiologic Measurement Tools

The holistic researcher will quickly discover the shortage of holistic instruments available to measure outcomes. If holistic and complementary therapies have the ability to affect an individual's body-mind-spirit, however, it is reasonable to believe that it should be possible to measure these effects. Yet, too often, researchers have studied body effects or mind effects, but rarely have they studied the interaction and relationship between the two.

The various physiologic instruments available to study the effects of holistic and complementary therapies are often used in combination to develop a physiologic profile of observed outcomes. Researchers tend to use psychologic instruments with less confidence, on the other hand, viewing them as less reliable and less valid than their physiologic counterparts. Many of the psychologic instruments currently available are not sensitive enough to demonstrate the subtle, yet significant, psychologic changes that occur with complementary therapies. The finding that a psychologic indicator is not significant does not necessarily disprove the existence of a significant psychologic effect. It may indicate that the wrong variable was studied or that the psychologic tool used was not sufficiently sensitive to measure the effect.

Holistic and complementary therapies influence many psychophysiologic parameters, but they do not necessarily influence the same variables in different individuals. Thus, a number of parameters must be used to evaluate the outcomes of these interventions satisfactorily.[38] Psychologic and physiologic outcomes should be used in combination and the effects of these outcomes should be correlated as a means of increasing the validity of the findings and discovering bodymind links. Psychologic and physiologic measurements should be combined in developing new psychophysiologic tools. More quantitative tools to study holistic phenomena such as health beliefs, functional status, comfort, dyspnea, dependency, and appraisal of stressors are appearing in the literature.[39-45] In addition, a variety of visual analog and numerical rating scales, diaries, logs, and graphs can be used to capture the holistic, longitudinal, and individualized perceptions of patient experiences.[46]

A current research mandate is to develop instruments that facilitate assessment, diagnosis, and selection of nursing interventions, as well as measure the effectiveness of interventions designed to enhance body-mind-spirit outcomes.[47] Nurses have the knowledge and ability to contribute significantly to this task by using both quantitative and qualitative research methodologies.

Multimodal Interventions

Quantitative intervention studies can be approached more holistically by taking into consideration the interactive nature of the patient's body-mind-spirit. Many of the holistic and complementary interventions, when used in combination as a multimodal intervention, may have a more powerful effect on outcomes than any one intervention used alone. For example, the combination of relaxation techniques and music therapy has been shown to be effective in producing the relaxation response, particularly in anxious patients; a head-to-toe relaxation script is used first to reduce muscle tension, and then soothing music is added to enhance relaxation.[48] A current study is evaluating the effects of distraction combined with positioning (i.e., child–parent chest-to-chest sitting position) on the pain and distress of small children undergoing venipuncture.[49] It was believed that distraction combined with positioning and parental support would be more effective than either one of these interventions alone. Likewise, much of the work in biofeedback has increasingly added abdominal breathing, the quieting response, progressive muscle relaxation, autogenic training, imagery, and music to the biofeedback protocol to enhance client outcomes.[50]

Ornish, a cardiologist, and associates conducted two landmark, controlled, randomized clinical studies to determine the effects of a holistic, comprehensive, lifestyle change intervention program for patients with coronary artery disease.[51,52] For the experimental group, current state-of-the-art knowledge on preventing heart disease related to diet, exercise, support groups, and stress reduction was the basis for the intervention. Subjects in the control group were treated with traditional medical approaches. Both groups were similar at the start of the study regarding demographic characteristics and disease severity. The outcomes of the study were determined by angiographic measurement of the size of coronary artery lesions after the first year of intervention and measurement of the size and severity of perfusion abnormalities using positron emission tomography after the fifth year of intervention. The results were astonishing. Patients in the experimental group demonstrated significant regression of their coronary artery disease during the first year following intervention, whereas those in the control group demonstrated a significant progression of their disease.[53] Likewise, after 5 years, the size and severity of the myocardial perfusion abnormalities documented by tomography improved in patients in the experimental group and worsened in control group patients.[54]

Until these studies were conducted, researchers had been unable to demonstrate regression of coronary artery lesions. Both studies were successful because the interventions used addressed the whole patient and the interactive nature of each patient's biologic, psychologic, sociologic, and spiritual dimensions. The researchers did not try to isolate the effects of diet, exercise, support groups, and stress reduction as is done in most investigations. Rather, Ornish put these elements together in a holistic, multimodal intervention package. Which part of the intervention was most effective? No one knows for sure. Could it be that the interactive nature of the interventions was more powerful than any one of the interventions alone in helping patients to repattern their pathways toward wellness? It appears that such holistic, multimodal, interactive interventions were responsible for reversing an outcome that had never before been changed.

Objectivity in Scientific Investigation

Most researchers accept the universal principle that objectivity must govern scientific inquiry. Heisenberg, who studied information obtained from an electron, has shaken this belief, however. His uncertainty principle states that it is impossible to look at a physical object without changing it,[55] which suggests that objects and clients change when researchers observe them. The holistic researcher realizes the enormous implications of this principle: researchers do not stand apart from the research or research subject, but rather are part of the research. They are not objective observers of the world, but rather participants in that world. This participation, in turn, affects the results that they obtain through research. Their participation may be a word, an action, a touch, an observation, or simply their presence. The researcher becomes an integral part of the experiment and its outcomes. The term *nonparticipant observer* in research is, therefore, meaningless.

Heisenberg also postulated that it is not possible to obtain a complete description of a physical object because describing it changes it. Thus, it is impossible to obtain all the data that describe an object; some information will always be unknown.[56] Observations verify research effects, but, if it is impossible to obtain a complete description of a physical object, some outcomes will be unknown. It is misleading to suggest that research can always be validated in terms of testable or observable effects. The effects of a certain experiment, whether they are observable or not, will ultimately affect the subject.[57]

Certain phenomena related to holistic research may not be accessible to scientific investigation because they cannot be objectively measured. The individual who experiences certain effects while using alternative therapies, for example, may be unable to conceptualize or express them or unable to translate or communicate these effects to another. Likewise, the researcher may be unable to interpret the effects because he or she lacks experience with these effects or because our language is inadequate for describing and communicating these phenomena.

The Placebo Response

Scientists have often viewed the placebo response as a nuisance and an unreliable factor that distorts research results. Many have assumed that a placebo is effective only when the illness is somehow unreal. Recently, however, we have begun to understand the power of the placebo effect and the mechanisms involved.[58]

Placebo means "I will please." The term refers to a medically inert preparation or treatment that has no specific effects on the body and is intended to have no therapeutic benefit. Yet, this medically inert substance or treatment can evoke a placebo response, relieving pain or dramatically affecting the patient's symptoms or disease.

The placebo response has been studied for several decades in a variety of patients. In an analysis of 15 double-blind studies, placebo medications were found to be effective in pain relief for 35 percent of patients with postoperative pain.[59] An analysis of 11 more recent double-blind studies in which 36 percent of the patients received at least 50 percent pain relief from placebos confirmed these findings.[60] In addition, the worse the pain or the more stressful the situation, the more effective the placebo.[61] The placebo effect may be even higher than these findings indicate. One study indicated that approximately 70 percent of patients in preliminary trials of five new promising medical treatments (for asthma, ulcers, and herpes) showed symptomatic improvements,[62] although later the treatments proved useless. It appears that, for more than one-third of clients, and probably for even more, the pharmacologically inert placebo is able to activate bodymind healing mechanisms.[63,64]

The placebo response also has been found to be present in the following conditions and therapeutic procedures, demonstrating the mind's ability to produce neurohormonal messenger molecules that alter the autonomic, endocrine, and immune systems:[65]

- hypertension, stress, cardiac pain, blood cell counts, headaches, pupillary dilation (suggesting the mind's ability to alter the autonomic nervous system)
- adrenal gland secretion, diabetes, ulcers, gastric secretion and motility, colitis, oral contraceptive use, menstrual pain, thyrotoxicosis (suggesting the mind's ability to alter the endocrine system)
- the common cold, fever, vaccinations, asthma, multiple sclerosis, rheumatoid arthritis, warts, cancer (suggesting the mind's ability to alter the immune system)

- surgical treatments (e.g., for reducing angina pectoris)
- biofeedback instrumentation and various medical devices
- psychologic treatments, such as conditioning (systematic desensitization) and perhaps all forms of psychotherapy
- making an appointment to see a physician

Thus, the placebo response, also called the general healing response, is a common mechanism that occurs because of a communication link between the body and the mind that is probably present in all clinical situations.[66] Furthermore, the placebo response probably exists, more or less, in each one of us.

It is known that how a drug is given or how a procedure is performed and by whom can affect the intensity of the placebo response. Therefore, the faith that the client has in the caregiver and the client's expectation that the drug or therapy will work greatly influence the placebo response. Likewise, the faith that the caregiver conveys to the client regarding the drug or therapy, as well as the trust and rapport established between the two, affects the placebo response.[67-69]

It is time to recognize the powerful effects of the placebo. Nurses must learn to incorporate the placebo response in their research and their clinical practice to maximize its potential. To enhance the placebo response when administering medications, for example, nurses can discuss with their clients the medication's known potency and effectiveness. When patients receive morphine intravenously for chest pain, nurses can ask them to visualize the molecules of this powerful, pain-killing medicine traveling through their veins to the source of the chest pain. Nurses can suggest that clients work to enhance the medication's effectiveness by allowing the relaxed, warm, and comfortable feeling associated with the morphine to flow throughout their bodies.[70]

The essence of the placebo response involves positive attitudes and emotions.[71] Many alternative therapies, such as imagery, music therapy, relaxation, and exercise, increase endorphin production.[72] When clients believe that they are doing something to enhance healing, their endorphin levels can rise. Therefore, clients can influence the course of their own illnesses and their responses to therapy by using their own consciousness.[73] Because basic nursing interventions such as touching, giving back rubs, teaching, positioning, and distracting all have the potential to raise endorphin levels, it is critical that nurses discuss with their clients the possible therapeutic benefits of each therapy as a part of research protocols and practice. When nurses realize that what they say to clients can augment the placebo response, they will develop new communication skills to enhance their clients' healing responses and maximize the benefits of their nursing interventions.

RESEARCH-BASED PRACTICE

Need To Conduct Research

The holistic care of clients must be based on the results of research for several reasons. Research provides the direction for selecting interventions with proved effectiveness. When nurses implement interventions that have been proved effective, patient outcomes are improved. In addition, in this day of cost containment, health care providers must ensure that the care provided makes a positive difference in the lives of their patients. Unfortunately, much of what nurses do is based on tradition, rituals, and the way they were taught, with little research evidence to support such actions.

One of the central arguments against using complementary and alternative therapies is that the efficacy of most of these therapies has not been proved.[74,75] Yet, many practitioners are surprised to learn that most conventional medical practices also have not been proved by research.[76,77] Smith estimated that only 15 percent of all biomedical interventions are validated by reliable scientific evidence and, in fact, most orthodox interventions have never been researched at all.[78] Interventions that are widely practiced, but have no research support, include episiotomy, laparoscopic vaginal hysterectomy, and radial keratotomy.[79] Thus, it is important to realize that research is needed in both the conventional and complementary domains of health care.[80]

In nursing, there is much work to do. Many holistic and complementary therapies have been used to treat a variety of problems in diverse settings, but their appropriateness and adequacy in various populations and settings have not been investigated fully. There is a great need to determine under what conditions holistic and complementary therapies are the treatment of choice, for which particular client/patient, and with what type of clinical problem.[81] Comparative outcome studies also are needed to determine the usefulness, indications, contraindications, and dangers of such therapies.[82] Moreover, the effectiveness of these interventions, as they are integrated with conventional treatments, requires evaluation not only in treating various illnesses, but also in promoting high-level wellness and preventing illness.

With the creation of the National Center for Complementary and Alternative Medicine (NCCAM) by the National Institutes of Health (NIH), many complementary and alternative therapies are now undergoing scientific evaluation to determine whether they affect the clinical course and outcomes of an illness or whether they enhance wellness.[83] Some traditional researchers are not happy that federal monies are being used to support this kind of research. Yet, approximately 40 percent of U.S. citizens use some form of alternative therapy, and they are spending enormous amounts of out-of-pocket money.[84–86] It appears that the public is looking for something more in health care—humanistic, holistic approaches that address their body-mind-spirit needs.[87] For these reasons, the time has come to determine which of these therapies are beneficial and effective in health care.

To date, the NCCAM has funded many studies to evaluate such therapies as acupressure, massage therapy, electrochemical treatment, hypnosis, music therapy, guided imagery, biofeedback, prayer, and administration of antioxidants. In addition, the NCCAM has established 13 research centers in complementary and alternative medicine to study the effects of such therapies on major health conditions (e.g., addictions, aging, asthma, allergy and immunology, cardiovascular diseases, cancer, chiropractic, general medical conditions, human immunodeficiency virus [HIV] and AIDS, pain, pediatric conditions, stroke and neurologic conditions, and women's health issues).[88] The results of these studies will provide the scientific basis for determining which complementary and alternative therapies work, which ones do not work, which ones are harmful, and, most important, which ones improve patient outcomes.

Research Utilization

Some areas of nursing practice do have research support. Unfortunately, often such findings are not incorporated into clinical practice. To ensure that nursing practice is based on research, clinical policies, procedures, and standards of practice need to reflect the results of valid and reliable studies and other up-to-date research-based information. Such information can be found from practice guidelines developed by expert consensus, federal and professional groups, journal and review articles, and current procedure manuals and books.[89]

Current state-of-the-art knowledge of several complementary and alternative therapies has been reviewed. For example, an NIH Technology Assessment Panel has evaluated the research supporting the use of behavioral and relaxation interventions in the treatment of chronic pain and insomnia.[90] The panel found strong evidence to indicate that the use of relaxation, meditation, and hypnosis is beneficial in the treatment of chronic pain. Likewise, there was strong evidence to support the use of behavioral techniques such as autogenic training, meditation, progressive muscle relaxation, and biofeedback for the treatment of insomnia. In addition, the NIH sponsored a Consensus Development Conference on Acupuncture, which found acupuncture effective in treating adult postoperative and chemotherapy nausea and vomiting, as well as postoperative dental pain.[91]

Systematic reviews also synthesize the evidence on a given topic, even if the results are inconclusive or conflicting, because such reviews generally point out where knowledge gaps exist.[92] In 1996, for example, the NCCAM funded a complementary medicine field within the Cochrane Collaboration, an international network of individuals and institutions committed to prepare, maintain, and disseminate systematic reviews on all topics of health care.[93] To date, systematic reviews (when possible, meta-analyses) have been completed on acupuncture, massage, homeopathy, and herbal medicine, with additional reviews planned in the future for acupuncture, herbs, manual therapies, music therapy, therapeutic touch, and yoga.[94]

Meta-analysis is a statistical technique that establishes an overall estimate of the therapeutic effectiveness of an intervention by combining the results of many experiments related to that intervention. The final conclusions generally are stronger than those provided in systematic reviews because meta-analysis takes into account factors such as sample size, strength of the experimental methods, and threats to internal and external validity, using both qualitative and quantitative interpretations.[95] Meta-analyses allow inferences to be made about the currently known effectiveness of a treatment and provide valuable information to researchers in planning future clinical studies. For example, nine studies were included in a meta-analysis on the effects of effleurage backrub on the physiologic components of relaxation. From this analysis it was concluded that effleurage backrubs of at least 3 minutes are an effective nonpharmacologic nursing intervention that promotes biologic and subjective relaxation. The findings were convincing enough for the authors to recommend that this traditional nursing activity be revitalized and implemented once again in clinical practice.[96]

Research-based information obtained from consensus and professional groups, systematic review articles, and meta-analyses is valuable for updating clinical policies and procedures, making decisions about clinical practice routines, changing clinical practice, and developing new clinical studies. Use of research findings alone, however, is not adequate in providing compassionate, effective care of patients. Decisions about the care of individual patients also must be based on the caregiver's educational knowledge and experience, as well as on patient preferences.[97]

CONCLUSION

Nurses have come to realize that the fit between traditional research methods and holistic nursing principles is not always a good one. The shift to the wellness model has caused the profession to take a new look at research priorities, methodologies, and findings. As a result, nurses have discovered that quantitative and qualitative strategies can be used in combination to gain a more complete understanding of human phenomena.

DIRECTIONS FOR FUTURE RESEARCH

1. Evaluate the complementary and alternative therapies that may potentially promote wellness behaviors in specific client populations.
2. Determine whether complementary and alternative therapies can be combined to augment their effectiveness in achieving desired client outcomes (e.g., combining relaxation with biofeedback or music therapy with imagery and progressive relaxation).
3. Determine the most effective way to integrate complementary and alternative therapies with traditional modes of therapy to achieve optimal client outcomes.
4. Identify the alternative therapies that are most complementary and effective for individuals with a specific problem or illness.

NURSE HEALER REFLECTIONS

After reading this chapter, the nurse healer will be able to answer or will begin a process of answering the following questions:

- How do I feel about the importance of research in advancing holistic nursing practice?
- What is my role in nursing research?
- How can I become more involved in holistic clinical research?

NOTES

1. P. Flynn, *Holistic Health: The Art and Science of Care* (Bowie, MD: Brady Co., 1980), 1–8.

2. N. Burns and S.K. Grove, *The Practice of Nursing Research: Conduct, Critique, and Utilization*, 2d ed. (Philadelphia: W.B. Saunders, 1993), 3.

3. L. Dossey, *Space, Time, and Medicine* (Boston: Shambhala, 1982), 12–14.

4. Burns and Grove, *The Practice of Nursing Research*, 26, 29–30.

5. A. Vickers, Old Myths Given New Voice: The Nuffeild Report: Researching and Evaluating Complementary Therapies: The State of the Debate, *Complementary Therapies in Medicine* 4 (1996):198–201.

6. R.J. Gatchell and A.M. Maddrey, Clinical Outcomes Research in Complementary and Alternative Medicine: An Overview of Experimental Design and Analysis, *Alternative Therapies in Health and Medicine* 4, no. 5 (1998):36–42.

7. D. Polit and B.P Hungler, *Essentials of Nursing Research: Methods, Appraisal, and Utilization* (Philadelphia: Lippincott-Raven, 1997).

8. A. Margolin et al., Investigating Alternative Medicine Therapies in Randomized Controlled Trials, *Journal of the American Medical Association* 280, no. 18 (1998):1626–1628.

9. Gatchell and Maddrey, Clinical Outcomes Research, 39.

10. D.F. Bockmon and D.J. Riemen, Qualitative versus Quantitative Nursing Research, *Holistic Nursing Practice* 2, no. 1 (1987):71–75.

11. D. Lukoff et al., The Case Study as a Scientific Method for Researching Alternative Therapies, *Alternative Therapies in Health and Medicine* 4, no. 2 (1998):44–52.

12. C.C. Clark, *Wellness Nursing: Concepts, Theory, Research, and Practice* (New York: Springer, 1986), 318.

13. M.A. Newman, *Health as Expanding Consciousness* (St. Louis: C.V. Mosby, 1986), 91–96.

14. M.C. Silva and D. Rothbart, An Analysis of Changing Trends in Philosophies of Science on Nursing Theory Development and Testing, *Advances in Nursing Science* 6, no. 2 (1984):1–13.

15. Burns and Grove, *The Practice of Nursing Research*, 27.

16. M. Sandelowski, "To Be of Use": Enhancing the Utility of Qualitative Research, *Nursing Outlook* 45 (1997):125–132.

17. Polit and Hungler, *Essentials of Nursing Research*, 200–205.

18. M. Sandelowski, Rigor or Rigor Mortis: The Problem of Rigor in Qualitative Research Revisited, *Advances in Nursing Science* 16, no. 2 (1993):1–8.

19. L. Mehl, *Mind and Matter: Foundations for Holistic Health* (Berkeley, CA: Mindbody Press, 1981), 74.

20. Clark, *Wellness Nursing*, 318.

21. Burns and Grove, *The Practice of Nursing Research*, 30–31.

22. N. Denzin and Y. Lincoln, eds., *Handbook of Qualitative Research* (Thousand Oaks, CA: Sage, 1994).

23. R.R. Parse et al., The Lived Experience of Health: A Phenomenological Study, in *Nursing Research: Qualitative Methods*, ed. R.R. Parse et al. (East Norwalk, CT: Appleton & Lange, 1985), 27.

24. R.R. Parse et al., The Lived Eperience of Health, 31.

25. C.E. Guzzetta, The Human Factor and the Ailing Heart: Folklore or Fact? (Editorial), *Journal of Intensive Care Medicine* 2, no. 1 (1987):3–5.

26. Bockmon and Riemen, Qualitative versus Quantitative Nursing Research, 71–74.

27. L.C. Dzurec and I.L. Abraham, The Nature of Inquiry: Linking Quantitative and Qualitative Research, *Advances in Nursing Science* 16, no. 1 (1993):73–79.

28. D. Weinholtz et al., Salvaging Quantitative Research with Qualitative Data, *Qualitative Health Research* 5 (1995):388–397.

29. W.D. Curtis and H.W. Wessberg, A Comparison of Heart Rate, Respiration, and Galvanic Skin Response among Meditators, Relaxers, and Controls, *Journal of Altered States of Consciousness* 2 (1975/76):319.

30. C.O. Boyd and P.C. Munhall, A Qualitative Investigation of Reassurance, *Holistic Nursing Practice* 4, no. 1 (1989):61–69.

31. Polit and Hungler, *Essentials of Nursing Research*.

32. D. Hamilton and G.A. Bechtel, Research Implications for Alternative Health Therapies, *Nursing Forum* 31, no. 1 (1996):6–10.

33. T.A. Meyers et al., Family Presence during Invasive Procedures and Resuscitation: Experiences of Family Members, Physicians, and Nurses, 1999 (unpublished).

34. B.J. Breitmayer et al., Triangulation of Qualitative Research: Evaluation of Completeness and

Confirmation Purposes, *Image* 25, no. 3 (1993): 237–243.

35. T.A. Meyers et al., Family Presence during Invasive Procedures and Resuscitation.

36. J. Astin, Why Patients Use Alternative Medicine: Results of a National Study, *Journal of the American Medical Association* 279, no. 19 (1998): 1548–1553.

37. Hamilton and Bechtel, Research Implications for Alternative Health Therapies.

38. P. Bohachick, Progressive Relaxation Training in Cardiac Rehabilitation: Effects of Psychologic Variables, *Nursing Research* 33 (1984):283–287.

39. K.Y. Kolcaba, Holistic Comfort: Operationalizing the Construct as a Nurse-Sensitive Outcome, *Advances in Nursing Science* 15, no. 1 (1992):1–10.

40. G.R. Parkerson et al., The Duke-UNC Health Profile: An Adult Health Status Instrument for Primary Care, *Medical Care* 19, no. 8 (1981):805–823.

41. V.L. Champion and C.R. Scott, Reliability and Validity of Breast Cancer Screening Belief Scales in African American Women, *Nursing Research* 46, no. 6 (1997):331–337.

42. S.C. Lareau et al., Development and Testing of the Modified Version of the Pulmonary Functional Status and Dyspnea Questionnaire, *Heart and Lung* 27, no. 3 (1998):150–168.

43. B. Riegel et al., Development of an Instrument To Measure Cardiac Illness Dependency, *Heart and Lung* 26, no. 6 (1997):448–457.

44. A.G. Gift and G. Narsavage, Validity of the Numeric Rating Scale as a Measure of Dyspnea, *American Journal of Critical Care* 7, no. 3 (1998):200–204.

45. M.A. Sevick et al., A Confirmatory Factor Analysis of the Caregiving Appraisal Scale for Caregivers of Home-Based Ventilator-Assisted Individuals, *Heart and Lung* 26, no. 6 (1997):430–438.

46. E.R. Giardino and Z.R. Wolf, Symptoms: Evidence and Experience, *Advances in Nursing Science* 7, no. 2 (1993):1–12.

47. Kolcaba, Holistic Comfort, 2.

48. C.E. Guzzetta, Effects of Relaxation and Music Therapy on Patients in a Coronary Care Unit with Presumptive Acute Myocardial Infarction, *Heart and Lung* 18 (1998):609–616.

49. K. Cavender et al., Effects of a Positioning-Distraction Intervention on Self-Reported Pain, Fear, and Behavioral Distress of Pediatric Patients Undergoing Venipuncture, Dallas, Texas: Children's Medical Center of Dallas, 1999.

50. M. Cowan et al., Self-Management Biofeedback Therapy for Sudden Cardiac Arrest Subjects: The Use of Process Variables, in *Nursing Research and Its Utilization*, ed. J.J. Fitzpatrick et al. (New York: Springer, 1994), 83–90.

51. D. Ornish, Can Lifestyle Changes Reverse Coronary Heart Disease? *Lancet* 336 (1990):129.

52. K.L. Gould et al., Changes in Myocardial Perfusion Abnormalities by Positron Emission Tomography after Long-Term, Intense Risk Factor Modification, *Journal of the American Medical Association* 274, no. 11 (1995):894–901.

53. D. Ornish, Can Lifestyle Changes Reverse Coronary Heart Disease?

54. Gould et al., Changes in Myocardial Perfusion Abnormalities.

55. W. Heisenberg, *Physics and Philosophy* (New York: Harper & Row, 1978), 42.

56. G. Zukav, *The Dancing Wu Li Masters: An Overview of the New Physics* (New York: William Morrow, 1979), 111–114.

57. C. Tart, *States of Consciousness* (New York: E.P. Dutton, 1975), 207–228.

58. C.E. Guzzetta and B.M. Dossey, *Cardiovascular Nursing: Holistic Practice* (St. Louis: Mosby-Year Book, 1992), 392–393.

59. H. Beecher, The Powerful Placebo, *Journal of the American Medical Association* 159 (1955):1602.

60. F. Evans, Expectancy, Therapeutic Instructions, and the Placebo Response, in *Placebo: Theory, Research, and Mechanism*, ed. L. White et al. (New York: Guilford Press, 1985).

61. L. Dossey, *Space, Time, and Medicine*.

62. A. Roberts, Placebo Therapies Spark "Improvement" for 7 of 10, *Brain Mind Bulletin* 18, no. 12 (1993):1.

63. J. Frank, Mind-Body Relationships in Illness and Healing, *Journal of Internal Academic Preventative Medicine* 2 (1975):46.

64. E. Rossi, *The Psychobiology of Mind-Body Healing* (New York: W.W. Norton, 1993), 15.

65. Rossi, *The Psychobiology of Mind-Body Healing*.

66. Rossi, *The Psychobiology of Mind-Body Healing*, 16.

67. A.H. Roberts, The Powerful Placebo Revisited: Magnitude of Nonspecific Effects, *Body/Mind Medicine* 1 (1995):35–43.

68. Frank, Mind-Body Relationships in Illness and Healing, 46.

69. L. Dossey, *Healing Words: The Power of Prayer and the Practice of Medicine* (San Francisco: HarperCollins, 1993), 134–135.

70. Guzzetta and Dossey, Cardiovascular Nursing: Holistic Practice, 392–393.

71. Rossi, The Psychobiology of Mind-Body Healing, 11–22.

72. C.B. Pert, Molecules of Emotion: Why You Feel the Way You Feel (New York: Charles Scribner's Sons, 1997).

73. L. Dossey, Space, Time, and Medicine, 36.

74. M. Angell and J.P. Kassirer, Alternative Medicine: The Risks of Untested and Unregulated Remedies, New England Journal of Medicine 339, no. 12 (1998):839–841.

75. P.B. Fontanarosa and G.D. Lundberg, Alternative Medicine Meets Science, Journal of the American Medical Association 280, no. 18 (1998):1618–1619.

76. L. Dossey, On Double-Blinds and Double Standards: A Response to the Recent New England Journal (Editorial), Alternative Therapies in Health and Medicine 4, no. 6 (1998):18–20.

77. D.A. Grimes, Technology Follies, Journal of the American Medical Association 269, no. 23 (1993):3030–3033.

78. R. Smith, Where Is the Wisdom, British Medical Journal 303 (1991):798–799.

79. Grimes, Technology Follies, 18.

80. W.B. Jonas, Alternative Medicine—Learning from the Past, Examining the Present, Advancing the Future, Journal of the American Medical Association 280, no. 18 (1998):1616–1617.

81. D.H. Shapiro, Overview: Clinical and Physiological Comparison of Meditation with Other Self-Control Strategies, American Journal of Psychiatry 139 (1982):267.

82. American Psychiatric Association, Position Statement on Meditation, American Journal of Psychiatry 134 (1977):720.

83. T. Cron, It's the Law: There Is an Office of Alternative Medicine, Alternative Medicine Newsletter 1, no. 1 (1993):1.

84. D. Eisenberg, Unconventional Medicine in the United States: Prevalence, Costs, and Patterns of Use, New England Journal of Medicine 328 (1993):246–252.

85. D.M. Eisenberg et al., Trends in Alternative Medicine Use in the United States, 1990–1997, Journal of the American Medical Association 280, no. 18 (1998):1569–1575.

86. Astin, Why Patients Use Alternative Medicine.

87. Astin, Why Patients Use Alternative Medicine.

88. Jonas, Alternative Medicine—Learning from the Past, Examining the Present, Advancing the Future.

89. M. Chulay, C.E. Guzzetta, B.M. Dossey, AACN Handbook of Critical Care Nursing (Stamford, CT: Appleton & Lange, 1997).

90. NIH Technology Assessment Panel on Integration of Behavioral and Relaxation Approaches into the Treatment of Chronic Pain and Insomnia, Integration of Behavioral and Relaxation Approaches into the Treatment of Chronic Pain and Insomnia, Journal of the American Medical Association 276, no. 4 (1996):313–318.

91. NIH, Consensus Development Statement on Acupuncture, NIH Consensus Statement Online, 15, no. 5 (1997):1–9.

92. J. Ezzo et al., Complementary Medicine and Cochrane Collaboration, Journal of the American Medical Association 280, no. 18 (1998):1628–1630.

93. L. Bero and D. Rennie, The Cochrane Collaboration: Preparing, Maintaining, and Disseminating Systematic Reviews on the Effects of Health Care, Journal of the American Medical Association 274, no. 24 (1995):1935–1938.

94. J. Ezzo et al., Complementary Medicine and Cochrane Collaboration, 1630.

95. Gatchell and Maddrey, Clinical Outcomes Research, 41.

96. S.E. Labyak and B.L. Metzger, The Effects of Effleurage Backrub on the Physiological Components of Relaxation: A Meta-Analysis, Nursing Research 46, no. 1 (1997):59–62.

97. G. Ellrodt et al., Evidence-Based Disease Management, Journal of the American Medical Association 278, no. 20 (1997):1687–1692.

CORE VALUE III
Holistic Nurse Self-Care

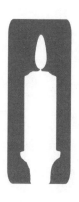

VISION OF HEALING
Toward the Inward Journey

The root word of healing and healer is "hael," which means to facilitate movement toward wholeness or to make whole on all levels—physical, mental, emotional, social, and spiritual. As sophisticated as our modern medical system is, there are no criteria for what constitutes healing. In fact, it often seems that there are two different sets of criteria for the evaluation of healing. One set of criteria looks at "the numbers" of biologic data; the other set is more subjective and assesses the experience of the client "feeling stronger" or "feeling better." If we use the root word in the true sense, healing incorporates both sets of criteria. The either/or—that is either a body problem or an emotional or spiritual problem—is a false dichotomy. There is no such thing, for the body-mind-spirit is a single integrated entity.

A healer is aware of the importance of understanding the belief systems of self and others. A healer recognizes that consciousness and the human spirit operates not only within a person, but also operates between and among individuals—between nurse and client, as well as among nurse, client, family, and colleagues. Nurses have the unique opportunity of being present to guide people in understanding meaning in their life, whether it be through wellness instruction, acute situational crisis intervention, chronic illness management, or the transition to peaceful death. Being present to guide and help the client in making connections of body-mind-spirit is healing. The clearest way to understand this interaction is through the concept of the nurse as a healer. The fundamental principle that a nurse follows to become a healer is skillfully bringing together inner resources of knowledge and intuition. The nurse healer must identify his or her own woundedness, the life polarities, and the purposes and meaning in life.

When nurses live and practice from a holistic perspective, they recognize that there is no separation between their personal and professional selves. As they expand their consciousness and repattern their lives with healing intention, they take into all aspects of their life and work a sense of sacredness. When nurses develop a sense of sacredness about their work and explore the state of "nurse as healing environment," then nurse healing is manifest at the highest level. As we challenge ourselves to understand more deeply the sacredness of our work and to understand ourselves as healing environments, we too are healed. We must reawaken our spirit and cultivate it if all the powers of our soul are to act together in perfect balance and harmony. There can never be any real opposition between spirituality and science, for one is the complement of the other. Self-knowledge brings us face to face with the mystery of our own being.

Chapter 10

The Nurse As an Instrument of Healing

Maggie McKivergin

NURSE HEALER OBJECTIVES

Theoretical

- Discuss the importance of the practice of presence as the essence of care on which to build nursing interventions.
- Compare and contrast different approaches to relationship-centered caring using the model of integrative theory.
- Assess the qualities and characteristics of an instrument of healing.

Clinical

- Identify opportunities in which to practice presence with self, clients, and colleagues.
- List the qualities that allow nurses to be most present with themselves and others.
- Discuss ways to create sacred space.
- Identify appropriate methods of intervention that will access an individual's inner healer/teacher.
- Assess one's personal skills as an instrument of healing and decide if there are areas that need improvement.

Personal

- Learn techniques to become more present and integrate these experiences into your daily life.

- Acknowledge your inner response when you are fully present with yourself and others.
- Align with qualities of becoming an instrument of healing for self and others, thus creating a healing environment that contributes to the overall good of the earth.

DEFINITIONS

Centeredness: a fine-tuned sensitivity to life's inner and outer patterns and processes;[1] a state of balance of self that allows optimum levels of attention and presence to the moment.

Chaos: a naturally occurring systemic pattern of uncontrolled activity whose direction cannot be predicted.[2]

Guide: one who helps others discover and recognize insights and healing awareness about their life journeys and priorities.[3]

Healing: the return of the integrity and wholeness of the natural state of an individual;[4] the emergence of right relationship at, between, and among all levels of the human being;[5] the process of bringing together parts of oneself (physical, mental, emotional, spiritual, relational) at deeper levels of inner knowing, leading to an integration and balance, with each part having equal importance and value.[6]

Healing Environment: one that facilitates the emergence of the Haelen effect, the synergistic, organismic, multidimensional response of the whole person in the direction of healing and wholeness;[7] the physical, emotional, social, kinesthetic, and energetic properties of the surroundings/field that can provide a climate of support for the healing process.

Intention: the conscious alignment with creative essence and divine purpose that allows the highest good to flow through a healing intervention or through life itself.

Intuition: a perceived inner knowing and insight into things and events without the conscious use of rational processes;[8] the ability to be present to another dimension of knowing.

Nurse As an Instrument of Healing: one who offers unconditional presence and helps remove the barriers to the healing process; one who creates the space, enhances the environment, and is present to the phenomenon of the unfolding of healing in another; a practitioner who opens the opportunity for another to feel safe and bring into alignment that which has been painful and out of relationship with the self, others, Creator, and creation.[9]

Presence: a multidimensional state of being available in a situation with the wholeness of one's individual being; the relational style and quality of "being with" rather than "doing to."[10]

Relationship: the nature, depth, and degree of connection and interaction between the self, others, Creator, and creation.

Transcendence: the ability to rise above circumstance and develop a broader perspective for experience that brings deeper meaning into and through the context of life.

Whole Person Assessment: a physical, intellectual, emotional, relational, spiritual, vocational, environmental, kinetic, and intuitive interpretation of another individual in relationship to himself or herself, others, Creator, and creation.[11]

THEORY AND RESEARCH

Healing does not occur in a vacuum. Life has its challenges and opportunities in which to learn, heal, and grow. An individual's response to each of those moments determines the effect of any given event upon his or her body, mind, spirit, relationships, work, and life. Understanding responses to life's challenges is critical, as people often are faced with decisions that tip the scales between life-giving or self-destructive behaviors.

People can think, feel, and behave in ways that are influenced by their perception of what is happening in their lives. Based on that perception, they can make sense out of what is going on, or they can respond with fear and confusion that can send their system into a stressed state. The choice depends on how they place a particular event into their lives and the meaning that they attribute to the ongoing story.[12] It is at this point that the healing presence offered by a nurse committed to nurturing the essence, wholeness, and integrity of the individual can be a support for clients and their families. This quality of presence can initiate a response from an individual that can bring perspective, discernment, alignment, balance, meaning, and healing.[13] The nurse has the opportunity to give the gift of relationship freely, helping to create the foundation from which all healing and interventions can be based.

The Concept of Healing

It is challenging to find truth and support for a healing lifetime in this world. Life is not always healing. As life begins, individuals encounter many challenges to the integrity of their systems. Family dysfunction, cultural influences, unhealthy systems in which they find themselves (e.g., schools, churches, communities, corporations) all affect the quality of their life and health. Such threats to one's system, either actual or perceived, make it necessary to protect oneself. The body has a wonderful system to build immunity and defense. The person, being sensitive in nature, is not always surrounded by an environment conducive to peace/harmony/loving; therefore, people are often subject to actual or perceived threats to the natural integrity and wholeness of their essence.

Understanding how to protect oneself helps in choosing responses to life's challenges. The system protects itself by closing down to varying degrees, some of which are healthy and some which can impede the degree of energy flow. Because a closed system does not have a healthy flow of life-giving energy and release of that which is toxic to the system, it can result in patterns of disease, pain, negative energy, and disconnection from the flow of life-giving energy. The picture of a patient in pain, lying in a hospital bed, contracted not only physically but also emotionally and spiritually, comes to mind when thinking of a closed system. Many times, nurses have attempted to reach out to these people who are so fragile, needing the gift of connection to help alleviate some of their suffering. As these individuals open up to share the stories of their lives, the dynamics of their unfolding story reflect much pain and put the physical pain within the context of life's pain. Part of the healing occurs through listening to this story and identifying cues that indicate more of the essence of disease.

Disease is often rooted in responses to life's challenges. Not only energetic blocks to flow, which are manifestations of responses to the patterns of life, but also an imbalance in many of the dimensions that encompass the human experience can produce disease. Changes in perceived levels of energy in relationship to areas of life, as well as the scanning of the energetic field, can be sensed earlier than the actual manifestation of physical symptoms.

Healing is defined as the return of the integrity and wholeness of the natural state of an individual.[14] It can occur across the continuum of illness through reaching one's highest potential at any moment in time. It can be defined as the emergence of the right relationship at, between, and among all dimensions of the human being. B.M. Dossey defined healing as the process of bringing together all parts of one's self (physical, mental, emotional, spiritual, relational) at deeper levels of inner knowing, leading to an integration and balance, with each part having equal importance and value.[15]

The process of healing is one in which the nurse exchanges energy, truth, and communication with clients to help those clients attune to their own healing capacities and implement the healthiest response possible for any given situation. The nurse serves as a mirror to another in helping reflect in a healing way the essence of the challenge and opportunity at hand. Connections are made in which a sensitive, selfless regard for another opens the door for meaningful relationship. The immense power evoked in the relationship between the nurse and client is instrumental in the therapeutic process of healing.[16] The essence of the healing relationship is the nature of the presence, which the nurse offers.

The Concept of Presence

Paterson and Zderad first described the concept of presence as "a mode of being with the wholeness of one's unique individual being: a gift of self which can only be given freely, invoked or evoked."[17(p.122)] They defined presence as a relational style within nursing interactions that involve "being with" as well as "doing with." Presence is generally defined as a multidimensional state of being available in a situation with the wholeness of one's individual being.[18] It is a holistic self-giving exchange, the acknowledgment of a sacred quality operating within one person that can intentionally connect with that sacred quality in others. This process results in an exchange and linking of authentic meaningful awareness and essence that can offer integration and balance in the healing relationship.[19]

Doona and associates described presence as "an intersubjective encounter between a nurse and a patient in which the nurse encounters the patient as a unique human being in a unique situation and chooses to spend herself on the patient's behalf while, at the same time, the patient invites the nurse into his experience."[20] The essence of presence, "being with," implies a conscious intention to appreciate the connection of the moment. A moment in time, the reality of the shared experience in the "now," creates an open container through which life, energy, and healing can flow. Letting go of past concerns or future fears, even for a moment, can create the space and opportunity for the system to open up and reveal what is needed to make it more whole.

Presence is an essential part of caring for a person who is transitioning into the next life. Many caregivers get busy with the tasks at hand and, in their fear, overlook opportunities in which to reframe the dying experience as one that is healing rather than just a physiologic event. Busyness and preoccupation serve the caregiver by offering distance from the dynamic at hand, rather than connection with the opportunity to experience the grace of the natural rhythm of life and death. Providing a peaceful, centered presence that connects with the essence of the other helps guide the dying person and the family into an experience that is meaningful, however.

Caregivers can encourage this presence and help to focus and bring forth the deepest desires for wholeness from another, creating the safe and nurturing environment that allows another to explore avenues of healing.[21] Doona and associates described the coexistence of nursing judgment and presence as so inextricably linked that one does not occur without the other.[22] There are many levels, dimensions, and ways in which to provide a whole-person approach that combines the skills of nursing judgment and presence. Three levels of presence are described in Table 10–1:

1. *Physical presence:* the nurse's "being there" for the patient in physical service. Many nursing interventions are carried out at this level, including the routine tasks that are prescribed for the patient. The way in which one person touches another communicates many meanings; love, anger, distress, or sadness can all be communicated nonverbally. The challenge for the caregiver is to let go of personal life issues in the caregiving experience to focus intentionally on caring for the client.

2. *Psychological presence:* the nurse's using self as an intervention tool; "being with" the client in a therapeutic milieu that meets the client's needs for help, comfort, and support. Recognizing belief systems and their effect on a person's response to life is critical in understanding the degree of presence needed from a cognitive standpoint. This relates to levels of knowing, which include intellectual thinking, rationalization, memory, and the mental component of health. Psychological presence provides understanding, interpretation, and meaning to life's events.

3. *Therapeutic presence:* the nurse's relating to the client as a whole being to whole being, using all the resources of body, mind, emotions, and spirit. The spiritual dimension of presence is ex-

Table 10-1 Levels of Therapeutic Presence

Levels of Interaction	Type of Contact	Skills
Physical presence	Body to body	Seeing, examining, touching, doing, hearing, hugging
Psychological presence	Mind to mind	Assessment, communicating, active listening, writing, reflecting, counseling, attending to, caring, empathy, being nonjudgmental, accepting
Therapeutic presence	Spirit to spirit Whole being to whole being Centered self to centered self	Centering, meditating, intentionality, at-one-ment, imagery, openness, intuitive knowing, communion, loving, connecting

Source: M. McKivergin and J. Daubenmire, The Essence of Therapeutic Presence, *Journal of Holistic Nursing*, Vol. 12, No. 1, pp. 65–81, © 1994. Reprinted by permission of Sage Publications, Inc.

perienced as unconditional love, the letting go of judgments and believing a person is doing his or her best in the situation. When a person is surrounded by unconditional love, which requires the caregiver's intention of presence, the person can access innate healing abilities and, thus, gain insights into self-healing.

Osterman and Schwartz-Barcott described four ways of "being there": (1) physically present with energy focused on the self; (2) physically present with energy focused on the task; (3) physically present and psychosocially focused (energy focused interpersonally); and (4) physically, psychosocially, and spiritually in relationship that is transforming (energy centered) and illuminates the oneness of nurse and patient.[23] The latter is defined as "transcendent presence" and is felt as peaceful, comforting, and harmonious. An outcome of this is positive change in the affective state, such as diminished anxiety, and a feeling of being connected to another and not being alone.

Natural cues can help nurses be more mindfully present with another. The breath is a natural cue for nurses personally as they practice presence to themselves. Holding the breath is an indicator of stress, and the ability to control one's response to an event, stress, or pain by becoming inspired literally through the breath helps one to be even more present to each moment. Nurses who work in the hospital can use the cue of the door to the room as a reminder to be centered and focused. A deep breath while standing outside the patient's door can help in the centering process as a reminder to be inspired in the moment. As the nurse prepares to leave the room, washing the hands can also be a conscious gesture on processing the dynamics of the connection and then moving on to the next moment of awareness with the next person. Presence inspires patient care and helps guide nurses in the mystery of each moment, yielding qualities of care described and felt by nurses and those with whom they share each moment.

Qualities of Presence

The nurse evolves the skill of being present to others. The initial focus for a new nurse is develping the adequate skill level to provide safe care through the acquisition and practice of basic skills and techniques. Maturity in the nursing profession increases the sensitivity of recognizing the connection between a person's life and health, as well as the perception of the person's body as metaphor. With each level of understanding, the nurse's attitude shifts from "What can I do?" to "How can I be with the person in this moment in a way that will provide the best possible outcome?"

As nurses have taken courses and explored the concept of presence, they have identified the qualities of presence to include unconditional acceptance, patience, lovingness, nonjudgmental attitude, understanding, good listening skills, honesty, empathy, and many other such descriptors.[24]

Five distinguishing features of nursing presence include

1. self giving to another at the moment at hand, being available and at the disposal of another
2. listening to the other
3. knowing the privilege in participating in the experience
4. giving of one's self
5. being with another in a way the other person perceives as full of meaning[25]

The nurse can encounter a patient in a variety of states that warrant the adoption of the qualities of presence. Patient experience can be chaotic, like a hurricane, swirling uncontrollably on a course beyond determination. Nurses can offer the gift of presence in the storm by being in the midst of the swirl with the patient, offering a groundedness that can help anchor the patient, providing a centering influence that is likened to being in the eye of the hurricane and is sensitive to its flow, or offering a transcendent quality that helps the patient to rise above the whole situation and put it into perspective, thus expanding consciousness.[26] To remain with a person in the midst of the storm, exposing one's humanness and offering comfort and healing

support is one of the greatest gifts nurses can offer. The journey with another helps promote a sense of well-being, offering silent presence or helping to understand and interpret the challenge at hand.

Blocks to Presence

Because it exposes one's vulnerability in the sometimes uncontrollable journey of being human, presence may be uncomfortable. Nurses may use defense mechanisms to avoid true connection with another. Manifestations of avoidance include turning and walking away, maintaining the integrity of an impenetrable defense system. Nurses often shield themselves under the guise of professionalism by using their role, counseling techniques, or communication skills as a protective wall to maintain distance.[27] Blocks to presence can be unintentional or intentional and are based on some of the following:

- Busyness/task focus
- Fear
- Concern over what other people will think
- Feelings of inadequacy ("I'm not ____ enough")
- Lack of desire/intent to be present
- Distractions
- Need to be in control
- Goal direction, responsibilities
- Lack of patience
- Lack of openness
- Personal or physical limitations[28]

At times, a nurse may be too tired, too busy, or unable to offer depth of presence and service to another. It is important for nurses to be aware of this and communicate limitations to their patients. Should this become a recurring pattern in which a nurse is running away from the cumulative effect of situations that are painful or uncomfortable or that make the nurse feel inadequate, it is essential for that nurse to process his or her own reactions and gain an insight into his or her own responses. The nurse may need the support of others in this process. It is thus that nurses become presence to the most important of relationships—the one with themselves—and have the ability to share learnings to help bring deeper meaning and healing to another's experience

Integrative Theory Supporting Relationship-Centered Care

In order to understand fully how to develop themselves as an instrument of healing, nurses need to recognize the importance of the dynamic quality of relationships. The essence of healing is one that is phenomenologic in nature, one that is intersubjective in the lived experience.[29] Being intersubjective implies relationship and, thus, the need for an understanding about the importance of the relationship of caring. An essential part of being human is the fact that people are not isolated entities, but are automatically in relationship with themselves, others, Creator, and creation.

In 1992, the Pew-Fetzer Task Force postulated that the foundation of care given by practitioners is the relationship between the practitioner and the patient, a relationship vitally important to both.[30] This relationship is a medium for the exchange of all forms of information, feelings, and concerns; a factor in the success of therapeutic regimens; and an essential ingredient in the satisfaction of both the patient and practitioner. For patients, the relationship with their provider is the most therapeutic aspect of the health care encounter.[31] The phrase "relationship-centered care" captures the importance of the interaction among people as the foundation of any therapeutic or healing activity.[32] The implications of this report are far-reaching.

Nurse theorists have an important perspective regarding the nature of health, disease, healing, and the dynamics of caring for another:

- Florence Nightingale—natural healing[33]
- Helen Erickson, Evelyn Tomlin, and Mary Ann Swain—modeling and role modeling[34]
- Madeleine Leininger—transcultural nursing[35]
- Betty Neuman—systems theory[36]
- Margaret Newman—health as expanding consciousness[37]
- Dorothea Orem—self-care[38]
- Rosemary Rizzo Parse—human-living-health, multidimensionality, co-creation[39]
- Martha Rogers—human energy fields[40]
- Sr. Callista Roy—the adaptation model[41]
- Jean Watson—caring[42]
- Josephine G. Paterson and Loretta T. Zderad—presence[43]
- Doris Hines—presence[44]

In addition to the theories derived directly from nursing, many theories from other disciplines, or borrowed theories, have concepts that contribute to the rich interpretation of the experience of caring. The integration of all of these theories provides support for the dynamic of relationship-centered care. When recognized as the foundation for practice, the relationship between the practitioner and the person emerges as an overlapping core surrounded by the essences of all the other theories (Figure 10–1). This mutuality of relationship provides the foundations of trust and reliability that can create a field for growth and healing to happen.

Theories can be integrated as appropriate throughout the continuum of care. Based on a whole-person assessment, the nurse can determine whether principles of self-care, energy field healing, learning through expansion of consciousness, or theories borrowed from another discipline can support the unfolding relationship of healing. In transforming health care, the focus should be on the nature of relation-

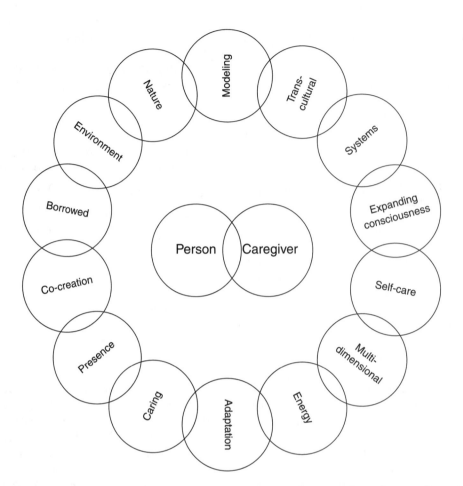

Figure 10-1 Integrative Theory Supporting Relationship-Centered Care. *Source:* Copyright © 1998, Maggie McKivergin.

ships that yield the dynamics of healing. Principles of presence are the essence of relationship-centered care and integral in nurturing the relationships with one's self, others, Creator, and creation.

Relationship with Self

A healing relationship with the self implies conscious and mindful approaches to being in the moment, recognizing the implications of life events on the self that then helps in understanding others. Focusing attention and care on what is bringing energy to or draining energy from one's life helps to guide the relationship with the self. Alignment with a personal process of healing and unfolding takes conscious intent, sensitivity, and awareness. Assessing the physical, emotional, intellectual, spiritual, vocational, environmental and relational dimensions of one's life, asking what in each of the areas is contributing to or diminishing the energy experienced in each of these areas, helps one to achieve deeper meaning and recognition of the unique gift of life and to nurture growth to the fullest capacity.

It is important to realize that there is a part of us that always needs healing, the wounded healer, yet we are tempted to ignore this woundedness.[45] Often, nurses find themselves caring for others at home, at work, in the community, within their marriages, and they do not take care of themselves. This leaves them drained, burned out, and fragmented, requiring a mindful approach to balance out the giving with the receiving, as well as the ability to introduce themselves as part of the equation of care.

Embracing one's perceived limitations provides guidance to increased wholeness. Making one's wounds a source of healing calls for a constant willingness to see the pain and suffering as rising from the depth of the human condition that is common to all and brings meaning to experience. Healing from one's woundedness creates strength and a growth from the alignment with healing that enhances a nurse's therapeutic capacity—the ability to hold another in deeper, broader, and more powerful ways.

Dossey and associates have described the characteristics of nurse healers that affect the relationship they have with themselves as instruments of healing:

- Awareness that self-healing is a continual process
- Familiarity with the terrain of self-development
- Recognition of strengths and weaknesses
- Openness to self-discovery
- Continued effort to develop clarity about life's purposes to avoid mechanical behavior and boredom
- Awareness of present and future steps in personal growth
- Modeling of self-care in order to help self and clients with the inward process
- Awareness that a nurse's presence is as important as technical skills
- Respect and love for clients regardless of who or how they are
- Willingness to offer the client methods for working on life issues

- Ability to guide the client in discovering creative options
- Presumption that the client knows the best life choices
- Active listening
- Empowerment of clients to recognize that they can cope with life processes
- Sharing of insights without imposing personal values and beliefs
- Acceptance of what clients say without judging
- Perception of time with clients as being there to serve and share with them[46]

To know the full truth of patients, to know them as they are present to themselves and to be a presence for them, a nurse must first recollect himself or herself, that is, be present to self, choose to participate in the experience of another, and make himself or herself available to the patient.[47]

Nurses should create their own team of support for their process of healing. They can then begin to understand how best to be present in relationship to others, enhancing their capacity to be therapeutic and to serve as instruments of healing for others. As they foster the characteristics listed, they form themselves through their intentions to know, love, and serve. They then have an abundance from which to share in their ministry to others.

Relationship with Others

Being in relationship with another is offering the multidimensional gift of interpersonal connection with another. The connection with another can be physical, emotional, psychologic, intuitive, spiritual, kinetic, or therapeutic in nature, with varying levels of depth and transcendence. The following story illustates connections on many levels:

Several years ago, I was visiting a Native American village in the Southwest where I immediately lost the party with whom I was traveling. Being aware that it felt out of the ordinary to be in this situation, I asked Spirit to guide me, and I was led through the village, across a bridge, and to an artist's studio. In the studio was a charming young Native woman who asked if I did healing work. In acknowledging my gift, she asked if I could help her with some back pain she had been experiencing. I was delighted to be of service.

I asked her how long she had been experiencing the low back pain, and she replied that it had been 1 year. I then asked her about what had been going on in her life at that time. She shared that her mother had died and her aunt, who was an elder of the tribe, had stolen her inheritance and lied about the incident. Afraid to challenge an elder, she let the incident go, but the pain in her back developed shortly thereafter.

Her intention for our time together was not only to be healed from her pain but also to forgive her aunt, as her feelings were hampering her spiritual essence. I reflected that what her aunt had done was wrong and that forgiveness for something that is wrong may not be the first step in healing. I suggested that we might want to try to understand why the aunt did what she did so that we might develop compassion for her, which eventually may lead to forgiveness.

With that, it was as if we both could see a movie screen, one that revealed to us a picture of the old days on the plains. The buffalo were roaming, and the Natives were quietly watching the peaceful scene of grazing under the big sky. White man entered the scene and proceeded to shoot the buffalo, stealing the Native's land and lying to the Native people with promises of payment and respect. With this vision, the Native woman and I looked at each other, and I stated, "Look, your aunt has become what she hates! It was wrong for the white man to do that, and it is wrong for your aunt to do this to you. We need to design a way to bring forth justice. I would suggest you find a woman on the council who can mentor you in regaining your property in a just and truthful way. Then I want you to climb to the top of that peak (which just so happened to be the tribe's holy mountain), look down on the village, and realize how small all of this is. Adopt the Spirit of the Eagle, and rise above the situation. Then you will free yourself."

By this time, most of the pain in her back had already subsided. I then smoothed out the energy in her lower back, and the woman was released from her pain, staying pain-free. She shared with me a present of a silver carving of her village so we would always be connected.

This story reflects presence to the many dimensions of physical, emotional, psychologic, intuitive, spiritual, and cultural healing, integrating and healing the many parts of the Native American woman's experience. She demonstrated the courage to heal and to address that which was painful to her.

With intention and practice, a nurse can learn to help bring people toward a more inclusive, unobstructed relatedness to life. Moss identified three qualities of relatedness:

1. Creative involvement: an original and spontaneous participation in life without judgment
2. Intensity: the quality of attention; the depth from which our involvement with life emanates
3. Unconditional love: the principle of inclusivity; an implicit sense of prior wholeness[48]

Presence implies relating to another person in the moment at hand in a way that the other person defines as meaningful. This presence is more powerful when connected with self, Creator, and creation. A healthy balance of relationship with each of these areas promotes well-being. When there is a deficit in any of these relationships, imbalances and voids can occur in that area. When individuals are unable to love themselves, for example, or be in relationship with themselves in ways that promote joy and happiness, they often depend on their relationship with others to fill that void. Increased expectations from others, whether from friends, spouse, or children, can create an unhealthy balance that can lead to codependence, or relationships with others that are dependent on needs rather than shared experience.

Qualities of a healthy relationship with others include reciprocity, the ability to give and receive respect; care for the unique path of the other; the ability to offer freedom for others to be themselves; openness to the wholeness of others without categorizing them; happiness in being together; trust; truth telling; freedom from physical or emotional abuse; willingness to tend to the connection with the other and self, to accept change in another without trying to stifle that growth, to share feelings, and to share relationships within the context of community; and the ability to honor the sacred within the other, as well as between the both. Key to quality relationships is they are heart-centered, offer-

ing unconditional love in each moment of presence to each other.

Relationship with Creator

As instruments of healing, nurses acknowledge that healing does not come from them, but through them. In their openness to the potential for healing that comes from the relationship not only between the caregiver and the individual, but also in relationship with the Creator and the energetic environment, they begin to experience the power and depth of the mystery of healing unfolding. Bringing the presence of the Creator into the many dimensions (e.g., physical, emotional) can bring a deeper understanding of wholeness, integrity, meaning, and truth of the moment/situation/self. The recognition of self as sacred integrates the essence of the Creator in this life through inspiration, transcendence, truth, grace, hope, and forgiveness and love. Openness to the unfolding of our lives in any moment, co-creating the unique expression of the gift of our lives with our Creator/Spirit, is the essence of our loving nature.

As an instrument of healing, a nurse develops an ear to listen for the themes of spiritual distress, namely, those areas in which a person feels unconnected; is yielding to emptiness or a lack of faith; has a diminished sense of trust in the process; or feels fear, hatred, and lack of forgiveness for self and others. Identifying areas of imbalance and helping the individual to recognize the spiritual essence that will help bring trust, forgiveness, courage, compassion, and love into his or her experience creates an openness that is healing and allows the wonders of the Creator to become manifest.

It is important to respect the definition that each individual brings to the concept of Creator/Spirit. Honoring the individual's belief system permits access to the individual's innate healing abilities and avoids imposing one agenda on another, thus diminishing the therapeutic potential of the dynamic of healing.

Relationship with Creation

Sensitivity to the essence of life and its seasons and rhythms, recognizing the message, meaning, and life-giving energy inherent in all of creation, heals us in many ways. In a healing interaction between two people, for example, the frequency of their different energies synchronizes with the same frequency of the earth.[49] The vibration between two people who are aligned in intention and open to the rhythm of healing produces a resonant vibration that is called entrainment. The mutuality of vibration that can be healing in nature helps to remove the blocks that inhibit the flow of energy.[50]

Nature teaches important themes related to the organic healing process. Seasonal themes hold rich metaphors in relating to the spectrum of life from the beginning of creation, new life, blossoming, fullness of life, letting go, changing, to recreation and rebirth. Metaphors of growth (e.g., the seed, planting, nurturing, harvesting, renewal) are instrumental in understanding the cycles of experience. In addition, rich messages lie within the phenomena of nature, such as flow, flexibility, and rootedness, all of which ground us to the earthly experience.

The native peoples from all around the world have a deep respect for the sacredness of natural healing and the importance of the healing essence of nature. They see themselves not as separate from the land, but as one with nature. In the Western culture, however, society is so fast-paced that people are losing touch with this inherent rhythm and are becoming divided from this natural, healing connection. As instruments of healing, it is important for nurses to be grounded within themselves, as well as to assist others in their healing process and to understand the wealth of beauty and energy that the earth has to offer. It is important to help people develop a sense of connection with the earth, its rhythms, and its seasons, as well as the healing energy that it has to impart through its essence and messages.

THE NURSE AS A HEALING ENVIRONMENT

There is immense power in the relationship between the nurse and the client that is instrumental in the therapeutic process of healing. Through the intention of unconditional presence, the nurse provides an environment of support and healing by patterning the environment to evoke the healing response. With attention and intention, the environment can become one in which the client can feel safe and explore the dimensions of self in the healing moment. The nurse who understands the nature of a healing environment can shape both the physical environment (external) and the personal environment (relationship-focused) to evoke the healing process. This environment is sacred in its essence and with focused intention can create an energetic climate to promote and enhance healing.

By connecting with the sacred within each person and accessing the person's inner healer, the alignment with the divine enhances and guides the healing process in a powerful way. In the process of expanding their consciousness and creating a sacred space in which healing can occur, nurses are also healed. Rogers postulated that the fundamental unity of the living system is an energy field that is coextensive with the environmental energy field; therefore, each one is affected by the other.[51]

The nurse not only is in the healing environment, but also offers himself or herself as an environment in which the individual can dwell.[52] Nelms related the gift of presence to the "creation of home being twofold, for in making a home for their patients, the nurse created homes for themselves; places where, as the nurse enables patient-being to be unconcealed, her own nurse-being is more fully revealed."[53]

The following enhance a nurse's capacity to develop greater depth, breadth, and height in becoming an instrument of healing:

- Self-care, not only physically, but also in all dimensions that remove the blocks to personal flow of energy and healing
- Personal interpretation of life's lessons and meaning
- Rootedness and expansiveness; an understanding of the art of balance between a grounded approach and the intuitive inspiration that creates a vision of health and wholeness and moves one in that direction
- Core dynamics; recognition of the holographic nature and metaphor of systems and the essential nature of life, health, and healing
- Expansion of consciousness; the ability to broaden one's thinking, shift perspectives, and encompass a new approach to life
- Growth in love; the ability to grow more and more in loving presence to self, others, and the world in a way that creates the highest level of healing
- Courage; the ability to overcome the fear that is encountered in the healing process as one walks through the fight or flight response with the clarity of intention to get through the block/pain
- Alignment with the Divine
- Openness to being an instrument of the Creator's healing grace
- Ability to detach oneself from the outcomes
- Groundedness and reliability
- Patience
- Authenticity
- Mindfulness
- Integrity[54]

The process of healing is one in which the nurse engages with the individuals in an authentic exchange of energy, truth, and communication in order to help them attune to their own healing capacities. By creating an environment of support and reflection, the nurse encourages them to reflect on past, present, and future perceptions and helps them to access their inner teacher, guide, and healer to reframe past experience, create a new reality which is healing, and release strong ties of belief, even at a cellular level in the process of becoming more whole. This process can have the effect of relaxation or actually demonstrate profound changes as one faces that which has been numbed, buried, or blocked because of its painful nature.

The emotional, social, and energetic properties of the surroundings/field have a profound effect on the individual. The physical properties of natural light, running water, plants, earth elements, fresh air, color, pleasant sounds, music, healing smells, comfortable temperature, and order contribute their therapeutic influence to a healing environment. Oftentimes, nurses involved with healing modalities cleanse and make sacred the energetic environment through a variety of blessings and rituals, possibly including the use of holy water, Epsom salts, and alcohol; smudging with sage; and prayer. The intention of creating an environment of healing is critical in providing a place where the client feels safe, light, and open.

HEALING INTERVENTIONS

Healing can occur in many ways, on many levels, and in many dimensions. Nurses can complement care by their presence, by the environment that they create, by the spectrum of interventions that they choose, guided by the individuals' need and response in the moment. It is important to address physical pain as a first priority in providing comfort, as pain relief can then help the individual to relax and be open and receptive to additional interventions and healing.

Preparation for a healing intervention is important to enhance the potential of the interaction. In addition to preparing the external environment, nurses prepare themselves through intention, centering, and alignment with the Divine. Part of the preparation is the degree of consciousness offered to a situation. There is a conscious awareness that is required in setting the intention of becoming an instrument of healing of self and others. Honoring the sacredness of the potential of the healing relationship, offering the gift of an unconditional loving presence, and connecting with the Divine is the essence of allowing oneself "to be" with another in a way that creates the environment for healing to occur.

Unknowing is a necessary foundation for openness within the dynamic of healing.[55] Approaching another or a new situation with the "beginner's mind" provides openness, freshness, and the opportunity to respect mutual knowing. This state evokes a mutual response rather than placing the patient in a dependent position, and it provides the access to the inner healer, teacher, and guide. The healing power of vulnerability comes as a result of the nurse's willingness to be present in the moment with the willingness to co-create the outcome rather than to impose a preconceived agenda for the moment.

Part of a nurse's intention is to protect himself or herself from some of the dynamics of the energetic interaction. As instruments of healing, nurses sometimes absorb the negative energy or patterns of others. Healthy ways in which they can protect themselves include

- having the intention to give and receive only love
- praying for protection from the Creator
- visualizing white light surrounding self and other

- being intentional about healthy boundaries
- being in a healthy, centered, energetic place themselves; determining if their own personal level of energy is adequate in considering being an instrument of healing to another

Preparing one's self as an instrument of healing and creating the container, whether physically or energetically, in which a person can experience healing is the most important component of a healing intervention, like preparing the ground for a seed to be planted.

Steps of the Holistic Caring Process

The nurse who serves as an instrument of healing goes through the steps of the holistic caring process, a circular process that involves six steps that may occur simultaneously. These steps are assessment, patterns/problems/needs, outcomes, therapeutic care plan, implementation, and evaluation. (See Chapter 14.)

Assessment includes

- interviews, involving the outline of the individual's story and the co-interpretation of responses to life's events
- whole person well-being
- functional capacity
- health risk indicators
- quality-of-life indicators
- process analysis/personal goals
- the openness or closure of the person as a system with identification of possible places that would indicate the direction of an intervention
- scanning of the energy field of the person
- interpretation with the person the meaning of the mutual exchange[56]

Assessment is a mindful process that assumes an approach that is deliberate and attentive to the many levels of being. In modulating the human energy field and its flow, facilitating an energy balance, the source of the pattern disturbance often comes into awareness, and the nurse helps to access the inner healer within the client so as to co-create a conscious repatterning of thought, memories, pain, anxiety, tension and energy flow.

Healers worldwide focus on the aspects of inner healing and provide deep inner work that has profound physical effects. Krieger and Kunz were first to describe and research the procedure of energy field intervention in nursing, referring to it as therapeutic touch.[57] Simultaneously, other schools of healing and individuals that help to provide understanding to the nurse and the individual have emerged:

1. Therapeutic touch
2. Healing touch
3. Hakoni
4. Reiki
5. Barbara Brennan's school
6. Inner Focus School of Energy Field Healing

Each of the different schools supplies a variety of actual approaches to healing work that nurses can use in the moment of shared experience:

- Center, align, and focus attention.
- Intend for the highest good of the client with detachment from ego needs of the healer and healee and outcomes.
- Be and create an environment within which the client feels safe and healing can emerge. Be conscious of giving and receiving only love.
- Assess the energy field intuitively as well as by running the hands over the different levels of the aura, meridians, and chakras.
- Note areas of energy congestion or stagnation, and provide feedback to the client in order to enhance synchrony and to ensure that the process is one of conscious awareness.

- Be present to the many levels of the client's being as energy is modulated, blocks to flow removed, and congestion dissipated.
- Encourage open communication in the healing process as it unfolds so as to enhance the depth of the healing experience.
- Apply different techniques as appropriate to help drain pain, chelate the energy, relax and smooth the area while helping the individual to breathe into the area and release unhealthy patterns. Adjunct modalities (e.g., massage, prayer, reflexology) can be used to enhance the experience.
- Provide grounding as the client explores new dimensions to his or her being by continuing to reflect truth while providing openness for reflection and exploration.
- Help the client in reframing experiences and memories in the release of what no longer serves the client's well-being so as to remove blocks that surface within the healing dynamic.
- Be aware of levels of energy patterning within the aura and field of the client, and facilitate the flow of energy as the healing emerges.
- Smooth out the whole field at the completion of the session, and help the person become grounded, conscious to the present, and oriented with the change.
- Ritualize the closure of the session by honoring the process as sacred (e.g., blow out the candle, give a gift of a flower).[58]

Techniques of healing are as varied as each individual's need. Skills of energy field healing coupled with the modalities of prayer, massage, reflexology, aromatherapy, music, and many others enhance the options for a full spectrum of care and whole person healing.

Outcomes of a Healing Intervention

Outcomes that reflect a change in a person's awareness, perception, behavior, and relationship to self, others, the Creator, and creation are assessed as they were before the healing intervention and may include the following:

- Whole-person outcomes
  1. Physical: decreased pain, enhanced wound healing, increased energy
  2. Emotional: enhanced ability to feel, name feelings, and express oneself; decreased anxiety; decreased sense of vulnerability; ability to give and receive more love
  3. Intellectual: perceptual reframing of an experience that influences the belief structure, attitudes, and ways of thinking about life and its influence; healing of a painful memory; increased enthusiasm and expression of self; expansion of consciousness
  4. Relational: improved relationship with self, self-esteem, and self-concept; deeper connection with others; sense of being supported by others; understanding of the reciprocal nature of relationships
  5. Spiritual: deeper sense of connectedness with all of life, self, Creator, creation; more hope, courage, trust, and wisdom; enhanced meaning regarding a life event; forgiveness of self or others
  6. Vocational: identification of and alignment with life's purpose and path of expression of gift in the world; improved excitement and creativity in work
  7. Environmental: in tune with harmony of nature and inherent healing rhythms; recognition of meaning and metaphor in the symbols of the earth

- Increased coping strength, even in the midst of unchanged circumstances; access to relaxation response; ability to maintain a flow state; decreased exhibition of self-destructive behavior; decreased perception of the impact of stress on daily life
- Increased sense of well-being/quality of life; demonstration of increased happiness, life satisfaction, and sense of security
- Functional capacity: increased ability to care for self, move, have less pain, enhanced range of motion
- Systemness: freer and more open feeling; establishment of healthy boundaries; feeling of connectedness in a healthier direction; lessened sense of isolation; sense of freedom to change and become less defined by external parameters[59]

Evaluation of a Healing Intervention

Scandrett-Hibdon and Freel have described five recurring elements of self-involvement that appear to be aspects of the natural healing process of a client:[60]

1. Awareness
2. Appraisal
3. Choosing/setting intention
4. Alignment
5. Acceptance

In terminating a session with a client, nurses should ask him or her to share the insights of the experience to see if these five elements are present. The release of chaotic patterns or the bringing of awareness and energy into areas that are stagnant yields a variety of outcomes as reported by the client. The nurse should

- note significant areas of change and energy balance
- have the client report the significance of this experience with implications for next steps

- support the shift of consciousness within the client by sharing the nature of the changes and insights gained with possible ways to approach life and health differently
- affirm positive self-care initiatives[61]

It is important to assist the client with the next steps and follow up as appropriate. For example, the nurse may advise the client to schedule a personal daily time of reflection as an opportunity to be present to the process of self unfolding, perhaps through journaling, art therapy, music therapy, and meditation. In addition, the nurse may help the individual access a team of support to help bridge and support the change as indicated. Such a team may include a therapeutic/pastoral counselor, physical support with fitness coach, body worker, chiropractor, physician, and significant family members or friends who can help nurture.

Follow-up with the client is important to ensure continuation of the healing process and to identify additional needs. It is also important to evaluate the personal interpretations that the nurse experiences as a result of the healing dynamic.

OTHER CONSIDERATIONS FOR INTEGRATION OF CONCEPTS

Educational Considerations

The concept of relating the essence of disease to the story of a person's response to life, not just caring for symptoms, is one of the most basic educational considerations. Using techniques for whole-person/whole-life assessment, studying the body as metaphor, and using energy field principles for assessment need to be the foundation for nursing education. Education programs should incorporate techniques for relaxation, energy field assessment and balancing, as well as courses in complementary pathways to enhance the current body of knowledge. Practicing techniques

of being present to patients, as well as self-care strategies, creates a nurturing environment that embodies the essence of nursing.

Practice Considerations

Hospital-based practice, outpatient clinics, schools, corporations, parish nurse programs, and private practice are all ways in which to integrate the concepts of whole-person assessment and healing. Holistic dimensions of physical, emotional, intellectual, relational, spiritual, vocational, and environmental can be assessed, as well as integrated into curricula that are school-, church-, or work-based. Nurses who offer their healing presence in each of these settings expand the role of the nurse as an instrument of healing, as they become more integral into the key systems of daily life. They can help advise and design programs that will help others understand the importance of personal interpretation and responses to life.

Themes of healing can be adapted to systems that are organic in nature, such as those found in families, schools, corporations, and communities. These systems represent the same dynamics as the human system, including the openness or closure of the system, areas of pain, and attributes on which to build. The nurse incorporates the skills of assessment of imbalances, scanning the energetic dynamics looking for blocks, as well as open doors for growth and healing. The nurse as an instrument of healing systems offers presence through relationship and knowledge of whole-person/whole-system dynamics to bring insight and outcomes that are healing to each of the arenas.

Research Considerations

There is limited research on the effectiveness of healing interventions, as well as on the integration of complementary therapies into care. Research has been essentially nonconclusive regarding the effectiveness of interventions such as therapeutic touch in that few measurement tools can capture the profound changes that happen during a healing intervention.[62–66]

A design that uses both qualitative and quantitative approaches is best for healing research. Qualitatively, the essence of healing is still being defined, still descriptive, and phenomenologic in nature. The research design should include a minimum investigation of the individual's experience with questions about how the individual defines the experience, what the experience means to him or her, and how he or she feels before and after the intervention. The key question is whether a person feels better as a result of the intervention. Reported outcomes of each intervention should be listed and clustered to identify the themes of healing. This approach creates a holographic model of systemic healing that permeates all systems. Descriptors would include the measurements of the openness or closure of the system, defined areas of pain relative to the system, attributes upon which to build, and directions for growth and healing.

Quantitative measures include such categories as demographic input, vital signs, diagnostic study findings, and cost implications. Types of patients can be grouped in a hospital by diagnosis or symptoms. For instance, ventilator-dependent comatose patients on intracranial monitors can be monitored pre– and post–therapeutic touch for changes in vital signs that could demonstrate a relaxing effect in a controlled study. State-trait anxiety tools can be used to identify level of stress experience pre- and post-intervention. Whole person qualities can be measured by the use of instruments that measure well-being.[67]

Future research should address the design of the tools and questionnaires that demonstrate the effectiveness of healing intervention. Effectiveness can be measured in patient satisfaction, decreased pain, decreased anxiety, enhanced well-being, increased functional capacity, as well as the demonstration of physical, intellectual, and emotional effects.

As instruments that scan the human energy field become refined, this diagnostic approach will become as commonplace as magnetic resonance imaging (MRI) is today and will demonstrate the effectiveness of energy field interventions such as healing touch, therapeutic touch, aromatherapy, reflexology, acupuncture, and biofeedback. In addition, scanning the energy field for the effect of negative thought patterns and their physiologic effects will demonstrate more strongly the bodymind connection and modifications that alter the field before they are actually manifested as symptoms. The challenge is to continue to refine the art of nursing, not only with what nurses do, but also by understanding the power of who they are. Researching qualitative and quantitative approaches and techniques to expand the spectrum of care is critical in demonstrating the healing effect of the qualities of caring, as well as the ways in which nurses use different techniques to heal others.

CONCLUSION

Nurses interested in becoming an instrument of healing must understand the nature of healing, the sources of healing, and the ways in which to offer their presence in relationship to self, others, the Creator, and creation that can promote the dynamic of healing. The nurse has the opportunity to give the gift of self freely to another to nurture this growth. The exchange of presence in any particular moment in time celebrates the privilege of conscious and intentional involvement with another. It is this relationship that forms the cornerstone of health care and provides the foundation for the practice of caring for others.

The skill of becoming an instrument of healing is one that can be cultivated. The ability to assess the multidimensional nature of another person in reference to that person's life experience is complex and requires an intuitive, spiritual, and skilled approach, as well as an understanding of the deeper meaning of human response to life.

As instruments of healing, nurses combine wisdom (what they know as well as do not know) with their skills (what they do), integrating these with the essence of who they are to form a holistic approach to caring for self, others, and creation. They partner in the journey of healing, offering new insights, new ways of coping, and a release from the bondage of fear and pain. Nurses offer the gift of walking with a person so that the person is not left alone to face the crossroads of healing and can emerge into new life—the manifestation of the powerful inner longing at every level to be whole. It is thus that life and health become a celebration of the unfolding of the essence and beauty of the human spirit, and the nurse truly becomes an instrument of healing.

DIRECTIONS FOR FUTURE RESEARCH

1. Study the effect of a particular type of healing intervention on a group of patients with a common symptom. Determine if the intervention has made a difference as measured by vital signs, well-being instrument, levels of anxiety.
2. Design a qualitative questionnaire to accompany a healing intervention that would include the questions:
   • What was your experience of this intervention?

   • How would you describe this experience?
   • What does health and healing mean to you?
   • Do you feel better as a result of this intervention?
3. Identify thought patterns and belief systems that affect a person's health negatively, and research the effectiveness of introducing new belief systems into a person's thinking.
4. Implement a standard of practice regarding presence on a patient care unit and measure patient and nurse satisfaction.

NURSE HEALER REFLECTIONS

After reading this chapter, the nurse healer will be able to answer or will begin the process of answering the following questions:

• How do I understand healing?
• What do I consider healing to be?
• What are ways in which I can enhance the relationship I have with myself? Others? Creator? Creation?
• What do I experience when I consciously practice presence to myself? To others?
• How can I create opportunities in which to heal myself and thus enhance my therapeutic capacity?
• What are the characteristics of my inner teacher/healer?
• What are ways in which I can be more of a healing presence for others?
• How can I contribute positively to the environment around me?
• How do I feel when I consider myself as an instrument of healing?

NOTES

1. B.M. Dossey, Nurse As Healer, in *Holistic Nursing: A Handbook for Practice*, 2d ed., ed. B.M. Dossey et al. (Gaithersburg, MD: Aspen Publishers, 1995), 62.

2. M.J. Wheatley, *Leadership and the New Science* (San Francisco: Berrett-Koehler, 1994).
3. B.M. Dossey, Nurse As Healer, 62.
4. M.J. McKivergin, *The Essence of Presence* (In

press, 2000).

5. J.F. Quinn, Holding Sacred Space: The Nurse As Healing Environment, *Holistic Nursing Practice* 6, no. 4 (1992):26–36.

6. B.M. Dossey et al., eds., *Holistic Nursing: A Handbook for Practice*, 2d ed. (Gaithersburg, MD: Aspen Publishers, 1995).

7. F. Nightingale, *Notes on Nursing* (Philadelphia: Lippincott, 1992).

8. B.M. Dossey, Nurse As Healer, 62.

9. M.J. McKivergin, The Nurse As an Instrument of Healing, in *Core Curriculum for Holistic Nursing*, ed. B.M. Dossey (Gaithersburg, MD: Aspen Publishers, 1997), 17–25.

10. J.G. Paterson and L.T. Zderad, *Humanistic Nursing* (New York: John Wiley & Sons, 1976).

11. McKivergin, *The Essence of Presence.*

12. M.J. McKivergin and A. Day, Presence: Creating Order out of Chaos, *Seminars in Perioperative Nursing* 7, no. 2 (1998):96.

13. McKivergin and Day, Presence: Creating Order out of Chaos, 96.

14. McKivergin, The Nurse As an Instrument of Healing, 17.

15. B.M. Dossey, Nurse As Healer, 62.

16. McKivergin, The Nurse As an Instrument of Healing, 21.

17. Paterson and Zderad, *Humanistic Nursing.*

18. McKivergin, The Nurse As an Instrument of Healing, 17.

19. McKivergin and Day, Presence: Creating Order out of Chaos, 98.

20. M.E. Doona et al., Nursing Presence: An Existential Exploration of the Concept, *Scholarly Inquiry for Nursing Practice: An International Journal* 11, no. 1 (1997):12.

21. McKivergin, The Nurse As an Instrument of Healing, 19.

22. Doona, et al., Nursing Presence: An Existential Exploration of the Concept, 6.

23. P. Osterman and D. Schwartz-Barcott, Presence: Four Ways of Being There, *Nursing Forum* 31, no. 2 (1996):28.

24. M.J. McKivergin and J. Daubenmire, *Essence of Therapeutic Presence: The Course*, Presented at Riverside Methodist Hospital, Columbus, Ohio.

25. J. Pettigrew, Intensive Nursing Care: The Ministry of Presence, *Critical Care Nursing Clinics of North America* 2, no. 3 (1990):503–508.

26. McKivergin and Day, Presence: Creating Order out of Chaos.

27. McKivergin, The Nurse As an Instrument of Healing.

28. McKivergin, The Nurse As an Instrument of Healing, 20.

29. P. Munhall, Unknowing: Toward Another Pattern of Knowing in Nursing, *Nursing Outlook* 41, no. 3 (1993):125–128.

30. Pew-Fetzer Task Force, *Health Professions Education and Relationship Centered Care* (San Francisco: Pew Health Professions Commission, 1994).

31. Pew-Fetzer Task Force, *Health Professions Education*, 9.

32. Pew-Fetzer Task Force, *Health Professions Education*, 11.

33. L. Selanders, *Florence Nightingale: An Environmental Adaptation Theory* (Menlo Park, CA: Sage, 1993).

34. H. Erickson et al., *Modeling and Role-Modeling: A Theory and Paradigm for Nursing* (Lexington, KY: Pine Press, 1983).

35. M. Leininger, *Cultural Care Diversity and Universality: A Theory of Nursing* (New York: National League for Nursing Press, 1991).

36. B. Neuman, *The Neuman Systems Model* (Norwalk, CT: Appleton-Century-Crofts, 1982).

37. M.A. Newman, *Health As Expanding Consciousness*, 2d ed. (New York: National League for Nursing Press, 1994).

38. D.E. Orem, *Nursing: Concepts of Practice*, 3d ed. (New York: McGraw-Hill, 1985).

39. R.R. Parse, Human Becoming: Parse's Theory of Nursing, *Nursing Science Quarterly* 1, no. 5 (1992):35–42.

40. M. Rogers, *The Theoretical Basis of Nursing* (Philadelphia: F.A. Davis, 1970).

41. C. Roy and H.A. Andrews, *The Roy Adaptation Model: The Definitive Statement* (Stamford, CT: Appleton & Lange, 1991).

42. J. Watson, *Nursing: Human Science and Human Care* (New York: National League for Nursing Press, 1988).

43. Paterson and Zderad, *Humanistic Nursing.*

44. D. Hines, *The Development of the Measurement of Presence Scale* (University Microfilms International, 1991).

45. H. Nouwen, *The Wounded Healer* (Garden City, NJ: Image Books, 1979).

46. B.M. Dossey, Nurse As Healer, 63–64.

47. Doona et al., Nursing Presence: An Existential Exploration of Concept, 10.

48. R. Moss, The Mystery of Wholeness, in *Healers on Healing*, ed. R. Carlson and B. Sheild (Los Angeles: Tarcher, 1989).

49. J. Zimmerman, Laying-on-of Hands and Therapeutic Touch: A Testable Theory. Unpublished research (Boulder, CO: Bio-Electro-Magnetics Institute, 1988).

50. E.L. Rossi, *The Symptom Path to Enlightenment: The New Dynamics of Self Organization in Hypnotherapy: An Advanced Manual for Beginners* (Pacific Palisades, CA: Palisades Gateway, 1997).

51. Rogers, *The Theoretical Basis of Nursing.*

52. Quinn, Holding Sacred Space.

53. T.P. Nelms, Living a Caring Presence in Nursing: A Heideggerian Hermeneutical Analysis, *Journal of Advanced Nursing* 24, no. 2 (1996):368–374.

54. McKivergin, The Nurse As an Instrument of Healing.

55. Munhall, *Unknowing.*

56. McKivergin, The Nurse As an Instrument of Healing.

57. D. Krieger, Therapeutic Touch: Searching for Evidence of Physiological Change, *American Journal of Nursing* 79, no. 4 (1979):660–662.

58. McKivergin, The Nurse As an Instrument of Healing.

59. McKivergin, The Nurse As an Instrument of Healing.

60. S. Scandrett-Hibdon and M.I. Freel, The Endogenous Healing Process: A Conceptual Analysis, *Journal of Holistic Nursing* 7, no. 1 (1989):66–71.

61. McKivergin, The Nurse As an Instrument of Healing.

62. J.R. Snyder, Therapeutic Touch and the Terminally Ill: Healing Power through the Hands, *American Journal of Hospice and Palliative Care* 14, no. 2 (1997):83–87.

63. B. Daley, Therapeutic Touch, Nursing Practice and Contemporary Cutaneous Wound Healing Research, *Journal of Advances in Nursing*, no. 6 (1997):1123–1132.

64. D.P. Wirth et al., Wound Healing and Complementary Therapies: A Review, *Journal of Alternative and Complementary Therapies* 4, no. 2 (1996):493–502.

65. E. Shuzman, The Effect of Trait Anxiety and Patient Expectation of Therapeutic Touch on the Reduction of State Anxiety in Preoperative Patients Who Receive Therapeutic Touch (University Microfilms International No. PUZ9423009, 1997).

66. P.P. Hughes et al., Therapeutic Touch with Adolescent Psychiatric Patients, *Journal of Holistic Nursing* no. 14 (1996):6–23.

67. M.J. McKivergin, *The Effects of a Non-Traditional Healing Intervention on Physiological and Qualitative Measures of Well-Being in Women* (University Microfilms International No. 1339540, 1990).

CORE VALUE IV

Holistic Communication, Therapeutic Environment, and Cultural Diversity

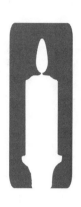

VISION OF HEALING

Human Care

The human care process between a nurse and another individual is a special, delicate gift to be cherished. The human care transactions make it possible for two individuals to come together and establish contact; one person's body-mind-spirit joins another's body-mind-spirit in a lived moment. The shared moment of the present has the potential to transcend time, space, and the physical world as we generally view it in the traditional nurse-client relationship.[1]

* * *

We nurses now find ourselves within a profession that ascribes to the holistic model. Because this model differs philosophically from the traditional biomedical model, it has been called a paradigm shift. Such a philosophic shift has monumental implications that are certain to change the profession forever. Not only does this paradigm make us realize that treating pathophysiologic problems with medical therapy is only half the answer, but also it weaves a tapestry of the interconnectedness of all human beings and suggests the presence of an undefined and powerful healing energy that remains to be harnessed. It challenges us to entertain new ideas that may conflict with our logic and science. It forces us to move away from a purely mechanistic view of the way in which human beings function.

Fashioning a new portrait of ourselves and our profession, this new paradigm alters the image of who we are and who we can become. It is also destined to alter the way in which we practice nursing. The challenge is to determine the course of this destiny. The boundaries within which we can assist patients to achieve wellness and help them to realize their own healing potential remain to be defined. Nonetheless, as we help patients facilitate their inner healing, we discover our own—and begin our journey as nurse healers. Each of us, however, must discover the path.[2]

NOTES

1. J. Watson, *Nursing: Human Science and Human Care* (New York: National League for Nursing Press, 1985), 47.

2. C.E. Guzzetta and B.M. Dossey, *Cardiovascular Nursing: Holistic Practice* (St. Louis: Mosby–Year Book, 1992), xvii.

Chapter 11

Therapeutic Communication: The Art of Helping

Sharon Scandrett-Hibdon

NURSE HEALER OBJECTIVES

Theoretical

- Describe the art of helping through therapeutic communication.
- Determine the differences between therapeutic communication and natural conversation.
- Compare differences between counseling and psychotherapy.
- Recognize when to refer clients for deeper work.

Clinical

- Integrate therapeutic communication skills into clinical practice.
- Evaluate the effects of helping skills on patient satisfaction and clinical outcomes.

Personal

- Refine personal communication skills to enhance personal clarity and effectiveness.
- Integrate therapeutic communication into daily life.
- Evaluate the quality of personal interactions when therapeutic communication skills are used.

DEFINITIONS

Therapeutic Communication: a systematic way of relating to another person that enhances self-discovery and ownership of personal issues; use of specific communication skills that support self-exploration and offer feedback to the client.

Therapeutic Communication Helping Model: a three-staged model of relationship that facilitates clear communication and self-discovery, and promotes change through constructive problem solving.

THEORY AND RESEARCH

Communication is constantly occurring, whether with words, silence, or behavior, one may or may not be conscious of the communication. Holistic in nature, includes many dimensions that influence one's ability to send and receive a message. One's perception and ability to take a message into account can be complex. "Taking into account" is considered to be the most important factor in the process of communication,[1] as a person experiences simultaneous information from radio, television, children talking, and a spouse requesting something. Communication occurs only when the receiver takes into

233

account a message from one of the sources or senders, when a message "gets through" to the receiver's consciousness. The receiver maintains control over which message will receive attention.

The process of communication is constant. What changes is the understanding of the process. In nursing, models of communication tend to be linear, reflecting a mechanistic approach in which the nurse develops a message to affect the client in a certain way so that the client will adopt a desired behavior, often around a healthier lifestyle. There is a feedback loop used; when the nurse asks the client how he or she is feeling, for example, the client's response is carefully attended to and reflected back in order to ensure clear understanding. This reflection is helpful to both the nurse and the client and offers a way for both parties to agree on a similar meaning. Using this technique, the client usually feels heard and "cared about," which builds rapport between the client and the nurse.

Nurses know, at some level, that much more is going on in exchanges with others than is being addressed. Often that sixth sense or "intuitive hit" nurses talk about is a form of covert communication with a client. To understand such covert communication, the communicator must expand personal awareness.

In the counseling field, there is a general debate as to the "helpfulness" of helping. Some take the position that "helping is never helpful," while others believe that "helping is always helpful." Evidence exists on both sides, but the general conclusion of most practitioners is that helping can be helpful.[2] Evidence suggests that competent helpers do make a difference. "Helping is not neutral; it is "for better or for worse."[3] Becoming a skilled, competent helper through the use of effective communication is imperative if holistic nurses are to make a significant contribution to healing.

THERAPEUTIC COMMUNICATION

A counseling approach that makes the client's self-discovery the key focus is the therapeutic communication process that builds a positive, supportive relationship so the client can explore his or her personal experience and behavior. The client can check the accuracy of perceptions immediately with the helper by the use of interpersonal skills. This provides the client with timely and constuctive feedback on personal issues. As a result of the obtained insights, the client can make the clearest decisions for desired changes.

The helper must use many personal skills to achieve focused interaction. The aspects of self involved in this process include accurate listening skills, personal feelings, solicitation of personal understanding about one's life and life themes, knowledge of the change process, and intuitive knowing.

Another important element of helping is keeping the majority of focus on the client's wholeness rather than on the dysfunctions that the client presents. This attention to the whole person provides the energetic emphasis for the client to attain the greatest possible growth. Often in medicine, however, focus on pathology dominates the energetic exchange.

In ordinary conversation, participants frequently use skills such as active listening, validation, and questioning. Each participant is usually invested in being heard, as well as in sharing his or her own story. The relationship is expected to be equal in that both parties benefit from the interaction. Often, painful feelings are "cut off" or diminished since many people have difficulty handling emotional issues. Advice is often solicited and given. Pleasing and judging each other are usually parts of the process.

In therapeutic communication, the helper focuses totally on the client. Initially, the helper puts his or her own reactions, feelings, and thoughts aside to affirm and assist in clarifying the client's personal expression and meaning. As the relationship develops, the helper begins to guide the client deeper into areas of behavior or patterns of which the client may not be fully aware, thus affording greater clarity, ownership, and the opportunity for change. In illuminating patterns, the helper uses personal awareness, such as reactions during the interaction or exploration of deeper feelings, to provide information for the client. All of these exchanges have the purpose of assisting the client in making desired changes in his or her life.

Helping skills used in psychotherapy are part of a deep process in which clients learn about their own personality and heal those aspects that are damaged. Corrective emotional experiences are important in psychotherapy so that clients can experience a healthier way of being than they ever have before. Shifting the personality is a key goal. Psychotherapy can take years and often addresses many issues.

The helper refers a client to a psychotherapist whenever the client seems to have a serious life problem that is causing depression, suicidal thoughts, or feelings of helplessness. Also, referrals are appropriate if the client seems to need inner child work, corrective emotional experiences, or deep inner work (e.g., hypnosis) to heal family wounds. Other problems that require psychotherapy or psychiatric care include personality disorders, physical or psychologic abuse, addictions, and psychoses. The helper can be a great support to these conditions, but further intervention is usually needed.

THERAPEUTIC COMMUNICATION HELPING MODEL

Having evolved from the study of master communicators in counseling and the ben-

eficial outcomes that they have produced for clients, the therapeutic communication helping model has three stages: (1) building of the relationship, (2) deeper exploration, and (3) implementation (Exhibit 11–1). Research on qualities of counselors who produced casualties in therapy were examined as well. Early researchers involved in this work were Kurt Truax and Robert Carkhuff.[4,5] Gerard Egan offers a problem management approach to helping based on the most effective of these skills.[6]

Stage 1 begins with a focus on building a relationship in which the client can choose a problem that will lead to some significant improvement in the quality of his or her life. The helper's task at this stage is to develop rapport with the client, support the client's self-discovery, self-exploration, and establish trust between the helper and the client. The client explores relevant experiences, behaviors, and feelings as concretely as possible. Self-defeating behaviors are identified. Personal participation in the helping process is facilitated and ownership of personal healing clarified. The four interpersonal skills used primarily in this stage—empathy, respect, genuineness, and concreteness—provide safety for the client to "cover the waterfront" of concerns. As the material shared becomes repetitive, the helper knows it is time to begin deeper exploration in an area of immediate concern for the client.

Stage 2 provides the client with the opportunity to clarify his or her life patterns. Some of these patterns are functional, and some are dysfunctional. As the helper listens to the client talk about life, the pattern pieces begin to emerge. The skill of additive empathy puts those patterns neatly together so the client can see what is occurring and what the reward is for continuing that pattern. Various resources and environmental conditions affecting the situation are explored. Patterns that the client may be reluctant to reveal may be explored

Exhibit 11-1 Therapeutic Communication Helping Model

Stage 1: Building of the Relationship

The helper's goal is to build rapport, positive regard, and trust by reflecting to the client at the level presented through use of the following skills:

Empathy
Respect
Genuineness
Concreteness

The client uses this relationship to explore the self.

Stage 2: Deeper Exploration

The helper's goal is to help the client to integrate understanding about personal patterns. The skills used include the following:

Additive empathy
Self-disclosure
Feedback
Confrontation
Immediacy

The client must listen nondefensively and attempt to understand the self through the dynamics of personal patterns.

Stage 3: Implementation

The helper's goal is to assist the client in taking action. The following skills are useful at this stage:

Problem solving
Support
Action plans

The client must collaborate with the helper, taking personal risks to make the desired changes and to take action in his or her life.

Source: Data from G. Egan, *The Skilled Helper*, © 1994, Brooks/Cole Publishing Co. and A. Turok, Interpersonal Skills Laboratory Experience, 1979, University of Iowa Mental Health Authority, Iowa City, Iowa.

---

by using the skills of feedback, confrontation, and immediacy. The helper uses personal life experiences and knowledge to help in identifying some of the patterns and underlying feelings. Self-disclosure is one skill in particular that leads the client deeper through the helper's sharing. Workable goals that will empower the client to manage the problem begin to emerge.

Stage 3 focuses on clarification of the goal and implementation of a plan to meet that goal. As the goal is clearly defined and owned by the client, the helper and the client together determine the plan. Mutual planning includes identification of potential obstacles and resources, as well as a discussion of the ways that the client may sabotage the goal. Ongoing evaluation of

progress toward the goal is done. As the client is empowered and progressing, the relationship is evaluated and plans are made for termination of the helping relationship. Often, the client learns how to cope with future difficult situations by experiencing this mutual problem-solving process.

Therapeutic Communication Skills

Stage 1: Building of the Relationship

Helpers must master specific skills to enhance therapeutic communication. Within Stage 1, *empathy* is the core skill to build rapport and trust between the helper and the client. This skill allows the helper to communicate to the client understanding and acceptance of the client's expressed feelings and the reasons for those feelings. Each time a thought is born, a feeling or emotion follows. In Western society, feelings have often been split from content so that only the reasons for reactions are shared. The skill of empathy reconnects these parts so the client can experience the full meaning of what is being shared.

The helper must complete several tasks to hear the client accurately. First, inner distractions must be avoided so the helper can listen to what is being said and how it is said. It is often helpful to repeat what the client says before responding. The client's dominant feeling is then identified and the reasons for that feeling considered. The helper responds with fresh words that reflect the same meaning as those offered by the client in a concise and incisive manner. The structured format to practice this skill is

You feel _____ because
_____.

In the first blank space, the helper inserts an incisive word that matches the general meaning and intensity of the client's described feeling. In the second space, the helper paraphrases the reasons for the feeling with fresh words.[7,8] For example, the client states, "I am afraid to leave my husband because I don't know if I can make it on my own." One empathic response the helper can offer to convey understanding would be, "You fear to leave him because you are not sure that you can live on your own." Other feeling words that the helper may use are scared, uneasy, threatened, intimidated, or apprehensive. The judge of the accuracy of the feeling description is the client. The client will correct the helper immediately by saying "no" if the feeling word is inaccurate and will then proceed to clarify the meaning. If the empathic response is accurate, the client will often delve deeper into the problem or

situation since the initial feelings were acknowledged by the helper.

With practice, the helper can adapt the format of this skill as long as both components (feeling and reasons) are included in the empathic response. The helper matches the level of intensity and with the meaning of the client. The helper's affirmation at each step of the way allows the client to lead the self-discovery process. The client knows exactly where important events or understandings need to go.

One mistake helpers often make is to jump ahead of the client or prematurely interpret what is being said. Premature interpretation adds another meaning to the exchange, which leaves the client in the "dust" and may reduce the trust level since the helper is no longer affirming the client's feelings at the rate the client feels safe to self-disclose. Another problem arises when the helper asks questions for more information, which leads the client and may distract the client from what is important in that moment.

Practice:

1. **I am feeling depressed since I cannot get ahead of the demands placed upon me.**

   Empathy statement: You feel _____ because
   _____.

   Example response: You feel down since you cannot catch up with the demands on you.

2. **I am excited about having time off to play during these holidays.**

   Empathy statement: You feel _____ because
   _____.

   Example response: You feel elated that you will have time to play during the holiday.

Formulate empathy statements in many situations and share those that feel appropriate.

The second core skill used in the first stage of the model is **respect.** Each client is a unique human being who is a precious whole being. Even when perceiving a client's many problems, the helper must see the innate wholeness within the person to actualize the client's maximum potential. In fact, one of the greatest things a helper can give another person is self-respect.[9] Clients usually know what they need for their healing and are capable of making decisions that are best for themselves. Helpers should encourage self-determination. Acknowledging one's resources is a way to build self-respect. Often, a person who is wrapped up in problems loses sight of the resources required to deal with the situation. Gentle reminders of skills used to cope with current or past problems can strengthen a client's coping. Helping the client to cultivate resources is another powerful tool that fosters self-respect. Accurate listening through the use of empathy is a skill that the helper can use to enhance self-respect even further.[10]

Genuineness enhances therapeutic interactions by allowing the helper to present himself or herself as a human being rather than as a role.[11] The helper may share some feeling directly with the client. For example, if the helper feels bored with some topic that has been shared previously, the helper may say, "We have discussed this topic before; what is going on right now?" If the behavior persists, then the helper may even say, "I feel tired of hearing about this topic because no movement is being made." The purpose of this transaction is to provide the client with a genuine response to the way he or she interacts. If such behavior occurs in the helping session, it most likely occurs elsewhere. Being genuine also means being spontaneous and free in communicating what is occurring in the helper.

Concreteness is the final core skill of this stage of the model which includes purposeful questioning and summarization.[12] *Purposeful questioning* is used when the client's statements are vague. Often, a client encodes or disguises an important issue (also called nominalization) by using one word to signify a larger issue. Asking for further concrete information on that issue is helpful. Often, the lead, "tell me more about this," can elicit more information. Other questions that can help are "What does _____ (vague word) mean?" or "describe what being in that situation is like." Using how, what, when, and describe encourages clients to detail further what they are experiencing. Avoid using why since this question requires the client to have a full understanding of what has happened. If the client just presents the content or facts with no feelings, then a good question to ask is, "What does that feel like?" "What is that experience like?" This technique adds to the holistic nature of the communication. The important thing is to continue connecting feelings with content.

Summarization is helpful when the client has presented a large amount of material. Stopping the client and offering a summary statement or two will let the client know that the helper is listening. Use of empathy conveys understanding. Frequent use of empathy will produce a similar response, which allows the client to move deeper into issues instead of trying to provide large amounts of information to make sure that the helper has "all the facts."

Practice:

Client: I feel so tired these days. I am working 70 hours a week, 7 days a week. There isn't enough time to complete the daily tasks that need to be done at home. I always feel I am behind.

Helper: You feel _____
because _____.

Client: I know that I must slow down. My teenage daughter gets upset when I am gone so much and that bothers me. I hate leaving her alone so much.

Helper: _____

Client: She has been a very responsible teen. I appreciate that she has been helping with cleaning the house.

Helper: _____

Client: I really want to have a different lifestyle in which I can be there for her more of the time. I know that talking is a problem here.

Helper: _____

As the helper uses the core helping skills in therapeutic communication, the client can easily learn some of them. Turock believed that teaching the use of the helping skills was therapeutic in that communications became clearer.[13] Learning to use the skill of empathy, for instance, forces the client to listen very carefully to others. Accurate listening can help to build positive connections between people.

The time to move to the **second stage** of the therapeutic communication model occurs when topics and emotions presented by the client begin to feel repetitive. The client is usually ready to begin deeper exploration of the issues. In nursing, the tendency at this point is to move directly to the third stage, that of problem solving. Yet the helper and the client may not have revealed the underlying patterns on which real changes must be based.

Stage 2: Deeper Exploration

There are five skills used in the second stage of the therapeutic communication model: additive empathy, self-disclosure, feedback, confrontation, and immediacy. The goal of this stage is to reveal the client's deeper patterns and let the client acknowledge how these patterns are maintained.

In **additive empathy,** the helper listens for and describes underlying feelings and behavioral themes. Usually, the client is not fully aware of these underlying feelings. Bringing these to the surface gives the client an opportunity to see clearly how such feelings operate and to decide whether to continue them. This skill has three parts: (1) focusing on surface and deeper feelings, as well as underlying fears; (2) identifying the themes and patterns of response that the client typically uses; (3) identifying the client's personalization of the pattern. The first part of this skill connects the surface feelings to the underlying deeper feelings. For example, "You feel angry at your son, yet I also sense you feel terrified that he will get hurt by pursuing this friend." Leading the client into the deeper feeling allows for exploration of more threatening feelings, such as fear, rage, vulnerability, a sense of being out of control, and failure. The transitional statement to underlying feelings is

> You say you feel _____
> (*expressed feeling*), but it sounds like you also feel _____
> (*underlying feeling*) because _____ (*cause of feeling*).[14]

The second part of the additive empathy skill is to identify the client's patterns and themes. Themes can occur in many dimensions. Emotional themes include feeling like a failure, being pessimistic or optimistic, feeling used, martyred, manipulative, or depressed. Behavioral themes may include sabotaging oneself, rising to opportunities, procrastinating, taking advantage of others, and being passive or aggressive. Cognitive themes include believing one is trapped, helpless, powerless, powerful, or successful. Experiential themes are less overt, as they involve perceiving things in certain ways (e.g., seeing life through rose-colored glasses or always looking at the negative side of events). The thematic part of the communication skill includes a triggering event or stimulus, the pattern of response, and the consequence of that pattern. For example, "When no one calls to remind you, you feel disrespected and withdraw from activities, and it leaves you feeling more alone." The thematic statement is

> When _____ (triggering event), you choose to _____ (pattern of response), and it leaves you _____ (consequence of behavior).[15]

The third part of additive empathy is called personalizing. The client may see the pattern, but it is essential that the client understand how this is maintained. Often a pattern is maintained to keep the client feeling "bad" about the self. An example of personalizing is, "You feel disgusted with yourself when you continue allowing your child to take advantage of you, and you want to assert yourself to put limits on his behavior."

The personalizing stem is

> You feel _____ (self-judgment) with yourself because you do not _____ (deficit behavior) and you want to _____ (goal behavior).[16]

Practice:

Bill complains that he feels unhappy with himself. He is constantly putting things off until the last moment; then he has to scramble to get caught up. He is

working toward a promotion, but feels unsure that it will come through this time since he has so many incomplete projects. He does feel that his work is very good, but wonders how long management will put up with his delayed deadlines.

Create an additive response to Bill. Make sure you include all three aspects of the skill.

_____.

_____.

_____.

An example of the whole additive empathy statements: "I sense you feel frustrated that you never feel caught up, yet I also hear that you fear failure to accomplish all that is being asked. When new requests are made of you, you readily accept them with no question, which leaves you feeling further behind. You despise yourself for continuing to accept more work when you would like to be assertive and plan a more reasonable work load."

The purpose of the *self-disclosure* skill is to lead the client into an exploration of deeper feelings. The helper uses his or her own life experience to assist in this process. It is most important to match the feeling area and to deepen the sharing about the underlying fears, although the life situation need not match exactly what the client shares. This skill quickly takes clients back to their own self-discovery. The format is

> When I _____ (life experience), I felt _____ (deeper feeling than client had shared), I wonder if that fits for you.[17]

If a client expresses despair about being alone and unable to meet anyone who holds similar interests, for example, the helper may say, "When I worked in a factory as a clinic nurse, I felt isolated and misunderstood. I wonder if that fits for you." This skill is often misused in that helpers talk about when they were in a similar situation and successfully survived. The message of this kind of sharing is embedded advice: Do what I did. Telling bigger and better stories of survival or trouble than the client is another error, as it diminishes the client's experience.

Feedback is a fairly familiar skill that provides a great deal of information to the client. This technique is commonly used in educational and training situations to assist learners gain information about their performance. Guidelines for this skill include making sure that the motivation for sharing information is to assist the other person, defining specific behaviors that can be changed, making no assumptions or interpretations about client behavior, conveying the impact of the behavior on others, giving feedback directly to the client as soon as the behavior occurs, and making sure that the client is in a receptive mode to hear the feedback. The format for this skill is

> May I share something with you? (*get permission*)
>
> When I _____ (*observed behavior*),
>
> I feel _____ (*reactive feeling*)
>
> I want to _____ (*desired behavior*)
>
> Right now I am _____ (*what actually will be done*).[18]

An example of this is

> "I would like to share something with you, Jane. (OK.)
>
> When I call and you always have me hold while you take care of something else,
>
> I feel unimportant,

> I want to hang up on you and say, "Get the information yourself,"
>
> Right now, I am letting you know how difficult this is for me."

Some believe that the desired behavior should be deleted, but this part demonstrates the intensity of the helper's response and provides the client with a great deal of information about the behavior's effect on others. Staying nonjudgmental is important, because the goal of this skill is to provide maximal information to the client about some aspect of behavior that the client may wish to change. Repeating the feedback received in the above format allows time to clarify any misunderstanding.

The skill of confrontation invites the client to examine *discrepancies* in behavior, in what is said, thought, felt, experienced, and done. Some of these behaviors may be in the consciousness of the client, and some may not. The format used for confrontation is

> On the one hand, you feel/say/do _____ (*give behavior*),
>
> and on the other hand, you feel/say/do _____ (*behavior*).[19]

For example, "You say you are excited about the upcoming visit, yet it looks to me like you are sad and depressed." Misuse of this skill often involves blame, punishment, "put downs," assumptions about motives, ambiguity, or dogmatic attitudes. Thus, the helper's motives must be examined before use of this fairly invasive skill. The client may deny the truth of the information initially. The helper then gently repeats the information in fresh words after the client has been acknowledged for the reaction through the use of primary empathy.

Immediacy means exploring the relationship at this moment. The occasions when immediacy is important are those in which the client's psychologic needs and intentions require the helper to take on a certain role that will satisfy those needs. The client may not be conscious of this influencing behavior, so bringing it into awareness can be very important for self-discovery and healing. Some of the roles that helpers may be influenced to assume are lover, protector, punisher, excuser, advocate, caretaker, victim, judge, comforter, and adversary.[20]

The helper must use immediacy carefully, since there is a risk of losing the relationship since immediacy is very confrontive and will jar a relationship. Guidelines in use of immediacy begin with the helper experiencing the influencing effort, noting the recycling patterns in communication that create the maneuver, and hypothesizing about what the client is trying to say that cannot be said directly, what the helper is feeling prompted to say, do, or feel, and what the client will gain from this maneuver. The fomat for delivering the immediacy statement is

> Right now I sense you expect or want me to _____ (desired action or role).[21]

For example, "Right now I sense you expect me to wait on you." After making this statement, the helper can use primary empathy to help the client examine the immediacy issues. The client may find these issues very threatening, and denial may surface initially. It is then helpful to share examples of when this influencing effort has occurred in the past.

Practice:

> Recall a time when you were interacting with a client and found yourself frightened. What did you fear might happen? What was the client saying that triggered your fear? What did you want to say/do, but chose not to? What did you say/do? Now do the same with a time when you were angry. Repeat the exercise with a situation in which you recognize a family's recurring pattern of communicating, "Here we go again."[22]

Stage 3: Implementation

The client who has identified a goal and seems ready to begin taking action has reached the problem-solving stage of the model, one of the most important stages to ensure successful change for a client. The first step is to clarify the exact goal. The helper and the client should set the goal together, and the helper must make certain that the client endorses the goal. Some helpful questions are: What does the client want now? What does the client want next year? What is the client invested in keeping? What are the client's resources and capabilities? Where can the client willingly begin? Can the client support this goal 100 percent? Will the client sabatoge this goal?

The goals need to be specific enough for the client to recognize the change or fulfillment. A guideline for setting goals is to ask if the goal would be visible, concrete, and specific enough to be observed by others.[23] Such goals are "I will relax daily," "I will reduce my stress by avoiding extra activities for the next month," "I will enhance my courage by saying yes when opportunities come that feel exciting to me."

Once a clear goal is set, the various options for the client should be examined. Often, the client sees only one or two options, both of which the client has probably already tried. By brainstorming possible ways to achieve the goal, the client and the helper may find many options. Brainstorming options should be done quickly, with no option rejected, and a list of all of the options presented should be recorded.

Once this list is compiled, the client is asked to **select three alternatives** that are most appealing or workable. The remainder of the list is kept for future reference. The client then sets about the task of taking each of the three alternatives and **evaluating** them by use of a **cost–gain analysis** to determine which one to use first. Once an alternative is selected, a **specific action** *plan* is developed by both the client and the helper.[24] Very *small, achievable steps* ensure success in reaching the goal. Since change is frightening for most people, it is important to make the steps small enough to guarantee success. Another approach is to ask clients if they can think of any possible barriers to fulfilling the desired goal. *Trouble shooting* action plans to overcome the rough spots can avert failure. Also, it is helpful to explore with the client what rewards would occur for failure. If a plan does not work as expected, how would the client respond?

Case Study

Helper: Mary, what is going on for you today?

Mary: I am distressed because I can't seem to get my son to help me.

Helper: You feel upset because you can't influence your son to help.

Mary: Yes, I really at this time need some support and help around the house. My job drains me badly. All he wants to do is stay out late, drink with his buddies, and play videogames.

Helper: You need assistance because your energy is low.

Mary: Yes, I am beginning to resent allowing him to live there. Yet I need to have some companionship.

Helper: You feel angry with him, yet you need him.

Mary: Yes, it's better than coming home to an empty house all of the time.

Helper: What would coming home to an empty house mean, Mary?

Mary: Well, I feel very vulnerable right now since the divorce, and my job really takes it out of me. Having someone there seems to give me a sense of security.

Helper: You feel more secure when someone is there.

Mary: Yes, although in reality, he is rarely there and is hostile whenever I ask him to do anything.

Helper: What is that like, Mary? To have someone rarely there and hostile?

Mary: Well, I feel guilty for taking his father away, and I want to help my son, but he sure does little to help me.

Helper: Mary, it seems like you feel responsible for your son, yet feel betrayed by him in that he uses you and continues to live there.

Mary: (*tears*): Yes.

Helper: When you ask for the help you need and nothing gets done, you allow the behavior to continue and abandon yourself, even though you really need support and nurturing.

Mary: (*crying harder*): Yes, I do need nurturing, and I do allow this to continue.

Helper: You blame yourself for your divorce and keep owing your son something, when you need to be taking better care of yourself.

Mary: That's exactly right. I do need to take better care of myself. I don't blame myself for the divorce; I did the best I could in the relationship. I do feel like I owe my son something, partly for contributing to the divorce at this time in his life. He's not on his feet yet either. But I do need help.

Helper: Mary, what would you like to do about this?

Mary: Well, it is imperative that I take care of myself, or I will become sick. So I need to begin working on that.

Helper: What would that be like, Mary?

Mary: Well, I want to feel that my home is a supportive place for me. That I don't have to wait on anyone else, even though I am willing to share space with him.

Helper: So what would be the specific goal?

Mary: I want to come to a peaceful, orderly home and not feel like I have to wonder where my son is and when he will be coming in or who he will drag in.

Helper: So coming in to a peaceful, orderly home and being informed of your son's plans?

Mary: Yes, that would be wonderful.

Helper: Let's play a bit and see if we to-gether can come up with some ideas on how these goals could be met.

Mary: OK.

Helper: You could have him pay rent and hire a housekeeper to clean once a week.

Mary: That would be great. Although get-ting him to pay rent would be a problem.

Both: You could tell him to move out unless he can afford to have a housekeeper come once a week.

I could make sure he has a beeper so I could contact him when he doesn't come in on time.

You could have him leave you a note each day.

I could make him call me at work before he leaves the house.

You could charge him for the meals he eats there.

You could have him move out and have a friend move in, charging them rent.

I could have weekly massages in my home.

You could make him pay for the mas-sages.

Helper: Mary, of all of the things suggested, what are three things that you could be-gin with knowing that you always have the option to come back to any of these.

Mary: Well, I like the idea of charging him rent and hiring a housekeeper. Also I want him to leave me a note daily. I like the idea of weekly massages as well.

Helper: This week I would like to have you work on assessing each of these options with a cost–gain analysis. You have two goals you are working on, and we have over 100 alternatives to choose from. Please take three of these and work with them, bringing them back to our next ses-sion so we can create a plan on the one you wish to start on.

(Next week)

Mary: I want to charge him rent and hire a housekeeper. I feel like that is a fair re-quest, even if I only charge him what a housekeeper would cost.

Helper: How would you like to do this, Mary?

Mary: I can call and find out housekeeper fees and then talk to him about my need for more help. If he cannot provide the help, then I can set the fee needed to hire the help I need and require him to pay that. If he won't do that, I can then tell him that he must find another place to live.

Helper: You have thought through this, haven't you?

Mary: Yes, I feel so good to be making plans to support me. I really needed this boost. Already I have a more positive outlook just by the possibility of having a change.

Helper: How would you undermine this happening, Mary?

Mary: If he throws a fit and I do my usual thing, which is to give in and make peace.

Helper: What can you do to prevent this be-havior from happening?

Mary: I can think of how bad I am feeling when I have no support. I can insist that I am as important in this house as he is and remember that I have been aban-doning myself.

Helper: Is that enough to hold you steady if he confronts you?

Mary: Yes, I really didn't look at how I al-ways put myself last. I did that in the marriage as well.

Helper: So the plan is that you will get com-petitive prices on a housekeeper, tell your son that he either will help with the cleaning or pay the cost of a house-keeper. If he refuses, you will tell him he must find another place to live?

Mary: Yes, I feel good about this.

Helper: How will you handle your feelings of responsibility and guilt?

Mary: I have realized as I listened to myself that I have nothing to feel guilty about. I provided well for him and gave him a good home for many years. Now it is my turn to at least be equally considered.

> **Practice:** Go back through the preceding interaction and highlight the stages of the therapeutic communication helping model and label the skills used.

CONCLUSION

Helping skills have consistently been proved to assist individuals to become more aware of their own issues. This model provides the client with maximal support for self-discovery and change. Holistic nurses are committed to empowering the client. Use of this approach provides a powerful way to enhance the client's self-healing. Teaching the client the skills also gives him or her the tools to build better relationships with others.

DIRECTIONS FOR FUTURE RESEARCH

1. Evaluate the outcomes of using the therapeutic communication helping model in various clinical settings.

2. Determine the effectiveness of using therapeutic communication with clients and nurses in achieving their desired change in lifestyle.

3. Document and quantify the coping changes clients make when they use the helping skills themselves.

NURSE HEALER REFLECTIONS

After reading this chapter, the nurse healer will be able to answer or begin the process of answering the following questions:

- How can these therapeutic communication skills become a long-term investment in my life?
- In what way would my personal and professional communications change if I incorporated these skills into my life?
- Do I hold a clear mirror for each client to see the majesty of his or her life?
- Do I recognize the privilege of being of service to others to help them empower their lives and to feel self-respect?
- While working with others, do I hold most of my vision on their wholeness or do I see mostly their disturbed patterns?

NOTES

1. L. Thayer, *Communication and Communication Systems* (Homewood, IL: Richard D. Irwin, 1968).
2. G. Egan, *The Skilled Helper* (Pacific Grove, CA: Brooks/Cole, 1994), 10.
3. Egan, *The Skilled Helper*, 11.
4. C.B. Truax and R.R. Carkhuff, *Toward Effective Counseling and Psychotherapy: Training and Practice* (Chicago: Aldine, 1967).
5. R. Carkhuff, *The Art of Helping IV*, 4th ed. (Amherst, MA: Amherst Resource Development Press, 1980).
6. Egan, *The Skilled Helper*.
7. A. Turok, *Interpersonal Skills Laboratory Experience* (Iowa City: University of Iowa Mental Health Authority, 1979).
8. Egan, *The Skilled Helper*, 111.
9. W. Stephenson, Professor, Lectureship in Communications, University of Iowa, 1970.
10. Turok, *Interpersonal Skills Laboratory Experience*.
11. Turok, *Interpersonal Skills Laboratory Experience*.

12. Turok, *Interpersonal Skills Laboratory Experience.*

13. Turok, *Interpersonal Skills Laboratory Experience.*

14. Turok, *Interpersonal Skills Laboratory Experience,* 12.

15. Turok, *Interpersonal Skills Laboratory Experience,* 12.

16. Turok, *Interpersonal Skills Laboatory Experience,* 12.

17. Turok, *Interpersonal Skills Laboratory Experience.*

18. Turok, *Interpersonal Skills Laboratory Experience.*

19. R.R. Carkhuff and R.M. Pierce, *Trainer's Guide the Art of Helping: An Introduction to Life Skills* (Amherst, MA: Human Resource Development Press, 1975), 113.

20. Turock, *Interpersonal Skills Laboratory Experience.*

21. A. Turock, Immediacy in Counseling: Recognizing Clients' Unspoken Messages, *Personnel and Guidance Journal* 59 (1980):168–172.

22. Turock, *Interpersonal Skills Laboratory Experience.*

23. A. Turock, Verbal Instruction in Training of Trainers Workshop, Iowa City, Iowa, 1974.

24. Turock, *Interpersonal Skills Laboratory Experience.*

VISION OF HEALING

Building a Healthy Environment

The use of the environment has become one of today's foremost issues. Nurses have risen to the occasion by proactively forming national organizations and sponsoring conferences to address environmental concerns. The American Holistic Nurses' Association (AHNA) has developed and propagates a statement on environmental issues.

American Holistic Nurses' Association Position Statement in Support of a Healthful Environment

The philosophy of the American Holistic Nurses' Association includes the belief that "health involves the harmonious balance of body, mind, and spirit in an ever-changing environment."

The environment involves both our immediate as well as global surroundings. Many of us are aware of a need to expand our consciousness regarding environmental issues and believe that this can have an effect on our own personal and community well-being.

Our concerns come from a reverence for the beauty and integrity of the earth which sustains us and is our home, our Mother Earth. Relevant environmental issues include preserving the integrity of the air, soil, and water as well as issues such as global warming, acid rain and other equally challenging situations. We believe as holistic nurses, we have a responsibility for increasing awareness regard-

ing these issues in others, through role modeling and educating within our communities.

The AHNA encourages self-responsible behavior as well as participation in socially responsible environmental groups, to protect and support improvement of the health of our environment.[1]

The reason that politicians, nurses, and most other segments of society are becoming involved in environmental issues is the growing awareness of the relationship between our physical reality and the earth. The twentieth century witnessed two dramatic events: a sudden, startling surge in human population and an abrupt acceleration of the scientific and technologic revolution.

From the beginning of humanity's appearance on earth to 1945, it took more than 10,000 generations to reach a world population of 2 billion people. Now, in the course of one human lifetime, the world population is increasing from 2 to more than 9 billion people.[2] All of us working with computers and hospital equipment can attest to the exponential explosion of technology during our careers. These factors and others have magnified our power to affect the world around us by burning, cutting, digging, moving, and transforming the physical matter that makes up the earth. As a society, we are straining under the burden of a burgeoning population that is demanding not only the fulfillment of basic needs, but also access to health care and space age technology. In trying to meet the ever-increasing demands, we have contaminated our air, soil, and waters with by-products, and we have attenuated our foods with herbicides, pesticides, and overprocessing. Urban and suburban areas reverberate with noise and violence, and frustrations mount as increasing numbers crowd into congested living areas.

Nurses are seeking to discover the best ways to utilize the environment to maximize the overall healing effort. All of us must aspire to develop global ecologic skills if we are to endure. Environmental scientists and nurses can cooperate in unique ways to promote a global healing ethic.[3]

On an individual level, the way in which people use their personal space affects not only the way that they feel, but also, in today's shrinking world, the space around others. For example, when we play our stereos or radios, the broadcast should fill only the short space between us and the speaker, not blare so loud that it reaches into the personal space of others who may not want to hear the program. In increasingly congested areas, we must take care to honor each person's right for quiet space. All of us need to work together to find individual and community solutions to the serious environmental issues that face us in the twenty-first century.

NOTES

1. Reprinted from *Environmental Philosophy* with the permission of the American Holistic Nurses' Association, 2733 East Lakin Drive, Suite #2, Flagstaff, AZ 86004, phone: 800-278-AHNA or 520-526-2196, FAX: 520-526-2752.

2. A. Gore, *Earth in the Balance: Ecology and the Human Spirit* (New York: Plume, 1993), 31.

3. J. Case, The Biosphere and the Healing Arts, *Holistic Nursing Practice* 6, no. 4 (1992): 10–19.

Nishmat Kol Chai (The Soul of All Living Things)—a Jewish morning prayer

Every day we find a new sky and a new earth
with which we are entrusted like a perfect toy.
We are given the salty river of our blood
winding through us, to remember the sea and our
kindred under the waves, the hot pulsing that knocks
in our throats to consider our cousins in the grass
and the trees, all bring scattered rivulets of life.

We are given the wind within us, the breath
to shape into words that steal time, that touch
like hands and pierce like bullets, that waken
truth and deceit, sorrow and pity and joy,
that waste precious air in complaints, in lies,
in floating traps for power in the dirty air.
Yet holy breath still stretches our lungs to sing.

We are given the body, the momentary kibbutz
of elements that have belonged to frog and polar
bear, corn and oak tree, volcano and glacier.
We are lent for a time these minerals in water
and a morning every day, a morning to wake up,
rejoice and praise life in our spines, our throats,
our knees, our genitals, our brains, our tongues.

We are given fire to see against the dark,
to think, to read, to study how we are to live,
to bank in ourselves against defeat and despair
that cool and muddy our resolves, that make us forget
what we saw we must do. We are given passion
to rise like the sun in our minds with the new day
and burn the debris of habit and greed and fear.

We stand in the midst of the burning world
primed to burn with compassionate love and justice,
to turn inward and find holy fire at the core,
to turn outward and see the world that is all
one flesh with us, see under the trash, through
the smog, the furry bee in the apple blossom,
the trout leaping, the candles our ancestors lit for us.

Fill us as the tide rustles into the reeds in the marsh.
Fill us as the rushing water overflows the pitcher.
Fill us as the light fills a room with its dancing.
Let the little quarrels of the bones and the snarling
of the lesser appetites and the whining of the ego cease.
Let silence still us so you may show us your shining
and we can out of that stillness rise and praise.

Marge Piercy

Chapter 12

Environment

Eleanor A. Schuster and Lynn Keegan

NURSE HEALER OBJECTIVES

Theoretical

- Name four ways in which substantive systems changes can diminish toxic exposures in life.
- Identify three principles that can direct human endeavors toward a sustainable future.
- Describe three characteristics of a learning community.
- Differentiate between the terms *schooling* and *education*.
- Increase awareness of environmental hazards, and make a commitment to reducing these hazards.

Clinical

- Subscribe, or arrange to have consistent access to, periodical literature specific to clinical application of environmental principles (e.g., *World-Watch*, a bi-monthly magazine of the Worldwide Institute).
- Identify and act on three ways to influence environmental accountability in the workplace.
- Consider joining an organization created to influence the direction of future sustainability.
- Become sensitive to the environmental space in the home, institution, health agency, or clinic.

Personal

- Seek out at least one other person for mutual support in examining ways to make a difference toward future sustainability.
- Make a consistent effort to eliminate, not just diminish, the concept of waste in your life.
- Assume a "beginner's mind," being open to knowing what is essential about environmental relationships in your life.
- Whenever possible, eliminate negative aspects of your personal environment (e.g., stale air, inadequate lighting, subliminal noises).
- Experiment with healing colors, scents, textures, sound, and lighting in your personal environment.

DEFINITIONS

Ambience: an environment or its distinct atmosphere; the totality of feeling that one experiences from a particular environment.

Anthropocentrism: the world view that places human beings as the central fact or final aim of the universe.

Chaos Theory: sometimes called the "new science," offers a way of seeing order and pattern where formerly only the random, the erratic, and the unpredictable had been observed.

Ecology: the scientific study of interrelationships between and among organisms, and between them and all aspects, living and nonliving, of their environment.

Ecominnea: the concept of an ecologically sound society.

Environment: everything that surrounds an individual or group of people: physical, social, psychologic, cultural, or spiritual characteristics; external and internal features; animate and inanimate objects; seen and unseen vibrations; and frequencies, climate, and not yet understood energy patterns.

Environmental Ethics: a division of philosophy concerned with valuing the environment, primarily as it relates to humankind, secondarily as it relates to other creatures and to the land.

Environmental Justice: a sub-branch of ethics examining the innate and relational value among organisms and all aspects of their environment.

Epistemology: the branch of philosophy that addresses the origin, nature, methods, and limits of knowledge.

Ergonomics: the study of and realization of the importance of human factors in engineering.

Personal Space: the area around an individual that should be under the control of that individual, including air, light, temperature, sound, scent, and color.

Restorative Justice: an ethical perception that directs that environmental damages be not only curtailed, but also repaired and recompensed in some meaningful way.

Superfund Sites: hazardous waste landfills or abandoned manufacturing sites, names of which appear on the Environmental Protection Agency's National Priorities List.

Sustainable Future: meet the needs of the present without compromising the needs of future generations.

Toxic Substance: a substance that can cause harm to a person through either short- or long-term exposure, as by (1) inhalation; (2) ingestion into the body in the form of vapors, gases, fumes, dusts, solids, liquids, or mists; or (3) skin absorption.

THEORY AND RESEARCH

To engage successfully with life in modern times, people are challenged to commit themselves to maturity as earth dwellers, earth citizens, who are willing to

- live in a world of vast complexity and unpredictability
- engage in their own grief work
- work with contradiction and paradox
- risk everything through the clarity of their values and convictions
- reside in joy of spirit and lightness of heart, the constants for everyone as children of the universe who are here because they are integral to the teeming fullness of life.

Environmental Education for Holistic Nurses

Since the term *environment* in its broadest sense can mean everything, both within and external to each person, it is a challenge to determine what "should be" provided to holistic nurses as a basic educational resource. Although many configurations are feasible and worthy, five themes can be used to form a constellation, a "mental map," to conceptualize the environmental world and the human place in it: (1) telling personal and collective life stories, (2) living in a toxic world, (3) choosing a sustainable future, (4) building learning communities, and (5) working from the inside out.

Theme 1: Telling One's Story

Admittedly, each nurse practices the profession of nursing as he or she sees fit. No one can tell nurses how to practice, nor can anyone do it for them. The profession is vastly fluid and creative. What was originally perceived as the premier practice role at one time may lose its appeal as a nurse continues in the profession. Each nurse has a unique and personal story to tell of the reasons that he or she is in nursing and the travails, rewards, and joys of the pathway. Sometimes, individuals tell themselves their story, in a reflective moment; sometimes, they share choice vignettes with others. Who has not reminisced with fondness about some shared early experiences when with colleagues? Nursing is for most practitioners, if not all, a joyous "soul-home," and they like to speak of this in the sacred circle of companions when circumstances are conducive to such disclosure.

Conventional wisdom has it that, in encouraging patients to tell stories, nurses have already engaged with them in a necessary part of the healing process. For example, "She heard me; I'm not crazy after all!" or "Oh, I feel better now!"

In a consideration of the environment, it is imperative to listen and respond to a larger story, not only as individual practitioners, but also as members of humankind. This reaffirms what we know through all the senses to be basic and important: What does it mean to be human? What does it mean to be an earth citizen? How can we face the great crises of our time: ecologic, political, social, economic, intellectual, psychologic, and spiritual? People cannot ignore the matrix of their own being if they are to understand and respond to contemporary needs. They must consider their existential context. Richard Tarnas, a philosopher and historian of Western thought, helped bring the human drama into consciousness.[1]

Two Stories of the Evolution. There are two versions of the evolution of human consciousness. Both are basic truths and deep patterns in the psyche that inform an individual's day-to-day experience in various ways. One is *progress and heroic advance,* characterized by gradual, progressive, and familiar milestones of discovery and accomplishment: the printing press, harnessing of electricity, the telephone, radio, computers, and so forth. These are learned in basic education. Generally, this version equates ever-increasing and refined knowledge with fulfillment and well-being. The scientific mind is the apex of this world view, having its roots in ancient Greece and the flourishing in the European enlightenment of the eighteenth century. The modern mind is known for individualistic democracy, power, and emancipation. Inventiveness, endurance, will to succeed, and adventuresome spirit are sources for pride. The "miracles of modern medicine" are found here.

The second version of the evolution of human consciousness is the *fall and tragic separation,* which is a deep wounding or schism that separates humankind from nature. Manifestations of this version include exploitation of the natural environment, devastation of indigenous cultures, and an increasingly unhappy state of the human soul. Through the lens of tragic separation, humanity and nature are seen as having suffered grievously under an increasingly dualistic domination of thought and society. The worst consequences of this development are directly derived from the hegemony of modern industrial society, empowered by science and technology.

All individuals are challenged, although they may not recognize it, to reconcile these perspectives in their day-to-day lives. Are we embroiled in progress? Are we victims of tragedy? The two perspectives are both correct in a certain way; the gestalt differs, while the data remain the same. For example, it is possible to maintain life support systems, equal to progress; however, the person may be maintained beyond all parameters of the natural dignity of dying, equal to tragedy. Both are readings, but only partial apprehensions of a deeper, larger, and more complex story. Gain and loss have been working together simultaneously until the dialectic has reached an almost climactic moment at present. Nurses are aware of pervasive and intense suffering, not only in their own inner work, but beyond, to the transpersonal and collective unconscious. The whole planet is in a transformative crisis.

The Core Elements Driving the Multidimensional Crisis. The modern mind, the mind of progress, originates in the world view that there is a radical and irreconcilable distinction between the human self as subject and the world as object. In contrast, the primal world view is that spirit or soul permeates the entire universe within which the soul is embedded. The human essence participates in a world soul or *anima mundi*. The modern mind condemns this as a naive epistemologic error, childish, immature, and to be outgrown. The wisdom of the modern mind asserts that the human self is the exclusive repository of conscious intelligence; all meaning in the universe comes from the human subject. This is the classic existentialist assumption that, without humankind, the universe is meaningless.

Typically, a modern person's allegiance is to science in the belief that science rules the cosmos and objective world, while poetry, music, and spiritual strivings inhabit the internal world. Our cherished Western autonomy, offspring of the progress perspective, has been purchased at a staggering price: gradual dilution and diminution of soul, meaning, and spirit. Thus, the purpose of the entire world is exclusive to the human self. Everything else is "out there," resulting in the demise of the metaphysical world and the disenchantment of the cosmos. Whether in conscious awareness or not, the greatest demand of modern time is to reconcile the imperatives of the two versions of what it means to be human. Must

everyone choose and align themselves with one or the other? Must everyone consign themselves to an existence where "progress" is purchased with the coin of soul loss?

Tarnas contends that modern culture itself is immersed in a rite of the most epochal and profound kind: the entire path of human civilization has taken humankind, the planet, and all its members into a trajectory of complete alienation that is part of the mythic death/rebirth story.[2] Something new is being formed, however, which is a new participative and holistic vision of the universe amply reflected by contemporary scientific and philosophic insights. In this emerging view, the human self is both highly differentiated, yet re-embedded in a participatory, meaning-laden universe.

Transformative Unfolding to a More Integral World. Expanding the epistemology from empiricism and rationalism, the paradigms of progress, to draw from the wider epistemologies of the heart is the first step toward a more integral world. There are ways of knowing that integrate imagination, intuition, aesthetic sensitivity, revelatory or epiphanic capacity, the abilities to love and be loved. Another powerful remedy against the pervasive ills of the modern world is a fundamental movement of remorse, a sustained weeping and grief for collective and individual offenses against humankind, other species, the innocent, the defenseless, the trusting. A self-overcoming, or metanoia, is our radical sacrifice integral to the shift of world view. Within the context of this evolving paradigm, there is an acknowledgment of a power greater than our own. It is the recognition that, when the self has been totally emptied in the moment of death, in the ego death, in the dark night of the soul, something else happens. That is when the Divine can come through and, finally, it is not other. It is within us. It is who we are.

There can be no responsible discussion and deliberation about the environment and the role of holistic nursing without knowing and honoring human history with all its triumph and terror, its puniness and majesty. Despite their various personal views of the world, what is real, and what is important, holistic nurses strive for clarity of meanings, values, and relationships about which they are impassioned! It is instructive, in this context, to hear what Macy related about a Tibetan Buddhist prediction of the twelfth century:

> In these days of misery, war, crises and economic collapse, and when the world itself is on the threshold of annihilation, there arises a multitude of Shambhala Warriors. These warriors are of every color, age, gender, from every culture and are found in all corners of the earth, in humble circumstances and in corridors of power. These men and women, elders and children wear no uniforms nor do they carry martial banners. Each wields two weapons: compassion and clear intent.[3]

Holistic nurses live the identical existential anguish of those they care for and care about. They are "wounded healers," a role that augments rather than diminishes their effectiveness. The role is reciprocal: they are healed as they heal. Additionally, they know the healing role is not confined to humankind, but is a common and shared attribute of all creation. Florence Nightingale, through her 13 canons, gave the most basic instruction of all: "the art of nursing requires us to alter the environment safely."[4] This simple injunction is the bedrock on which rests all environmental aspirations, values, thought, and activity, for today and for any foreseeable future.

At this juncture, it is helpful to reflect on the wisdom of the I Ching, "The superior man (our essential self) eats, drinks, is joyous and of good cheer."[5] We are not ordinarily accustomed to prolonged apocalyptic reflection so may become ill at ease in its presence. We are children of the universe, however. We belong here as part of the wondrous greening of things. We exist! That alone is cause for joyous celebration!

Theme 2: Living in a Toxic World

A guaranteed formula for depression is to make a list of "problems," thus dwelling energetically and metaphorically in a room without sunlight or exit. A more life-affirming exercise is to clarify individual and collective goals and then work toward those goals. Although grief and remorse are appropriate responses to ubiquitous planetary degradation, which has its genesis with humankind, they are counterproductive within themselves. Grief and remorse alone, without action, lead inexorably into downward emotional spirals or into diversionary escapes. Human beings are characterized by the ability to choose and change; the past need not be perpetuated. Human beings have the ability to elect life-affirming ways, relinquishing that which kills them, in both body and spirit.

Environmentalism evolved in several stages, all of which coexist today.[6] The U.S. conservation movement began in the late nineteenth century in reaction to the devastation of what had seemed an inexhaustible wilderness. The national park system arose from this new awareness. Wilderness advocates such as anglers, hunters, and hikers still represent a large percentage of environmentalists. Carson exposed the dangers of DDT, introducing a second stage of the environmental movement.[7] Activists of the 1960s and 1970s targeted other hazardous materials—polychlorinated biphenyls (PCBs), mercury, lead, and other heavy metals. Environmental legislation that created state and federal protection agencies widened the focus from preservation to protection.

The discovery in the 1980s of the hole in the ozone layer over Antarctica, along with escalating concern over global warming, introduced a third phase of environmentalism. Rather than focusing on dangers from toxic substances, this stage emphasizes sustainability, which is protecting future generations from the dangers of exceeding nature's ability to restore itself. A fourth stage addressed the notion of environmental equity—a determination of a safe global quota for emission of gases that cause the greenhouse effect and the allotment of an equal share of that quota to each human inhabitant of the planet. Other evolving perspectives speak of environmental justice and environmental ethics and, even more recently, restorative justice. The main thrust of the first two categories is preventing toxic wastes from endangering others, such as factory emissions close to neighborhoods or the export of radiologically active by-products to Third World countries. Restorative justice means not only curtailment of environmentally eroding practices, but taking conscious and deliberate steps toward repair of damages.

The configuration of stages or perspectives has two commonalities. First, it is anthropocentric in that virtually all efforts are directed to the well-being of humankind. Only tangentially are other creatures considered; they have no inherent "rights." Second, popular literature rarely addresses the imperative to alter lifestyles, even though the difficulties that abound are immediately attributable to living in collective excess in collusion with a market-driven economy. Macy noted, "While the agricultural revolution took centuries, and the industrial revolution took generations, this ecological revolution has to happen within a matter of a few years. It also has to be more comprehensive—involving not only the political economy but the habits and values that foster it."[8]

We inhabit a toxic world.[9] The products and by-products of industrial society are poisoning the earth and its inhabitants. Caring, inventive people know that a very different community could be created by using alternative strategies to provide the same essential services that chemicals provide, however. The world's most gifted

engineers have gathered in places like Silicon Valley, formerly Santa Clara Valley, of the San Francisco Bay area; Silicon Desert in Arizona; Silicon Glen in Scotland; and Silicon Plateau in India over the past 20 years. An immense infrastructure has developed to support this high-technology world.[10] Silicon Valley is a particularly poignant example of the "progress" versus the "tragedy" metanarrative. Before "clean" industrialization, few places in the world equaled the fertility of this agricultural mecca. In some places, the topsoil of fine loam was 40 feet deep, alluvial fans laid down by two mountain stream systems. Below that were huge fresh water aquifers of gravel and clay, permitting irrigation through a vast system of artesian wells. When industries entered the valley, however, at the peak of computer chip manufacturing, a highly water-intensive process, Santa Clara county was forced to import water.

Industries have struggled to maintain a positive image despite the endemic proliferation of poisoned wells, leaking chemical tanks, and illegal sludge dumps. The once pristine valley now has 29 Superfund sites, the most dense concentration of highly hazardous waste dumps in the United States. Even the most sophisticated clean-up methods cannot remove the toxic solvents (such as the trichloroethylene [TCE] used in chip production) from aquifers. Studies by IBM and the Semiconductor Industry Association have linked the use of solvents to problems in workers' reproductive health and to birth defects.[11] High concentrations of heavy metals in sewage emissions have had a disastrous impact on San Francisco Bay. Shoreline communities harvested 15 million pounds of oysters annually at the turn of the century; since 1970, the entire oyster population has been too contaminated to eat.[12]

Through hindsight, it is becoming evident that even the economic bottom line must address quality-of-life issues. Furthermore, only from a broad bioregional base can planners consider the complex interactions among jobs, profits, housing, farmland and water quality, parks and playgrounds, ethnic diversity, class tensions, and freeway build-ups. Now in Silicon Valley, actions are under way to preserve strips of open land and stop further expansion; private sector coalitions are forming to protect farms, open land, and wildlife. Natural soaps and citrus solutions are replacing toxic manufacturing processes, and light rail lines are improving the rapid transit system. Perhaps the clearest indicator that change is essential is the fact that more engineers are declining positions in this prestigious location because of quality-of-life issues.

In less than one lifetime, production of synthetic organic chemicals (e.g., dyes, plastic, solvents) has increased more than 1,000-fold in the United States alone.[13] There are roughly 70,000 different synthetic chemicals on the global market, with more in continuous production. In addition, many chemicals are emitted as by-products of production or incineration (particularly relevant to the hospital industry). Some chemicals, such as antihistamines, have direct health benefits. Others, such as pesticides and herbicides, are designed to be usefully lethal (many developed as military offense measures during the Vietnamese war). The most pernicious and pervasive were not meant to come into human contact. When PCBs were created in 1929, for example, they were intended for use only in electrical wiring, lubricants, and liquid seals. Today, PCBs, along with 250 other synthetic chemicals can be found in the bodies of almost everyone in the industrial world.[14]

According to the most recent tally, 40 carcinogens appear in drinking water, 60 are released by industry into the ambient air, and 66 are sprayed on crop food as pesticides.[15] Whatever a person's past exposure, often bioaccumulative, this is the current situation. An issue yet to be examined in any depth is the interactional effect of all these substances. It is known that one pharmacologic substance may potentiate the action of another; the same dynamic is logical for industrial chemicals and by-products. A specific cause of alarm, as a result of evidence that began to appear in the early 1990s, is the role of 50 or more chemicals as endocrine disruptors and, more particularly, as hormone mimics with likely linkages to breast cancer.[16] A narrow focus on genetic roots, as well as an emphasis on lifestyle obscures cancer's environmental roots, as well as the underlying genesis of other illnesses.

Clearly, the hazards that Carson noted 50 years ago have flourished.[17] They are a robust presence among us despite vast concern, legislation, grassroots actions, and deep-down engagement with the problem by many people and organizations. For the most part, even the best intentioned activities are temporary stopgap measures that can only delay the demise of the natural world as presently known; much like the fleeting relief offered by some of contemporary biomedical regimens, they provide alleviation and management of symptoms, not systemic change. A way of life, a conscious choice, is possible if we are willing to work, really work, to change from the industrial growth society to a life-sustaining society. It is possible to meet our needs without destroying our life support system.

> To choose life in this planet time is a mighty adventure. As people in all countries and walks of life are discovering, this adventure elicits more courage and enlivening solidarity than any military campaign. From high school students restoring streams for salmon spawning, to inner city neighbors creating community gardens on vacant lots, from forest activists delaying logging until environmental impact studies are done, to windmill engineers bringing their technology to en-

ergy-hungry regions—countless groups are learning, organizing, taking action.[18]

Part of the wonderment is that engaging in the life-affirming healing work transforms us into a microcosm of the new paradigm.

Three Key Principles. As with any major enterprise, basic guidelines provide parameters and rationale to illumine the path. The removal of all carcinogens or other noxious substances is unlikely, but elimination of some would reduce the physiologic and bioregional burden, thus preventing considerable suffering and loss of life. Steingraber offered three principles based on the ideal that it is every person's right to live in a nonpolluted environment:[19]

1. *Precautionary Principle.* Public and private interests should act to prevent harm before it occurs; an indication of harm rather than proof of harm should trigger for action. Current methods rely on the "dead body" approach: wait until damage is proved before action is taken (e.g., definitive remedial steps taken 11 years after the first discovered evidence of ozone layer depletion).
2. *Principle of Reverse Onus.* Safety rather than harm should necessitate demonstration. Those who seek to introduce chemicals should demonstrate that what they propose to do will not hurt anyone. This is the current standard for pharmaceuticals, but most industrial chemicals have no firm requirement for advanced demonstration of safety.
3. *Principle of the Least Toxic Alternative.* Toxic substances should not be used as long as there is another way of accomplishing the task. Society in general proceeds on the assumption that toxic substances will be used; the only question is how much.

Life-Affirming Trends. As consumers' awareness and knowledge of the effects of chemical and other exposures in the workplace and homes increase, so does their influence on industry as well as retail outlets. Public awareness, especially if it is organized, can revolutionize both industry and the marketplace. As evidence, the organic food industry has increased 20 percent each year since 1990.[20]

Health care organizations have also become more environmentally aware. Health Care Without Harm is a collaborative campaign for environmentally responsible health care in which more than 140 organizations and individuals work together to eliminate pollution in health care practices without compromising safety or care.[21] Health care practices, especially medical waste incineration, are leading sources of dioxin and mercury emissions. The emissions are airborne or water-borne and eventually contaminate fish, meat, and dairy products. The singular intent of this group is directed toward making hospitals models of environmental accountability, a remarkable ambition substantially different from meeting basic codes and standards.

Shaner, a nurse, and her colleagues provide professional consulting worldwide concerning the responsible and effective management of the waste stream in hospitals. This vast sphere of influence grew from her original awareness, as a staff nurse in a community hospital, of unnecessary waste and misidentification of what needed special handling. The manual of which she is a principal author, *An Ounce of Prevention*, is available through the American Hospital Association and is a primary resource for health care agencies in relation to waste management.[22] Likewise, the medical community formed the Consortium for Environmental Medicine to advance human health by understanding its relationship to environment.[23]

These efforts are part of a general societal thrust to have a habitable planet, now and in years to come. Many of these efforts, in the aggregate, are pragmatic and based on economic interests; others are derived from a philosophic outlook such as environmental justice. Many, if not most, of the movements remain human-centered, addressing impacts as they relate to humankind. Any benefit for the rest of the biotic community is a by-product from that frame of reference. The holistic outlook, as has been stated, recognizes all systems as interacting. If one part is affected, change of a greater or lesser magnitude occurs everywhere.

The ultimate purpose of this way of thinking is to weave the human economy back into the earth economy. Cowan, a building and landscape architect, noted that toxicity, waste, and extravagant resource use are all symptoms of poor design and production processes.[24] Around the world, innovative companies and product designers are taking ecology as the basis for design, thus phasing out toxicity, cutting waste, and increasing resource efficiency. Other companies such as Andropogon, are restoring the ecologic integrity of the landscape by restoring native vegetation, reestablishing water flow, and reconnecting wild areas.[25]

Unsatisfied with scientific and regulatory approaches to the symptoms of systemic failure—in his medical practice, bizarre tumors among his patients could be traced to underlying environmental toxicity—Karl-Henrik Robert, a Swedish oncologist and founder of *The Natural Step*, elected to set aside his medical practice to address the issue with zeal and vigor.[26] With the help of the Swedish scientific community, he established a guide toward sustainability based on four rigorous systems conditions that must be satisfied for any company, municipality, or nation to move toward a more healthy environment:

1. Substances from the earth's crust must not systematically increase in nature (e.g., cessation of dispersion of heavy metal contaminants by industries through the waterways, soil, and/or by incineration).
2. Synthetic compounds must not systematically increase in nature (e.g., use of natural substances to accomplish the tasks formerly accomplished by herbicides and pesticides).
3. The physical basis for the productivity and diversity of nature must not be systematically allowed to deteriorate (e.g., stringent guidelines for land use and human population mobility to safeguard the ability of the bioregion to sustain itself).
4. There must be fair and efficient use of resources with respect to meeting human needs (e.g., social justice issues, such as not stripping the rain forest acreage to make way for cattle grazing).

While these principles are based on impeccable science and are "easy" to state, they have vast implications and relationships. Increasingly, industries both large and small are implementing the principles, finding that "doing good" can result in "doing well."

Cowan proposed strategic questions for use in evaluating which products, companies, and initiatives will lead to a less toxic world.[27] Four major categories of questions can be asked when potential products are considered for use: substitution, stewardship, ecology, and simplicity (Exhibit 12–1).

Theme 3: Choosing a Sustainable Future

The World Commission on Environment and Development (the Brundtland Commission) stated, "Sustainable development is development that meets the needs of the present without compromising the ability of future generations to meet their own needs."[28] In the United States, the President's Council on Sustainable Develop-

Exhibit 12-1 Strategic Questions To Evaluate Products, Companies, and Initiatives for a Less Toxic World

---

1. Substitutions of Materials
- Is it synthetic? Does it biodegrade? Does it accumulate in living tissues?
- Is it a known carcinogen, mutagen, teratogen, endocrine disrupter, or acute toxin?
- When it degrades, off-gases, combusts or reacts, does it pose any of the above threats?

2. Substitution of Less Toxic or Nontoxic Products
- How toxic is this product during its extraction, manufacturing, use, recycling, or disposal?
- Is this product durable, easy to maintain, repair, reuse, remanufacture, or upgrade?
- Does it have replaceable or reusable components, parts and materials?
- Will the manufacturer take responsibility for this product and packaging?
- Will the manufacturer completely recycle the product and packaging?
- Can the benefits of this product best be provided by turning it into a service product?

3. Industrial Ecology
- If "waste equals food," what processes does this chemical or product feed during its entire life cycle?
- Can this entire class of chemicals or products be phased out by reconfiguring industrial ecosystems?
- At the most basic level, what services does this product provide?
- Can these services be provided by healthy ecosystems instead?

4. Voluntary Simplicity
- Despite all efforts, does this product remain unacceptably toxic? If so, is it truly essential?
- Does the product have other purposes? Does it meet basic needs?
- What level of this product or service genuinely contributes to the quality of my life?
- Can this level of service be best supplied through my own initiative and that of my local community?

*Adapted with permission from Stuart Cowan, *A Design Revolution* in *Yes! A Journal of Positive Futures*, No. 6, p. 30, © 1998.

---

ment was convened in 1993 to find ways to meet people's needs without jeopardizing the future. In its vision statement, the 30-member Council stated, "Our vision is of a life-sustaining earth. We are committed to the achievement of a dignified, peaceful and equitable existence. A sustainable United States will have a growing economy that provides equitable opportunities for satisfying livelihoods, and a safe, healthy, high quality of life for current and future generations. Our nation will protect its environment, its natural resource base, and the function and viability of natural systems on which all life depends."[29]

Grant advised caution regarding the term *sustainable development,* which is regularly used in the sense of *sustainable growth,* a self-contradictory concept supporting growth as a solution to all problems.[30] The simple fact is that growth, de-mographic or economic, is ultimately *un*sustainable; perpetual growth is mathematically impossible in a finite space such as the earth. Sustainability demands a redefinition of consumption goals, such as use of renewable resources at a rate that does not exceed their rates of regeneration and use of nonrenewable resources at a rate that does not exceed the rate at which sustainable, renewable substitutes are developed. The task is to confine human activity so that it can be pursued without damage to the natural systems. No goal including sustainability is absolute, however. For every contemplated policy or action, it is essential to consider what the threat to sustainability is and whether the anticipated gains are so overwhelming that they justify the action.

Support for "sustainability" is worthless unless it is translated into policy. The

President and Congress do not address sustainability directly.[31] They advance or set it back through policies or legislation that are ostensibly directed to other ends, such as welfare, health, employment, trade, land use, or agricultural price supports. Because of systems interactions, decisions in these areas affect the rate of resource use, the environment, immigration, and U.S. population growth, among other considerations. In U.S. population growth, two principal variables drive the demographic future: fertility and migration.[32] Population restraint is central to long-term environmental sustainability. Yet, suggestions to bring human fertility in line with replacement level, rather than above it as it is presently, are judged racist or elitist, and limiting immigration is perceived as xenophobia. As sensitive and incendiary as these issues are and will remain, they are intimately bound to present and future sustainability and quality of life.

Orr, an environmental studies professor, presented sustainability from another perspective.[33] He claimed that much of academic communities' ennui in the face of the environmental crises is a combination of denial coupled with the conviction that money and technology hold all the answers. Colleges and universities continue to equip students for short-term success in an extractive economy, not for long-term success in a sustainable and resilient community. If administrators and trustees are aware of the reality of global change, that awareness rarely influences institutional policy. For Orr, denial coupled with lack of imagination prevent us from educating ourselves and others in "love of life." "Denial is not just a way of avoiding the future; it is also a way to avoid discussing our own complicity in the larger problems of our time."[34]

Part of being a sustainable and resilient community is the conscious intent to bring all stakeholders into future planning. On one university campus, a full design team was engaged from the inception of an idea for a new ecologic center building.[35] Students, faculty, and administrators, as well as architects, were integral to this rich, real-life experience of planning and implementation. The basic building program emerging from a 1-year planning phase demonstrates decisions based on principles of sustainability. Most, if not all, the project goals are generalizable to other building or renovation projects. The building

- discharges no waste water (i.e., "drinking water in; drinking water out")
- generates from sunlight more electricity in the course of a year than it uses
- uses no material known to be carcinogenic, mutagenic, or endocrine disruptors
- uses energy and materials efficiently
- uses products or materials grown or manufactured sustainably
- is landscaped to promote biologic diversity
- promotes analytic skills in assessing full costs over the lifetime of the building
- promotes ecologic competence and mindfulness of place
- is genuinely pedagogical in its design and operations
- meets rigorous requirements for full cost accounting.

This is a building that permits no ugliness, either human or ecologic, at this or any other time or place.

Supporting and providing leadership for devising pathways to a sustainable future is the Green Design Initiative of Carnegie Mellon University.[36] This is a major interdisciplinary research effort to make an impact on environmental quality through green design (environmentally sensitive in planning and execution). The central idea is to form partnerships among companies, government agencies, and foundations to develop pioneering design, management, manufacturing, and regulatory processes. The intent is to improve environmental quality while enhancing economic development.

The University of Virginia's Institute for Sustainable Design was also created to develop viable alternatives to conventional design and practice in human production.[37] This is another interdisciplinary creative endeavor. While advocating innovative design and restorative action, this group stresses the interdependence of ecology, equity, and economy. The work of William McDonough, Dean of the School of Architecture, is closely aligned with the new, but ever-ancient notion, that nature provides premier models for both process and product.[38] McDonough proposed a strategy for change requiring a new and enriching vision of taking, making, using, and consuming. Three principles have guided his work:

1. *Waste equals food.* In nature, there is no such thing as waste, so the concept of "waste" is eliminated (not minimize waste but eliminate the concept).
2. *Current solar income should be used.* Nature does not mine the past, nor does it borrow from the future. It meets its needs from what is available right now (including all solar technologies, geothermal power, wind power, hydroelectrics).
3. *It is important to respect diversity.* Everyone, every project, every place has its differences and needs; honor the differences rather than homogenize.

Along with the three guiding principles are design criteria. Historically, these have been

- cost (Can I afford it?)
- performance (Will it do what I want it to?)
- aesthetics (Does it please me?)

Sustainable design, according to McDonough, calls for an additional three questions:

1. Is it ecologically intelligent?
2. Is it just?
3. Is it fun?

Historically, there are five major categories of organization and influence in the world: (1) business, (2) education, (3) religion, (4) the military, and (5) government. The fact that health care arose from the religious and military spheres is responsible for some of the earlier traditions in nursing, such as uniforms and reliance on a rigorous chain of command. Where is the weighting of influence now? Observation indicates three: business, education and government. Despite this considerable shift in emphasis from earlier times, each of the five categories has a pervasive history and role that influence contemporary outlooks. Business, a major polluter and exploiter on many fronts, is beginning to make contributions to future sustainability in terms of clean design and production. Education has pockets of excellence, but has shown no obvious leadership; too often, it serves the needs of business. Religion is beginning in many quarters to move from a "dominator" model toward stewardship and, more recently, into partnership, co-creating, with the Creator or Life Force. The military remains the greatest source of large-scale pollution and destruction of life support systems, virtually exempt from any regulation or sanction beyond itself. Government provides guidelines and safeguards for the environment but they are frequently diluted or diverted by partisan and/or specific interest groups. There remain, of course, grass roots activists, citizens who have clear vision with zest, caring, and drive to see something better.

Because the emerging world paradigm is a participative one, a community's environmental sustainability depends in large measure on how well it is able to recruit and retain citizen involvement at all levels. America Speaks, a not-for-profit organization committed to linking citizen voices to governance in new ways, has distilled nine criteria characteristic of communities that have successfully mobilized citizen engagement at all levels:[39]

1. Political, corporate, and civic leadership listen to all voices in the community.
2. Community activists focus on the common good.
3. Media (print, television, radio, and Internet) value and commit resources to building community.
4. Technology, hardware, and software are of sufficient quantity and quality to enable community and regional deliberation processes.
5. Projects reflect natural ecologic and economic regions; they are not bound by traditional political jurisdictions.
6. Citizen involvement in a project can continue for the long term.
7. Resources are committed to enhancing community members' skills for the short and long term.
8. There is an established sense of trust and mutual valuing among community members.
9. Leaders recognize that needed changes are systemic, not isolated, and that both individuals and institutions are responsible for making them.

Over a decade prior to any formal call for sustainability, an Australian group formed the Permaculture Institute as a demonstration site and a central information base.[40] Their aim is to create systems worldwide that are ecologically sound and economically viable, provide for their own needs, do not exploit or pollute the environment, and are, therefore, sustainable in the long run.

The concept of sustainability is complex and intertwined because it has to do with all systems interrelated. The bottom line is wonderfully simple and straightforward, however: to live as if we belong here and are planning to stay a while.

Theme 4: Building Learning Communities

A learning community is a group of people who choose to enter into a discovery mode, meaning that each person is willing to teach or learn, depending on what he or she has to contribute. Characterized by safety, support, and openness, the learning community focuses on personal and societal learning. Within the context of seeking a sustainable future, the search for humankind's rightful and responsible place in the natural world fuels learning.

A glance at the history of public education in the United States reveals that, at the height of the Industrial Revolution from 1886 to 1920, financiers, industrialists, and their private charitable foundations spent more money on required schooling than did the government itself, with the aim of binding schooling to the service of business and the political state.[41] Thus, a system of modern schooling was constructed without public comprehension or participation. The trend was magnified following World War II when virtually everyone went to school courtesy of the G.I. Bill. Higher education changed; the economy and industry boomed with a vast supply of educated workers. Geographic mobility increased, largely from rural to urban settings. The individual's worth was frequently weighted on the scales of economic value and productivity, making him or her a cog in a well oiled machine.

Gatto made a clear distinction between schooling and education.[42] Schooling takes place in an environment controlled by others and often for the purposes of others. Schooling is never adequate, even when offered by those who care about and strive to understand the student. Education describes largely self-initiated efforts to take charge of life with wisdom and understanding. Education is a process more than a state, a tapestry woven from information, mistakes, experiences, commitments, and risk taking. Growth and mastery come to those who are vigorously self-directed: initiating, being alone, working within group or community, reflecting, creating, doing. Schooling can help or hinder education, and it requires individuals to respond collectively. While there are excellent educational opportunities regarding a sustainable future in established public and private institutions, the topic is not consistently valued or available.

People are learning and teaching all of the time by virtue of being human. A combination of yearning, searching, concern, curiosity, and a need for community draws increasing numbers of individuals into learning communities such as the Buddhist Alliance for Social Engagement.[43] The community bond for such groups is the opportunity to honor deeply held values that integrate personal, social, and spiritual lives. Members enrich their inner lives while selectively engaging in some form of service work. A particular and often painfully difficult challenge is addressing immediate social concerns (sometimes called the Band-aid approach or even "help-me-not-feel-so-guilty" approach) while acting on behalf of structural transformation (the "upstream" approach involving commitment to identify and change causative factors). These small grass roots efforts are conducting much of future sustainability work, however.

A wondrous paradox has surfaced. In some select instances, business communities are assuming leadership in striving toward sustainability. The trend engenders a different type of learning community, one that is integral to the preferred corporate image. Perhaps the most remarkable contemporary example is Interface, a global manufacturing enterprise that produces 40 percent of the world's carpeting.[44] Because of a personal, radical commitment to sustainability, its founder and chief executive officer, Ray Anderson, committed his company to becoming a zero-waste enterprise. It is well on its way to realizing this goal. To accomplish this immense task, involving 26 manufacturing sites delivering to 110 outlets worldwide, a very specific educational process has been initiated to engage the conscious commitment of employees at all levels over time, as well as that of stockholders. Increasingly, businesses are seeing that "green is good"—economically, socially, and sustainably.

Many facilitative and reliable resources are available to seekers and learners, from neighborhood wise persons to the Internet (Appendix 12–A). Highly authoritative avenues for learning and practicing sustainability include, but are not limited to, the three named here because of their excellence and widespread recognition over time: (1) *Co-op America*,[45] an organization dedicated to creating a just and sustainable society throgh economic means; (2) World Watch Institute,[46] which provides in-depth analysis of environmental issues and trends; and (3) *Yes! A Journal of Positive Futures*,[47] which fosters the evolution of a just, sustainable, and compassionate future.

Observation of the natural world has long been a source of discovery, inspiration, and healing of one form or another. Herbal remedies, for example, were and are discovered by observing the actions of animals in their natural habitat. Humans are the newcomers in the evolutionary unfoldment; eons of wisdom precede us and can inform us if we are wise enough, and humble enough, to seek that knowledge.[48–50] A concerned informal learning group, Friends Committee on Unity with Nature/Sustainability Committee provided a sense of the whole:

> Sustainability includes a resolve to live in harmony with biological and physical systems, and to work to create social systems that can enable us to do that. It includes a sense of connectedness and an understanding of the utter

dependence of human society within the intricate web of life; a passion for environmental justice and ecological ethics; an understanding of dynamic natural balances and processes; and a recognition of the limits to growth due to finite resources. Our concern for sustainability recognizes our responsibility to future generations, to care for the earth as our own home and the home of all who dwell herein. We seek a relationship between human beings and the earth that is mutually enhancing.[51]

Palmer, a renowned contemporary educator, presented a cogent argument for education in these matters: "no punishment can be greater than conspiring in one's own diminishment."[52]

Theme 5: Working from the Inside Out

As holistic nurses who are sensitive to environmental issues, we know, at least intuitively, that the sole thing we have to offer is the way we live our lives. The way we live our lives is crafted from our day-to-day choices.

We live in a world of vast complexity and diversity. Our choice is to do whatever it takes to commit to and maintain our basic values, whatever we determine them to be. Only we can arrive at the personal meanings and understanding of relationships that provide coherence to our existence. While we may have models, support, and assistance, each of us is called to make this determination. In our holistic practice, we assist others in examining their options and encourage them to make life-affirming choices. Our primary task is to be with our clients within their life circumstances. Often, our greatest contribution is to walk freely with our clients as they face their ordeals, joys, and transitions.

We engage in our own grief work. We acknowledge and choose to make amends for our complicity, whether conscious or unintended, in the seemingly insurmountable environmental degradation observed today. We are not immobilized or demoralized by grief, however. We use it to fuel our resolve to "make it right." Because humankind has brought us to today's apparent impasse, we as members freely claim accountability. We have a heightened sense of belonging as we walk this path, for we know in some way that the ills we see through our nursing practice derive in large measure from the pervasive sense of alienation and loneliness of our clients and, indeed, of communities and larger societies. We have a heightened awareness that the emotions attendant to "not belonging" give rise to disease states with innumerable manifestations.[53]

We work with contradiction and paradox. As humans, we often seek a state of entropy or comfort; we tend to cling to familiar patterns and routines. Yet, contradiction and paradox are so commonplace that we cannot always be sure what should command our attention. For example, what does it take to be a health care system rather than an illness care system? Why do we call artery-clogging foods, "treats"? Why do we solicit research funding for health projects from industries that manufacture illness-causing chemicals? We see holistic practitioners working consciously to restore sanity and balance in all settings.

We risk everything through the clarity of our values and convictions. Being human is not for the fainthearted. Being human calls for every shred of body, mind, and spirit that we can muster. Before we can take a stand or set a direction on an issue, we must reflect long and carefully about what counts the most in our lives. One approach is to seek clarity, within ourselves, about our purpose for existence. Some people believe that we have a four-fold purpose: to learn, to serve, to love, to be loved. If this or something else is a personal credo, certain choices follow: we have direction and anchor, a lifestyle. Williams, a naturalist, suggested that we invoke the archetype of bear: fierce, not neat, not bloodless, and not cozy.[54] The bear is free to roam, stripped of society's musts, oughts, and shoulds. The bear relentlessly shreds and devours illusions, and is never so domesticated that it turns away from the life-giving work at hand.

We reside in joy of spirit and lightness of heart. Although the universe could unfold without us, we are here. Again, we have choices: to founder in the mire of impotent rage, fear, and confusion in the face of our planetary peril; to claim our birthright; or, as the new paradigm proposes, to be integral to the development of a new way. All the universe conspires to give us our heart's deepest desire. Holistic nurses are uniquely positioned to access the fountainhead of wisdom and strength within ourselves and to assist others to reclaim their own inner strength. The work, as in all authentic endeavors, is born in silence and stillness. Striving with joy and equanimity for an environmentally impeccable life means aspiring to be part of a larger whole, our inner life a seamless garment with its outer manifestation.

Environmental Conditions and Health

One of the reasons that it is difficult to study the link between environmental conditions and illness or disease is that there are so many intervening variables. Hundreds of substances and lifestyle factors are involved. Furthermore, not all toxic substances and environmental conditions induce immediate untoward reactions; many toxins seem to cause disease later, perhaps years after the period of exposure. Breathing asbestos fibers, for example, seldom causes immediate symptoms, but has often resulted in serious chronic disease many years later. Other environmental elements now known to be hazardous include lead, cigarette smoke, silica, benzene, mercury, chlorine, poor lighting, stress, and noise.[55]

Since the 1970s, national attention has focused on efforts to clean up the nation's environment and ensure workers' safety. Two federal agencies, the Environmental Protection Agency (EPA) and the Occupational Safety and Health Administration (OSHA), were formed to monitor environmental concerns. In the 1980s, several states enacted right-to-know laws that require employers to notify employees of health hazards; to provide formal education regarding the safe use of toxic substances; and to keep medical records of those workers routinely exposed to specific toxic substances.[56] In 1991, the Ecological Society of America published the Sustainable Biosphere Initiative (SBI), calling for a coordination of ecologic research, environmental education, and policy making. The project focuses on global change, loss of biodiversity, and sustainability. Its purpose is to gain a full understanding of the interactions of the biotic and the abiotic worlds in space and time.[57]

Internationally, the England Health and Safety Executive launched a huge campaign in 1991 to peak British awareness of health concerns at work. Called Lighten the Load, one program is designed to raise awareness of work-related musculoskeletal disorders and encourage employers to adopt programs that will reduce the frequency with which these disorders occur. Occupational health nurses play a major part in implementing this program, which includes assessment, intervention, evaluation, and prevention of stresses emanating from environmental working conditions.[58]

Environmental concerns range from eating contaminated poultry, hormone-fed beef, and irradiated fruits and vegetables to living near high-voltage power lines, understanding the Antarctic atmospheric ozone hole, and coping with other new high-technology hazards that we are only now recognizing (Figure 12–1). Noise, lighting, air quality, space allocation, and workplace toxins have gained increasing attention as chronic stressors.

Noise

Although its danger is still for the most part unrecognized, noise pollution may be the most common modern health hazard. Studies have repeatedly demonstrated that a high noise level is the single most important factor in diminishing office productivity.[59] Yet, more than 20 million workers in the United States are exposed to hazardous levels of noise every year, and the majority of them are in the white-collar work environment. Other studies here and in Europe have shown that high noise levels constrict

blood vessels; increase blood pressure, pulse, and respiration rates; and release extra fats into the bloodstream.[60]

The danger posed by noise pollution is a function of the volume of sound heard over a period of time. Sound and its intensity are measured in decibels, abbreviated dB (Table 12–1). Because the scale is logarithmic, rather than linear, each 10-dB increase is equivalent to multiplying the intensity by 10. The arbitrary zero is the weakest sound that a young, sensitive human ear can hear. Humans begin to perceive irritation around 50 to 90 dB and actually feel pain around 120 dB. At levels above 70 dB, the autonomic nervous system can become aroused, often without the person's awareness. When exposed for 8 hours to noise at 70 dB, which is the sound level of many typing pools or cafeterias, people may become

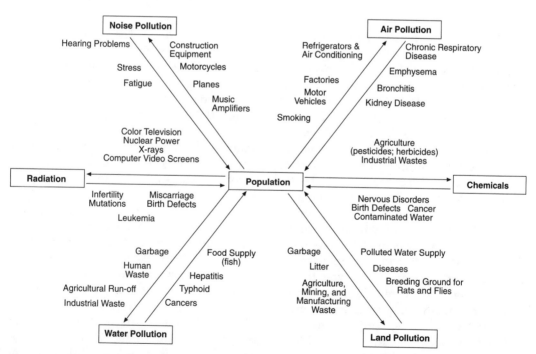

Figure 12–1 Current Environmental Concerns. *Source:* Reprinted with permission from the *Journal of Health Education,* August/September 1986, pp. 26–27. The *Journal of Health Education* is a publication of the American Alliance for Health, Physical Education, Recreation and Dance, 1900 Association Drive, Reston, VA 20191.

Table 12-1 Decibel Levels of Various Sounds

Decibel (dB) Level	Generating Sound
120–140	Jet engine at take-off Amplified rock band at close range
100–110	Power lawn mower Oncoming subway train Chain saw Jackhammer
80–100	Alarm clock Screaming child Truck traffic at close range Cocktail party
60–80	Electric kitchen aids Washing machine
40–60	Normal conversation Refrigerator hum
20–40	A cat's purr
0–10	Threshold of hearing

irritable, distracted, or tense.[61] With prolonged exposure to noise levels higher than 75 dB, gradual hearing loss can occur.

People are disturbed not only by loud sound, but also by dissonant or inharmonic sound.[62] Random, unstructured noises, even those below the threshold of awareness, can foster an irritating tension. In most hospitals and health care settings, the "quiet" areas are actually flooded with random noises and subtle, tension-promoting sounds that interfere with restfulness. Varied patterns of auditory input are more restful than quiet ambience. Healthy subjects who were confined to bed in a varied harmonic environment perceived themselves to be more rested than did those subjects confined in a quiet ambient environment.[63] This finding supports the concept that it is better to pattern the auditory input for those confined to bed.

To study the effect of noise exposure on vasoconstriction, Dengerlink and associates measured plasma concentrations of the vasoconstrictor angiotensin II in subjects before and after either rest or exposure to 100-dB white noise (noise with no discernible language or music, with sounds that are a cross between static and a waterfall).[64] Plasma angiotensin II concentrations decreased for subjects in the no-noise condition, but remained high for those in the noise condition, suggesting that noise may stimulate the production of angiotensin II. Elevated levels of angiotensin II may be partially responsible for the reported vasoconstriction and blood pressure increases that appear to accompany noise exposure.

An Australian group monitored noise levels in six intensive care units.[65] The measuring instruments included a Brugel and Kjaer microphone and measuring amplifier. After noting the high baseline or ambient noise level, the researchers found that there were three primary sources of noise: people (i.e., patients, staff, and visitors), equipment, and furniture. People-generated noise was in the range of 70 to 76 dB. The variety of noises generated from equipment included the random beeping alarms. Noise levels were as high as 80 dB when plastic chairs were being moved and 85 dB when garbage was removed. Noise from other routine tasks, such as disposing of used needles, tearing paper from monitors, and wheeling in stretchers, were commonly 10 to 20 dB above the baseline noise levels of the continuously operating machinery.

Considerable empirical evidence supports the claim that advances in hospital technology have led to increased sound levels in the critical care unit. In one study, 70 patients were randomly assigned to a noise or quiet controlled environment while attempting to sleep overnight in a simulated critical care unit. Researchers sought to determine if the sound levels suppress rapid eye movement (REM) sleep. Subjects in the noise group heard an audiotape recording of critical care unit nighttime sounds. These subjects showed poorer

REM sleep on 7 of 10 measures. Thus, there appears to be a causal relationship between critical care units and suppression of REM sleep.[66] In a related study of 105 females, a comparison with subjects in quiet environments showed that subjects in noise-simulated conditions had poorer sleep efficiency, more difficulty falling and staying asleep, more intrasleep awakenings, and less time in REM.[67]

Hospital noise has been associated with sleep deprivation, sensory overload, increased perception of postoperative pain, and intensive care unit psychosis.[68] A controlled study of 28 surgical intensive care unit patients indicated that noise not only was disturbing, but also caused the heart rate to accelerate.[69] A degree of hearing loss has occurred in newborns placed in incubators with ultrasonic nebulizers.[70] In addition, there is concern about the impact of the nursery environment on the development of low-birthweight infants. In contrast to the uterine environment, the neonatal intensive care unit is characterized by bright, often continuous lighting; loud, sharp, unpredictable sound; limited, unpredictable, and often noxious tactile stimulation; and severe limitations on mobility. It has been suggested that such an environment, which differs markedly from the expected, may irrevocably alter neonatal development in ways not yet clearly understood.[71]

Food Irradiation

The stated purpose of food irradiation in plants is to kill larval infestation, thereby (1) increasing the shelf-life of foods; (2) eliminating insects, bacteria, and other organisms; and (3) preventing sprouting. Even though the Food and Drug Administration (FDA) has pronounced it safe, this new technique has been controversial from the time of its first use.

Irradiation raises controversy for three reasons. First, it partially depletes nutrients from the food, with vitamins C, A, B complex, and E being the most vulnerable. In several studies, Temple oranges lost up to 28 percent of their ascorbic acid, corn lost up to 29 percent of its ascorbic acid and 44 percent of its carotene, and whole milk lost up to 61 percent of its vitamin E.[72] The transportation of highly radioactive materials (cobalt-60 and cesium-137) through communities for use in irradiation has also raised concern. Finally, the process creates radioactive products in the form of trace chemicals in the irradiated food product.

Meat irradiation is also controversial, causing *The Wall Street Journal* to print the following:

Meat Irradiation Facts

- **What Is It:** Short bursts of gamma rays from the radioactive isotopes cobalt-60 or cesium-137, or from electron beams.
- **What It Does:** Removes almost all traces of *E. coli* in beef, *Salmonella* in poultry, cholera in fish, trichinosis in pork and bacteria that spoil produce.
- **Proponents of Beef Irradiation:** The National Food Processors Association, the American Medical Association, the World Health Organization, and the American Meat Institute. All say beef irradiation will help reduce deaths from *E. coli.*
- **Critics of Beef Irradiation:** Food and Water, Inc. They say nutrients are lost in the process, and not enough is known about the stray molecules that result from it.[73]

A study by the U.S. Army found that irradiated beef contained 65 volatile trace chemicals that had not been present before irradiation. Some nuclear chemists contend that the radiolytic particles and substances may be carcinogenic.[74] The safety of irradiation is still under investigation, and nurses need to be aware of the debate and stay abreast of the issues.

Meat and Poultry Supplementation

For a number of years, cows, pigs, and chickens have been treated with both hormones and antibiotics. The purposes of these treatments are to increase the size and weight of the animal and to prevent *Salmonella* contamination. In 1993, after 9 years of scrutiny, the FDA approved the use of bovine somatotropin (BST). This hormone became commercially available in February 1994. The FDA concluded that the drug, which boosts milk production by more than 10 percent, is safe despite its association with an increase in udder infection common among lactating cows.[75] Like irradiation, supplementation has raised safety concerns among critics because it introduces a new element of pharmacologic intervention into a population that was previously free of disease. Its long-range effects are yet to be determined.

Passive Smoking

Everyone is aware of the health hazards related to smoking tobacco products, but a new at-risk population has been identified: nonsmokers. Exposure to tobacco smoke produced by others, referred to as passive smoking, places individuals at the same risk for illnesses as their smoking counterparts.[76] In fact, new studies reveal that sidestream smoke contains higher concentrations of carcinogens and other toxic substances than does mainstream smoke.[77] Nonsmokers who are chronically exposed to the pollutants in tobacco smoke scored lower on tests of small airway function than did nonsmokers who had not been exposed.[78] Nonsmoking women exposed to their husbands' smoking are now showing a 2:1 increase in mortality from lung cancer as compared to control groups.[79] Such data should alert nurses and other health care professionals to the con-

tinual unfolding of new hazards to public environmental health and safety.

Violence, Dehumanization, and the Technologic Age

Life in the modern age has built-in inherent environmental dangers. For many, the very act of getting to and from the workplace is an encounter with smog, noise, congestion, stench, and debris. In addition, many people spend numerous hours a week in front of television screens, vicariously engaging in violence and corruption. Being exposed to constant news and commercial programming may in part shift our focus to deploring the negative aspects of our world rather than creating a more positive environment for ourselves or for those with whom we live and work.

In the past, people and their environments were harmoniously intertwined. When people worked, they walked from their dwelling to their field, toiled with the elements, and directly reaped the benefits of their labors. In today's technologic era, however, the nature of our relationship with the environment has changed to one of use rather than an exchange with the elements. We have become increasingly alienated from the natural world. The artificial environment of the technologic society has replaced nature as the all-encompassing environment. Technology evokes from us the emotions of fascination and dread that nature once did.[80] Searching for security, fulfillment, and meaning from our technologic civilization, we unconsciously surrender our freedom and autonomy and replace it with efficiency. For many, the result is dehumanization, demoralization, and victimization. For those who are knowledgeable and able to make choices effectively, the technologic age can heighten the positive effects of the environment and thereby enhance the overall quality of life. In either case, there are specific interventions that the individual nurse can do.

Nurses' Working Environment

Over the past three decades, a growing body of literature has indicated that nursing is a stressful profession. Improved technology and a greater turnover of acutely ill patients are two factors that have increased nurses' work pressure.[81] The constant caring for acutely ill patients with a myriad of physical and emotional needs occurs within an often complex organizational system.[82] Hospital work environment stressors include limited control of tasks, ongoing job changes, and continual technologic change.[83] Based on this and additional data, many nurses are proactively addressing this issue. For example, nurses at Kaiser Permanente in California designed a program to create a better work environment for their staff. Before strategic changes were implemented, only 32 percent of the staff felt the hospital did a good job of making nurses feel important. After management had been restructured and a more participative decision-making style adopted, 62 percent felt that they had an opportunity to influence decisions about their professional practice environment.[84]

Rationales for the workplace as a primary site for environmental health promotion activities include the large amount of time spent there by the majority of the population, the economic and other incentives for employers to invest in employee health promotion, the opportunity to mobilize peer pressure to help employees make desirable changes in health habits, and the many reports of workplace success in making health promotion changes.[85]

HOLISTIC CARING PROCESS

Assessment

In preparing to exercise environmental control, assess the following parameters:

- the client's personal space for comfort, lighting, noise, ventilation, and privacy

- the client's environment for people or objects that induce anxiety
- the client's awareness that environmental concerns affect individual and family coping skills
- the client's awareness of objects or other environmental factors in the physical space that induce comfort or discomfort
- the client's environmental concerns, as well as the family's environmental concerns
- the client's possible environmental fears (e.g., a feeling of claustrophobia from being confined to a hospital intensive care bed or intravenous lines, or a fear of death because the patient in the next bed just died)
- the client's grief and its relationship to environmental factors (e.g., Is the client in the same home atmosphere in which the spouse just died? Are others around the client sad and depressed? Are the colors in the environment dark and heavy?)
- the client's personal health maintenance in relation to environmental factors (e.g., Can the client easily reach self-care hygiene items? Are throw rugs anchored? Are sunglasses worn outside to prevent glare?)
- the client's ability to maintain and manage his or her own home
- the client's risk of injury associated with factors in the environment
- the client's activity deficits as a result of environmental factors
- the client's home environment for its potential impact on effective parenting
- the client's potential noncompliance because of environmental factors
- the client's risk of impairment in physical activity because of environmental factors
- the client's risk of impairment in respiratory function because of environmental factors, such as feather pillows, polluted or stale air, cigarette

smoking, known or suspected allergens, or overexertion with chronic respiratory conditions
- the client's possible sleep deficit because of agents in the environment, such as lighting, noise, overstimulation, overcrowding, or allergenic pillows
- the client's alterations in thought processes that may be influenced by environmental factors, such as sensory bombardment with noise, lack of sleep, and transient living patterns

Patterns/Problems/Needs

The patterns/problems/needs compatible with environmental interventions and related to the nine human response patterns (see Chapter 14) are as follows:

- *Exchanging:* All diagnoses
- *Choosing:* Potential for ineffective choices
- *Moving:* Altered self-care
  Altered growth and development
- *Perceiving:* Potential for sensory perceptual alteration
- *Knowing:* Impaired environmental interpretational syndrome
  Potential for knowledge deficit
- *Feeling:* Altered comfort
- *Relating:* Altered role performance

Outcomes

Table 12–2 guides the nurse in client outcomes, nursing prescriptions, and evaluation for the use of the environment as a nursing intervention.

Therapeutic Care Plan and Implementation

Before the Session

- Become aware of personal thoughts, behaviors, and actions that may contribute to the teaching, counseling, or caring environment.
- Prepare the physical environment for optimal lighting, seating, air quality, and noise control.
- Consider your internal environment. Is it calm, centered, and ready to interact with others?
- Clear your mind of other matters or personal encounters in order to be fully present when meeting with the client.

Beginning the Session

- Allow the client to express specific environmental concerns.
- Guide the client to consider changes that would improve his or her personal and employment environment.
- Encourage the client to write down areas of concern or improvement.

During the Session

- Encourage the client to initiate specific intervention ideas in his or her personal or professional work environment.
- Suggest to clients that they can serve on the environmental control committee at their place of employemnt or if their agency does not have one, that they volunteer to form one.
- Urge clients to consider the areas of sound (e.g., noise, music, machinery), air (e.g., quality, smell, circulation), and aesthetics (e.g., art, color, design, texture), as well as other topics specific to the overall environment.
- Educate hospitalized clients about the deleterious effects of too much noise.
- Encourage hospitalized clients to limit the time spent watching television and

Table 12–2 Nursing Interventions: Environment

Client Outcomes	Nursing Prescriptions	Evaluation
The client will demonstrate awareness of environment.	Assist the client in shaping his or her own personal space environment.	The client personalized his or her own environment.
	Assist the client with choices that contribute to a positive, safe environment for those who share his or her personal and community space.	The client monitored and controlled the noise that he or she contributed to the surrounding area.
		The client respected the rights of others by not polluting air, water, and public places with wastes.
		The client did not violate the personal space of others with tobacco smoke.
	Provide the client with information that helps in expanding concern for the concept of a healthy global environment.	The client participated in discussions, committees, or programs to work for a safe global environment.
The client will avoid contact and exposure to toxic substances and/or hazardous materials.	Give the client ideas for how to participate in safety education programs at his or her place of employment.	The client participated in his or her workplace offerings of environmental safety programs.
	Teach the client the importance of not handling unnecessary toxic substances.	The client did not handle unnecessary toxic substances and educated himself or herself about the dangers of hazardous materials.

instead listen to their own personal cassette players with headphones.
- Create mechanisms whereby music, imagery, relaxation, color, aromas, and the like can be introduced into the workplace settings.

At the End of the Session
- Be aware that you function as a role model. As such, modulate your voice. Speak audibly, but softly during the session.
- Help clients learn practical ways to cope with hazards in the environment (Table 12–3).
- Work together to write down goals and target dates.

- Give handout material to support established goals.
- Schedule follow-up sessions.

Specific Interventions

Personal Environment. Strategies to heal the environment abound on both a personal and a professional level. Personally, we begin to modify our own internal environment. The ability to regulate our state of consciousness, thought patterns, and reactive behaviors gives us the power to move smoothly through external crises both at work and at leisure. Approaching a hectic external environment with internal composure and tranquillity makes it possible

Table 12–3 Coping with Environmental Hazards

Problem	Solution
Too much noise	1. Turn off radios and televisions. 2. Lower your voice. 3. Ask your colleagues to quiet down. 4. Ask to serve on the agency's environmental control committee.
Inadequate lighting	1. Add more lights. 2. Use incandescent bulbs instead of fluorescent tubes whenever possible. 3. Open curtains and blinds whenever possible. 4. Go outdoors for full-spectrum light breaks, rather than taking cafeteria coffee breaks.
Stale air	1. Make sure agency ventilation systems work. 2. When doing home health visits, open the doors and windows and get fresh air in the home when appropriate. 3. Request that broad-leaf green plants be stationed in the workplace. They are aesthetically pleasing and give off oxygen. 4. Wear masks or protective gear if there is any risk of toxic inhalants.
Long periods at computer video display terminal	1. Use a shield that cuts down glare and radiation and grounds the field of electrostatic charge. 2. Learn some relaxation exercises to do at your desk. 3. Ask your institution or agency to have minimassage available on the premises. 4. Take frequent eye and movement breaks away from the screen. 5. Use properly designed chairs.
Space allocation	1. Try to find some personal space in the workplace. 2. Respect others' personal space. Ask before entering the client's room, closet, or dresser. 3. Make the space you are allocated as pleasant as possible. Decorate with colorful objects, soothing scents, and aesthetic objects.

to transform crises into manageable situations. Clean, clear internal environments can influence all the external environments in which we work and live.

As we develop the optimal workplaces and living areas to foster self-actualizing conditions and maximize bodymind responses, we must be aware of the impact of all aspects of the environment on human health. Many nurses find that the following exercise increases their sensitivity to the environment and its impact:

At different times during the day, close your eyes, and take a few moments to listen carefully to all the sounds in your environment.

- Jot down the many different sounds you hear, noting which are pleasant and which are distracting or disturbing noises.
- Become aware of all the sounds that you ordinarily hear, such as the air conditioner, radios and televisions, the hum of fluorescent lights, the beeping and buzzing of hospital machinery, or the incessant MUSAK that some institutions play over the speaker system.

- Notice new smells, feelings of temperature, etc. There will be many sounds, smells, and sensations of which you may not have previously been aware.

Workplace Noise. Noise seems to be a major area of environmental concern that nurses can control for the most part. It is the accumulation of noises that adds up in decibels and adds up to stress. By becoming increasingly sensitive to all potential environmental stressors, the nurse becomes more attuned to the opportunities for specific interventions.

One researcher taught progressive muscle relaxation to coronary care unit patients who were disturbed by hospital noise. This technique significantly decreased noise sensitivity in these patients.[86] This study suggested that nurses should not only eliminate noise whenever possible, but also use creative ways to help patients to deal with noise when they cannot remove its source.

Some specific recommendations to reduce workplace noise include

- developing staff education programs about noises, their source, and ways to quiet them
- setting telephones and alarms to low volumes or replacing sound devices with flashing lights
- installing buffers in open space areas to minimize impact noise
- closing the patient's door whenever feasible
- using bedside chairs with wheels in patient rooms with hard floors
- choosing quieter equipment
- placing computer printers away from patient rooms and/or installing sound-proof covers
- giving patients headphones to listen to television or radio so that they do not disturb others
- lowering our voices when we speak

Planetary Consciousness. Schuster suggested that there is an impetus and underlying reason for our developing environmental consciousness. She noted that we are all hoping to foster and sustain our fullest conscious participation in the ongoing web of interrelationships.[87] Three points emerge as most salient within the context of nursing, in general, and holistic practice, in particular.

1. It is important to address the nature of being human and, in our Western mode, the pervasive influence of the self–other dichotomy.
2. We must be aware that we have viable choices of how we want to be and how we represent ourselves in the world.
3. An integration of items 1 and 2 develops a personal orientation to all environmental concerns. With such an orientation, we can act from internal conviction, relatedness, rather than from institutional directives.[88]

The most enduring and far-reaching environmental work originates with individuals as consumers and practitioners, not with organizations, however enlightened.[89] Thus, it is up to each of us to develop an environmental sensitivity in our daily lives and become increasingly cognizant of our opportunities to institute positive change.

Case Study

Setting:	Outpatient clinic, or private visit
Client:	A.B., a 55-year-old married man
Patterns/ Problems/ Needs:	1. Altered comfort related to recurrent headaches
	2. Ineffective individual coping related to environmental stress

A.B. visited the occupational health nurse because of recurrent headaches and chronic fatigue. A physical examination and laboratory tests revealed no pathology or disease, but his subjective declaration of feeling stress in the workplace warranted a closer examination of his workplace environment. A detailed history of his work hours, commuting travel, and work setting yielded evidence of environmental imbalance. A.B. began his day with a 45-minute automobile commute through a suburban area to the inner city; he finished the day the same way. He had made this commute for years, but the traffic had lately increased and road repairs frequently slowed his pace. When he arrived at work, he went to his office, an interior room with no windows and fluorescent ceiling lights. The office walls were the standard institutional beige color; A.B. had done nothing to decorate or personalize his office. Instead of a secretary outside his office, he now had his own computer inside his office. During the company's modernization process, middle managers had been taught computer skills, and many secretarial positions had been eliminated. Each manager was now responsible for developing reports and interacting with others via personal computer terminals. A.B.'s work routine had little variation. It consisted of meetings, telephone work, and online computer time.

This information suggested that A.B. was experiencing environment-related stress, and the nurse worked with him to develop a five-step plan of action:

1. Vary the commuting time. Begin the commute 15 minutes earlier to decrease the rushed feeling of getting to work on time. Join a health club in the city, and stay after work to exercise. The traffic would be considerably less 1 hour later, and the commute would then take only 30 minutes. Total morning and evening commute time would remain the same as before, but more would have been accomplished with less environmental stress.
2. Implement and practice computer protection skills (see Table 12–3).

3. Mount a shoulder rest on the telephone to prevent neck strain after long periods on the telephone.
4. Personalize the office with soft soothing colors. Add a wall picture of a mountain valley and stream that have a personal significance.
5. Put an incandescent lamp on the desk, and use that rather than the overhead fluorescent lights for desk work.

A copy of this plan was posted in a prominent place in A.B.'s home. Along with a plan for exercise and weight management (see Chapters 19 and 27) and a plan for the development of relaxation and imagery skills (see Chapters 21 and 22), this program incorporated A.B.'s need for motivation, lifestyle change, and values clarification.

When A.B. returned for his follow-up visit 2 months later, his headaches had abated, and he had made some progress toward his weight loss. He and his wife had redecorated his office, and on his own he had added a small cassette player to play his favorite classical music.

Six months later, A.B. was free of headaches. He had spearheaded a no-smoking policy for his workplace and asked the company director to install full-spectrum lights on all ceiling overhead panels. He felt he had regained some sense of control over his environment and was working on improvement in the other areas for which he and the nurse had developed plans.

Evaluation

Each environmental intervention should be measured. The nurse can evaluate with the client the outcomes established before the implementation of any interventions (see Table 12–2). To evaluate the results further, the nurse can explore the subjective effects of the experience with the client, based on the evaluation questions in Exhibit 12–2. Nurses have always been sensitive to environmental issues. Historically, nurses have been the health care providers

Exhibit 12–2 Evaluating the Client's Subjective Experience with Environmental Concerns

1. Were you aware that noise, lighting, air quality, space allocation, and workplace toxins could be chronic stressors?
2. Are there any of these potential stressors in your environment? If so, can you do anything to reduce or remove them?
3. Do you realize that you can contribute to a healthier planet by virtue of changing elements in your own personal space?
4. Do you have an environmental sensitivity group at your workplace? If one existed, would you like to be a part of it?
5. Do you feel empowered to be the person who initiates change in your work setting?
6. What are some specific things that you would like to do to create a healthier environment in your personal space or work setting?
7. What is your next step (or your plan) to integrate these changes in your life?

primarily concerned with health promotion, sanitation, and improvement in the quality of life for all people. Our technologic society has raised new issues and concerns, ranging from the use of increasingly toxic substances to high-technology machinery. Last year's methods of handling laboratory specimens and chemotherapy preparations, for example, may be outdated next year. Nurses keep abreast of the changing face of the environment in order to equip themselves with the newest strategies to counteract hazards. Future nurses would be well advised to remember and recall some of the basic nursing tenets of yesteryear that are still most relevant today. These interventions include fresh air, control for a comfortable climate, cheerful colors and sights, and noise reduction.

Much of how we relate to and what we do about environmental issues is based on the development of our personal philosophy. We continue to become increasingly aware that each of the small things that we do for or against the environment has short- and long-term ramifications. Nurses want to be alert for ways to contribute to positive environmental changes for their own lives, their clients' lives, and the overall health of the planet. Environmental concerns are important to all of us, and one person's actions can have a ripple effect on many other lives. Nurses can be key agents to ensure that the environment is held sacred, supported, and tended as it supports and gives life to all of the earth's people.

DIRECTIONS FOR FUTURE RESEARCH

1. Evaluate the perception of quality of rest by subjects with different types of auditory stimulation.
2. Study the relationship between environmental hazards (e.g., artificial lighting, working on video display terminals, unventilated air, shift work, high noise levels) and the rise in infertility rates, conditions affecting unborn fetuses, and neonate abnormalities.
3. Investigate the use of tactile, auditory, and/or olfactory stimuli on wound healing, rate of complications, length of recovery, and other health-related factors.
4. Study the effect of the environment on the reduction of stress and/or anxiety in ambulatory clients.

NURSE HEALER REFLECTIONS

After reading this chapter, the nurse healer will be able to answer or begin a process of answering the following questions:

- How does the environment affect my job satisfaction?
- What are the environmental stressors at work and at home?
- What strategies can I incorporate in my environment to be healthier?

- What things can I do to improve my own personal and workplace environment?

- How can I be involved with environmental issues at work and in my community?

NOTES

1. R. Tarnas, The Great Initiation, *Noetic Sciences Review*, no. 47 (1998):24–31, 57–59.

2. Tarnas, The Great Initiation, 28.

3. J. Macy, *Coming Back to Life: Practices To Reconnect Our Lives, Our World* (Gabriola Island, B.C., Canada: New Society Publishers, 1998), 60–61.

4. L. Selanders, *Florence Nightingale: An Environmental Adaptation Theory* (Newbury Park, CA: Sage Publications, 1993), 19.

5. C. Anthony, *A Guide to the I Ching*, 3d ed. (Stow, MA: Anthony, 1988), 21.

6. E. Schuster, Environment Needs Nurses Who Care, *The American Nurse* 24, no. 4 (1992):25.

7. R. Carson, *Silent Spring* (Boston: Houghton Mifflin, 1962).

8. J. Macy, *Coming Back to Life*, 17.

9. J.D. Mitchell, Nowhere To Hide: The Global Spread of High Risk Synthetic Chemicals, *World-Watch* 9, no. 2 (1997):27–36.

10. A. Sachs, Virtual Ecology: A Brief Environmental History of Silicon Valley, *World-Watch* 12, no. 1 (1999):12–21.

11. Sachs, Virtual Ecology.

12. T. Colburn, *Our Stolen Future* (New York: Penguin Books, 1996), 19.

13. Mitchell, Nowhere To Hide, 28.

14. L.C. Oliver and B.W. Shackleton, The Indoor Air We Breathe: A Public Health Problem of the '90s, *Public Health Reports* 113, no. 5 (1998):398–409.

15. S. Steingraber, *Living Downstream: An Ecologist Looks at Cancer and the Environment* (New York: Addison-Wesley, 1997), 270.

16. T. Colburn, *Our Stolen Future*, 73–75.

17. Carson, *Silent Spring*.

18. Macy, *Coming Back to Life*, 16–17.

19. Steingraber, *Living Downstream*, 254–272.

20. Mitchell, Nowhere To Hide, 28–29.

21. See Http://www.noharm.org/hcwh/about.cfm

22. G. McRae et al., *An Ounce of Prevention: Waste Reduction Strategies for Health Care Facilities* (Chicago: American Society for Healthcare Environmental Services, 1993), 213–214.

23. See Http://www.ceem.org/

24. S. Cowan, A Design Revolution: *Yes! A Journal of Positive Future*, Summer no. 6 (1998):27–30.

25. Cowan, A Design Revolution.

26. Cowan, A Design Revolution.

27. Cowan, A Design Revolution.

28. The World Commission on Environment and Development, *Our Common Future* (London: Oxford University Press, 1987), 43.

29. The President's Council on Sustainable Development, *Sustainable America: A New Consensus for Prosperity, Opportunity and a Healthy Environment* (Washington, DC: U.S. Government Printing Office, 1996), iv.

30. L. Grant, Sustainability: Part I. On the Edge of an Oxymoron, *Negative Population Growth Forum*, March (1997):1–6.

31. L. Grant, Sustainability, Part II. A Proposal to Foundations, *Negative Population Growth Forum*, March (1997):6.

32. Grant, Sustainability, Part II, 1.

33. K. deBoer, David Orr and the Greening of Education, *Earthlight* 7, no.1 (1996):1, 23.

34. D. Orr, Transformation or Irrelevance: The Challenge of Academic Planning for Environmental Education in the 21st Century, 3. Address to the North American Association for Environmental Education, Florida Gulf Coast University, March 4–8, 1998. See Http://www.2nature.org/programs

35. Orr, Transformation or Irrelevance, 5.6.

36. Carnegie Mellon University, About the Green Design Initiative. See Http://www.ce.cmu.edu/Greendesign/about.html

37. Institute for Sustainable Design. See Http://www.virginia.edu/~sustain/home-mainpage.html

38. J.M. Benyus, *Biomimicry: Innovation Inspired by Nature* (New York: William Morrow, 1997).

39. America Speaks, How Sustainable Is Your Community's Citizen Involvement? *Wingspread* 19, no. 2 (1997):18.

40. B. Mollison, *An Introduction to Permaculture, The Ecology of Health: Identifying Issues and Alternatives* (Newbury Park, CA: Sage Publications, 1996), 308–311.

41. J.T. Gatto, Universal Education, *Yes! A Journal of Positive Futures* 3, no. 1 (1998/99):14–18.

42. Gatto, Universal Education.

43. D. Rothberg, Spiritual Practice and Social Service: The Buddhist Peace Fellowship BASE Program, *The Inner Edge* 1, no. 3 (1998):12–13.

44. Interface, *Sustainability Report* (Atlanta: Interface Research Corporation,1996).

45. Co-op America, 1612 K Street, #600, Washington, DC 20006.

46. Worldwatch Institute, 1776 Massachusetts Avenue, N.W., Washington, DC 20036. See www.worldwatch.org

47. *Yes! A Journal of Positive Futures*, P.O. Box 10818, Bainbridge Island, WA 98110.

48. Benyus, *Biomimicry*.

49. J.E. Lauck, *The Voice of the Infinite in the Small* (Millspring, NC: Swan Raven, 1998).

50. E.F. Keller, *A Feeling for the Organism: The Life and Work of Barbara McClintock* (New York: W.H. Freeman, 1983).

51. Friends Committee on Unity with Nature/Sustainability Committee, Ecological Sustainability as a Witness, *Friends Journal* 45, no. 2 (1999):26–27.

52. P.J. Palmer, Integral Life, Integral Teacher, *Yes! A Journal of Positive Futures* 8, no. 1 (1998/99):44–47.

53. C.B. Pert, *Molecules of Emotion: Why You Feel the Way You Feel* (New York: Charles Scribner's Sons, 1997).

54. S. Abercrombie, Faith, the Feminine and Bear, *Earthlight* 30, no. 3 (1998):8–9.

55. B. Thomson, Health Hazards in the Workplace, *East West* 17, no. 1 (1987):35.

56. K. Doxsey, Toxic Substances in the Hospital Environment, *Journal of Nursing Staff Development* 3 (1987):41–42.

57. J. Lubchenco et al., The Sustainable Biosphere Initiative: An Ecological Research Agenda, *Ecology* 72, no. 2 (1991):371–412.

58. C. Meusz, The Nurse's Role in Workplace Assessment, *Nursing Standard* 6, no. 49 (1992):29–32.

59. K. Pelletier, The Hidden Hazards of the Modern Office, *Holistic Medicine Newsletter* 1 (1987):13.

60. Thomson, Health Hazards in the Workplace.

61. Pelletier, The Hidden Hazards of the Modern Office.

62. S. Halpern and L. Savary, *Sound Health* (San Francisco: Harper & Row, 1985):3–9.

63. M. Smith, Human-Environment Process: A Test of Rogers' Principle of Integrality, *Advances in Nursing Science* 9, no. 1 (1986):21–28.

64. J. Dengerlink et al., Changes in Plasma Angiotensin II with Noise Exposure and Their Relationship to TTS, *Journal of the Acoustical Society of America* 72 (1982):276–278.

65. A. White and M. Burgess, Strategies for Reduction of Noise Levels in ICUs, *The Australian Journal of Advanced Nursing* 10, no. 2 (1992–1993):22–26.

66. M. Topf and J. Davis, Critical Care Unit Noise and Rapid Eye Movement (REM), *Heart and Lung* 22 (1993):252–258.

67. M. Topf, Effects of Personal Control over Hospital Noise on Sleep, *Research in Nursing and Health* 15, no. 1 (1992):19–28.

68. J.P. Griffin, The Impact of Noise on Critically Ill People, *Holistic Nursing Practice* 6, no. 4 (1992):53–56.

69. C. Baker, Discomfort to Environmental Noise, *Critical Care Nursing Quarterly* 15, no. 2 (1992):75–90.

70. R.W. Beckham and S.C. Mishoe, Sound Levels inside Incubators and Oxygen Hoods Used with Nebulizers and Humidifiers, *Respiratory Care* 35, no. 12 (1990):1272–1279.

71. M.J. Lotas, Effects of Light and Sound in the Neonatal Intensive Care Unit Environment on the Low-Birth-Weight Infant, *NAACOG's Clinical Issues in Perinatal & Women's Health Nursing* 3, no. 1 (1992):34–44.

72. G. Harrington, The Nuclear Pantry, *New Age Journal*, November/December 1987, 25–30.

73. R. Gibson, *The Wall Street Journal*, February 4, 1994, B1.

74. Harrington, The Nuclear Pantry, 30.

75. *Temple Daily Telegram*, February 4, 1994, 6C.

76. N. Schlapman, Concerns about Passive Smoking, *Nursing Success Today* 3, no. 6 (1986):26–28.

77. T. Hirayama, Passive Smoking and Lung Cancer: Consistency of Association, *Lancet* 2 (1983):1425–1426.

78. J.R. White and H.F. Froeb, Small Airways Dysfunction in Nonsmokers Chronically Exposed to Tobacco Smoke, *New England Journal of Medicine* 13 (1980):720–723.

79. P. Correa et al., Passive Smoking and Lung Cancer, *Lancet* 2 (1983):595–596.

80. J. Ellul, *The Technological Society* (New York: Alfred A. Knopf, 1964), ix.

81. G.A. Baker et al., The Work Environment Scale: A Comparison of British and North American Nurses, *Journal of Advanced Nursing* 17 (1992):692–698.

82. N.R. Tommasini, The Impact of a Staff Support Group on the Work Environment of a Specialty

Unit, *Archives of Psychiatric Nursing* 6, no. 1 (1992):40–47.

83. G. Thomas, Working Can Be Harmful to Your Health, *Canadian Nurse* 89, no. 6 (1993):35–38.

84. M.B. Townsend, Creating a Better Work Environment, *Journal of Nursing Administration* 21, no. 1 (1991):11–14.

85. J.E. Fielding and P.V. Piserchia, Frequency of Worksite Health Promotion Activities, *American Journal of Public Health* 79, no. 1 (1989):16–20.

86. J.P. Griffin, The Effect of Progressive Muscular Relaxation on Subjectively Reported Disturbance Due to Hospital Noise (Doctoral dissertation, New York University, 1988).

87. E. Schuster, Earth Dwelling, *Holistic Nursing Practice* 6, no. 4 (1992):1–9.

88. Schuster, Earth Dwelling.

89. Schuster, Earth Dwelling.

APPENDIX 12–A

Web Site Resources

Architectural Projects
www.archrecord.com

Bovine Growth Hormone in Milk
www.foxbghsuit.com

Boycotts
www.coopamerica.org/boycotts/
bancover.htm

The Center for Health Design
www.healthdesign.org/oracle/chdwho.htm

Center for Non-Violent Communication
www.loveandcommunity.com/NFNC

Committee for the National Institute for
the Environment
www.cnie.org

Consortium for Environmental Education
in Medicine
www.ceem/org/

Co-op America: Just and Sustainable
Society
www.coopamerica.org

Ecopsychology
www.ecopsych.com

Encyclopedia of Environmental
Contaminants
www.aqd.nps.gov/toxic/index.html

Endocrine Disruptors
www.osf-facts.org

Endocrine Disruptors
www.wwfcanada.org/hormone-disruptors

Environmental Toxicology Encyclopedia
Listings
aqd.nps.tov/toxic/index.html

Fact Sheets Chlorine, PVCs and Dioxins
www.Greenpeace.org

Greens/Green Party
www.greens.org

Green Design Initiative-Carnegie Mellon
University
www.ge.cmu.edu/greendesign/

Health and Light
www.ottbiolight.com

Health Care without Harm
www.sustain.org/hcwh

Health Care without Harm
www.noharm.org

ICN, Nursing and Medical Waste
www.icn.ch/news.htm#11

Indoor Air Quality
www.envirosense.org

Information Clearinghouse and Referral Center Promoting Alternatives to Toxic Chemicals
www.accessone.com/~watoxics

Institute for Sustainable Design
www.virginia.edu/~sustain

Mothers and Others for a Livable Planet
www.mothers.org/mothers

National Patient Safety Partnership
www.aamc.org/newsroom/pressrel/
971006/htm

New American Dream: Reduced Shift Consumption
www.newdream.org

Nightingale Institute
www.NIHE.org

Positive Futures Network
www.futurenet.org

President's Council on Sustainable Development
http://sunsite.utk.edu/neighborhoods/FINS/
sustainable_Development/

Resource Hub for Promoting Sustainable Consumption
www.newdream.org/cgi-bin/AT-
cnadsearch.cgi

Seeds of Simplicity—Voluntary Simplicity and Planetary Well Being
www.slnet.com/cip/seeds

Simple Living Network
www.slnet.com

Strategies for Better Environment
www.informing.org

Sustainable Alternatives to Pesticides
www.igc.org

"Toolkit" of Resources
www.Amherst.edu/~loka

Update & Dangers of Toxic and Endocrine-Disrupting Chemicals
www.monitor.net/Rachel/

VISION OF HEALING

Sharing Our Healing Stories

In each moment, we nurses have many levels of story; some heal, and some do not. Transforming our own healing, the healing of health care, and developing innovative practice models begin with dialogue. We must begin the dialogue that envisions, builds trust, and establishes community in the deepest sense. A healthy dialogue means that an individual does not hold a fixed position, but listens to others explore diverse realities. No one can change in isolation.

To transform our hospitals, clinics, outpatient rehabilitation programs, and schools of nursing into healing environments, we must share our stories, visions, and desires in a healthy dialogue that can lead to creative action. Most nurses are very modest and take their skills and interactions for granted. Sometimes they do not value or even recognize the profound healing that often takes place in the ordinariness, such as the way that a nurse touches a patient in taking a blood pressure, sits with a patient, and is present in the unknowing.

Nurses can learn to become open and comfortable in talking about healing. Common comments by nurses are "Well, that is what I do because I am a nurse," or "It is expected that I help patients." Frequently, nurses do not give themselves credit for healing moments, which can contribute to burnout. Nurses must create time within themselves to affirm the value of their actions and their presence both for themselves and for others. They must say to themselves, "I did a wonderful job," and then feel inspired about their work and healing interactions.

As nurses become active listeners and support each other in the change process, their skills and awareness of love, respect, and trust will increase. Trust levels can mobilize and enhance the healing journey. There are many ways to benefit from a trusting dialogue at work or in our personal relationships. We can meet to share healing moments. The group can define some new areas of healing to be explored for use in the clinic, hospital, school, or community. Then in-service education may offer different topics and teach new skills in healing presence, therapeutic and healing touch, establishment of healing environments, and use of complementary and caring–healing interventions.

Another way to build trust and share visions among nurses is to adopt a council process. This is part of a Native American tradition that creates a state of focused listening. The group sits in a circle. One person serves as a leader for the session to keep the group on track. The rules of the council process are simple: speak honestly, be brief, and speak from the heart. Each person speaks when given the "talking stick," which can be literally a stick or another object that the group has selected for special meaning. The challenge for the council members is to focus on who is speaking rather than on what they wish to say when it is their turn. Planning ahead what one wants to say hinders or eliminates much of the spontaneity of speaking from the heart. The council process is transformative and helps build trust. A profound healing experience occurs when a person is silent within and is focused on another person's ideas, visions, or fears.

Joining colleagues to do a critical analysis about the future of health care, case management, advanced skills, and healing interactions, as well as identifying the essential qualities of healing expertise is inspiring. It also brings together the minds of creative nurse thinkers who have the ability to institute healing practices within nursing.

Chapter 13

Cultural Diversity and Care

Joan C. Engebretson and Judith A. Headley

NURSE HEALER OBJECTIVES

Theoretical

- Compare common value orientations associated with cultures.
- Describe the influence of technology on cultural development and communication systems.
- Analyze components of cultural diversity.
- Describe the components and principles of cultural competence.
- Discuss cultural influences on beliefs and explanatory systems related to health and illness.

Clinical

- Discuss the role of culture in interactions with clients.
- Use components of transcultural assessment in caring for clients.
- Identify appropriate nursing diagnoses in the cultural domain.
- Explore with a colleague interventions that reflect cultural competence.
- Discuss ways in which nursing interventions may be evaluated in relation to cultural competence.

Personal

- Clarify your own values, beliefs, and ideas related to your cultural heritage.
- Identify barriers in your own life to acceptance of cultural diversity.
- Explore activities to increase your awareness and acceptance of cultural differences.

DEFINITIONS

Acculturation: the process of the adaptation, assimilation, or accommodation of an individual immigrant or immigrant group to a new culture.

Assimilation: the process of integration, or taking as one's own, of a new culture by an individual immigrant or immigrant group.

Culture: "the complex whole, which includes knowledge, belief, art, morals, laws, custom and any other capabilities and habits acquired by man as a member of society."[1]

Culturally Competent Health Care: the ability to deliver health care with knowledge of and sensitivity to cultural factors that influence the health and illness behaviors of an individual client or family.

Ethnicity: designation of a population subgroup sharing a common social and cultural heritage.

Ethnocentrism: a world view that is based to a great extent on the socialization of individuals within their own culture, to the extent that such individuals believe that all others see the world as they do.

Race: a social classification that denotes a biologic or genetically transmitted set of distinguishable physical characteristics.

Stereotyping: consigning cultural attributes to a group of people based on assumptions, opinions, or attitudes.

Xenophobia: an inherent fear or hatred of cultural differences.

THEORY AND RESEARCH

Culture is the whole of ideas, customs, skills, arts, and other capabilities of a people or group, although as a whole, it is more complex than any one of these elements. Culture is learned from birth through language acquisition and socialization, the process by which an individual adapts to the group's organized way of life. This process also provides for the transmission of culture from one generation to another. Members of the cultural group share cultural beliefs and patterns of behavior that create a group identity, which has a powerful influence on behavior, usually on a subconscious level. Culture is largely *tacit*, that is, generally unexpressed or discussed at an unconscious level. Most culturally derived actions are based on implicit cues rather than written or spoken sets of rules.

While many of the underlying belief and value systems of a culture are stable, all cultures are inherently dynamic and changing; therefore, it is difficult to generalize from one situation or time to another. Cultural practices are continually adapting to the environment, historical context, technology, and availability of resources. Therefore, the context in which people live influences and is influenced by cultural practice. Anthropology is one of the few disciplines that describe a theoretical holistic focus, an approach that it shares with nursing.

Culture has a significant impact on health and illness behaviors and patterns of response. It directly influences health behaviors such as diet and exercise. Cultural beliefs and practices also affect the types of health problems that are attended to and the actions taken to deal with them. Activities taken to promote, maintain, or restore health must all be performed in a cultural context. As the client may engage in many of these activities, an understanding of the client's perceptions and the context in which he or she lives is necessary for optimal client care.

Culture also determines much of the relationship and communication between a client and a health care provider. Given that the United States is a culturally diverse nation, nurses and other health care providers encounter individuals and groups whose habits of health maintenance, reactions to illness or disease, and use of health care services may differ from their own. An awareness of and accommodation to the cultural aspects of health and illness behaviors enable the nurse to blend professional knowledge skillfully with the individual's or group's beliefs to promote health. Culturally competent care is the delivery of health care with skill, knowledge, and sensitivity to cultural factors. With the increase in cultural pluralism in North America, it is essential that nurses develop cultural competency to deliver holistic care.

Cultural Competency

Health care must be provided within the context of a client's cultural background, beliefs, and values related to health and illness to attain optimal client outcomes. Nurses should gain knowledge of various cultural practices related to health and illness, and they should integrate this knowledge into their interventions. Bernal has identified five components of culturally competent care: (1) open-mindedness, (2) awareness of one's own cultural values, (3) understanding, (4) knowledge, and (5) adaptation skills.[2]

1. Awareness and acceptance of cultural differences require an open-minded attitude about other world views. Competency starts with the attitude that providing care based on one's own world view may not be in the best interest of the client. Nurses who use a nonjudgmental approach in learning about a client's cultural belief system will not only gain a wealth of information, but also will readily establish mutual trust in their nurse–client relationships.

2. An awareness of one's own biases and attitudes that create barriers to direct interaction with a group or groups makes it possible to overcome them. Recognition of personal cultural attitudes requires conscious effort; most people are unaware of their cultural beliefs because their beliefs are so integrated into their perception of the world. Personal reflection and values clarification are useful strategies to facilitate awareness.[3] Values clarification facilitates self-understanding, focuses on what is meaningful to the individual, and includes values that are both fixed and changing. Clarification of values is a critical thinking process that involves making choices from a variety of alternatives that are consistent with one's own beliefs. As nurses become more aware of their own values, they can enable clients to clarify and express what is important for them. Nurses must not assume that their own values are right, nor should they judge a client's values according to their own values, for such action might lead to ethnocentrism. Knowledge and understanding of the values, beliefs, and behaviors of a culture enable a nurse to individualize nursing interventions.

3. It is essential to understand dynamic differences and to recognize basic differences among cultures without promoting the superiority of one culture over the other. Many people, in an effort to connect with people of other cultures, assume that there are no differences among cultures and focus only on fundamental similarities. Al-though this is useful for connecting with other cultures, it can obscure some basic differences that must be understood for cultural understanding. For example, a European-American cannot fully understand an African-American without recognizing the legacy of slavery in the African-American culture.

4. With a basic knowledge about a client's culture, nurses can develop and share knowledge and skills in a straightforward manner. The best way to learn about diverse cultures is to interact with people from that culture, as participation and communication provide opportunities to discuss and experience cultural variances. Opportunities to become immersed in another culture are not always available, however. Culturally focused literature, films, and music can be used to enhance cultural understanding. Stories by and about a specific cultural group can provide a microscopic view of factors that have shaped lives, have influenced values, and reflect beliefs related to health and illness. The false notion of a single monolithic culture can be dispelled through reflections of literature, such as the depiction of the concept of health and related underlying beliefs, values, and behavior patterns of life in an African-American community in *The Color Purple*.[4]

5. Adaptation skills include being receptive to different cultures, actively seeking advice and consultation from individuals of that culture, and incorporating those ideas into one's practice. Skills include the ability to articulate an issue from another's perspective, as well as to recognize and reduce resistance and defensiveness. The ability to admit errors is important, as resolving errors in interacting with someone from another culture allows for the exploration of cultural issues that enhance understanding and communication. It is better to risk a confrontation than to avoid the issue, resulting in continued misperception or lost opportunity for better cultural understanding.

Cultural Diversity

White Anglo-American mainstream (WAAM) denotes the dominant culture in North America. Historically and socially, Latinos have often been considered part of the white population. According to census data, however, Latinos are a separate classification. The ratio of minority group members to the non-Latino white population is increasing every year. It is estimated that the non-Latino white group will constitute only 52 percent of the population by the year 2050, as compared to about 75 percent in 1992.[5]

Ethnicity refers to values, perceptions, feelings, assumptions, and physical characteristics associated with ethnic group affiliation. Often, ethnicity refers to nationality, a group sharing a common social and cultural heritage. In contrast, race typically refers to a biologic, genetically transmitted set of distinguishable physical characteristics. In medical literature, however, race has often been misused to describe differences in people that have no basis in biology or science. Demographic data are commonly gathered with no differentiation of ethnicity or definitions of race. Both skin color and country of origin have been used to classify race. For example, many natives of India (considered racially Caucasian) have darker skin than do many natives of Africa.

Race and culture have a significant relationship to illness states, as biologic differences may make certain groups of people vulnerable to specific diseases. For example, genetic predisposition for sickle cell disease affects people of African and Mediterranean descent; predisposition for Tay–Sachs disease affects Ashkenazi Jews. Also, certain diseases that may be attributable to a combination of genetic predisposition and lifestyle, including nutritional patterns, are more prevalent in some groups. One example is the disproportionately high prevalence of diabetes in Native Americans and Hispanics. Some diseases are connected to lifestyle risks, such as substance abuse and human immunodeficiency virus (HIV) infection, which are related to particular social behaviors.

Cultural grouping is not limited to ethnicity or race, but can be attributed to multiple factors that determine values, beliefs, and behaviors. Ethnicity is the most common cultural demarcation, but intra-ethnic variations may be more differentiating than inter-ethnic variations, especially in a culturally pluralistic society. Other variables that have been proposed as influencing cultural groupings are religion, socioeconomic status, geographic region, age, common beliefs, and professional orientation.

Factors Related to Culture

Religion is an important factor in determining the values and beliefs of a culture. An organized system of beliefs, religion is differentiated from spirituality, which is born out of each person's unique life experience and efforts to find meaning and purpose in life.[6] Religious faith and the institutions derived from that faith have a powerful influence over human behavior. All religions have experiential, ritualistic, ideologic, intellectual, and consequential dimensions. Religious views have historically served as a unifying force for groups of people according to a set of core values and beliefs.

Socioeconomic status refers to one's social status, occupation, education, economic status, or a combination of these. Socioeconomic explanations have often been discounted in determining the relationships between ethnicity or race and the risk of health conditions such as acquired immune deficiency syndrome (AIDS), violence, and drug abuse. It is necessary to distinguish between cultural identification and the common experience of being poor in our society. By illustration, the experience of being poor in our society is different from that of being Hispanic and must be further distinguished from being both poor and Hispanic. The impact of socioeconomic status on both morbidity and mortality measures of specific groups is highly significant; lower socioeconomic status groups have higher morbidity and mortality rates.[7]

The local or regional manifestations of the larger culture address such distinctions as rural, urban, Southern, or Midwestern. For example, African-Americans living in the Southern region of the United States may have different beliefs and behaviors than those in the Northern region, based somewhat on their heritage of slavery and exposure to the civil rights movement.

Age of the individuals within a cultural group has a profound influence over their beliefs and behaviors. Value systems are tied to historically shared events that occur in childhood; therefore, each generation develops a unique value system. For example, persons born in the United States prior to the 1940s generally maintain traditional values, while those born in 1940s, 1950s, and particularly the generation of the 1960s often consciously strive to reject those values.[8]

Common beliefs or ideologies may unite a cultural group, and differentiate that group from the larger culture. These value systems may be related to religion (e.g., the Amish), lifestyle (e.g., communal groups), sexual orientation (e.g., gay and lesbian groups), or political ideologies (e.g., feminist separatist groups). Social or professional orientations often constitute a type of cultural grouping. For example, the biomedical culture of many hospitals constitutes an unfamiliar culture for many lay people. Health care teams use a unique and esoteric language, as well as rituals, roles, expectations and patterns of behavior, and symbolic communication that are alien to the lay person.

Common Myths and Errors

Errors of stereotyping are common among those who define the world by strict categories of ethnicity or race and presume that all members of another culture conform to a common pattern without regard to individual characteristics or the variety found within one cultural grouping. For example, some people assume that all African-Americans eat soul food or all Hispanics are Catholic. Failure to recognize that values from a particular cultural group can vary across time and location can lead to stereotyping cultures with values that no longer guide the group's thinking or behaviors. Stereotyping is less obvious in some cases, such as a nurse manager's assigning all Hispanic clients to the Mexican-American nurse. Such action does not take into account the differences within the Hispanic group, presumes that all Hispanics are alike, and disregards the individual.

The heterogeneity of ethnic groups is often underestimated, but as mentioned earlier, the variations within ethnic groups may be as great or greater than those between ethnic groups. For example, the Hispanic culture includes persons of Puerto Rican, Cuban, Spanish, and South and Central American origins. These people are from many different socioeconomic backgrounds and represent the Caucasian, Mongoloid, and Negroid racial groups. Sometimes Asians from different countries and backgrounds are grouped together and treated as generic Asians, an attitude that totally ignores the historical differences among Asians. Kipnis related a clinical incident that occurred in Hawaii, in which a Korean gentleman with a serious medical condition refused a treatment that promised a better than 50 percent recovery with minimum risks.[9] The ethical and cultural consultant was called when the patient requested full support when asked about his preference for treatment of a cardiopulmonary arrest. Clinical staff were puzzled by his refusal of treatment for his disease coupled with his request for life support if he experienced cardiopulmonary arrest. On further investigation, he mentioned that all his physicians were Japanese. In the early 1900s, Japan had ruthlessly tyrannized Korea, much as the Nazis in Germany tyrannized Poland prior to and during World War II. Thus, the Korean gentleman very much wanted to live, but his cultural history caused him to refuse treatment directed by the Japanese physicians.

Ethnocentrism is the tendency, usually unconscious, for individuals to take for granted that their own values are the only objective reality and to look at everyone else through the lens of their own cultural norms and customs. Ethnocentric views often result from a lack of knowledge of other cultures and the presumption that one's own behavior is not influenced by culture and is correct. Many people of the dominant culture falsely assume that they have no culture practices and beliefs. This restrictive view of the world perceives people and cultures with different beliefs and behaviors as culturally inferior. An extreme and more conscious form of ethnocentrism is xenophobia, an inherent fear of cultural differences, which often leads people to bolster their security in their own values by demeaning the beliefs and traditions of others. This attitude often takes the form of prejudice or racism.

Cultural imposition is the perception that successful cultural adaptation involves a change to the cultural views of the dominant group, regardless of an individual's cultural heritage. This posits an inherent view that the dominant culture is superior, and its values are imposed upon others.

Often disguised as equal treatment for everyone, cultural blindness ignores cultural differences as if they did not exist. This view overlooks real diversity and the importance of other perspectives. The concept of the "melting pot" assumes that, in the process of acculturation and assimilation, everyone takes on significant aspects of the dominant culture such that the original culture is largely lost. This assimilation or "melting pot" view is being challenged by concepts of heritage consistency, which is the degree to which one maintains practices and beliefs that reflect one's own heritage.[10]

Development of Cultural Patterns and Behaviors

Anthropologists have studied the similarities between cultures related to the universal experience of being human. Their major focus has been on the variations in the ways that humans organize and structure their social world. Some of the factors that contribute to the development of cultural patterns and behavior are geography and migration, gender-specific roles, value orientations and cultural beliefs, and technology.

Geography and Migration

Social groups evolve in interaction with the climate, availability of food, and resources. The persistence of dietary patterns reflects the types of food available in a particular region. For example, fish constitutes a large portion of the traditional diet of people from Norway and the Philippines, whereas dairy products and meats are dominant in food patterns in Finland and Denmark.

Social organization has followed these geographic patterns; for example, the social structure of a fishing village differs from that of a nomadic group that hunts for food or a settled agrarian culture. Urbanization and industrialization are important in the way society organizes and social roles develop. Social roles become patterned and often institutionalized into hierarchical structures that reflect social, economic, and political power. These social structures and roles greatly alter people's daily life and the economics of providing for families.

Climate, environmental conditions, political and economic factors are very important in migration patterns. Climate change, famine, political upheaval, or overpopulation beyond the immediate environment's resources have been responsible for migration. For example, a large wave of Irish immigrants came to the United States in the late 1840s following a potato famine that was causing starvation, disease, and death in Ireland. Many immigrants came to the United States to flee political unrest in El Salvador in the 1980s. Many Vietnamese and Southeast Asians sought political refuge and opportunities in the United States following the Vietnam War. A large number of nurses moved to the mainland United States from the Philippines in the 1980s seeking professional and economic opportunities. Even in the 1990s, a large number of immigrants have steadily come to the United States seeking economic opportunities.

Cultural patterns further develop through the sharing of ideas, beliefs, and practices that follow trade or migration. Immigrants bring cultural patterns, values, and beliefs with them. Along with their adaptation to the new host culture, they expose the host culture to a different set of cultural beliefs and practices. Both cultures assimilate aspects of the other.

In culturally pluralistic societies such as the United States, the historical context of the immigration of groups and individuals is important. Many African-Americans arrived involuntarily and endured a lengthy history of slavery; Hispanics may be immigrants seeking economic opportunity, refugees from political upheavals, or descendants of people living in the Southwest before it became a part of the United States. The fact that many Asian immigrants find it necessary to take a job with lower status than they had in their country of origin creates cultural and economic hardship for the family. In many Hispanic families, the father immigrates alone to establish a better economic future for the family. Estranged from the family, he may be at risk for such behavioral health risks as AIDS

and alcohol abuse. Health issues may also arise because of low income and low self-esteem.

Acculturation is an important process in the adaptation, assimilation, or accommodation of immigrant groups to a new culture. Often, acculturation is a process of assimilation, in which immigrants integrate the new culture into their beliefs and lifestyle and yet retain heritage consistency, maintaining pride in and adhering to their parent culture. According to the theory of orthogonal cultural identification, this process does not take place along a single continuum, but has numerous dimensions that operate independently from each other. Intergenerational gaps frequently develop within the traditional culture in the process of acculturation. As youth become more quickly acculturated to the dominant society, they challenge the more traditional values, beliefs, and customs of their parents; this, in turn, may threaten the integrity and lines of respect in the family and roles within the family and society, particularly the role of women. Conflicts that arise from intergenerational gaps can lead to the alienation of young people and families from both the ethnic culture and the general dominant culture.

Gender Roles

Over the past century, in the United States, the social role for women has undergone many changes. The role of women has expanded from its traditional focus on childbearing and child rearing to include participation in the workplace and marketplace. The feminist movement has championed this expanded role and has heightened consciousness about full opportunities consistent with the American values of individualism, equality, and political freedom. Furthermore, it has challenged the values and structures developed by a masculine power elite, such as competition, strong focus on objectives and goals, harnessing and control of nature, principle-based ethics, and productive activities. Feminists have promoted cultural practices and organizations that espoused more feminine values such as teamwork, focus on social process, working in harmony with nature, relationship-based ethics, and social connections. As people from other cultures move into the United States, these differing and expanded roles for women may be very challenging for the traditional family roles.

Women have played significant roles in the healing arts as well. Historically and cross-culturally, women have discovered and preserved information about healing herbs and plants. In the Middle Ages, women were often persecuted for their knowledge of plants and other healing arts that were deemed mysterious and suspicious. As medicine became more scientific and moved into a professional and scientific status, women were disengaged from the official healing roles.[11] Women were associated with nature, and men, with developing technology to tame and control nature. Women's roles in the healing arts reflected this dichotomy. With the establishment of medical professions, women's roles even in midwifery—a traditional role for women—were reduced, and physicians took over the practice and moved it into hospitals. Women who worked in medical professions were often in nonphysician roles or positions of lower power and social status, such as nurses, social workers, and physical therapists. Women have a strong presence among complementary healers and users of complementary therapies, however.[12]

Value Orientations and Beliefs

All cultures hold certain values in high regard, and these values are central to cultural patterns of behavior. These values can be either implicit or explicit. They influence an individual's perception of others; direct that individual's responses to others; reflect his or her identity and are the basis for self-reflection; serve as the foundation for positions on personal, professional, social, political, and philosophic issues; motivate behavior and direct goals; and give meaning to life.[13] In the United States, for example, the public generally perceives values as having a strong moral orientation and an emphasis on active instrumental mastery over the world according to external standards. Individual and peer relationships rather than hierarchical relationships are stressed. The focus is on progress and change with a rationalistic rather than traditional approach. Orderliness and attention to structure and form are important.

Value Orientations. Variants of value orientations have been outlined following Kluckhohn's five categories.[14] They reflect the way in which a culture solves the universal problems of human nature:

1. **Innate human nature.** Cultures' dominant views of human nature range from seeing human beings as basically evil, or perfectible only with discipline and effort, to seeing human beings as good and being unalterable or incorruptible. Some see human nature as mixed, a combination of good and evil, but with the capacity for self-control. Individuals' views of human nature have implications for their trust in the medical establishment.

2. **Relationship to nature.** Various cultures are fatalistic, seeing humans as subjugated to nature in their destiny.

Some believe that humans coexist with nature in harmony. Mastery over nature is the perspective that natural forces are to be overcome and put to human use. A culture's view of the cause of disease often is based on the perceived relationship of humans to nature.

3. **Relationship to time.** Past-oriented people value tradition and have a great respect for the wisdom of ancestors and elders. They may first seek guidance for health problems from older family or group members or from folk healers. Present-oriented people live in the moment and may be late for appointments, have trouble making ends meet financially, and delay educational goals to meet immediate needs of self or family. In future-oriented cultures such as that in the United States, most middle-class individuals tend to delay gratification to pursue education or career and set high future goals. They value punctuality and efficiency and plan actions to save time and money. They may alter their lifestyle to promote health, and the emphasis is on youth and new ideas.

4. **Purpose of being.** Cultures oriented toward "being" express impulses and desires spontaneously and are not focused on development. "Being-in-becoming" cultures are oriented toward self-development and self-realization wherein the self is contained and controlled within. This detachment from the outer world brings enlightenment. In "doing" cultures, people actively strive to meet goals, and they evaluate their accomplishments competitively against externally applied standards of achievement. Individuals' culturally determined interpretations of their purpose for being affect their responses to illness and disability.

5. **Relationship to other persons.** Lineal relationships have continuity through time and are expressed in heredity, kinship ties, and orderly succession. Emphasis on the welfare of society, group goals, and family orientation is the hallmark of the collateral value. Individual orientations, where personal autonomy and independence are primary, subject group goals to individual goals. The type of relationships among members of a particular culture often influence how health care decisions are made and by whom, and how individuals respond to dependency on others.

Cultural Beliefs. A group's beliefs are tenets with a shared meaning. They are a set of metaphorical explanations used to explain the phenomenon of nature and form a world view or a paradigm. Spiritual teachings and the social codes of behavior stem from these world views. Often formalized into religious systems that are the institutionalization of a belief set, these world views are the source of many of the assumptions that people have about creation, reality, behavior, and rituals.

Three dominant cosmology assumptions essential to world views held by Western Judeo-Christian-Islam beliefs differ from those in some of the other world religions.[15] Monotheism, the belief in one God Creator who is separate from humans, contrasts with the beliefs common in many agrarian societies whose members believe in polytheism, multiple gods with different attributes, or pantheism (i.e., the locus of the sacred in all living things). The Western view of transcendence, or relating to God as separate from humans and knowing God through prayer, supplication, and rituals to connect to the Divine, can be contrasted with the Eastern view of immanence, or finding God by looking inward and doing other spiritual exercises to discover the sacred. Finally, Western dualism, separation of material from nonmaterial aspects of being, is in contrast to *monism*, or the essential unity found in both the pantheistic and Eastern belief systems.

Technology and Culture

In contemporary Western culture, technology is highly valued. Technology began with early "tool-using" societies in which tools were invented and used to solve specific problems.[16] Societies then progressed in their development of technology and used it to improve the human condition and better society. When tools play a central part in the "thought world" of the culture, the society becomes a technocracy. The coexistence, tension, and dialogue between science, technology, philosophy, and values characterize a technocracy, epitomized by the Industrial Age.

Technopoly, according to Postman,[17] occurs when technocracy becomes totalitarian and eliminates alternatives. Postman expressed some concern that the United States is moving to this state in which technology defines values, art, religion, politics, and medical issues. This pattern is particularly prominent in health care. The use of technology in medicine began with solving physical problems. For example, the stethoscope was invented to better locate areas of pulmonary congestion related to pneumonia, a common medical problem at the time. Medical technology progressed in its development to complex instruments that allow for more complex procedures, such as electrocardiograms, amniocenteses, and gene mapping. The development of these technologies poses new ethical

and cultural questions related to how, when, and what impact this technology may have. Once the technology is available for use, it becomes the focus of many ethical debates and necessitates the formation of ethical committees to make specific decisions. The fear, issued in Postman's warning, is that the next step will be a technopoly in which the cultural values and ethical questions are no longer considered. In this situation, technology's development is inevitable. It drives the system, and the uses or ethical applications are no longer questioned or debated.

Technology has held a powerful influence on culture through its use in communication. Linguistics, a study of cultural ideation, is the form in which members of the culture communicate thought and meaning. Many forms of communication may coexist in a culture. These forms have become more sophisticated with industrialization and education. The actual form of communication often dictates the type of information that can be conveyed. For example, many people can recognize a picture of George Washington or Napoleon, but would be hard-pressed to describe those individuals in words. Thus, the medium of communication, to some extent, determines the content.

Traditionally, knowledge was passed on by oral means in stories, parables, and poetry. Essential knowledge (e.g., cultural wisdom) was distilled through a process of discourse and discussion over time. The tone, timbre, rhetoric, and sounds of the words were just as important as the message they conveyed. Many cultures today are based primarily in oral traditions.

With the advent of the printing press and written communication, the Western world became a different culture in a fundamental way based on the type of knowledge that was conveyed and developed. Written culture allows for "frozen speech" that can be referred to across time and space. It can be scrutinized for accuracy and precision in a way that oral speech cannot. It facilitates lengthy discussions of logic and rational argument, as it allows time for the formation of complex thoughts and new ideas. It also permits the recording of large amounts of detailed factual data in a precise fashion that was not possible in an oral culture. This medium is the heart of academic and rational discourse. The demand for precision and verification is congruent with the development of scientific methods and quantification in modern scholarship.

Today's electronic culture is dependent on telephones, radio, television, and computers to communicate information. Electronic media allow for fast and democratic dispersal of information. The primary concerns are speed and image. Lengthy scholarly discourses have been replaced by short messages meant to capture the attention of the viewer and convey a message. These messages, however, are generally without context and, as a result, often have little relevance or coherence for the viewer. Pictures with visual and auditory images in story format are extremely persuasive in conveying messages related to lifestyle and behaviors; thus, they influence cultural values as well as health behaviors.

Changing Beliefs and Values

In the late twentieth century, people in the developed and industrialized world have been exposed to a number of different cultures, as a result of both immigration and electronic technology. Scientific and technologic advances, as well as global, political, social, and economic changes, have challenged existing cultural systems and increased the velocity of cultural change. Some cultural critics have predicted a major cultural change in the United States. They believe that concern for the quality of life, personalization, and a reverence for nature will replace modernism, which focuses on materialism, scientific progress and objectivism, and the role of humans in controlling and exploiting nature.[18,19] Anderson described a shift in contemporary culture as evidenced by the emphasis on the environ-ment, religion and spirituality, and post-modern multiculturalism.[20]

A recent large marketing survey indicated that the U.S. population can be divided into three groups according to values. Ray identified Cultural Creatives as those who are on the leading edge of change, comprising nearly one-quarter of the population.[21] This group holds a holistic philosophy of health; values ecologic preservation, spirituality, relationships, and self-actualization; and expresses interest in other cultures and new ideas. The largest group (47 percent), the Moderns, place a high value on success, consumerism, materialism, and technologic rationality. A third group (approximately 29 percent), the Traditionalists or Heartlanders, believe in the nostalgic images of small towns and strong churches that define the "Good Old American Way."

In a recent survey of more than 1,000 adults, Astin found that those who use alternative/complementary therapies have a higher education and a more holistic orientation to health, were more likely to have had a chronic health problem or other recent illness, and often had been through a transformational experience that changed their world view.[22] This group expressed a set of values, beliefs, and philosophic orientations that included commitment to environmentalism, feminism, and interest in spirituality and personal growth. Other studies have described these users as generally well educated and affluent members of the middle class.[23–25] The use of complementary therapies and the search for holistic approaches to health care is consistent with the cultural beliefs of the Cultural Creatives. This percentage of the population is substantial and, according to Ray,[26] is growing while the Traditionalist groups are generally older and not growing as fast.

Ethnic Groups in North America

Culturally diverse groups in the United States have grown to substantial proportions of the population. In their practice, nurses are likely to encounter representatives of several different cultures. They should read and engage in cultural discussions and experiential learning with members of these cultural groups to avoid stereotypic interpretations of individuals or families who represent these groups and to develop cultural competency.

Native American

The indigenous peoples of the Americas number nearly 2 million and live across the United States, Alaska, and the Aleutian Islands.[27] They cluster in tribal groups with the largest concentrations located in the Pacific and Western Mountain regions of the United States. There is considerable variation among the tribes regarding language, beliefs, customs, health practices, and rituals. Tribes or clans constitute a social unit in which members may or may not be blood relatives, and both family and clan are powerful sources of the Native American's identity and support. Largely because of the respect for the wisdom accrued with aging, elders are the leaders. Value orientations center on harmony with nature, a present time orientation, and an integration of rituals and religion into everyday life. Many Native Americans still adhere to folk healing practices, seeking out the medicine man before going to a health care clinic. Folk healing practices may fall into the shamanic category or often be understood in a supranormal paradigm. Common health problems include diabetes, obesity, infectious disease, alcohol abuse, and diseases associated with poverty.[28] Years of racism, dehumanization, and oppression have left a legacy in which many Native Americans may mistrust white health care providers.

European-Americans

The largest ethnic group in North America is made up of the European-Americans. They constitute the dominant culture and comprise approximately 83 percent of the population of the United States.[29] The largest emigrations from various regions in Europe occurred in the late 1700s, all through the 1800s, and into the first half of the twentieth century. Many immigrants to the United States carried the European ideas of the Age of Reason, dominance over nature, and the belief in progress and technologic advancement. Their quest for freedom enhanced an abiding value of individualism. They were generally action-oriented, future-directed, and focused on progress and productivity. Families are an important social unit among European-Americans, but the value of individualism is pervasive. Although this group is diverse, the values are consistent with dominant values of the culture. Therefore, members of this group may not be as aware of the role that culture plays in their lives as members of other cultural groups.

African-Americans

The 1990 Census estimated the number of African-Americans in the United States to be 31 million, or 12 percent of the population, and this is anticipated to increase to 61 million by 2050.[30] One-third of this population was under the age of 18 in 1990. This group is very heterogeneous and varies in economic status, religion, education, and regional background. Many African-Americans are descendants of slaves who were brought to the United States; others are recent immigrants from Africa and the Caribbean Islands. Within the social structure of slavery, families were dispersed and individuals were not allowed to read. Thus, a tradition of strong matriarchal family units with a rich oral tradition developed. Social organization centers on the family, kinship bonds, and the church. Health problems of high morbidity and mortality may be related to the disproportional rate of poverty. Many African-Americans have absorbed much of the dominant culture, but some hold to ancestral beliefs of illness as disharmony with nature and supranormal healing rituals or folk healing. The history of slavery and the Tuskegee atrocities have made some African-Americans mistrustful of receiving health care from the health care system or participating in clinical research studies.

Asian-Americans

Constituting 3 percent of the total US population or approximately 7.5 million people in 1990, Asian-Americans, including Pacific Islanders, are expected to represent 8 percent of the population by 2050.[31] Approximately two-thirds reside in the Western part of the United States. This group is composed of immigrants and refugees from the Pacific Rim countries: China, Japan, Korea, Thailand, Laos, Vietnam, Cambodia, the Philippines, and other Asian countries. Some include people from India in this group as well. There is wide diversity in language, customs, and beliefs. Traditional Asian families tend to be patriarchal, to revere their elders, and to value achievement and honor. Certain infectious diseases, such as tuberculosis and hepatitis, are common among Asian-Americans, depending on the country from which they emigrated. Stress-related diseases and suicides are high, as many do not seek mental health care because of an associated stigma and a threat to honor. Asians' traditional health practices are often oriented around the balance paradigm in which health is equated with balance and unimpeded flow of energy or "chi." Traditional healing includes the use of herbal preparations, and many families practice traditional self-care procedures such as coining, pinching, or rubbing.

Hispanic or Latino Americans

The Hispanic population in the United States includes more than 22 million people, or 9 percent of the U.S. population, and is predicted to reach 24 percent by 2050.[32] The majority of these immigrants come from Mexico, with others from Puerto Rico, Cuba, and Central and South America. This is the fastest growing group in the United States. Although the Spanish language is a common factor, there is much diversity in dialects and cultural practices. This group comprises indigenous peoples of the Americas, Spanish and other European settlers, and some African-Caribbean groups. Predominant religions are Catholicism and Pentecostalism. The family and extended family are important, and the family unit is traditionally patriarchal. Many believe that illness may be punishment for sins or the result of witchcraft *brujería* or the evil eye. Traditional health beliefs regarding hot and cold remedies for various maladies reflect humoral balance beliefs. Healing also incorporates many spiritual elements, such as worship of saints and use of talismans.

Impact of Culture on Health Care

Cultural understandings of health and illness reflect larger philosophic world views or paradigms that provide a way of understanding the body and the forces that influence health and illness. According to Andrews and Boyle,[33] three major types of cross-cultural paradigms operate: magicoreligious, holistic, and scientific. Although aspects of all three are found in most cultures, one usually predominates.

In the magicoreligious health paradigm, the fate of the world depends on God, gods, or supernatural forces. Events such as sorcery, breach of taboo, intrusion of a disease object, intrusion of a disease-causing spirit, or loss of soul are considered responsible for illness. This paradigm relates to a psychic or metaphysical need of humanity for integration and harmony.[34] For example, people from some African-Caribbean cultures believe that parts of a person such as hair, fingernails, or blood represent the person and can be used in healing.

Also, they may believe that lack of protection for these body parts can make the person vulnerable to illness.

In the holistic health paradigm, the forces of nature must be kept in harmony according to natural laws and the larger universe. These systems often have a strong emphasis on health rather than on the treatment of disease.[35] In Ayurvedic medicine from India, for example, health results from being in harmony with oneself, others, and the environment. Diet and activity are adapted according to the individual's doshas (i.e., forces of the human body whose composition varies among individuals) and the seasonal variations in the environment. In Western culture, this idea appears in humoral theories, such as the concepts of balancing hot and cold held by Hispanic, Arab, African, Caribbean, and other societies. Holistic health care is regaining some popularity in developed countries, bastions of the scientific paradigm, as the focus begins to shift to promoting health.

The scientific or biomedical paradigm is characterized by four main concepts:

1. **Determinism.** A cause-and-effect relationship exists for all natural phenomena.
2. **Mechanism.** The relationship of life to the structure and function of machines suggests the possibility of control through mechanical or engineered interventions.
3. **Reductionism.** The division of all life into isolated smaller parts, such as the dualism of mind and body, facilitates the study of the whole.
4. *Objective materialism.* That which is real can be observed and measured.[36]

This paradigm is the basis for acute health care systems in Western society, where the disease is viewed as the "enemy," the body is the "battlefield," and the physician is the "general." Great effort, expense, and technology are invested in determining the underlying cause of disease. The "system at fault" is isolated, and the most medical attention is directed toward measuring the functions of and repairing this faulty part. Persons are often placed in foreign environments (e.g., hospitals) in which limited attention is given to individual needs and cultural beliefs.

Cultural Sectors

Health care systems in most cultures have certain sectors in common. Kleinman identified three sectors that are generally present: professional, popular, and folk.[37] Cultures vary widely in the way that they combine these three systems. Usually, one is dominant, although simultaneous use is common.

In the United States, the professional, or orthodox biomedical, sector of health care has held a legal/political and ideologic monopoly for most of this century. This sector corresponds to the scientific paradigm described earlier. Nurses and other organized health care professionals are part of this sector.

The popular sector, in the broadest sense, includes all the personal and social networks that lay people use to understand their health and plan their health care. Individuals, family, and social networks determine whom to consult, when to seek a consultation, whether to adhere to suggested treatments, when to switch treatments, and how to evaluate the usefulness of treatments. Nearly all persons are active in their own health care decisions and practice some form of private or self-prescribed health care.

All secular and sacred healers that are generally outside the professional sector make up the folk sector. This sector also includes healing devices and practices used to promote health and treat illness. According to Giger and Davidhizar,[38] folk medicine frequently classifies diseases or illnesses as natural or unnatural. Natural events arise from the way that a higher power made the world and intended it to be. The basic principle is that everything in nature is connected and events can be explained in terms of this relationship. In some folk sectors, disease represents a disturbance in that relationship with nature. A natural disease or illness results from a disturbance in the person's relationship or balance with nature, and recovery requires the restoration of this relationship. This view is common among Native Americans, whose concept of medicine embraces the forces of nature. Because death is seen as part of the life cycle, a component of natural harmony, a cure for illness is not necessarily sought. Unnatural illnesses are usually attributed to punishment from a higher power for one's sins or improper behavior. The origin of unnatural illnesses in folk medicine is based on the continuous battle between good and evil forces. Witchcraft and breaking of a taboo are sometimes considered the origin for unnatural illnesses.

Explanatory Models of Health and Illness

Concepts of health and healing are rooted in culture. The concept of disease generally refers to the diagnostic label used to describe a particular disorder, while the concept of illness incorporates the personal, social, and cultural aspects of the experience. Some cultural principles influence an individual's behavior to promote, maintain, and restore health; others help the individual cope with illness or dying.

The beliefs of an individual or group about the causes, symptoms, and treatments of illness is an explanatory model. Culturally specific explanatory models are interpretations of the culture's world view as it pertains to health and healing, and generally provide an understanding of disease and direct treatment. Explanatory models of health and healing are used to recognize, interpret, respond to, cope with, and make sense of an illness experience.[39] For example, a client who believes that the cause of his or her illness is related to committing a sin or breaking a taboo may not accept medication as a cure. Some form of

catharsis, forgiveness, or ritual may be necessary. The questions in Exhibit 13–1 may be used to elicit a client's explanatory model.[40]

Multiparadigm Model of Healing

As Western culture is becoming increasingly culturally pluralistic, a number of alternative and complementary healing practices and beliefs are surfacing. The meaning of the word "holistic" is related to the word "health," which stems from the root word "hale," the same root as "to make whole." This definition would necessarily incorporate multiple approaches to support health. One effort to place diverse modalities into a unified model is illustrated in Exhibit 13–2.[41] Paradigms of health and healing are based in underlying philosophy, cultural beliefs, and explanatory models of health and illness. Hence, there is resonance between the biomedical model and the technologic development of mod-

---

Exhibit 13–1 Questions To Elicit Explanatory Models

- What do you call your problem? What name does it have?
- What do you think has caused your problem?
- Why do you think it started when it did?
- What does your sickness do to you? How does it work?
- How severe is it? Will it have a short or long course?
- What do you fear most about your sickness?
- What are the chief problems your sickness has caused you?
- What kind of treatment do you think you should receive?
- What are the most important results you hope to receive from the treatment?

Source: Adapted with permission from Kleinman et al., Culture, Illness, and Care: Clinical Lessons from Anthropologic and Cross-Cultural Research, *Annals of Internal Medicine*, Vol. 88, pp. 251–258, © 1978, American College of Physicians—American Society of Internal Medicine.

Exhibit 13-2 Multiparadigm Model of Healing

	Positivist ◄────────────────────────────────► Metaphysical				
Material ▲	**Modalities**	**Mechanical**	**Purification**	**Balance**	**Supranormal**
	Physical manipulation	Biomedical Surgery	Colonics Cupping	Magnetic healing Polarity	Drumming Dancing (Dervishes)
	Applied and ingested substances	Pharmacology	Chelation	Humeral medicine	Flower remedies Hallucinogenic plants
	Energy	Laser/radiation	Bio-energetics	T'ai chi Qigong Acupuncture Acupressure	Healing touch Laying-on of hands
	Psychological	Mind-body	Self-help (confessional type)	Mindfulness	Imagery
▼ **Nonmaterial**	Spiritual	Attendance at organized religious functions	Forgiveness Penance	Meditation Chakra balancing	Primal religious experience Prayer

Source: This figure originally appeared in *Advances in Nursing Science*, volume 20, number 1, pages 22–34. Reprinted with permission. © 1997 Aspen Publishers, Inc.

ern society. In this unified model, modalities or healing activities are suggested based on the explanation that healers have given for their use.

The unified model illustrated in Exhibit 13-2 uses four paradigms across the horizontal axis: mechanical, purification, balance, and supranormal. The mechanical paradigm best describes the biomedical model or the professional sector, in which the prevailing views are that the body is a system of structure and function, disease is a disruption of its mechanism of action, and the purpose of treatment is to restore or replace that function. The mechanical paradigm is self-correcting and produces increasingly sophisticated understandings of the mechanics of the function of the human body.

The purification paradigm underlies many illness/disease healing and religious healing practices. The general intention is to cleanse and rid the body of polluting influences. This approach to healing is evident as far back as the early Egyptians, who understood and used some of the concepts of purification in the process of mummification. This paradigm was very dominant in European medicine as late as the nineteenth century and was the rationale behind purges, bloodletting, and other cathartic treatments.

Evident in many cultures, the balance paradigm is epitomized in many of the Oriental healing practices that balance yin and yang and the harmonious flow of "chi." "Chi" is defined as "matter on the verge of becoming energy, or energy at the point of materializing."[42] This concept also was part of Hippocratic medicine in the balancing of the humors and is still evident in Mexican food patterns used to balance disorders with cold or hot foods.

The final paradigm, supranormal, corresponds to some of the magicoreligious healing practices and has been used cross-culturally to explain phenomena that physical laws cannot explain. Many paradoxical healings that defy a scientific understanding of physiology may be more clearly understood from this paradigm. Many of the more mystical spiritual practices of ritual, pilgrimages, prayer, and other activities of religious discipline related to healing mind, body, and spirit stem from this paradigm. The explanation for spontaneous healing that has no medical explanation may be attributed to divine intervention, miraculous synergy, vital energies, or capabilities of living organisms beyond the current understanding of medicine. Many of the explanations refer to abilities acquired in an altered state of consciousness by the healer or healee or both. Several complementary modalities of healing, such as visual imagery, healing touch, or prayer, are best understood through this paradigm. This paradigm is the most distant from the mechanical paradigm, which may contribute to some individuals' resistance to these types of healing activities.

In the multiparadigm model, the healing activities are classified as physical manipulation, applied or ingested substances, uses of energy, psychologic modalities, and spiritual modalities. Each of the paradigms contains all types of healing activities. As one moves to the right in the model (see Exhibit 13–2), however, all healing is conceptualized as more holistic; all activities affect the entire human. For example, a physical manipulation in the supranormal paradigm is assumed to have spiritual effects and vice versa.

Healing activities are inserted in the model as examples; other modalities can be added. Among the examples that are useful to illustrate healing activities is the practice of cupping, which involves placing heated cups on parts of the body. The cooling of the air creates a suction, superficial capillaries break, and blood collects in the cup. Cupping exemplifies physical manipulation in the purification paradigm, a healing modality that removes toxins or impurities from the body. Bach flower remedies are viewed as an ingested or applied substance in the supranormal paradigm, as their action is understood through a more spiritual or essential manner than a biochemical mechanism. Acupuncture is an energy activity in the balance paradigm because it is the energy that is being acted on, not physical manipulation of the needles or the physical body. Mindfulness is a mental discipline based on Eastern thought. This practice is a process of becoming detached and observing thoughts, feelings, and perceptions while remaining fully attentive and in the present. This is a psychologic activity in the balance paradigm. Spiritual practices extend through all paradigms; however, attendance at organized religious functions is an example of spiritual activities in the mechanical paradigm. Epidemiologic research has indicated that attendance at religious events or membership in religious organizations has a salutary effect on health.[43] Some proposed explanatory mechanisms are that these individuals have healthier lifestyles, better genetic factors, benefit from social support, or have better stress-coping abilities. This example illustrates the link of mental and spiritual activities to physical outcomes. This breakthrough understanding has promoted the legitimacy of many of the psychologic and spiritual activities that holistic nurses use in promoting physical health within the mechanical paradigm.

In many cultures, systems of healing combine many levels of activities. For example, shamanism includes physical manipulation, applied and ingested substances, use of vital energy, psychologic aspects of belief, and spiritual practices that cluster in the supranormal paradigm. Contemporary complementary healers may use modalities from several paradigms. An understanding of the paradigm from which the modality was developed is important for appropriate use in conducting research.

NURSING APPLICATIONS FOR DEVELOPING CULTURAL COMPETENCY

Members of minority groups may distrust and fear the Western biomedical health care system, of which nurses are a part. As the element of trust is essential to the formation of a therapeutic nurse–client relationship, clients need to know that nurses are receptive and nonjudgmental regarding their differences. Nurses must approach cultural competency through knowledge of self and knowledge of other cultures. To develop the ability to interact with clients appropriately, nurses should clarify their personal values, recognize the health care system as a culture, learn about the specific culture of each client, interact and intervene in a culturally consistent manner, and elicit feedback regularly from the client and family. Skills such as listening, explaining, acknowledging, recommending, and negotiating facilitate a nonjudgmental perspective toward the client's cultural beliefs. Nurses and clients should validate their perceptions and discuss similarities and differences in their perceptions to formulate health-related goals and interventions.

Cultural competency is a dynamic, challenging process faced by all health care providers, regardless of their cultural background or association. Members of minority cultural groups also encounter situations in which cultural competency is desirable. Various principles are important in developing cultural competency.[44] The process of sharing information in a straightforward manner demystifies other cultures and makes it possible for the nurse and client to find common ground and understand the context of differences, for example. To find common ground, it is necessary to consider terminology. Many individuals may consider some terms such as *Negro, Black,* or *foreigner* inappropriate and possibly offensive. The terms *Hispanic, Latino,* and *Chicano* all are used to describe people from Spanish-speaking cultures. The terms may be used by the individual themselves in some cases or, in other cases, may be considered an insult. Individuals working together in provider–client interactions need to ensure that the terminology used is mutually understood and acceptable. Researchers and scholars need to strive for consensual cultural terminology so that research findings can be appropriately applied and compared.

Communication

Interactions between the health care provider and client are based on the communication between the two and reflect their respective cultures. Both the provider and the client bring their personal beliefs, values, and cultural backgrounds to the interaction. These factors then affect the transfer of information, decision making, adherence to treatment, and healing outcomes. The professional nature of the encounter brings the culture of the health care system into the exchange. Even if the meeting occurs in the client's home or community setting. An understanding of the cultural world of the client and the cultural world of the health care system enables the provider to deliver culturally appropriate care. Nurses often act as cultural brokers between the client and the biomedical culture.

All health care providers of the professional sector in the United States have acculturated to the biomedical model and accompanying technology by virtue of their education and the sociology of the health care institution where they practice. Each institution has its own culture that defines the norms, protocols, and hierarchy, both formal and informal. Most health care institutions are based on the biomedical model and accept clients into the system because of a perceived physical or mental disease or illness. In contrast, healers in the folk sector approach health from a holistic perspective and usually attend to the psychologic and spiritual domains, as well as the physical domain. Such healers have become acculturated to the holistic model through education, which is often based on an apprenticeship with a more experienced practitioner.

The purposes of communication in the health care environment are to create an interpersonal relationship, exchange information, and allow for decision making. Specific barriers may impede the achievement of these goals. First, communication between the provider and client generally involves individuals of nonequal positions, with the provider assuming a higher rank to some extent simply by virtue of greater medical knowledge. Second, communication related to health care is often not planned, involves vitally important issues, and is emotionally laden. Finally, differences in language, both verbal and nonverbal, may isolate the client and the family. Nonverbal aspects of oral communication, such as voice tone, eye contact, and body positioning, are often as significant as verbal communication. If the cultural backgrounds of the provider and the client are significantly different, these communication factors may make it difficult to obtain and provide health care without misunderstandings.

Roles in the relationship between provider and client are frequently derived from cultural norms and can enhance or impede communication. Such roles can be seen as a spectrum of control ranging from paternalistic to mutualistic.[45] In a paternalistic (provider-centered) relationship, the provider has the control, directs care, makes decisions about treatment, and is authoritative. A mutual (client-centered) relationship involves shared decision making and is egali-

tarian. Problems can arise in communication if the expectations of the client do not match those of the provider with respect to control and decision making.

Problems can also arise if communication style, both nonverbal and verbal, differ. Such expectations are often culturally related, and nurses can avoid some problems by developing sensitivity to various communication styles. Table 13–1 depicts common communication styles associated with various ethnic groups.[46]

Use of Translators

The increasing number of languages and dialects in the United States requires that nurses, even those who are bilingual, often rely on translators or interpreters to communicate with clients. Translators play powerful roles in the exchange of valuable information between nurses and their clients.[47] A translator not only may provide misinformation to the client, but also may use words, tones, or gestures that emphasize the translator's own personal preferences, omit portions of a message deemed irrelevant, or diminish the importance of the intended message. Indeed, translators may dominate the conversation, nearly usurping nurses' roles. It is best to avoid using family members as translators whenever possible, as they are likely to filter information based on what they want the client to hear and it might be culturally inappropriate for the client to discuss certain health matters with certain family members. When they must use translators, nurses should attempt to

1. orient the client to the process and the purpose of using a translator.
2. orient the translator to the topics to be covered, the client's situation, and the degree of accuracy required.
3. avoid standing; sit so that the client can observe the nurse's body language and make eye contact; avoid placing the translator between them and the client.

Table 13–1 Communication Style Differences (Overt Activity Dimension—Nonverbal/Verbal)

American Indians	Asian-Americans— Hispanics	Whites	Blacks
1. Speak softly/slower	1. Speak softly	1. Speak loud/fast to control listener	1. Speak with affect
2. Indirect gaze when listening or speaking	2. Avoidance of eye contact when listening or speaking to high-status persons	2. Greater eye contact when listening	2. Direct eye contact (prolonged) when speaking, but less when listening
3. Interject less/seldom offer encouraging communication	3. Similar rules	3. Head nods, nonverbal markers	3. Interrupt (turn taking) when can
4. Delayed auditory (silence)	4. Mild delay	4. Quick responding	4. Quicker responding
5. Manner of expression low-keyed, indirect	5. Low-keyed, indirect	5. Objective, task oriented	5. Affective, emotional, interpersonal

Source: D.W. Sue and D. Sue, *Counseling the Culturally Different: Theory and Practice,* 2nd ed., p. 67, Copyright © 1990, John Wiley & Sons, Inc. Reprinted by permission of John Wiley & Sons, Inc.

4. observe the client for nonverbal communication that does not match the message intended and request clarification.
5. slow down the communication process.
6. encourage the translator to let the nurse know when something is difficult to translate so that they can reword it.
7. limit the use of medical jargon, slang, and metaphors to reduce the chances for errors.
8. consider the impact of differences in gender, educational level, and socioeconomic status between the client and translator. This is particularly important when topics of a sensitive or personal nature are to be discussed.
9. ask translators to translate in the client's own words and ask clients to repeat the information communicated to increase accuracy.[48,49]

HOLISTIC CARING PROCESS

When engaged in the holistic caring process, nurses need to understand concepts that are affected by cultural background. Six phenomena evidenced in all cultural groups have variations that are relevant to the provision of culturally competent nursing assessment and care:[50]

1. **Communication.** There are cultural variations in expression of feelings, use of touch, body contact, gestures, and verbal and nonverbal communication. Language shapes experiences and influences perceptions and actions. Warmth and humor are two communication factors that are interpreted differently through various cultures.
2. **Personal space.** Spatial behavior refers to the comfort level related to personal space, the area that surrounds a person's body. Spatial territoriality is the need to have and to control personal space. Cultures vary in the level of proximity to others that is acceptable. For example, Western culture has three zones: intimate zone (less than 18 inches), personal zone (18 inches to 3 feet), and social zone (3 feet to 6 feet). Cultural background also in-

fluences aspects of objects within space, such as orderliness, cleanliness, and structural boundaries of furniture and architecture.

3. **Time.** Cultures vary in their orientation toward time, both social time and clock time. Social time refers to patterns and orientations related to the ordering of social life, whereas clock time represents an objective, ordered approach of viewing time in a linear fashion that infers causality. Some cultures orient around cyclic approaches that attach time to natural events that repeat, such as seasons or migration patterns. In mystical thought, magic or ritual may negate the temporal order of causality and reverse a bad event. All cultures contain the three orientations of future, present, and past, with one being dominant.

4. **Social organization.** Families, religious groups, kinship groups, and special interest groups are social organizations. Families vary by structure, dynamics, roles, and organizational patterns. Kinship structures and the relative geographic location of family members have cultural implications. Religious organizations provide not only social connections, but also a context in which to understand one's relationship to the world, the cosmos, and meaning in life.

5. **Environmental control.** Different cultures have different perceptions of the ability of an individual to control nature, the environment, and personal relationships. The locus of control may be external (i.e., an event contingent on luck or fate), internal (i.e., an event contingent on one's own behavior or characteristic), or outside (i.e., an event in harmony with nature, as in some Asian cultures). In folk medicine, events are perceived as natural and unnatural. Natural events have to

do with the world as God intended and the laws of nature. Unnatural events upset the harmony of nature and are outside the world of nature.

6. **Biologic variations.** In a pluralistic culture, it is important to determine those factors that are strictly biologic (i.e., genetic) and those that are ethnic adaptations related to living in a particular environment (e.g., availability of certain types of food) or in certain social conditions (e.g., socioeconomic status or lifestyle). Biologic factors to be considered are body size and structure, including variations in teeth, facial features, and skin color; variations in metabolism and enzyme production that result in drug reactions, interactions, and sensitivities; susceptibility to disease (e.g., hypertension, diabetes, sickle cell anemia); and nutritional issues, including food preferences, habits and patterns, and deficiencies such as lactose intolerance.

These six components of human environmental responses are incorporated into Table 13–2 depicting cultural variation among Asian-Americans, Native Americans, Black Americans, and Hispanics.[51]

Assessment

Leininger has defined a cultural nursing assessment as "a systematic appraisal or examination of individuals, groups, and communities as to their cultural beliefs, values, and practices to determine specific needs and interventions within the cultural context of the people being evaluated."[52] A cultural assessment should be performed during the initial contact with a client; it may be brief, with questions about ethnic background, religion, family patterns, food preferences, and health practices.[53] Data from a brief assessment can be used to determine the need for a more in-depth assessment that focuses on more specific pa-

Table 13–2 Cultural Variation in Human-Environmental Responses (Four Examples)

Response Variants	Asian-American (Hmong)	Native American	Black American	Hispanic
Communication	Oral tradition. Gender- and age-specific patterns. Group learning. Spiritual link. Taboos guiding topics. Conversation focus to promote harmony. Language barrier—interpreter.	Oral tradition. Storytelling. Group learning. Spiritual foundation of life. Only able to speak for self, nonaggressive. Role of elder.	Black English. Specific dialect. Significance of names/terms. Nonverbal: talk-look at, listening-look away, prolonged eye contact, frequent touch, emotional sharing. Group learning.	Language barrier—interpreter. Verbal: privacy, avoid conflict, emotional expressive. Nonverbal: touch, handshake, avoid prolonged eye contact. Group learning.
Space	Avoid eye contact. Sacred parts of body. Avoid public display of affection and extreme emotions.	Avoid eye contact, limit touch. Negative significance rt handshake.	Often space much closer than "Anglos."	Familial closeness—demonstrative.
Time	Cyclical, present oriented, holistic, fatalistic. Social time vs. clock time.	Circular, holistic, present oriented, fatalistic.	Wide variation. Social time vs. clock time.	Present-oriented, "Latin Time," polychronic.
Social Organization	Clan structure. Decision-maker: elder male, clan leader. Family-patrilineal. Male dominant in affairs extending beyond the home. Female more active role within the home. Clearly defined roles/responsibilities—age and gender. Children indulged until the age of five then more strict discipline—"communal focus."	Clan/family/tribes. Role of elder. Role definition. Social relations—wheel of life. Core values: thanks, harmony, sharing, and hospitality.	Disruptive influence of slavery and discrimination on the family structure. Today variance, a link with social economic status (SES). Lower SES: matrifocused—present focused. Mid/Upper SES: egalitarian. Children—socialized to be in control, independent at earlier age. Importance of extended kinship.	"La familia": patrilineal, extended, gender significance. Machismo: decision-maker, protector. Marianismo: nurturer, mediator. Respect elders. Children a priority, dependency. Family value: respect, pride, responsibility, spirituality (Catholic).
Environmental Control	Explanatory Model of Health/Illness (H/I): H: Mandate for life, predetermination, maintain harmony. I: Supernatural, soul loss, spiritual disharmony, imbalance, sins of ancestors, self in relation to others. Curers: Herbalist,	Explanatory Model of Health/Illness (H/I): Beliefs—balance with mother nature, predetermination—Creator. I: lack of harmony, failure to live according to code of life, evil spirits, fear and jealousy of other	Explanatory Model of Health/Illness (H/I): I: an inability to function due to a hex, sins, disharmony, natural or supernatural. Curers: family first, "Old lady" or "Granny," voodoo priest, spiritualist, root doctor. Tx:	Explanatory Model of Health/Illness (H/I): I: Severity rt pain or blood, unable to perform roles/ADLs. Illness: mild or severe, lg of time. Causes: sins, will of God, "evil eye," "nerves," "bad blood"—loss of

continues

Table 13–2 Continued

Response Variants	Asian-American (Hmong)	Native American	Black American	Hispanic
	Shaman. Tx: foods, maintain harmony with the forces, spiritual divination, massage, herbs, foods, coining, pinching, cupping. Special Tx for certain conditions, e.g., childbirth.	nations. Curers: Shaman/ faithkeeper, Midwiwin, False Face Society, Herb specialist. Tx: herbs, ceremonies, e.g., sweat and medicine lodge, vision quest, talking circle, etc. Significant elements.	includes use of teas, cod liver oils, dietary choices, laxatives for purging, wearing of garlic, amulets, copper or silver bracelets. Folk practices include: silver dollar to navel, oil—baby's bath, cradle cap, prayer cloth to diaper, PICA.	respect, imbalance of humors or hot and cold. Direct re between certain illnesses—supernatural intervention. Many folk illnesses. Curers: family, curandero herbalist, spiritualist. Tx: prayer, massage, ceremonies rt specific illnesses.
Biological	Small stature, small bone structure, Mongolian spots, eye. Disease susceptibility: Hepatitis, TB, lactase deficiency, hemoglobinopathies, altered drug metabolism.	Taller, bigger, heavier bone structure. Cheek bones, dark eyes. Disease susceptibility: Diabetes mellitus, ETOH abuse, TB, SIDS, AIDS. Health Risks: Pneumonia, malnutrition, adolescent suicide, MVA, homicide.	Skin variance: Mongolian spots, keloids, vitiligo, nigra. Heavier/ denser bones, shorter trunk, longer legs. Body fat link to economics. Disease susceptibility: TB, hypertension/CV, sickle cell anemia, enzyme disorders, diabetes. Health Risks: Obesity, ETOH abuse, infant mortality, homicide, AIDS.	Skin color. Susceptibility to disease: Diabetes, TB, AIDS. Health risks: Obesity, alcoholism, adolescent pregnancy.

Source: Copyright © 1994, American Nephrology Nurses Association.

rameters, such as nutritional patterns, social support networks, and coping (Exhibit 13–3).[54]

Tripp-Reimer and colleagues recommended that an in-depth assessment be conducted in two phases: a data collection phase and an organization phase.[55] During the data collection phase, it is essential to obtain details that are specific enough to develop culturally appropriate interventions related to healing and identify cultural factors that may influence the effectiveness of the interventions. Depending on the individual situation, it may be important to ask for information related to developmental milestones, such as puberty, or rituals and customs related to birth and death. As the community passes cultural tradition through the family, frequently through women, it is helpful to ask about the practices or beliefs of the client's mother or grandmother. During the organization phase, data are systematically examined to identify areas of incongruence between the client's needs and the goals of Western medicine. Patterns, problems, and

Exhibit 13–3 Cultural Areas Critical to a Nursing Assessment.

- Nutritional patterns
- Exercise and physical activities
- Decision making: how made, who is involved, and why
- Health and healing practices
- Family organization, structure, and role differentiation and child care practices
- Social support networks and relationships
- Spiritual beliefs, rituals, and practices
- Cognitive attributive style and personal/ family coping approaches
- Demographics and socioeconomic status, employment patterns
- Immigration and cultural history
- Communication style and relationship toward authority

From: J. Engebretson, "Cultural Diversity and Care" in Core Curriculum for Holistic Nursing, ed. B.M. Dossey (Gaithersburg, MD: Aspen Publishers, 1997), 114.

needs related to culture can then be formulated, based on the areas of incongruence. For example, a difference in time perception between an individual who is present-oriented and thus has little concern for health consequences and the future orientation of American culture may lead to a disregard for dietary restrictions. The problem of noncompliance related to noncongruent value systems could be formulated, and one nursing intervention would be to focus on the immediate benefits of health promotion strategies.

Patterns/Problems/Needs

In the cultural domain, patterns, problems, and needs involve primarily biophysical and psychologic disturbances, alterations, impairments, and distresses. These patterns, problems, and needs are largely derived from the conceptual areas of normalcy based on North American culture and heavily influenced by biomedicine. The patterns, problems, and needs as-

sociated with cultural differences and related to the nine human response patterns are as follows:

- **Communicating:** Altered or impaired communication related to language differences or communication style. Even with the aid of translators, language and dialect differences may exist based on the region in which the client was born (e.g., China).
- **Relating:** Altered or impaired social interaction related to sociocultural dissonance. Difficulties in relating with members of the health care team may occur when there are socioeconomic or educational gaps.
- **Choosing:** Noncompliance related to incongruent value systems between provider and client. Clients may be considered noncompliant with follow-up appointments when differences in the perception of time is at the root of missed or late appointments.
- **Feeling:** Anxiety related to culturally unusual expectations for behavior and treatment; fear related to unknown environment or customs. The biomedical health care system may be particularly anxiety-provoking for clients whose custom is to be cared for in the home during an illness.

Outcomes

Culturally appropriate outcomes would be developed with the client for each culturally related pattern, problem, or need.

Therapeutic Care Plan and Implementation

Knowledge and acceptance of the client's right to alternative solutions and modalities should be incorporated into the plan of care so that the plan is mutually designed. Explanatory models and the meaning of illness must be determined with the client in order for interventions to be presented and negotiated in a culturally acceptable manner. The focus should be on the concept of engagement rather than compliance, as the concept of compliance implies an authoritative relationship in which the provider is active and in control while the client is in a passive, accepting role.[56]

Cultural healing practices should be part of the client's care unless contraindicated. Nurses should convey respect for the practice and should make every effort to acquire appropriate foods, people, artifacts, and so on, as well as to secure space and time for such practices. Three modes of intervention involving clinical decision making incorporate the client's cultural practices:[57]

1. Cultural preservation and/or maintenance refers to professional actions that retain relevant care values in health promotion, restoration, management of disabilities or chronic illness, and death. Nurses using cultural preservation can support those aspects of the client's culture that positively influence his or her health care.

2. Cultural accommodation and/or negotiation refers to professional actions to bridge the gap between the client's culture and biomedicine for beneficial health outcomes. Nurses using cultural accommodation recognize the cultural relevance of a practice and assist the client to integrate it into the planned treatment, even though the cultural practice has no scientific basis for health promotion or disease prevention.

3. Cultural repatterning and/or restructuring refers to professional actions that help a client improve his or her life pattern while respecting cultural values and beliefs. Nurses using cultural repatterning assist clients to make changes in, but not discard, cultural behaviors that are harmful, negative, or maladaptive to their well-being.

A variety of healing modalities may be used, depending on the illness and cultural preferences. Touch as communication has culturally specific meaning. In some Arab and Hispanic cultures, male providers may be prohibited from examining or touching parts of the female body. Some Asians believe that the center of strength lies in the head, and touching the head is a sign of disrespect or threat. Thus, the process of shaving the head preoperatively may be viewed very negatively. Gentle touch may be seen as a caring gesture. Many cultures have traditions of healing touch or laying on of hands. Touch can be instrumental, but healing touch should be viewed from an energetic or spiritual framework. Clients in Western cultures are often unfamiliar with such techniques of healing.

Foods or herbs may be used for many different purposes with respect to illness. The use of hot or cold foods may remedy an imbalance in the body. Many preparations are used to purify and remove toxins from the body, such as emetics and colonic irrigations. For the treatment of specific illnesses, herbs used in traditional healing have antiseptic and healing properties. Herbs such as *Echinacea* or foods such as garlic may also be used to prevent illness. Other herbs facilitate body processes. Chamomile and mint teas are used to aid digestion, and barley water is used to promote lactation.

Many cultures approach healing from a spiritual perspective. Rituals and practices to protect one from evil, disease, or danger include the use of amulets, talismans, ritualistic behavior, the avoidance of taboos, exorcism, and purification or cleansing rituals. Rituals may be positive in nature, including those related to spiritual growth, redemption, and life transitions, such as initiations into adulthood or birth.[58] Often viewed as having divine gifts, healers are believed to be able to negotiate with the spiritual world through prayer, meditation, blessings, chants, and other primal religious experiences, many incorporating altered states of consciousness. Individuals also may seek healing forces by sacrifice, penance, and pilgrimages.

Evaluation

Together, the nurse, the client, and any member of the extended family or social group whom the client feels is significant should evaluate desired client outcomes. Evaluation must be woven throughout the entire holistic caring process, as it is essential to obtain validation through mutual understanding when there are differences between the cultural backgrounds of nurse and client. It is important to note the purpose of the activity in evaluating its effectiveness. A massage that is given for the purpose of comfort needs to be evaluated on the basis of comfort, for example, not its medical effect on the disease process. A healing activity that is understood by the client as having multiple effects (e.g., spiritual benefits, psychologic benefits, and better health) should be evaluated on many levels and should not be discounted if the physical benefits are not comparable to those of a pharmaceutical product. Each component of the health care plan and each nursing intervention should be carefully examined to ensure that it is understandable and acceptable to the client, effective for achievement of short- and long-term goals, and appropriately revised as necessary during the evaluation process. Cultural modifications can be made upon careful evaluation.

DIRECTIONS FOR FUTURE RESEARCH

1. Survey patterns of usage of healing modalities from various paradigms and cultural backgrounds.
2. Develop efficient and effective ways of assessing the degree of acculturation in clients with various cultural backgrounds.
3. Analyze effective models for interaction between biomedical and traditional health care systems.
4. Evaluate the degree to which health care goals are achieved when nurses deliver culturally competent care.
5. Analyze various methods for teaching nursing students or staff how to provide culturally competent care.

NURSE HEALER REFLECTIONS

After reading this chapter, the nurse healer will be able to answer or begin a process of answering the following questions:

- What are my values and beliefs regarding health and illness in relationship to models of healing?
- How do I feel when caring for clients whose cultural backgrounds differ from my own?
- What are my biases and attitudes toward clients with various cultural backgrounds?
- How can I determine if I am offering culturally competent care in a holistic manner?

NOTES

1. M.M. Andrews and J.S. Boyle, eds., *Transcultural Concepts in Nursing Care* (Philadelphia: J.B. Lippincott, 1995).

2. H. Bernal, Delivering Culturally Competent Care, in *Psychosocial Nursing: Care of Physically Ill Patients and Their Families*, ed. P.D. Barry (Philadelphia: J.B. Lippincott, 1996), 78–99.

3. S.M. Steele and V.M. Harmon, *Values Clarification in Nursing*, 2d ed. (Norwalk, CT: Appleton-Century-Crofts, 1983).

4. G.M. Bartol and L. Richardson, Using Literature To Create Cultural Competence, *Image: Journal of Nursing Scholarship*, 30 (1998): 75–79.

5. Resident Population of the United States: Esti-

mates by Sex, Race, and Hispanic Origin, with Median Age (Consistent with the 1990 Census), www.census.gov/population/estimates/nation/intfile3-1.tx (Accessed December 1998).

6. Andrews and Boyle, *Transcultural Concepts in Nursing Care.*

7. R.G. Evans et al., eds., *Why Are Some People Healthy and Others Not? The Determinants of Healthy Populations* (New York: Aldine de Gruyter, 1994).

8. M. Massey, *What You Are Isn't Necessarily What You Will Be* (Videotape No. 3123.03) (Farmington, MI: Magnetic Video Corp., 1977).

9. K. Kipnis, Quality Care and the Wounds of Diversity (Paper presented at the meeting of the American Society for Bioethics and Humanities, Houston, TX, November 18, 1998).

10. R.E. Spector, *Cultural Diversity in Health and Illness* (Stamford, CT: Appleton & Lange, 1996).

11. J. Achterberg, *Woman As Healer* (Boston: Shambhala, 1991).

12. J. Engebretson, Comparison of Nurses and Alternative Healers, *Image: Journal of Nursing Scholarship* 28 (1996):95–99.

13. Andrews and Boyle, *Transcultural Concepts in Nursing Care.*

14. F.R. Kluckhohn, Dominant and Variant Value Orientations, in *Transcultural Nursing: A Book of Readings*, ed. P.J. Brink (Englewood Cliffs, NJ: Prentice Hall, 1976), 63–81.

15. J. Engebretson, Considerations in Diagnosing in the Spiritual Domain, *Nursing Diagnosis* 7 (1996):100–107.

16. N. Postman, *Technopoly* (New York: Vintage Books, 1993).

17. Postman, *Technopoly.*

18. F. Capra, *The Turning Point: Science, Society and the Rising Culture* (New York: Bantam Books, 1982).

19. H. Smith, *Beyond the Post-Modern Mind* (New York: Crossroad Publishing Co., 1982).

20. W.T Anderson, *The Truth About the Truth* (New York: G.P. Putnam's Sons, 1995).

21. P.H. Ray, The Emerging Culture, February, 1997. American Demographics: www.demographics.com (Accessed June 1998).

22. J.A. Astin, Why Patients Use Alternative Medicine, *Journal of the American Medical Association* 279 (1998):1548–1553.

23. Engebretson, Comparison of Nurses and Alternative Healers.

24. D.M. Eisenberg et al., Unconventional Medicine in the United States: Prevalence, Costs, and Patterns of Use, *New England Journal of Medicine* 328 (1993):252–256.

25. M.B. McGuire, *Ritual Healing in Suburban America* (New Brunswick, NJ: Rutgers University Press, 1988).

26. Ray, The Emerging Culture.

27. Resident Population of the United States: Estimates.

28. Resident Population of the United States: Estimates.

29. Resident Population of the United States: Estimates.

30. Resident Population of the United States: Estimates.

31. Resident Population of the United States: Estimates.

32. Resident Population of the United States: Estimates.

33. Andrews and Boyle, *Transcultural Concepts in Nursing Care.*

34. Andrews and Boyle, *Transcultural Concepts in Nursing Care.*

35. Andrews and Boyle, *Transcultural Concepts in Nursing Care.*

36. Andrews and Boyle, *Transcultural Concepts in Nursing Care.*

37. A. Kleinman, *Patients and Healers in the Context of Culture* (Berkeley, CA: University of California Press, 1980).

38. J.N. Giger and R.E. Davidhizar, eds., *Transcultural Nursing: Assessment and Intervention*, 2d ed. (St Louis: Mosby, 1995).

39. J. Engebretson, A Multiparadigm Approach to Nursing, *Advances in Nursing Science* 20 (1997):22–34.

40. Kleinman, *Patients and Healers in the Context of Culture.*

41. Engebretson, A Multiparadigm Approach to Nursing.

42. T.J. Kaptchuk, *The Web That Has No Weaver: Understanding Chinese Medicine* (New York: Congdon & Weed, 1983).

43. J.S. Levin, Religion and Health: Is There an Association, Is It Valid and Is It Causal, *Social Science in Medicine* 29 (1994):589–600.

44. M.A. Orlandi, ed., *Cultural Competence for Evaluators* (Washington, DC: U.S. Department of Health and Human Services, 1992).

45. D.W. Sue and D. Sue, *Counseling the Culturally Different: Theory and Practice*, 2d ed. (New York: John Wiley & Sons, 1990).

46. Sue and Sue, *Counseling the Culturally Different.*

47. C. Degazon, Cultural Diversity and Community Health Nursing Practice, in *Community Health Nursing: Promoting Health of Aggregates, Families and Individuals*, 4th ed., ed. M. Stanhope and J. Lancaster (St. Louis: Mosby, 1996), 117–134.

48. Degazon, Cultural Diversity and Community Health Nursing Practice.

49. Bernal, Delivering Culturally Competent Care.

50. Giger and Davidhizar, *Transcultural Nursing: Assessment and Intervention*.

51. J. Engebretson, Cultural Diversity and Care, in *Core Curriculum for Holistic Nursing*, ed. B.M. Dossey (Gaithersburg, MD: Aspen Publishers, 1997), 108–118.

52. M.M. Leininger, *Transcultural Nursing: Concepts, Theories and Practices* (New York: John Wiley & Sons, 1978), 85–86.

53. T. Tripp-Reimer et al., Cultural Assessment: Content and Process, *Nursing Outlook* 32 (1984):78–82.

54. B.M. Dossey et al., eds., *Holistic Nursing: A Handbook for Practice*, 2d ed. (Gaithersburg, MD: Aspen Publishers, 1995).

55. Tripp-Reimer et al., Cultural Assessment: Content and Process.

56. Dossey et al., *Holistic Nursing: A Handbook for Practice*.

57. Leininger, *Culture Care Diversity and Universality: A Theory of Nursing* (New York: National League for Nursing, 1991).

58. D. Kinsley, *Health, Healing, and Religion: A Cross-Cultural Perspective* (Upper Saddle River, NJ: Prentice-Hall, 1996).

CORE VALUE V

Holistic Caring Process

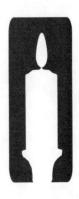

VISION OF HEALING
Working with Others

As we engage in holistic nursing and embark on our inward journey for self-change, what we communicate by word, act, attitude, and setting will affect our potential for change. We must consciously learn the skills to stay in the present moment because change takes place in the present, not in the past or future. Everything affects our clients, our choice of words, our presence, and our greeting. Our beliefs are important and affect our self-image, which, in turn, affects our actions. It also influences our capacity for self-healing.

Our beliefs are conveyed to our clients. We must perceive ourselves and the client as whole. When we perceive the cancer patient as a person with cancer, we release the label and learn to focus primarily on the person's healing potential. Every part is connected to every other part, and every part in the system affects every other part. We form a network in which everyone participates. There is no such thing as an independent observer. Nurse and client are always creating change in one another.

We must consider all the client's life potentials—physical, mental, emotional, spiritual, relationships, and choices. Only when we consider the whole client and his or her significant others do we have a chance to direct the client toward wholeness. We must continue to gain new skills and become self-experienced in all modalities that we offer to the client. We cannot guide clients down new paths to new experiences if we do not know the path from experience. The more we know from experience, the more we know that change is possible. We must remind the client to acknowledge all changes, however slight, because each change leads to another and each slight change is progress.

When we teach from experience, we are in a better position to help the client learn without judgment. We also teach in such a manner that the client cannot fail because goals are realistic and measurable. For example, nurses should encourage a person with migraine headaches to "be with the process"—not to blame himself or herself for the headache symptoms, but to focus on stress management skills to decrease the headache pattern. The client must learn that the body is not the problem, but part of the solution. As we teach clients to reframe experiences positively, their internal thoughts create new beliefs that most often lead to new, healthier response patterns. If failure is not reframed, it leads to more failure. Instead of "the glass is half-empty," the client reframes it by saying, "the glass is half-full." We must also encourage the client to involve friends and family in the learning. Learning is an ongoing process and new skills must be practiced, shared, and integrated into all aspects of life.

Chapter 14

The Holistic Caring Process

Pamela J. Potter and Cathie E. Guzzetta

NURSE HEALER OBJECTIVES

Theoretical

- Define the terms *nursing process* and *holistic caring process.*
- Outline the steps of the holistic caring process.
- Explore the ways in which conceptual models of nursing inform and guide the holistic caring process.
- Discuss the ways in which standards of holistic nursing practice are incorporated into the holistic caring process.

Clinical

- Analyze the assessment tool that you are using in clinical practice to determine whether the tool is consistent with a holistic nursing perspective.
- Explore the possible ways to incorporate nursing diagnoses, the Nursing Interventions Classification, and the Nursing Outcomes Classification within a holistic nursing practice.
- Identify the nursing diagnoses and interventions most relevant to your nursing practice.
- Submit a "You Make the Diagnosis" case study to the journal *Nursing Diagnosis*, and frame the diagnosis in terms of the holistic caring process.

- Determine whether the system of nursing diagnosis you use is organized in terms of the nine human response patterns or in terms of functional health patterns.
- Incorporate wellness diagnoses into practice.
- Use the trifocal model of nursing diagnosis as an organizing structure for a visual composite of the three levels of a person's health patterns in prioritizing and planning nursing interventions and patient outcomes within the nurse–person interaction.
- Implement the Standards of Holistic Nursing Practice of the American Holistic Nurses' Association (AHNA) in your work and life.

Personal

- Observe the pattern appraisal-identification process in your everyday life as you walk into a new situation.
- Identify the four patterns of knowing (empirical, ethical, aesthetic, and personal knowledge) as they guide you within the nurse–person interaction.
- Develop and trust your intuitive thinking processes when assessing clients' conditions.
- Evaluate the impact of intuitive thinking in both your professional and personal life.

- Explore your own beliefs and values regarding the concepts of holistic nursing.
- Write down specific examples of holistic nursing at each step of the holistic caring process.

DEFINITIONS

Functional Health Patterns: a system for organizing nursing assessment and diagnosis based upon 11 areas of human functioning.

Holistic Caring Process: an explication of the nursing process within the paradigm of holism, the holistic caring process is a circular process that involves six steps which may occur simultaneously. These steps are assessment, patterns/problems/needs, outcomes, therapeutic care plan, implementation, and evaluation.

Holistic Nursing: see Chapter 1.

Intuition: the perceived knowing of things and events without the conscious use of rational processes; the use of all the senses to receive information.

Nursing Diagnosis: a clinical judgment about the individual, family, or community responses to actual and potential health problems/life processes. A nursing diagnosis is the basis for the selection of nursing interventions to achieve outcomes for which the nurse is accountable.

Nursing Interventions Classification (NIC): a standardized comprehensive classification of treatments that nurses perform, including both independent and collaborative, as well as direct and indirect.[1]

Nursing Outcomes Classification (NOC): "a comprehensive taxonomy of patient outcomes influenced by nursing care."[2]

Nursing Process: the original model describing the "work" of nursing, defined as steps used to fulfill the purposes of nursing, such as assessment, diagnosis, client outcomes, plans, intervention, and evaluation.

Paradigm: a model for conceptualizing information.

Patterns/Problems/Needs: a person's actual and potential life processes related to health, wellness, disease, or illness, which may or may not facilitate well-being.

Person: an individual, client, patient, family member, support person, or community member who has the opportunity to engage in interaction with a holistic nurse.

Standards of Practice: a group of statements describing the level of care expected from a holistic nurse.

Taxonomy I: a classification schema for the organization of the accepted list of nursing diagnoses based on the nine human response patterns.

Unitary Person Framework: a framework created by the North American Nursing Diagnosis Association (NANDA) to guide the identification and development of nursing diagnoses.

THEORY AND RESEARCH

The holistic caring process is an adaptation and expansion of the nursing process that incorporates holistic nursing philosophy. It is a systematic, dynamic, living framework for discovering, describing, and documenting health patterns unique to a person. These patterns, identified within the nurse–person relationship, provide the foundation for mutual goals and responses to actions initiated in the nurse–person caring process.

Even the contemporary definition of nursing from the American Nurses' Association incorporates the concept of caring for the whole person. This definition of nursing acknowledges four essential features of practice:

- Attention to the full range of human experiences and responses to health and illness without restriction to a problem-focused orientation;

- Integration of objective data with knowledge gained from an understanding of the person's or group's subjective experience;
- Application of scientific knowledge to the processes of diagnosis and treatment; and
- Provision of a caring relationship that facilitates health and healing.[3(p.6)]

Focused on establishment of health and well-being within the person, the holistic caring process is a circular process that includes six steps: assessment, patterns/problems/needs, outcomes, therapeutic care plan, implementation, and evaluation. The original concept of "nursing process" can be traced to the late 1950s and early 1960s, when nursing in the United States sought to identify itself as a distinct, autonomous profession within health care. Kreuter first formally identified the conceptualization of the nursing process as an orderly approach to the conduct of independent nursing activities in 1957.[4] Proponents of the nursing process saw it as a tool for unifying the language of nursing, systematizing nursing practice and education, and enhancing independent practice.

Frisch and Frisch noted that there are two definitions for the nursing process. The first defines it as a step-by-step linear process for solving problems. The second, more compatible with holistic nursing, defines the nursing process as "a means of reflecting on the entire process of the nurse–client interaction;" furthermore, "process means a series of actions leading to an end"[5] (Figure 14–1). Intervention begins with the first nurse–person interac-

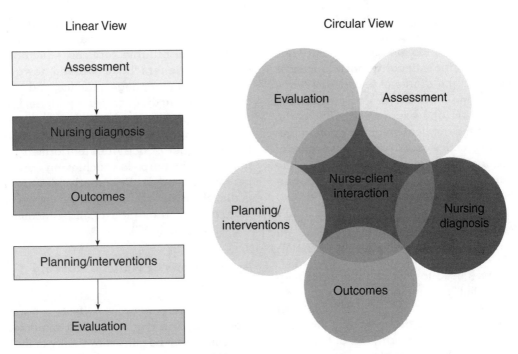

Linear View

Assessment

Nursing diagnosis

Outcomes

Planning/interventions

Evaluation

Circular View

Evaluation

Assessment

Planning/interventions

Nurse-client interaction

Nursing diagnosis

Outcomes

Figure 14–1 Two Views of the Nursing Process. *Source:* Reprinted by permission. *Psychiatric Mental Health Nursing: Understanding the Clients as Well as the Condition* by Frisch, Delmar Publishers, Albany, New York, Copyright © 1998.

tion, while evaluation is continuous and does not merely come at the end of the process. Within the circular view of the nursing process, the steps become organizing principles for documenting and describing nursing care and the person's response to that care.

Gradually, the circular view of the nursing process faded when the first definition of nursing process as a problem-solving model based on the scientific method became the generally accepted definition. This model was accepted without question as the foundation for nursing practice and education until the early 1980s when nursing scholars began to focus on philosophy and theory in nursing.[6] Emphasizing holistic care in their theory of modeling and role modeling, Erickson and associates reclaimed the circular view and described the nursing process as "the ongoing, interactive exchange of information, feelings, and behavior between the nurse and client(s), wherein the nurse's goal is to nurture and support the client's self care."[7]

Critics of nursing process theory say it is reductionistic, too steeped in positivism and a scientific rationality that emphasizes science as the source of knowledge while disallowing other ways of knowing, such as intuition and experience. Those who criticize the application of the nursing process in practice assert that it serves the interests of the nursing profession over the interests of the person and results in burdensome, time-consuming, reductionist jargon that de-emphasizes the patient's role and labels the patient. The problem may not lie in the nursing process per se, but rather in the differing philosophic perspectives used to describe it. Varcoe suggested that "the nursing process is compatible with a variety of philosophical positions, and that the critique of the nursing process is really criticism of a positivist-philosophical orientation which has been illogically identified with the process itself."[8]

The origins of the nursing process reside within the concept of pattern recognition, an innate tendency found among humans. Pattern recognition may be observed even in young infants who, early on, recognize and react to familiar as well as unfamiliar patterns (facial, vocal, and kinesthetic) in their caregivers. When nurses encounter a patient for the first time, they observe the state of the patient's health. They notice the patient's color (pale or cyanotic), affect and eye contact, respiration depth and rate, rate and volume of speech, body odor, scars, wounds, and more. Within 60 seconds, they notice if something is different from the expected and whether any nursing action is necessary. This is pattern appraisal and pattern recognition. Using all their nursing knowledge, nurses apply the patterns they observe to known patterns, make decisions about those patterns, and then act upon those decisions. After doing so, they reappraise and react based on the response of the person.

In an effort to establish nursing as a distinct, recognizable health care profession with distinct billable services, educators and practitioners have worked toward standardizing language, practice, and outcomes. Nursing diagnoses are patterns frequently appraised by nurses in giving care. The Nursing Interventions Classification (NIC) is a list of activities performed by nurses for the purpose of achieving nurse–person care goals. Frequently identified goals, observable throughout the course of care, are listed as the Nursing Outcomes Classification (NOC).

Applications of Holistic Nursing Theory

Like the nursing process itself, nursing diagnoses, interventions, and expected outcomes must be guided by theory in their application to nursing care. Certainly, the theoretical context of the nurse, as well as the nursing institution, can constrain the nursing process as a framework for nursing practice. Nurses who contend that they work "without a theory" very likely base their practice unquestioningly on a rational, biochemical, mechanical, medical model. Application of holistic nursing philosophy to the nursing process emphasizes a holistic perspective and yet remains incomplete without a nursing theoretical framework compatible with holism. There are many conceptual models of nursing, such as Nightingale's theory of environmental adaptation,[9] Roy's adaptation model,[10] Erickson's theory of modeling and role modeling,[11] Rogers' unitary human being theory,[12] King's systems model,[13] Leininger's theory of cultural care,[14] Orem's self-care model,[15] Watson's human care model,[16] Parse's human becoming theory,[17] and Newman's health as expanding consciousness model.[18] The theory that guides nursing practice will be identifiable in the application of nursing process. (See Chapter 8 for a discussion of nursing theories.) Adaptation and expansion of the nursing process based on holistic nursing philosophy includes the person as a co-participant in nursing care. The holistic caring process adds emphasis to the understanding that the person is primary in the nurse–person relationship. This has not always been the case. Historically, the disease or the problem was foremost. In today's managed care environment, sometimes the insurance "payer" appears to be more important than the person in the health care relationship.

The holistic caring process incorporates both the problem-solving components of natural science methodology and the caring dimension of the human science approach, which emphasizes the unmeasurable human side of the traditional art of nursing.[19] It accommodates the whole person—as a bio-psycho-social-spiritual being within the environmental context. Thus, the advantages of a holistic caring process parallel those delineated for the nursing process in general—with the addition of the whole-person perspective. The holistic framework is a person-centered process. This approach examines a person's reality, perceptions, and life meanings for insight into the lived experience of health and well-being. The holistic caring process is a relational process. Through mutual relationship, the nurse collaborates with the person to identify and pursue goals for health enhancement. As a synthesis of natural and human sciences, the holistic caring process reflects an equal valuing of qualitative and quantitative dimensions of the person's health patterns.

A systematic process for the practice of holistic nursing acts as a guiding structure for the novice and as internalized ballast for the experienced nurse; it "unifies, standardizes, and directs nursing practice."[20] Standardization of language about nurses' activities and responsibilities affords a unified structure for the application of nursing theory and subsequent nursing research. The holistic caring process lends itself to theory application. Within the holistic caring process, information relevant to the person's care is gathered and processed according to a theoretical model. Nurses must choose a theoretical practice model that is realistic, useful, and consistent with their professional values and philosophy. Patterns, desired outcomes, and nursing actions are identified through a synthesis of the theory base and information gathered from the person in mutual process with the nurse. Care is evaluated and documented in the language of the theory.

Four Patterns of Knowing

Insights derived from the four patterns of knowing identified by Carper guide the nurse's process within the nurse–person interaction.[21] Empirical or scientific knowledge is based on objective information measurable by the senses, including scientific instrumentation. Ethical knowledge flows from the "basic underlying concept of the unity and integral wholeness of all people and of all nature."[22] Aesthetic knowledge draws on a sense of form and structure, beauty and creativity, for discerning pattern and change. Personal knowledge incorporates the nurse's self-awareness and knowledge, as well as the intuitive perception of meanings based on personal experiences, and is demonstrated by the therapeutic use of self.

Within the holistic caring process, the unitary person framework, as developed by the North American Nursing Diagnosis Association (NANDA),[23] is used for organizing data. Each person is considered to be an open system in constant interaction with the environment; each person's unique organization is manifested by nine human response patterns. These patterns are believed to demonstrate all aspects of the whole person and to indicate the person's state of health. Taxonomy I organizes all NANDA-approved nursing diagnoses according to these nine human response patterns (Exhibit 14–1).[24]

Because these human response patterns are not necessarily mutually exclusive, some nurses encounter difficulty when using them as a structural framework for documentation. Yet, this taxonomy yields itself quite well to the holistic perspective. The words are gerunds, neither noun nor verb, lending them to a more fluid understanding of the nurse–person interaction. This level of organization has been chosen for organizing the holistic nursing assessment tools (Appendixes 14–A and 14–B). Functional health patterns are another way to organize data gathered in the nursing process (Exhibit 14–2).[25] A more concrete level of the taxonomy, functional health patterns are found in many institutional practice settings.[26] They are easily adaptable to the holistic caring process.[27]

Exhibit 14–1 Nine Human Response Patterns

1. Exchanging: a human response pattern involving mutual giving and receiving
2. Communicating: a human response pattern involving sending messages
3. Relating: a human response pattern involving establishing bonds
4. Valuing: a human response pattern involving the assigning of relative worth
5. Choosing: a human response pattern involving the selection of alternatives
6. Moving: a human response pattern involving activity
7. Perceiving: a human response pattern involving the reception of information
8. Knowing: a human response pattern involving the meaning associated with information
9. Feeling: a human response pattern involving subjective awareness of information

Source: Reprinted with permission from C. Roy, Framework for Classification Systems Development: Progress and Issues, in *Classification of Nursing Diagnoses: Proceedings of the Fifth Conference,* M.J. Kim et al., eds., pp. 40–45, © 1984, Mosby.

HOLISTIC CARING PROCESS

Nurses who adhere to the holistic caring process focus on the care of the whole unique person, respecting and advocating for the person's rights and choices. Based on a holistic assessment of the person's health patterns, decisions about care flow from collaboration with the person, other health care providers, and significant others. The person assumes an active role in health care planning and decision making by seeking the professional expertise of the nurse via various nurse–person interaction. Facilitated by the nurse in the healing relationship, the person expresses health concerns and strengths, a unique health pattern, which the nurse identifies and documents in the health care record. The person is encouraged to participate as actively as possible,

Exhibit 14–2 Functional Health Patterns

1. *Health perception–health management pattern:* perceptions about one's health and how those perceptions shape personal health practices
2. *Nutritional–metabolic pattern:* one's biopsychosocial status in relation to the food and water supply and to nutrient and food intake
3. *Elimination pattern:* relates to elimination through the gastrointestinal tract, urinary tract, and skin
4. *Activity–exercise pattern:* motivation and capability to engage in energy-consuming activities
5. *Sleep–rest pattern:* one's perceptions of rest and sleep practices
6. *Cognitive–perceptual pattern:* one's ability to perceive, understand, remember, make decisions, and process information from both the internal and external environment
7. *Self-perception:* one's attitudes toward self and self-competency
8. *Role–relationship pattern:* one's need for and actual interactions with others (e.g., co-workers, family, community)
9. *Sexuality–reproductive pattern:* one's actual and perceived satisfaction or dysfunction in sexuality or reproduction
10. *Coping–stress intolerance pattern:* one's adaptive or maladaptive responses to stress and change
11. *Value–belief pattern:* one's beliefs and values guiding life choices and lifestyle

Source: Reprinted with permission from G.K. McFarland and E.A. McFarlane, *Nursing Diagnosis & Intervention: Planning for Patient Care,* © 1993, Mosby.

taking responsibility for personal health choices and decisions for self-care. The nurse must remember that the holistic caring process is merely a tool, a framework for ordering, documenting, and discussing the nurse–person interaction. Excessive reliance on structure and objectivity may reduce the person to a mere object.[28]

Assessment

Each person is assessed holistically using appropriate traditional and holistic methods while the uniqueness of the person is honored.[29]

Assessment is the information-gathering phase in which the nurse and the person identify health patterns and prioritize the person's health concerns. A continuous process, assessment provides ongoing data for changes that occur over time. Each nurse–person encounter provides new information that helps to explain interrelationships and validates previously collected data and conclusions. A key to a holistic assessment is to appraise the overall pattern of the responses.[30] The nurse gleans information about the person's patterns via interaction, observation, and measurement. Each pattern identification taps into the hologram of the person, contributing to the revelation of the whole. Interpersonal interaction reveals perceptions, feelings, and thoughts about health patterns/problems/needs as identified by the person. Nursing observation relies on information perceived by the five senses and intuition, while measurement provides quantifiable information obtained from instruments. The client is the primary source and interpreter of the meaning of information obtained by the assessment process. Family, significant others, other health care professionals, and measurable data provide supplemental information.

During assessment of the person's bio-psycho-social-spiritual patterns, the holistic nurse looks for the overall pattern of interrelationships, uses appropriate scientific and intuitive approaches, assesses the state of the energy field, and identifies stages of change and readiness to learn. The nurse also collects pertinent data from previous client records and other members of the health care team, if appropriate. All pertinent data are documented in the person's record.

The holistic nurse views the person as a whole and listens for the meaning of the current health situation to the person within the environment. While acknowledging his or her own patterns and their potential influence on the healing relationship, the nurse reflects to the person patterns recognized from the assessment. In response, the person validates the meanings of these identified health patterns. Assessment and documentation are continuous within the nurse–person interaction, as changes in one pattern always influence the other dimensions. A lack of awareness about one's own personal beliefs and patterns may subtly influence the nurse–client interaction (e.g., communication barriers relative to culture, class, age, gender, sexual orientation, education, or physical limitation) and impede holistic assessment.

Holistic Nursing Assessment Tools

In a holistic nursing assessment, it is critical that the appropriate data be collected and evaluated. A holistic nursing assessment tool has been developed for use with hospitalized patients to help nurses formulate nursing diagnoses (Appendix 14–A). It also can be adapted for use with clients in a wellness or health care clinic setting (Appendix 14–B). Based on the nine human response patterns, these tools facilitate assessment of all facets of a person.[31] In developing the tools, the nine response patterns were rearranged and became the tools' skeleton.[32] The term *transcending* was added to the valuing pattern and changed the definition of this pattern to one involving spiritual growth because the term *valuing* did not fully reflect the spiritual dimension. Three subcategories of transcending (i.e., meaning and purpose in life, inner strengths, and interconnections) were added to this pattern to elicit the information necessary to assess spirituality. (See

spiritual assessment tools in Chapter 5.) The Standards of Holistic Nursing Practice were incorporated into these assessment tools (see Appendix 1–A),[33] and specific assessment parameters (signs and symptoms) related to most nursing diagnoses were added to the appropriate nine human response patterns in the tools.[34]

The holistic nursing assessment tools group parameters for a particular problem so that the nurse can determine whether a specific nursing diagnosis is appropriate. Subjective data are followed by objective data within each major category of the tool. Summary assessment parameters (e.g., "willingness to comply with future health care regimen" under the choosing pattern) help in the evaluation of each nursing diagnosis. Relevant nursing diagnoses associated with the data appear in the right-hand column of the assessment tools, and each may appear in more than one place. They are intended as a guide to focus thinking and direct more detailed attention to the collection of data relative to a possible problem. This column is not meant to be static or absolute.

When assessing signs and symptoms that suggest a particular diagnosis, the nurse circles that diagnosis in the right-hand column. The circled diagnosis does not confirm the presence of that particular problem, but alerts the nurse to a possible problem or alteration. After completing the assessment, the nurse scans the possible problems in the right-hand column visually, synthesizes the data to determine whether other clusters of signs and symptoms also suggest that the problem is present, and formulates a nursing diagnosis.

The benefits of using the holistic nursing assessment tools are multiple. Because the data measure human response patterns, they are pertinent to nursing diagnoses made from a holistic nursing point of view.[35] Furthermore, because the tools permit evaluation of specific signs and symptoms, they assist the nurse in validating the presence of a particular nursing diagnosis. When the tools are used in practice, the data are so rich that nursing diagnoses appear to "fall out" after the assessment.[36] Continued use of these tools in various practice settings will be beneficial in easing problems with nursing diagnoses.

Intuitive Thinking

Holistically assessing the status of a person involves evaluation of data not only from a rational, analytic, and verbal (or left brain) mode, but also from an intuitive, nonverbal (right brain) mode. Unfortunately, we in nursing have not placed much value on "soft" data that cannot be measured and validated through scientific methods. Intuitive perceptions have been seen as opposing the empirical knowledge base of practice.[37] The idea that only quantifiable data are important in science is changing, however (see Chapter 9). Intuitive thinking does not conflict with analytic reasoning.[38] It is simply another dimension of knowing. There are multiple ways of knowing and assessing the status of clients, and intuition is a desirable component of the nursing process.[39] In addition to analysis, scientific exploration is now known to involve a qualitative, yet undefinable, process that scientists use to organize fragmented findings into meaningful wholes.[40] This undefinable process is called intuition, the tacit dimension, which is fundamental to all knowing.[41] It is a process whereby people know more than they can explain.

Intuitive perception allows one to know something immediately without consciously using reason.[42] Clinical intuition has been described as a "process by which we know something about a client which cannot be verbalized or is verbalized poorly or for which the source of the knowledge cannot be determined."[43] It is a "gut feeling" that something is wrong or that we should do something, even if there is no real evidence to support that feeling. The most experienced and technically proficient nurses have been found to be intuitive thinkers. Within the caring relationship between nurse and person, intuitive events emerge as the nurse is open and receptive to the person's subtle cues, such as color, activity, movement, tone, and posture. [44]

Intuition functions both as a process and as a product.[45] The intuitive process involves a nurse–person encounter in which cues, feelings, and past experience become integrated with the current event. The intuitive product is a conclusion in the form of knowing something, doing something, or both. In the majority of intuitive incidents, information emanates from "feeling" cues. Highly accurate, intuitive cues are useful in deciding upon a particular course of action.

Certain conditions or attributes facilitate intuitive thinking.[46] For example, direct person/client contact and nursing experience have been shown to be associated with intuitive perceptions.[47] In addition, the nurse must be emotionally able and willing to receive information. Personal and emotional problems reduce receptivity. For example, the nurse's energy level influences his or her readiness to receive, perceive, and interpret information. A nurse whose energy level is low, as in times of illness or stress, is less intuitive. Self-confidence also facilitates intuitive thinking by enabling the nurse to believe in the validity of his or her intuition.

Benner's work has been enormously useful in clarifying why the novice nurse can never view the world of nursing from the same perspective as the expert.[48,49] She described a hierarchy of thinking, judgment, behavior, and experience that clearly differentiates the novice from the expert. Novice nurses cling to rules and checklists to guide their practice and often miss the big picture. Because of the richness of their experience, expert nurses have an intuitive grasp of the situation and are able to focus on the real problem.[50] They are able to recognize patterns, understand the problem, and know instinctively when the situation is urgent and warrants immediate action. Moreover, they are skillful in convincing others to change the treatment plan when necessary. Their practice is person-driven.[51]

In summarizing the research and rhetoric on intuition, King and Appleton observed that "the attributes of intuition in nursing can be defined as the integration of forms of knowing in a sudden realization. This then precipitates an analytical process which facilitates action in patient/client care."[52] Intuitive judgment appears to increase proportionately with nursing experience. Although clinical experience is a significant common denominator for the most proficient application of nursing intuition, intuition is not limited to the expert and can be observed and cultivated in the novice as well. The research suggests that intuition can be taught through mentoring and role modeling by expert nurses. Within an educational environment that stresses a linear approach to nursing care, however, cultivation of intuition in the novice nurse is an ongoing concern for those educators who value a holistic approach to nursing education and practice.

Another important discovery related to nursing intuition is that the expert nurse gives significant credence to the patient's perceptions/intuitions.[53] Intuitive nurses acknowledge and follow up on those vague descriptions a person may give about how he or she is feeling; they perceive that the patient is often the first to know when something is not right. Based upon nurses' descriptions, nursing intuition may be categorized as cognitive, gestalt, or precognitive.[54] Cognitive inference evolves from the rapid processing of cues. Gestalt intuition perceives the situational pattern as a whole and fills in the gaps. Intuition functions precognitively, suggestive of an energy field interaction, when the nurse perceives a change before it happens.

Although research supports intuition as an aspect of all levels of nursing, King and Appleton recommended further research to explore intuition at each of the various levels of nursing expertise, particularly the relationship between intuition and cognitive processes in clinical judgment. They expressed the dilemma of many nurse researchers and educators: intuition is strongly linked to the skill of nursing judgment, but the contemporary nursing environment with its standardized procedures and plans for care may ignore the role of intuition. They noted that "intuitive feelings appear to act as a trigger within the linear problem-solving approach of the nursing process" and recommended that nursing research be directed toward discovering the intricacies of this relationship.[55(p.200)]

Intuition is refined in the crucible of experience. Benner's work makes it clear that intuitive events occur more often in the expert than in the novice.[56,57] Expert nurses should become mentors who help novice nurses cultivate and develop their intuitive skills.[58] Within the context of the educational setting, Beck developed a teaching strategy for explicating the intuitive moments within the nursing practice of graduate students and then framing them as a teaching tool for undergraduate nursing students.[59] As a lesson in concept analysis, the graduate students were asked to write in detail about an experience in which they had used intuition in their clinical practice. Beck then did a concept analysis of the experienced nurses' descriptions and identified four themes:

1. A "gut" feeling swept over the nurses as they knew something was not right.
2. Listening to their intuition involved nurses' conscious commitment to be persistent in following up on the patient's status.
3. Intuition involved astute observation of subtle nonverbal cues and changes in a patient's normal pattern of behavior.
4. Intuitive experiences resulted in positive, as well as some negative, consequences.[60]

These stories and the results of the concept analysis were then presented to the undergraduate nursing students with a threefold purpose: (1) to show the steps of concept analysis, (2) to give actual examples of intuitive thinking in nursing practice, and (3) to validate intuitive knowledge as a way of knowing within the nursing process. The undergraduate students responded enthusiastically to this learning experience. Like the Gray Gorilla Syndrome described by Pyles and Stern in which the older and more experienced gorilla mentors the younger ones,[61] Beck recommended a future program of direct interaction and mentoring between the two groups.

Novice nurses can learn the skills necessary to recognize subjective data and to verbalize feelings, cues, and decisions in order to enhance their intuitive perceptions.[62] Various exercises to enhance intuition and open a beginner's awareness to intuitive and spiritual experiences include listening to music, participating in physical exercise, progressive muscle relaxation, writing in a journal, and using a technique to cluster ideas (e.g., brainstorming). Exercises to deepen the intuitive process for more advanced intuitive thinkers include meditation, contemplation of harmonic symbols, directed drawing, guided imagery, and dialogue with the transpersonal self.[63] Educators and clinicians can also cultivate intuitive processes by

- emphasizing the value of intuitive thinking combined with analytic thinking in nursing and continuing education (e.g., by taking this position in nursing articles, textbooks, and conferences)
- encouraging nurses to use their intuition and senses in combination with analytic, objective thinking when assessing the clinical status of patients
- providing inexperienced nurses with subtle, repeated cue patterns that will assist them in recognizing intuitive information, thereby increasing their confidence about interpreting the cues and acting on their decisions
- encouraging nurses to trust their intuition
- using educational strategies that encourage pattern recognition (e.g., case studies, role playing, interactive videos)
- systematically evaluating the usefulness of the cues in making correct decisions
- sharing intuitive experiences with students and colleagues
- supporting nurses who have experienced intuitive events and encouraging them to review and analyze the process
- creating a climate of openness, curiosity, and the yen to discover.[64,65]

In the midst of a database approach to diagnosis, intervention, and outcomes in nursing with standardized names and numbers to describe nursing observations and activities, one may wonder how intuition can ever play a role. A completely intuitive approach may forgo labels and descriptors for a more individualized picture of each unique human being. At the other extreme is the theory that, if an observation about a person cannot be measured or categorized, it does not exist. A holistic, intuitive approach, as suggested by the holistic caring process, incorporates the best of both perspectives: application of the common language of nursing diagnoses, interventions, and outcomes within the context of both the intuitive and analytic practice of nursing. Such an approach requires creating new language where necessary and deviating from the path as the situation dictates, thus fostering a living, growing body of nursing knowledge.

Patterns/Problems/Needs

Each person's actual and potential patterns/problems/needs and life processes related to health, wellness, disease or illness which may or may not facilitate well being are identified and prioritized.[66]

Within the second step of the holistic caring process, the nurse describes a person's patterns/problems/needs based on a standardized language that is understandable to nurses, other health care professionals, the managed care provider, and the person receiving nursing care. Depending on the nurse's theoretical framework as well as institutional policy, nursing diagnosis as delineated by NANDA provides the most universal descriptor language for common patterns identified by nurses giving care[67] (Exhibit 14–3).

A nursing diagnosis can be defined as a "clinical judgment about the individual,

---

Exhibit 14–3 NANDA-Approved Nursing Diagnoses

This list represents the NANDA-approved nursing diagnoses for clinical use and testing.

Pattern 1: Exchanging

1.1.2.1	Altered Nutrition: More Than Body Requirements
1.1.2.2	Altered Nutrition: Less Than Body Requirements
1.1.2.3	Altered Nutrition: Risk for More Than Body Requirements
1.2.1.1	Risk for Infection
1.2.2.1	Risk for Altered Body Temperature
1.2.2.2	Hypothermia
1.2.2.3	Hyperthermia
1.2.2.4	Ineffective Thermoregulation
1.2.3.1	Dysreflexia
1.2.3.2	Risk for Autonomic Dysreflexia
1.3.1.1	Constipation
1.3.1.1.1	Perceived Constipation
1.3.1.1.2	Colonic Constipation (deleted in 1998)
1.3.1.2	Diarrhea
1.3.1.3	Bowel Incontinence
1.3.1.4	Risk for Constipation
1.3.2	Altered Urinary Elimination
1.3.2.1.1	Stress Incontinence
1.3.2.1.2	Reflex Urinary Incontinence
1.3.2.1.3	Urge Incontinence
1.3.2.1.4	Functional Urinary Incontinence
1.3.2.1.5	Total Incontinence
1.3.2.1.6	Risk for Urinary Urge Incontinence
1.3.2.2	Urinary Retention
1.4.1.1	Altered Tissue Perfusion (Specify type: Renal, Cerebral, Cardiopulmonary, Gastrointestinal, Peripheral)
1.4.1.2	Risk for Fluid Volume Imbalance
1.4.1.2.1	Fluid Volume Excess

1.4.1.2.2.1	Fluid Volume Deficit
1.4.1.2.2.2	Risk for Fluid Volume Deficit
1.4.2.1	Decreased Cardiac Output
1.5.1.1	Impaired Gas Exchange
1.5.1.2	Ineffective Airway Clearance
1.5.1.3	Ineffective Breathing Pattern
1.5.1.3.1	Inability to Sustain Spontaneous Ventilation
1.5.1.3.2	Dysfunctional Ventilatory Weaning Response
1.6.1	Risk for Injury
1.6.1.1	Risk for Suffocation
1.6.1.2	Risk for Poisoning
1.6.1.3	Risk for Trauma
1.6.1.4	Risk for Aspiration
1.6.1.5	Risk for Disuse Syndrome
1.6.1.6	Latex Allergy Response
1.6.1.7	Risk for Latex Allergy Response
1.6.2	Altered Protection
1.6.2.1	Impaired Tissue Integrity
1.6.2.1.1	Altered Oral Mucous Membrane
1.6.2.1.2.1	Impaired Skin Integrity
1.6.2.1.2.2	Risk for Impaired Skin Integrity
1.6.2.1.3	Altered Dentition
1.7.1	Decreased Adaptive Capacity: Intracranial
1.8	Energy Field Disturbance

Pattern 2: Communicating

2.1.1.1	Impaired Verbal Communication

Pattern 3: Relating

3.1.1	Impaired Social Interaction
3.1.2	Social Isolation
3.1.3	Risk for Loneliness
3.2.1	Altered Role Performance
3.2.1.1.1	Altered Parenting
3.2.1.1.2	Risk for Altered Parenting

continues

Exhibit 14–3 continued

3.2.1.1.2.1	Risk for Altered Parent/Infant/Child Attachment
3.2.1.2.1	Sexual Dysfunction
3.2.2	Altered Family Processes
3.2.2.1	Caregiver Role Strain
3.2.2.2	Risk for Caregiver Role Strain
3.2.2.3.1	Altered Family Process: Alcoholism
3.2.3.1	Parental Role Conflict
3.3	Altered Sexuality Patterns

Pattern 4: Valuing

4.1.1	Spiritual Distress (Distress of the Human Spirit)
4.1.2	Risk for Spiritual Distress
4.2	Potential for Enhanced Spiritual Well-Being

Pattern 5: Choosing

5.1.1.1	Ineffective Individual Coping
5.1.1.1.1	Impaired Adjustment
5.1.1.1.2	Defensive Coping
5.1.1.1.3	Ineffective Denial
5.1.2.1.1	Ineffective Family Coping: Disabling
5.1.2.1.2	Ineffective Family Coping: Compromised
5.1.2.2	Family Coping: Potential for Growth
5.1.3.1	Potential for Enhanced Community Coping
5.1.3.2	Ineffective Community Coping
5.2.1	Ineffective Management of Therapeutic Regimen: Individuals
5.2.1.1	Noncompliance (specify)
5.2.2	Ineffective Management of Therapeutic Regimen: Families
5.2.3	Ineffective Management of Therapeutic Regimen: Community
5.2.4	Effective Management of Therapeutic Regimen: Individual
5.3.1.1	Decisional Conflict (specify)
5.4	Health-Seeking Behaviors (specify)

Pattern 6: Moving

6.1.1.1	Impaired Physical Mobility
6.1.1.1.1	Risk for Peripheral Neurovascular Dysfunction
6.1.1.1.2	Risk for Perioperative Positioning Injury
6.1.1.1.3	Impaired Walking
6.1.1.1.4	Impaired Wheelchair Mobility
6.1.1.1.5	Impaired Transfer Ability
6.1.1.1.6	Impaired Bed Mobility
6.1.1.2	Activity Intolerance
6.1.1.2.1	Fatigue

6.1.1.3	Risk for Activity Intolerance
6.2.1	Sleep Pattern Disturbance
6.2.1.1	Sleep Deprivation
6.3.1.1	Diversional Activity Deficit
6.4.1.1	Impaired Home Maintenance Management
6.4.2	Altered Health Maintenance
6.4.2.1	Delayed Surgical Recovery
6.4.2.2	Adult Failure to Thrive
6.5.1	Feeding Self-Care Deficit
6.5.1.1	Impaired Swallowing
6.5.1.2	Ineffective Breastfeeding
6.5.1.2.1	Interrupted Breastfeeding
6.5.1.3	Effective Breastfeeding
6.5.1.4	Ineffective Infant Feeding Pattern
6.5.2	Bathing/Hygiene Self-Care Deficit
6.5.3	Dressing/Grooming Self-Care Deficit
6.5.4	Toileting Self-Care Deficit
6.6	Altered Growth and Development
6.6.1	Risk for Altered Development
6.6.2	Risk for Altered Growth
6.7	Relocation Stress Syndrome
6.8.1	Risk for Disorganized Infant Behavior
6.8.2	Disorganized Infant Behavior
6.8.3	Potential for Enhanced Organized Infant Behavior

Pattern 7: Perceiving

7.1.1	Body Image Disturbance
7.1.2	Self-Esteem Disturbance
7.1.2.1	Chronic Low Self-Esteem
7.1.2.2	Situational Low Self-Esteem
7.1.3	Personal Identity Disturbance
7.2	Sensory/Perceptual Alterations (Specify: Visual, Auditory, Kinesthetic, Gustatory, Tactile, Olfactory)
7.2.1.1	Unilateral Neglect
7.3.1	Hopelessness
7.3.2	Powerlessness

Pattern 8: Knowing

8.1.1	Knowledge Deficit (Specify)
8.2.1	Impaired Environmental Interpretation Syndrome
8.2.2	Acute Confusion
8.2.3	Chronic Confusion
8.3	Altered Thought Processes
8.3.1	Impaired Memory

Pattern 9: Feeling

9.1.1	Pain
9.1.1.1	Chronic Pain

continues

Exhibit 14-3 continued

9.1.2	Nausea		9.2.3.1	Rape-Trauma Syndrome
9.2.1.1	Dysfunctional Grieving		9.2.3.1.1	Rape-Trauma Syndrome: Compound Reaction
9.2.1.2	Anticipatory Grieving			
9.2.1.3	Chronic Sorrow		9.2.3.1.2	Rape-Trauma Syndrome: Silent Reaction
9.2.2	Risk for Violence: Directed at Others			
			9.2.4	Risk for Post-Trauma Syndrome
9.2.2.1	Risk for Self-Mutilation		9.3.1	Anxiety
9.2.2.2	Risk for Violence: Self-Directed		9.3.1.1	Death Anxiety
9.2.3	Post-Trauma Response		9.3.2	Fear

Source: Reprinted with permission from North American Nursing Diagnosis Association (1999). *NANDA Nursing Diagnoses: Definitions and Classification 1999–2000,* Philadelphia: NANDA.

family, or community responses to actual and potential health problems/life processes. Nursing diagnoses provide the basis for selection of nursing interventions to achieve outcomes for which the nurse is accountable."[68] After nursing diagnoses are identified and prioritized, they become the basis for the remaining steps of the nursing process.

North American Nursing Diagnosis Association

Although patterns/problems/needs identification has always been an important function of nursing practice, there was little effort to standardize the terminology used until NANDA evolved more than 25 years ago out of the First National Conference for the Classification of Nursing Diagnoses in 1973.[69] By defining, explaining, classifying, and researching summary statements about health concerns related to nursing, NANDA has worked to standardize the labels for identified patterns/problems/needs, facilitate communication, and encourage research so that specific potential outcomes and nursing interventions can be developed for each diagnosis.[70] As clinical practice and scientific research continue to validate it, the nursing diagnosis movement has the potential for enhancing the quality of nursing care and identifying those patterns/problems/needs and activities that are unique to nursing.

What began out of a concern for systematically defining and describing nursing decision making and process has evolved into a language suitably adaptable to the computer-based patient record and inclusion in standardized multidisciplinary vocabularies. The North American Nursing Diagnosis Association has asserted that the standardized language of nursing diagnosis places nursing in timely flow with future trends: "As we move to a true multidisciplinary, patient-focused care environment, the standardized vocabularies and nomenclatures of all disciplines are being scrutinized for inclusion into an overall standardized vocabulary for the CPR [computer-based patient record]."[71] Furthermore, NANDA has established a liaison with the International Council of Nursing (ICN) and the World Health Organization for developing the International Classification of Nursing Practice, a global effort to standardize nursing language.

Types of Nursing Diagnoses

In addition to arranging all approved nursing diagnoses by the relevant human response patterns, NANDA has divided nursing diagnoses into three categories: actual nursing diagnoses, risk nursing diagnoses, and wellness nursing diagnoses.[72]

Actual Nursing Diagnoses. A description of an individual's actual health problems in terms of a pattern of related cues (e.g., energy field disturbances related to slowing or blocking of energy flows secondary to surgical procedure[73]) is the actual nursing diagnosis. These diagnoses describe human responses to health conditions/life processes in an individual, family, or community. The diagnostic label is a "concise phrase or term which represents a pattern of related cues" that defines the diagnosis in practice.[74] The diagnostic qualifiers outlined in Exhibit 14–4 are used with the diagnostic label; other qualifiers may also be used.

Related factors are those "factors that appear to show some type of patterned relationship with the nursing diagnosis."[75]

Exhibit 14–4 Qualifiers for Diagnoses

(Suggested/not limited to the following)

Acute: Severe but of short duration

Altered: A change from baseline

Chronic: Lasting a long time, recurring, habitual, constant

Decreased: Lessened; lesser in size, amount, or degree

Deficient: inadequate in amount, quality, or degree; defective; not sufficient; incomplete

Depleted: Emptied wholly or in part, exhausted of

Disturbed: Agitated, interrupted, interfered with

Dysfunctional: Abnormal, incomplete functioning

Excessive: Characterized by an amount or quantity that is greater than necessary, desirable, or useful

Impaired: Made worse, weakened, damaged, reduced, deteriorated

Increased: Greater in size, amount or degree

Ineffective: Not producing the desired effect

Intermittent: Stopping or starting again at intervals, periodic, cyclic

Source: Reprinted with permission from North American Nursing Diagnosis Association (1999). *NANDA Nursing Diagnoses: Definitions and Classification 1999–2000,* Philadelphia: NANDA.

They may be antecedent to, associated with, related to, or abetting the problem. They help identify what is maintaining the problem and what is preventing improvement. Related factors guide the plan of care, because they indicate the changes necessary for the client to achieve a state of health.[76] An actual nursing diagnosis and related factors are connected by the phrase *related to,* forming a two-part diagnostic statement,[77] such as "knowledge deficit about acute myocardial infarction related to newly diagnosed health problem." (The phrase *related to* is preferable to the phrase *caused by* because cause and effect have not yet been established for most nursing diagnoses.[78]) The diagnostic statement should be specific enough to guide the remaining steps of the nursing process.

Before making a specific nursing diagnosis, the nurse assesses the defining characteristics of the diagnosis, those behaviors or signs and symptoms (observable cues and inferences) that cluster together as manifestations of the diagnosis.[79] They are necessary to identify the diagnostic entity and to differentiate between various nursing diagnoses. These characteristics, which should be measurable, can be divided into three categories: (1) critical indicators, (2) major defining characteristics, and (3) minor defining characteristics. A critical indicator must be present before the diagnosis can be made. A major defining characteristic is usually present when the diagnosis exists (i.e., it is present in 80 to 100 percent of the clients who experience the condition). A minor defining characteristic provides supporting evidence for the diagnosis, but may not be present in all clients who experience the condition (i.e., it is present in 50 to 79 percent of clients). Although minor defining characteristics are not always present, they help complete the clinical picture.

Partial lists of defining characteristics have been published to assist nurses in verifying a particular nursing diagnosis.[80,81] After assessing a client's condition and formulating the possible nursing diagnoses, a nurse refers to the list of defining characteristics to determine if there were sufficient critical indicators to confirm the diagnosis. Although a particular diagnosis may have quite specific defining characteristics, nurses must use their knowledge, education, experience, and intuition to determine if the signs and symptoms observed during the nursing assessment are sufficient to confirm the existence of the actual health problem.

For many diagnoses, research has not yet validated the defining characteristics. NANDA has established a formal process for research and validation of these diagnoses. Sometimes, when none of the available nursing diagnoses appear to fit the person's circumstances, the nurse must develop a diagnosis. If such a diagnosis appears to recur in the nurses' practice, she or he may consider a formal submission of the diagnosis to NANDA. The American Nurses' Association Psychiatric Mental Health Nursing Group has submitted an extensive list of labels for development as specialty nursing diagnoses.[82]

Risk Nursing Diagnoses. As of 1992, all NANDA-approved diagnoses that were designated as "potential" were changed to "risk" diagnoses.[83] A risk nursing diagnosis is a diagnosis that "describes human responses to health conditions/life processes which may develop in a vulnerable individual, family, or community. It is supported by risk factors that contribute to increased vulnerability."[84] The qualifiers listed in Exhibit 14–4 are also used with risk nursing diagnoses.

Risk nursing diagnoses are associated with risk factors, "environmental factors and physiologic, psychologic, genetic, or chemical elements that increase the vulnerability of an individual, family, or community to an unhealthful event."[85] The risk factors guide nursing interventions to reduce or prevent the occurrence of the problem. The diagnosis and the risk factors are connected by the phrase *related to* and written as a two-part statement, for example, "risk for altered nutrition: less than body requirements related to nausea, vomiting, fatigue, and activity intolerance associated with chemotherapy."

Specifically stating which clients are at risk for a particular problem is essential to providing quality nursing care. Moreover, nursing will be better able to demonstrate and document its contribution to desired client outcomes when the quality of nursing care prevents or reduces problems in clients at risk. Also, the risk category is beneficial in justifying allocation of resources and personnel, as well as in obtaining third-party reimbursement.

Wellness Nursing Diagnoses. The North American Nursing Diagnosis Association defines a wellness nursing diagnosis as one that "describes human responses to levels of wellness in an individual, family, or community that have a potential for enhancement to a higher state."[86] The diagnoses listed in Exhibit 14–3 are used together with the phrase *potential for enhanced* in wellness nursing diagnoses. Such diagnoses are written as one-part statements, such as "potential for enhanced adjustment to illness or potential for enhanced spiritual well-being."[87] Wellness and health promotion have become national priorities, and wellness nursing diagnoses broaden nursing's perspective from an illness-dominated framework to one that incorporates a positive, wellness orientation.

There is a distinction between the concepts of illness prevention (or risk reduction), health maintenance, and health promotion. Illness prevention or risk reduction involves behaviors aimed at actively protecting against or reducing the chances of encountering disease, illness, or accidents.[88,89] The risk nursing diagnoses are directed toward prevention. Nursing interventions associated with these diagnoses are actively selected to reduce or prevent the particular problem.[90] Health maintenance focuses on sustaining a neutral state of health. For example, the nursing diagnosis for people who are unable to identify, manage, or seek help to maintain health would be altered health maintenance (Exhibit 14–5).[91] For these clients, nursing interventions would include activities not only to prevent illness, but also to protect health (e.g., eating a balanced diet, stopping smoking, having regular medical examinations, sleeping 6 to 8 hours per night).

A trifocal model for nursing diagnosis as developed by Kelley and associates organizes the person's problems/patterns/needs in a wellness pyramid[92] (Figure 14–2). The base of the pyramid represents actual health problems for each of the nine human response patterns. The next level, representing a higher level of wellness than manifest problems, identifies areas where the person is at risk for developing problems. The apex of the pyramid represents areas/patterns that may be potentially enhanced, thus facilitating a state of harmony and balance.[93] Frisch and Frisch observed that this model "gives the nurse a framework to use the diagnostic language in all aspects of nursing care."[94] The flexibility of the trifocal model allows the nurse to identify and map a multidimensional picture of the person who always has strengths that may be substantially enhanced in the midst of moving through potential or manifest illness. The trifocal model may also serve as a motivational communication device to use with the person in creating a mutual plan of care.

Health promotion goes beyond illness prevention or health maintenance. Because it involves a personal responsibility for their health, individuals strive actively to improve their lifestyle to achieve high-

Exhibit 14–5 Altered Health Maintenance

Definition

Inability to identify, manage, and/or seek out help to maintain health

Defining Characteristics

History of lack of health-seeking behavior; reported or observed lack of equipment, financial, and/or other resources; reported or observed impairment of personal support systems; expressed interest in improving health behaviors; demonstrated lack of knowledge regarding basic health practices; demonstrated lack of adaptive behaviors to internal/external environmental changes; reported or observed inability to take responsibility for meeting basic health practices in any or all functional pattern areas

Related Factors

Ineffective family coping; perceptual/cognitive impairment (complete/partial lack of gross and/or fine motor skills); lack of, or significant alteration in, communication skills (written, verbal, and/or gestural); unachieved developmental tasks; lack of material resources; dysfunctional grieving; disabling spiritual distress; lack of ability to make deliberate and thoughtful judgments; ineffective individual coping

Source: Reprinted with permission from North American Nursing Diagnosis Association (1999). *NANDA Nursing Diagnoses: Definitions and Classification 1999–2000,* Philadelphia: NANDA.

level wellness.[95] The diagnosis of health-seeking behaviors (i.e., health-promoting behaviors) is consistent with the concept of health promotion (Exhibit 14–6). Health-seeking behaviors may include such activities as requesting additional information and recipes to enhance a low-cholesterol, low-fat, low-salt, low-sugar, and high-fiber diet; practicing daily relaxation techniques; and participating in aerobic exercises three to five times per week.[96] The category of wellness nursing diagnoses using Taxonomy I with the qualifier of *potential*

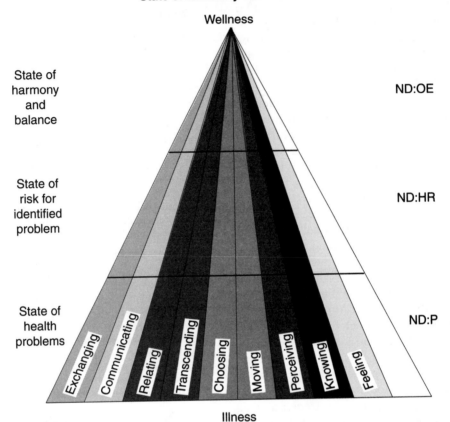

Integration of Human Response Patterns to the State of Harmony and Wellness

Legend
ND: Nursing diagnosis
OE: Opportunity for enhancement
HR: High risk
P: Problem

Figure 14–2 Trifocal model of nursing diagnosis. *Source:* Reprinted with permission from J. Kelley, N. Frisch, and K. Avant, A Trifocal Model of Nursing Diagnosis: Wellness Revisited, *Nursing Diagnosis,* Vol. 6, pp. 123–128, © 1995, North American Nursing Diagnosis Association.

for enhanced also addresses health promotion activities and allows the nurse to focus on wellness, facilitate responsibility for self-care, and promote healthy behaviors.

Essential to the holistic caring process is the understanding that nursing diagnosis is a means for describing a person's health pattern manifestation; nursing diagnoses are not the pattern. They are merely a descriptive tool for articulating patterns identified in the nurse-person relationship, rather than a rigid, limiting diagnostic label that might constrict and stereotype care. The person's value system, not the nurse's, is the basis for holistic nursing decisions and diagnostic labeling. Setting aside preconceived notions about health enhancement for the person, the nurse chooses diagnoses that most accurately reflect the person's perceptions about his or

Exhibit 14-6 Health-Seeking Behaviors

Definition

A state in which an individual in stable health is actively seeking ways to alter personal health habits and/or the environment in order to move toward a higher level of health

Defining Characteristics

Expressed or observed desire to seek a higher level of wellness; demonstrated or observed lack of knowledge in health-promotion behaviors; stated or observed unfamiliarity with wellness community resources; expression of concern about current environmental conditions on health status; expressed or observed desire for increased control of health practice

Related Factors

To be developed

Note: Stable health states is defined as age-appropriate, illness-prevention measures achieved; client reports good or excellent health; and signs and symptoms of disease, if present, are controlled.

Source: Reprinted with permission from North American Nursing Diagnosis Association (1999). *NANDA Nursing Diagnoses: Definitions and Classification 1999–2000,* Philadelphia: NANDA.

Outcomes

Each person's actual or potential patterns/problems/needs have appropriate outcomes specified.[97]

An outcome is a direct statement of a nurse–person identified goal to be achieved within a specific time frame; the person's significant others and other health care practitioners may participate in goal setting. An outcome indicates the maximum level of wellness that is reasonably attainable for the person in view of objective circumstances and the person's perceptions.[98,99]

After the person's patterns/problems/ needs have been identified, one or more specific and concisely stated outcomes are written for each. Outcome criteria must be measurable and may fall into the following categories:

- circumstances that should or should not occur in the client's status
- the level at which some change should occur
- the client's verbalizations about what he or she knows, understands, or feels about the situation
- specific client behaviors or signs/ symptoms that are expected to occur as a result of intervention
- specific client behaviors that are expected to occur as a result of adequate management of the environment[100,101]

Outcome criteria outline the specific tools, tests, observations, or personal statements that determine whether the patient outcome has been achieved. They reflect the goals of the nurse–person intervention. The holistic nurse selects interventions on the basis of desired outcomes, discussing with the person possible ways for achieving these desired outcomes. The person helps to establish observable milestones for knowing whether desired changes have occurred and makes a commitment to move toward those desired changes. Client outcomes direct the plan of care.

her health patterns. Whenever possible, the nurse collaborates with the person to validate and prioritize nursing diagnoses. Impediments to a holistic nursing diagnosis result from neglecting to make the person the focus of the process and failing to have a continual focused awareness of the person as a whole. Fitting the pattern of a dynamic, changing human being into an arbitrary diagnostic statement rather than reflecting the actual pattern of the person limits the effectiveness of the holistic caring process. Also, the language of nursing diagnosis leans heavily on a biomedical perspective and may not always reflect other nursing theoretical paradigms.

Similar to the attempt to classify and codify nursing diagnoses, there has been major effort to standardize outcome measures. The Nursing Outcomes Classification (NOC) developed by the Iowa Outcomes Project at the University of Iowa provides a comprehensive taxonomy of more than 200 outcomes organized into six domains and 24 classes. Within this classification system an "outcome is stated as a variable concept representing a patient or family caregiver state, behavior, or perception that is measurable along a continuum and responsive to nursing interventions."[102]

Using variable concepts allows for measurement of change as positive, negative, or no change in the person's situation, behaviors, or perceptions. Indicators and a measurement scale are listed with each outcome.

The six NOC domains are (1) Functional Health, (2) Physiologic Health, (3) Psychosocial Health, (4) Health Knowledge and Behavior, (5) Perceived Health, and (6) Family Health. (See Exhibit 14–7 for an example of the classes for the domain of Psychosocial Health and Exhibit 14–8 for measurable indicators for the nursing outcome Self-Es-

Exhibit 14–7 Classes for the Domain of Psychosocial Health

Level 1	3) Domain III—Psychosocial Health Outcomes That Describe Psychological and Social Functioning			
Level 2	**M-Psychological Well-Being**	**N-Psychosocial Adaptation**	**O-Self-Control**	**P-Self-Interaction**
	Outcomes that describe an individual's emotional health	Outcomes that describe an individual's psychological and/or social adaptation to altered health or life circumstances	Outcomes that describe an individual's ability to restrain behavior that may be emotionally or physically harmful to self or others	Outcomes that describe an individual's relationships with others
Level 3	1200-Body Image 1201-Hope 1202-Identity 1203-Mood Equilibrium 1204-Self-Esteem 1206-Will to Live	1300-Acceptance: Health Status 1301-Child Adaptation to Hospitalization 1302-Coping 1303-Dignified Dying 1304-Grief Resolution 1305-Psychosocial Adjustment: Life Change 1306-Suffering Level	1400-Abusive Behavior Self-Control 1401-Aggression Control 1402-Anxiety Control 1403-Distorted Thought Control 1404-Fear Control 1405-Impulse Control 1406-Self-Mutilation Restraint 1407-Substance Addiction Consequences 1408-Suicide Self-Restraint	1500-Parent–Infant Attachment 1501-Role Performance 1502-Social Interaction Skills 1503-Social Involvement 1504-Social Support

Note: The numbers represent the numeric code assigned by the Nursing Outcomes Classification.
Source: M. Johnson and M. Maas, *Nursing Outcomes Classification,* © St. Louis, Mosby, 1997. Reprinted by permission.

Exhibit 14–8 Measurable Indicators for the Nursing Outcome of Self-Esteem

Self-Esteem (Personal judgment of self-worth)	Never Positive	Rarely Positive	Sometimes Positive	Often Positive	Consistently Positive
Indicators:					
Verbalizations of self-acceptance	1	2	3	4	5
Acceptance of self-limitations	1	2	3	4	5
Maintenance of erect posture	1	2	3	4	5
Description of self	1	2	3	4	5
Regard for others	1	2	3	4	5
Open communication	1	2	3	4	5
Fulfillment of personally significant roles	1	2	3	4	5
Maintenance of grooming/hygiene	1	2	3	4	5
Balance of participation and listening in groups	1	2	3	4	5
Confidence level	1	2	3	4	5
Acceptance of compliments from others	1	2	3	4	5
Expected response from others	1	2	3	4	5
Acceptance of constructive criticism	1	2	3	4	5
Willingness to confront others	1	2	3	4	5
Description of success in work or school	1	2	3	4	5
Description of success in social groups	1	2	3	4	5
Description of pride in self	1	2	3	4	5
Feelings about self-worth	1	2	3	4	5
Other_____ (specify)	1	2	3	4	5

Source: M. Johnson and M. Maas, *Nursing Outcomes Classification,* © St. Louis, Mosby, 1997. Reprinted by permission.

teem.) As with NANDA nursing diagnoses, the NOC provides common nursing language for communicating about the effectiveness of nursing actions, a language that can be recognized by providers, payers, and other health care professionals.

If outcomes are to be achieved, the nurse must establish them with the assistance of the patient and family. The person must be motivated to establish healthy patterns of behavior. Assumptions made by the nurse concerning desired outcomes without collaboration with the person impede outcome achievement. Rigid adherence to specific outcomes by the person or the nurse may make it impossible to recognize the value of the journey with its myriad of other paths and other possible outcomes.

Therapeutic Care Plan

> Each person engages with the holistic nurse to mutually create an appropriate plan of care that focuses on health promotion, recovery, restoration, or peaceful dying so that the person is as independent as possible.[103]

During the planning stage, nurses who use the holistic caring process help the person identify ways to repattern his or her behaviors to achieve a healthier state. The planning process reveals interventions that will achieve outcomes. The plan outlines nursing prescriptions, which are the specific actions that the nurse performs to help the person solve problems and accomplish outcomes.[104] Nursing prescriptions direct the implementation of care.

A nursing intervention has been defined as "any direct care treatment that a nurse performs on behalf of a client. The treatments include nurse-initiated treatments resulting from nursing diagnoses, physician-initiated treatments resulting from medical diagnoses, and performance of the daily essential functions for the client who cannot do these."[105] During the planning phase, the nurse generally chooses interventions by

- determining whether the intervention will be useful in helping the client achieve the desired outcome
- identifying the characteristics of the patterns/problems/needs (i.e., whether the intervention is aimed at the etiology, at signs/symptoms, or at potential problems)
- evaluating the research base that validates the effectiveness of the intervention, its clinical significance, and the nursing control associated with the intervention
- determining the feasibility of implementing the intervention in terms of any other diagnoses and their respective priorities, and the cost and time involved with the intervention
- evaluating the acceptability of the intervention to the client in terms of his or her own goals and priorities related to the treatment plan
- ensuring the nursing competency necessary to implement the intervention successfully.[106,107]

Efforts have been under way to develop a classification of nursing interventions that parallels the classification of nursing diagnoses. The Iowa Intervention Project has developed the Nursing Interventions Classification (NIC), which contains an alphabetic list of 336 interventions.[108] Each intervention is listed with a label, a definition, a set of related activities that describe the behaviors of the nurse who implements the intervention, and a short list of background readings. The NIC includes all direct care interventions that nurses perform for patients, both independent and collaborative interventions. Holistic nurses frequently select noninvasive nursing interventions to complement standard nursing care, such as guided imagery to help the person visualize healing during a dressing change. (See Exhibit 14–9 for a list of noninvasive nursing interventions.)

The organization of the holistic care plan reflects the priority of identified opportunities to enhance the person's health. Priorities for intervention are based on an assessment of the urgency of the threat to the person's life and safety. The holistic nurse chooses interventions based on utility, relationship to the person's patterns/problems/needs, effectiveness, feasibility, acceptability to the person, and nursing competency. Holistic nursing interventions reflect acceptance of the person's values, beliefs, culture, religion, and socioeconomic background. Any revision of the care plan reflects the person's current status or ongoing changes. This plan is documented in the person's record.

Implementation

> Each person's plan of holistic care is prioritized and holistic nursing interventions are implemented accordingly.[109]

Nurses who are guided by a holistic framework approach the implementation phase of care with an awareness that (1) people are active participants in their care; (2) nursing care must be performed with purposeful, focused intention; and (3) a person's humanness is an important factor

Exhibit 14–9 Noninvasive Nursing Interventions

4920 Active Listening	7150 Family Therapy	8120 Research Data Collection
4310 Activity Therapy	1660 Foot Care	6610 Risk Identification
1320 Acupressure	5290 Grief Work Facilitation	5370 Role Enhancement
Addictions Counseling*	5300 Guilt Work Facilitation	5390 Self-Awareness
AMMA Therapy*	Hakomi Counseling*	Enhancement
4320 Animal-Assisted Therapy	Healing Presence*	5400 Self-Esteem
5210 Anticipatory Guidance	Healing Touch*	Enhancement
5820 Anxiety Reduction	7960 Health Care Information	4470 Self-Modification
Aroma Therapy*	Exchange	Enhancement
4330 Art Therapy	5510 Health Education	Self-Reflection*
4340 Assertiveness Training	Herbal Remedies*	4480 Self-Responsibility
6710 Attachment Promotion	Holistic Self-	Facilitation
5840 Autogenic Training	Assessments*	Sexual Abuse
Back Remedies*	6520 Health Screening	Counseling*
1610 Bathing	7400 Health System Guidance	5248 Sexual Counseling
4360 Behavior Modification	5310 Hope Instillation	Shen Therapy*
4680 Bibliotherapy	5320 Humor/Laughter	6000 Simple Guided Imagery
5860 Biofeedback	5920 Hypnosis	1480 Simple Massage
Biomagnetic Healing*	Journaling*	6040 Simple Relaxation
5220 Body Image	5244 Lactation Counseling	Therapy
Enhancement	5520 Learning Facilitation	1850 Sleep Enhancement
0140 Body Mechanics	5540 Learning Readiness	4490 Smoking Cessation
Promotion	Enhancement	Assistance
5880 Calming Technique	2380 Medication Management	5420 Spiritual Support
7040 Caregiver Support	5960 Meditation	Spirituality Counseling*
4700 Cognitive Restructuring	4400 Music Therapy	6340 Suicide Prevention
5230 Coping Enhancement	4410 Mutual Goal Setting	5430 Support Group
5240 Counseling	5246 Nutritional Counseling	5440 Support System
Craniosacral Therapy*	1400 Pain Management	Enhancement
6160 Crisis Intervention	4420 Patient Contracting	7500 Sustenance Support
5250 Decision-Making Support	7710 Physician Support	5604 Teaching: Group
7370 Discharge Planning	4430 Play Therapy	5606 Teaching: Individual
7920 Documentation	Polarity Therapy*	8180 Telephone Consultation
5270 Emotional Support	5340 Presence	5465 Therapeutic Touch
6480 Environmental	1460 Progressive Muscle	5450 Therapy Group
Management	Relaxation	5460 Touch
0200 Exercise Promotion	5360 Recreation Therapy	5470 Truth Telling
7110 Family Involvement	8100 Referral	5480 Values Clarification
7130 Family Process	Relationship Counseling*	Violence Counseling*
Maintenance	4860 Reminiscence Therapy	1260 Weight Management
7140 Family Support		Wellness Counseling*

*Not yet recognized by the Nursing Interventions Classification Code.

Note: The numbers represent the numeric code assigned by the Nursing Interventions Classification.

Source: Data from J.C. McCloskey and G.M. Bulechek, *Nursing Interventions Classification (NIC),* © 1996, Mosby–Year Book, Inc.

in implementation. Within the holistic framework, anything that produces a physiologic change causes a corresponding psycho-social-spiritual alteration. Conversely, anything that produces a psychologic change causes a corresponding physio-social-spiritual alteration. Thus, a nurse's encounter with a person, be it for the purpose of talking to the person, touching the person, or taking a blood pressure, produces psychophysiologic outcomes. The encounter changes the consciousness and the physiology of both the nurse and the person. Because human emotions can be translated into physiologic responses, the greatest tool/intervention for helping and healing clients is the therapeutic use of self.[110]

Evaluation

> Each person's responses to holistic care are regularly and systematically evaluated and the continuing holistic nature of the healing process is recognized and honored.[111]

Evaluation is a planned review of the nurse–person interaction to identify factors that facilitate or inhibit expected outcomes. Within the holistic caring process, evaluation is a mutual process between the nurse and the person receiving care. Data about the client's bio-psycho-social-spiritual status and responses are collected and recorded throughout the holistic caring process. The information is related to the person's patterns/problems/needs, the outcome criteria, and the results of the nursing intervention. Measures from the NOC may be used to document the effectiveness of the nursing interventions received by the person in the course of care.

The goal of evaluation is to determine if outcomes have been successful and, if so, to what extent. The nurse, person, family, and other members of the health care team all participate in the evaluation process. Together, they synthesize the data from the evaluation to identify successful repatterning behaviors toward wellness. During the evaluation, the person becomes more aware of previous patterns, develops insight into the interconnections of all dimensions of his or her life, and sees the benefits of repatterning behaviors. For example, does the person understand that his or her current job and level of stress have a direct impact on the current illness?

The evaluation of outcomes must be continuous because of the dynamic nature of human beings and the frequent changes that occur during illness and health. It may be necessary to develop new outcomes and revise the plan of care. Factors facilitating effective outcomes or preventing solutions to problems must also be explored. The failure to recognize that all measurable outcomes may not be immediate, but are in a process of becoming, is an impediment to evaluation.

CONCLUSION

By definition, any nurse in any setting can practice holistic nursing. Because the Standards for Holistic Nursing Practice (Appendix 1–A) are based on the universal language of the nursing process, they may be easily combined with other more physiologically based standards, such as those for cardiovascular and critical care nursing. Thus, the Standards for Holistic Nursing Practice can be incorporated into all subspecialty standards of care to ensure not only quality physiologic care, but also quality holistic nursing care to these specialty populations. Table 14–1, which lists nursing interventions central to differing specialty practices, provides an interesting opportunity for speculating about ways in which the holistic nursing perspective may contribute to nursing care in two different practice realms—critical care nursing and psychiatric nursing—thus enhancing nursing practice.

Standards of Holistic Nursing Practice necessitate the application of a whole new lens to the nursing process. Although standardized language is beneficial for the acknowledgment and documentation of nursing expertise and practice, such labels do not always communicate adequately the person's health situation and need for care. Standardized nursing diagnoses, nursing interventions, and nursing outcomes when

Table 14–1 Nursing Interventions and Core Use by Specialty Organizations

American Association of Critical-Care Nurses	American Holistic Nurses' Association	American Psychiatric Nurses Association
Acid–Base Monitoring	Acupressure	Abuse Protection
Airway Management	Active Listening*	Active Listening*
Airway Suctioning	Animal Assisted Therapy	Anger Control Assistance
Analgesic Administration	Anticipatory Guidance	Assertiveness Training
Anxiety Reduction*	Anxiety Reduction*	Anxiety Reduction*
Artificial Airway Management	Art Therapy	Behavior Management
Cardiac Care	Autogenic Training	Behavior Modification
Cardiac Care: Acute	Bibliotherapy	Body Image Enhancement
Cardiac Precautions	Calming Technique	Complex Relationship Building
Caregiver Support*	Caregiver Support*	Delusion Management
Code Management	Cognitive Restructuring*	Cognitive Restructuring*
Conscious Sedation	Coping Enhancement*	Coping Enhancement*
Delegation	Counseling*	Counseling*
Decision-Making Support*	Diet Staging	Decision-Making Support*
Electrolyte Management	Energy Management	Dementia Management
Discharge Planning*	Discharge Planning*	Eating Disorders Management
Documentation*	Documentation*	Elopement Precautions
Emergency Care	Environmental Management*	Environmental Management*
Emotional Support*	Emotional Support*	Family Therapy
Fluid/Electrolyte Management	Exercise Promotion	Grief Work Facilitation
Family Involvement*	Family Involvement*	Guilt Work Facilitation
Hyperglycemia Management	Health Education	Hallucination Management
Intravenous Therapy	Health Screening	Impulse Control Training
Mechanical Ventilation and Weaning	Hope Instillation	Limit Setting
Medication Administration	Humor	Milieu Therapy
Multidisciplinary Care Conference	Meditation	Mood Management
Oxygen Therapy	Music Therapy	Physical Restraint
Pain Management	Mutual Goal Setting	Play Therapy
Patient Rights Protection	Nutritional Counseling	Reality Orientation
Physician Support*	Physician Support*	Reminiscence Therapy
Positioning	Presence	Seclusion
Respiratory Monitoring	Progressive Muscle Relaxation	Suicide Prevention
Teaching: Procedure/Treatment	Self-Awareness Enhancement*	Self-Awareness Enhancement*
Technology Management	Self-Modification Assistance	Support Group
Visitation Facilitation	Self-Responsibility Facilitation	
Vital Signs Monitoring	Simple Guided Imagery	
	Simple Massage	
	Simple Relaxation Therapy	
	Spiritual Support	
	Teaching: Group	
	Teaching: Individual	
	Therapeutic Touch	
	Touch	
	Truth Telling	
	Values Clarification	

*Interventions in common across two or three disciplines

Source: Data from J.C. McCloskey, G.M. Bulechek, and W. Donahue, Nursing Interventions Core to Specialty Practice, *Nursing Outlook,* Vol. 46, No. 2, pp. 67–76, © 1998.

viewed through the lens of holistic standards for practice would benefit from the refinement of the holistic perspective.

DIRECTIONS FOR FUTURE RESEARCH

1. Evaluate each nursing diagnosis, nursing intervention, and nursing outcome for compatibility with holistic nursing practice standards.
2. Explore whether writing nursing diagnoses related to holistic nursing standards (e.g., potential for enhanced nutrition) enhances outcomes.
3. Evaluate the effectiveness and nature of intuitive judgments used by holistic nurses.
4. Investigate whether incorporating the holistic caring process into practice positively affects subjective and objective client outcomes.
5. Determine the effects of incorporating the holistic caring process into practice on nurse work satisfaction and turnover.

NURSE HEALER REFLECTIONS

After reading this chapter, the nurse healer will be able to answer or will begin a process of answering the following questions:

- How am I guided in my everyday life and work by the holistic caring process?
- How do I reconcile what I know about health and healing with whatever beliefs and realities that might be held by the people to whom I give care and by my co-workers?
- How can I systematically begin to apply the holistic caring process in terms of standardized nursing taxonomies for diagnoses, interventions, and outcomes?
- How can I cultivate my intuitive processes?
- How do I react when clients indicate that they are not motivated to change health patterns and behavior?
- How do I feel when I incorporate the principles of holistic nursing into my nursing practice?

NOTES

1. J.C. McCloskey and G.M. Bulechek, *Nursing Interventions Classification (NIC)*, 2d ed. (St. Louis: Mosby, 1996).
2. M. Johnson and M. Maas, The Nursing Outcomes Classification, *Journal of Nursing Care Quality* 12, no. 5 (1998):9–20.
3. American Holistic Nurses' Association, *Nursing's Social Policy Statement* (Washington, DC: AHNA, 1995), 6.
4. F.R. Kreuter, What Is Good Nursing Care? *Nursing Outlook* 5 (1957):302–304.
5. N.C. Frisch and L.E. Frisch, *Psychiatric Mental Health Nursing: Understanding the Client As Well As the Condition*, ed. L. Keegan (Albany, NY: Delmar Publishers, 1998), 97.
6. C. Varcoe, Disparagement of the Nursing Process: The New Dogma? *Journal of Advanced Nursing* 23 (1996):120–125.

7. H.C. Erickson et al., *Modeling and Role-Modeling: A Theory and Paradigm for Nursing* (Englewood Cliffs, NJ: Prentice Hall, 1983), 103.
8. Varcoe, Disparagement of the Nursing Process, 123.
9. L.C. Selanders, The Power of Environmental Adaptation: Florence Nightingale's Original Theory for Nursing Practice, *Journal of Holistic Nursing* 16, no. 2 (1998):247–263.
10. C. Roy, *Introduction to Nursing: An Adaptation Model* (Englewood Cliffs, NJ: Prentice Hall, 1976).
11. H. Erickson et al., *Modeling and Role-Modeling: A Theory and Paradigm for Nursing* (Lexington, SC: Pine Press, 1983).
12. M. Rogers, *Introduction to the Theoretical Basis of Nursing* (Philadelphia: F.A. Davis, 1969).

13. I. King, *Toward a Theory of Nursing* (Boston: Little, Brown and Company, 1981).

14. M. Leininger, *Cultural Care Diversity and Universality: A Theory of Nursing* (New York: National League for Nursing, 1991).

15. D. Orem, *Nursing Concepts of Practice* (New York: McGraw-Hill, 1980).

16. J. Watson, *Nursing: Human Science and Human Care* (Norwalk, CT: Appleton-Century-Crofts, 1985).

17. R.R. Parse, Human Becoming: Parse's Theory of Nursing, *Nursing Science Quarterly* 5 (1992): 35–42.

18. M. Newman, *Health As Expanding Consciousness* (St. Louis: C.V. Mosby, 1986).

19. Watson, *Nursing: Human Science and Human Care.*

20. J.W. Kenney, Relevance of Theory-Based Nursing Practice, in *Nursing Process: Applications of Conceptual Models*, ed. P.J. Christensen and J.W. Kenney (St. Louis: Mosby, 1995), 9.

21. B.A. Carper, Fundamental Patterns of Knowing in Nursing, *Advances in Nursing Science* 1, no. 13 (1978).

22. American Holistic Nurses' Association, Position Statement on Holistic Nursing, in *Code of Ethics for Holistic Nurses* (Raleigh, NC).

23. C. Roy, Framework for Classification Systems Development: Progress and Issues, in *Classification of Nursing Diagnoses: Proceedings of the Fifth Conference*, ed. M.J. Kim et al. (St. Louis: Mosby, 1984), 40–45.

24. R.M. Carroll-Johnson and M. Paquette, eds., *Classification of Nursing Diagnoses: Proceedings of the Tenth Conference* (Philadelphia: J.B. Lippincott, 1994).

25. M. Gordon, *Manual of Nursing Diagnosis 1997–1998* (St. Louis: Mosby, 1997).

26. L.J. Carpenito, *Nursing Diagnosis: Application to Clinical Practice*, 7th ed. (Philadelphia: Lippincott-Raven, 1997).

27. G.K. McFarland and E.A. McFarlane, *Nursing Diagnosis & Intervention: Planning for Patient Care*, 2d ed. (St. Louis: Mosby, 1993).

28. M. Leininger, *Care: The Essence of Nursing and Health* (Thorofare, NJ: Charles B. Stack, 1984).

29. American Holistic Nurses' Association, Standards of Holistic Nursing, (Flagstaff, AZ: AHNA, 1998).

30. B. Dossey et al., Nursing Diagnoses Use and Issues: American Holistic Nurses' Association, in *Classification of Nursing Diagnoses: Proceedings of the Tenth Conference*, ed. R.M.

Carroll-Johnson and M. Paquette (Philadelphia: J.B. Lippincott, 1994), 160–166.

31. C.E. Guzzetta et al., *Clinical Assessment Tools for Use with Nursing Diagnoses* (St. Louis: Mosby–Year Book, 1989).

32. C.E. Guzzetta et al., Unitary Person Assessment Tool: Easing Problems with Nursing Diagnoses, *Focus on Critical Care* 15 (1988):12.

33. American Holistic Nurses' Association, Standards of Holistic Nursing, (Raleigh, NC: AHNA, 1994).

34. North American Nursing Diagnosis Association, *Nursing Diagnoses: Definitions and Classification, 1992–1993* (St. Louis: NANDA, 1992).

35. Guzzetta et al., *Clinical Assessment Tools for Use with Nursing Diagnoses.*

36. Guzzetta et al., *Clinical Assessment Tools for Use with Nursing Diagnoses.*

37. C.E. Young, Intuition and Nursing Process, *Holistic Nursing Practice* 1, no. 3 (1987):54.

38. C. Jung, *Psychological Types* (New York: Harcourt Brace, 1959).

39. P. Benner, *Novice to Expert: Excellence and Power in Clinical Nursing Practice* (Reading, MA: Addison-Wesley, 1985).

40. M. Polanyi, *Personal Knowledge* (New York: Harper & Row, 1958).

41. Polanyi, *Personal Knowledge.*

42. B.D. Schraeder and D.K. Fisher, Using Intuitive Knowledge in the Neonatal Intensive Care Nursery, *Holistic Nursing Practice* 1, no. 3 (1987):47.

43. Young, Intuition and Nursing Process, 52.

44. Schraeder and Fisher, Using Intuitive Knowledge in the Neonatal Intensive Care Nursery.

45. Young, Intuition and Nursing Process.

46. Young, Intuition and Nursing Process.

47. Schraeder and Fisher, Using Intuitive Knowledge in the Neonatal Intensive Care Nursery.

48. Benner, *Novice to Expert.*

49. P. Benner et al., *Expertise in Nursing Practice: Caring, Clinical Judgment and Ethics* (New York: Springer, 1996).

50. L.A. Ruth-Sahd, A Modification of Benner's Hierarchy of Clinical Practice: The Development of Clinical Intuition in the Novice Trauma Nurse, *Holistic Nursing Practice* 7, no. 3 (1993): 10.

51. P. Benner et al., From Beginner to Expert: Gaining a Differentiated Clinical World in Critical Care Nursing, *Advances in Nursing Science* 14 (1992):13–28.

52. L. King and J.V. Appleton, Intuition: A Critical Review of the Research and Rhetoric, *Journal of Advanced Nursing* 26 (1997):195.

53. King and Appleton, Intuition: A Critical Review of the Research and Rhetoric.

54. L. Rew, Intuition in Decision-making, *Image* 20, no. 3 (1988):150–154.

55. King and Appleton, Intuition: A Critical Review of the Research and Rhetoric.

56. Ruth-Sahd, A Modification of Benner's Hierarchy of Clinical Practice.

57. V.E. Slater, Modern Physics, Synchronicity, and Intuition, *Holistic Nursing Practice* 6, no. 4 (1992):20–25.

58. L. Rew, Intuition: Nursing Knowledge and the Spiritual Dimension of Persons, *Holistic Nursing Practice* 3, no. 3 (1989):60.

59. C.T. Beck, Intuition in Nursing Practice: Sharing Graduate Students' Exemplars with Undergraduate Students, *Journal of Nursing Education* 37, no. 4 (1998):169–172.

60. Beck, Intuition in Nursing Practice, 171.

61. S. Pyles and P. Stern, Discovery of Nursing Gestalt in Critical Care Nursing: The Importance of the Gray Gorilla Syndrome, *Image* 15 (1983): 51–58.

62. Young, Intuition and Nursing Process.

63. Rew, Intuition: Nursing Knowledge and the Spiritual Dimension of Persons.

64. Young, Intuition and Nursing Process, 61.

65. Ruth-Sahd, A Modification of Benner's Hierarchy of Clinical Practice, 13.

66. American Holistic Nurses' Association, Standards of Holistic Nursing (1998).

67. North American Nursing Diagnosis Association, *Nursing Diagnoses: Definition and Classification, 1999–2000* (Philadelphia: NANDA, 1999), 1–7.

68. North American Nursing Diagnosis Association, *Nursing Diagnoses: Definitions & Classification, 1999–2000*, 149.

69. North American Nursing Diagnosis Association, *Nursing Diagnoses: Definitions & Classification, 1999–2000*.

70. A.M. McLane, *Classification of Nursing Diagnoses: Proceedings of the Third and Fourth National Conference* (New York: McGraw-Hill, 1992–1993).

71. North American Nursing Diagnosis Association, *Nursing Diagnoses: Definitions and Classification, 1997–1998*, 7.

72. North American Nursing Diagnosis Association, *Nursing Diagnoses: Definitions & Classification, 1999–2000*, 149.

73. Carpenito, *Nursing Diagnosis: Application to Clinical Practice.*

74. North American Nursing Diagnosis Association, *Nursing Diagnoses: Definitions and Classification, 1999–2000*, 150.

75. North American Nursing Diagnosis Association, *Nursing Diagnoses: Definitions & Classification, 1999–2000*, 150.

76. North American Nursing Diagnosis Association, *Taxonomy I: Revised* (NANDA, 1990).

77. C.E. Guzzetta and B.M. Dossey, Nursing Diagnoses, in *Cardiovascular Nursing: Holistic Practice*, ed. C.E. Guzzetta and B.M. Dossey (St. Louis: Mosby–Year Book, 1992).

78. M.D. Mundinger and G. Jauron, Developing a Nursing Diagnosis, *Nursing Outlook* 23 (1975): 94.

79. North American Nursing Diagnosis Association, *Nursing Diagnoses: Definitions and Classification, 1999–2000*, 150.

80. Gordon, *Manual of Nursing Diagnosis 1997–1998.*

81. M.J. Kim et al., *Pocket Guide to Nursing Diagnoses* (St. Louis: Mosby, 1997).

82. North American Nursing Diagnosis Association, *Nursing Diagnoses: Definitions and Classification, 1997–1998*, 89.

83. North American Nursing Diagnosis Association, *Nursing Diagnoses: Definitions and Classification, 1999–2000*, 83–88.

84. North American Nursing Diagnosis Association, *Nursing Diagnoses: Definitions and Classification, 1999–2000*, 149.

85. North American Nursing Diagnosis Association, *Nursing Diagnoses: Definitions and Classification, 1999–2000*, 150.

86. North American Nursing Diagnosis Association, *Nursing Diagnoses: Definitions and Classification, 1999–2000*, 149.

87. North American Nursing Diagnosis Association, *Nursing Diagnoses: Definitions and Classification, 1999–2000*, 149.

88. C.J. Allen, Incorporating a Wellness Perspective for Nursing Diagnosis in Practice, in *Classification of Nursing Diagnoses: Proceedings of the Eighth Conference*, ed. R.M. Carroll-Johnson (Philadelphia: J.B. Lippincott, 1989), 37–42.

89. N.J. Pender, Languaging a Health Perspective for NANDA Taxonomy on Research and Theory, in *Classification of Nursing Diagnoses: Proceedings of the Eighth Conference*, ed. R.M. Carroll-Johnson (Philadelphia: J.B. Lippincott, 1989), 31–36.

90. G.M. Bulechek and J.C. McCloskey, Nursing Interventions: Treatments for Potential Nursing Diagnoses, in *Classification of Nursing Diagnoses: Proceedings of the Eighth Conference*, ed. R.M. Carroll-Johnson (Philadelphia: J.B. Lippincott, 1989), 23–30.

91. North American Nursing Diagnosis Association, *Nursing Diagnoses: Definitions and Classification, 1999–2000*, 94–95.

92. J. Kelley et al., A Trifocal Model of Nursing Diagnosis: Wellness Reinforced, *Nursing Diagnosis* 6, no. 3 (1995): 123–128.

93. Kelley et al., A Trifocal Model of Nursing Diagnosis.

94. Frisch and Frisch, *Psychiatric Mental Health Nursing*, 81.

95. North American Nursing Diagnosis Association, *Nursing Diagnoses: Definitions and Classification, 1999–2000*, 83.

96. Guzzetta and Dossey, Nursing Diagnoses.

97. American Holistic Nurses' Association, Standards of Holistic Nursing (1998).

98. J.C. McCloskey and G.M. Bulechek, Classification of Nursing Interventions: Implications for Nursing Diagnoses, in *Classification of Nursing Diagnoses: Proceedings of the Tenth Conference*, ed. R.M. Carroll-Johnson and M. Paquette (Philadelphia: J.B. Lippincott, 1994), 116.

99. C.F. Capers and R. Kelly, Neuman Nursing Process: A Model of Holistic Care, *Holistic Nursing Practice* 1, no. 3 (1987):23.

100. Guzzetta and Dossey, Nursing Diagnoses.

101. G.M. Bulechek and J.C. McCloskey, Nursing Interventions: What They Are and How To Choose Them, *Holistic Nursing Practice* 1, no. 3 (1987):43.

102. Johnson and Maas, The Nursing Outcomes Classification, 11.

103. American Holistic Nurses' Association, Standards of Holistic Nursing (1998).

104. Guzzetta and Dossey, Nursing Diagnoses, 116.

105. McCloskey and Bulechek, Classification of Nursing Interventions: Implications for Nursing Diagnoses.

106. Bulechek and McCloskey, Nursing Interventions: What They Are and How To Choose Them, 40.

107. McCloskey and Bulechek, Classification of Nursing Interventions: Implications for Nursing Diagnoses, 114.

108. Iowa Intervention Project, *Nursing Interventions Classifications* (St. Louis: Mosby–Year Book, 1992).

109. American Holistic Nurses' Association, Standards of Holistic Nursing (1998).

110. D. Krieger, *Foundation of Holistic Health Nursing Practice* (Philadelphia: J.B. Lippincott, 1981).

111. American Holistic Nurses' Association, Standards of Holistic Nursing (1998).

Holistic Nursing Assessment Tool for Hospitalized Patients

Name: _____ Age: _____ Sex: _____
Address: _____ Telephone: _____
Significant other: _____ Telephone: _____
Date of admission: _____ Medical diagnosis: _____
Allergies: _____ Dyes: _____

Nursing Diagnosis
(Altered/High Risk for/
Potential for Enhanced)

Communicating—A pattern involving sending messages
Read, write, understand English (circle) _____   Communication
Other language _____   Verbal
Intubated _____ Speech impaired _____   [Nonverbal]
Alternate form of communication _____

"Valuing/Transcending"—A pattern involving spiritual growth
Religious preference _____   [Spiritual state]
Important religious practices _____   Spiritual
Cultural orientation _____   well-being
Cultural practices _____   Spiritual distress
Meaning and purpose in life _____   Hopelessness
Inner strengths _____   Powerlessness
Interconnections (self, others, universe, higher power) _____

Relating—A pattern involving establishing bonds
[Alterations in role]
    Marital status _____   [Role performance]
    Age and health of significant other _____   Parenting
                                                                                Sexuality patterns
    Number of children _____ Ages _____
    Responsibilities in home _____
    Financial support _____   Family processes
    Occupation _____
    Job satisfaction/concerns _____
    Physical/mental energy expenditures _____
    Sexual relationships (satisfactory/unsatisfactory) _____
    Physical difficulties related to sex _____

Source: Adapted with permission from C.E. Guzzetta, S.D. Bunton, L.A. Prinkey, A.P. Sherer, and P.C. Seifert, *Clinical Assessment Tools for Use with Nursing Diagnoses,* pp. 15–22, © 1989, Mosby-Year Book, Inc.; 1999.

Nursing Diagnosis
(Altered/High Risk for/
Potential for Enhanced)

[Alterations in socialization]
Quality of relationships with others _____

   Patient's description _____   Impaired social
   Significant other's description _____   interaction
   Staff observations _____
   Verbalizes feelings of being alone _____   Loneliness
   Attributed to _____   Social isolation

Knowing—A pattern involving the meaning associated with information

Previous hospitalization/surgeries _____
_____   Knowledge deficit

Educational level _____
History of the following diseases:
  Heart _____
  Lung _____
  Liver _____ Kidney_____
  Cerebrovascular _____ Rheumatic fever_____
  Thyroid _____
  Diabetes _____
Medication _____
Current health problems _____
_____

Current medications _____
_____

Risk factors	Present	Knowledge of
1. Hypertension	_____	_____
2. Hyperlipidemia	_____	_____
3. Smoking	_____	_____
4. Obesity	_____	_____
5. Diabetes	_____	_____
6. Sedentary living	_____	_____
7. Stress	_____	_____
8. Alcohol use	_____	_____
9. Oral contraceptives	_____	_____
10. Family history	_____	

Altered family process:
Alcoholism

Knowledge of planned test/surgery _____
_____

Misconceptions _____
Readiness to learn _____   [Learning]
  Learning impeded by _____   Thought processes

Feeling—A pattern involving the subjective awareness of information

[Alterations in comfort]
Pain/discomfort
   Onset _____ Duration_____
   Location _____ Quality_____Radiation_____   Pain
   Associated factors _____   Chronic
   Aggravating factors _____   [Acute]

Alleviating factors _____

[Alterations in emotional integrity]

Recent stressful life events _____

_____

Verbalizes feelings of fear or anxiety _____

Source _____

Physical manifestations _____

[Discomfort]
Chronic
Acute
Anxiety
Chronic sorrow
Nausea
Fear
Post-trauma response
Rape-trauma syndrome

Moving—A pattern involving activity

[Alterations in activity]

History of physical disability _____

_____

Limitations in daily activities _____

_____

Exercise habits _____

[Alterations in rest]

Hours slept/night_____Difficulties _____

Sleep aids (pillows, medications, food) _____

[Alterations in recreation]

Leisure activities _____

Social activities _____

[Alterations in activities of daily living]

Home maintenance management_____

Size and arrangement of home (stairs, bathroom) _____

_____

Housekeeping responsibilities _____

Shopping responsibilities _____

Health maintenance

Health insurance _____

Regular physical checkups _____

[Alterations in self-care]

Ability to perform ADL:

Independent_____ Dependent _____

Specify deficits _____

Discharge planning needs _____

Impaired physical
mobility
Activity intolerance
Fatigue
Impaired walking
Impaired bed mobility
Impaired transfer
ability
Sleep pattern
disturbance
Sleep deprivation

Deficit in diversional
activity

Impaired home
maintenance
management

Health maintenance
Adult failure to thrive
Self-care
Feeding
Bathing
Dressing
Toileting
Delayed surgical
recovery

Perceiving—A pattern involving the reception of information

[Alterations in self-concept]

Patient's description of himself/herself _____

Effects of illness/surgery on self-concept _____

_____

[Sensory/perceptual alterations]

Vision impaired _____ Glasses _____

Visual examination _____

Auditory impaired _____ Hearing aid _____

Auditory examination _____

Kinesthetics impaired_____ Romberg _____

Body image
Self-esteem
Personal identity

Visual

Auditory

Gustatory impaired _____

Tactile impaired_____   Examination _____   Kinesthetic

Olfactory impaired_____   Examination _____   Gustatory

Reflexes: Biceps   R ___ L ___   Triceps   R ___ L ___   Tactile

         Brachio-   Olfactory

           radialis   R ___ L ___   Knee   R ___ L ___   Reflexes

         Ankle   R ___ L ___   Plantar   R ___ L ___

Choosing—A pattern involving the selection of alternatives

[Alterations in coping]

Patient's usual problem-solving methods _____

_____   Ineffective individual

Family's usual problem-solving methods _____   coping

_____   Ineffective family coping

Patient's method of dealing with stress _____

_____

Family's method of dealing with stress _____

_____

Patient's affect _____

Physical manifestations _____

[Alterations in participation]

Compliance with past/current health care regimen _____   Noncompliance

_____   Ineffective management

Willingness to comply with future health care regimen _____   of therapeutic regimen

_____   Family

    Individual

    Community

Exchanging—A pattern involving mutual giving and receiving

[Alterations in nutrition]

Teeth, gums, lesions _____   Altered dentition

Dentures _____   Oral mucous membrane

Ideal body weight _____   Altered nutrition

Height_____Weight _____   More than body

Eating patterns   requirements

   Number of meals per day _____

   Special diet _____

   Where eaten _____   Less than body

   Food preferences/intolerances _____   requirements

   Food allergies _____

   Caffeine intake (coffee, tea, soft drinks) _____

   Appetite changes _____

   Presence of nausea/vomiting _____   Nausea

Current therapy

   NPO _____ NG suction _____

   Tube feeding _____

   TPN _____

Laboratory results

   Na _____ K _____ Cl _____ Glucose _____

   Cholesterol_____ Triglycerides_____ Fasting _____

[Alterations in physical regulation]

[Immune]

Lymph nodes enlarged_____ Location _____   Infection

WBC count _____ Differential _____   Hypothermia

Alteration in body temperature   Hyperthermia

Temperature_____ Route _____   Ineffective
thermoregulation

[Alterations in physical integrity]

Skin integrity _____ Rashes _____ Lesions _____   Impaired skin integrity

Petechiae_____ Surgical incision _____   Impaired tissue integrity

Bruising_____ Abrasions_____   Latex allergy response

[Alterations in circulation]

Cerebral (circle appropriate response)

Pupils	Eye opening	Cerebral tissue
L 2 3 4 5 6 mm	None (1)	perfusion
R 2 3 4 5 6 mm	To pain (2)	
Reaction: Brisk _____	To speech (3)	
Sluggish _____	Spontaneous (4)	
Nonreactive _____		Fluid volume

Best verbal	Best motor	Deficit
Intubated (0)	Flaccid (1)	Excess
Mute (1)	Extensor response (2)	Imbalance
Incomprehensible sound (2)	Flexor response (3)	
Inappropriate words (3)	Semipurposeful (4)	Cardiac output
Confused conversation (4)	Localized to pain (5)	
Oriented (5)	Obeys commands (6)	

Glasgow coma scale total   Confusion

_____   Impaired memory

Neurological changes/symptoms _____

[Cardiac]

Apical rate and

rhythm _____

PMI _____   Cardiopulmonary tissue

Heart sounds/murmurs _____   perfusion

Dysrhythmias_____

Pacemaker _____

BP: Sitting   Lying   Standing   Fluid volume

R_____ L_____   R_____ L_____   R_____ L_____   Deficit

A-Line reading _____   Excess

Cardiac index _____ Cardiac output _____

CVP _____PAP _____ PCWP_____   Cardiac output

IV fluids _____

IV cardiac medications _____

_____

Serum enzymes _____

Peripheral   Peripheral tissue

Pulses: A = absent   B = bruits   D = Doppler   perfusion

+ 3 = bounding + 2 = palpable + 1 = faintly palpable   Peripheral

Carotid	R ___ L ___	Popliteal	R ___ L ___	neurovascular
Brachial	R ___ L ___	Posterior tibial	R ___ L ___	dysfunction

Nursing Diagnosis
(Altered/High Risk for/
Potential for Enhanced)

Radial   R ___ L ___   Dorsalis pedis   R ___ L ___

Femoral   R ___ L ___

Jugular venous distention   R ___ L ___

Skin temperature_____ Color _____

Edema _____ Capillary refill _____

Clubbing _____ Claudication _____

Fluid volume
  Deficit
  Excess
  Imbalance
Cardiac output

Gastrointestinal

Liver: Enlarged _____ Ascites _____

GI tissue perfusion

Renal

Urine output: 24 hour _____ Average hourly _____

Renal tissue perfusion

BUN _____ Creatinine _____ Specific gravity _____

Urine studies _____

[Alterations in oxygenation]

Rate _____ Rhythm _____ Depth _____

Fluid volume
Cardiac output

Labored/unlabored (circle) Chest expansion _____

Use of accessory muscles _____

Orthopnea _____

Breath sounds _____

Complaints of dyspnea _____ Precipitated by _____

Cough: Productive/nonproductive _____

Sputum: Color _____ Amount _____ Consistency _____

LOC _____ Splinting _____

Arterial blood gases/O$_2$ sat. _____

Oxygen percent and device _____

Ventilator _____

Ineffective airway
  clearance
Ineffective breathing
  patterns
Ineffective gas exchange
Inability to sustain
  spontaneous
  ventilation

[Alterations in elimination]

Bowel

Abdominal physical examination _____

Usual bowel habits _____

Alterations from normal _____

Urinary

Bladder distention _____

Color _____ Catheter _____

Usual urinary pattern _____

Alteration from normal _____

Dysfunctional
  ventilatory weaning
  response
Bowel patterns
  Constipation
  Diarrhea
  Incontinence
Urinary patterns
  Incontinence
  Retention

ADL = activities of daily living; A-line = arterial line; BP = blood pressure; BUN = blood urea nitrogen; CVP = central venous pressure; GI = gastrointestinal; IV = intravenous; LOC = level of consciousness; NG = nasogastric; NPO = nothing by mouth; PAP = pulmonary artery pressure; PCWP = pulmonary capillary wedge pressure; PMI = point of maximal impulse; TPN = total parenteral nutrition

Energy Field Patterns

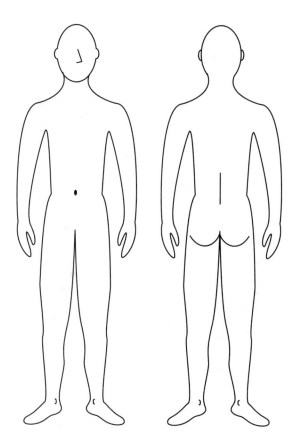

Nursing Diagnosis
(Altered/High Risk for/
Potential for Enhanced)

Energy field
   disturbance

Holistic Nursing Assessment Tool for Outpatients

Name _____ Date of Birth _____ Sex _____
Address _____ Telephone _____
Significant Other _____ Telephone _____
Date _____ Education _____ Employment _____
Medical Diagnosis _____
Reason for Seeking Holistic Nursing Care _____
_____

Height _____ Weight _____ B/P _____ T _____ P _____ R _____

Nursing Diagnosis
(Altered/High Risk for/
Potential for Enhanced)

Communicating—A pattern involving sending messages
Verbal: _____
Nonverbal: _____

[Communication,
    altered]
    Verbal
    Nonverbal

"Valuing/Transcending"—A pattern involving spiritual growth
Meaning and Purpose in Life: _____
Inner Strengths: _____
Interconnections (Self, Others, Universe, Higher Power): _____

[Spiritual State]
    Spiritual well-being
    Spiritual distress
        Hopelessness
        Powerlessness

Relating—A pattern involving establishing bonds
Role (Marital Status, Children, Parents): _____
_____
_____
_____
_____
_____
Occupation: _____
Sexual Relationships: _____
Socialization: _____
_____
_____
_____
_____
_____
_____
_____

Role performance,
    altered
    Parenting, altered
    Parental role conflict
    [Work]
    Sexual dysfunction

Family process, altered
Sexuality patterns,
    altered
[Socialization, altered]
    Social interaction,
        impaired
    Social isolation
    Loneliness

Source: Adapted with permission from C.E. Guzzetta, S.D. Bunton, L.A. Prinkey, A.P. Sherer, and P.C. Seifert, *Clinical Assessment Tools for Use with Nursing Diagnoses,* © 1989, Mosby-Year Book, Inc.; Revised 1999.

Nursing Diagnosis
(Altered/High Risk for/
Potential for Enhanced)

Knowing—A pattern involving the meaning associated with information

Orientation: _____
_____
_____
_____

Thought processes,
   altered
   [Orientation]
   Confusion

Memory: _____
_____
_____

Impaired memory

Previous Illnesses/Hospitalizations/Surgeries: _____

Identified Health Problems (Present/History): _____

Current Medications (Medication Allergies): _____

Risk Factors (Smoking, Family History, etc.): _____
_____

Altered family process
   Alcoholism

Perception/Knowledge of Health/Illness: _____
_____

Knowledge deficit
   (Specify)

Expectations of Holistic Health Intervention: _____
_____

Readiness to Learn (Ready, Willing, Able): _____
_____

[Learning]

Feeling—A pattern involving the subjective awareness of information

Comfort: _____
_____
_____
_____
_____

[Comfort, altered]
   Pain, chronic
   Pain, acute
   [Discomfort, chronic]
   [Discomfort, acute]
Nausea

Emotional Integrity States: _____
_____
_____
_____
_____
_____
_____
_____
_____
_____
_____
_____

[Grieving]
   Anticipatory
   Dysfunctional
Anxiety
Fear
[Anger]
[Guilt]
[Shame]
[Sadness]
Chronic sorrow
Post-trauma response
Rape-trauma syndrome

Moving—A pattern involving activity

Activity (Physical Mobility Limitations): _____
_____
_____
_____

[Activity, altered]
   Activity intolerance
   Impaired physical
     mobility

Nursing Diagnosis
(Altered/High Risk for/
Potential for Enhanced)

Rest: _____

Impaired walking
Impaired transfer
  mobility
Fatigue
Sleep pattern
   disturbance
Sleep deprivation
   [Hypersomnia]
   [Insomnia]
   [Nightmares]

Recreation: _____

Diversional activity
  deficit

Environmental Maintenance: _____

Impaired home
  maintenance
  management
   [Safety hazards]

Health Maintenance: _____

Health maintenance,
  altered

Self-Care: _____

Adult failure to thrive
Bathing/hygiene deficit
Dressing/grooming
  deficit
Feeding deficit
Toileting deficit
Delayed surgical
  recovery

Perceiving—A pattern involving the reception of information

Sensory Perception: _____

[Sensory perception,
  altered]
  Visual
  Auditory
  Kinesthetic
  Gustatory
  Tactile
  Olfactory
  Unilateral neglect

Self-Concept: _____

[Self-concept, altered]
  Body image
   disturbance
  Personal identity
   disturbance
  Self-esteem
   disturbance
   —Chronic low
   —Situational

Nursing Diagnosis
(Altered/High Risk for/
Potential for Enhanced)

Choosing—A pattern involving the selection of alternatives

Coping: _____
_____
_____

Judgment/Decisions: _____
_____
_____

Participation: _____
_____

Family Coping: _____
_____
_____
_____
_____
_____
_____
_____

Individual coping,
    ineffective
    Adjustment: impaired
    Conflict: decisional
    Coping: defensive
    Denial: impaired
    Noncompliance

[Family coping,
    ineffective]
    Compromised
    Disabled

Ineffective management
    of therapeutic regimen
        Family
        Individual
        Community

Exchanging—A pattern involving mutual giving and receiving

Nutrition: _____
_____
_____
_____
_____
_____
_____
_____

Elimination: _____
_____
_____
_____
_____
_____
_____

Renal/Urinary: _____
_____
_____
_____
_____
_____

Physical/Tissue Integrity: _____
_____
_____
_____
_____

[Nutrition, altered]
    [Nutritional deficit]
    < or > Body
    requirements
Oral mucous membranes,
    impaired
Altered dentition
Nausea
[Bowel elimination,
    altered]
    Bowel incontinence
    Constipation: colonic
    Constipation:
        perceived
    Diarrhea
GI tissue perfusion
[Urinary elimination,
    altered]
    Incontinence (specify)
    Retention
    [Enuresis]
Renal tissue perfusion
[Tissue integrity,
    impaired]
    Impaired skin
        integrity
Latex allergy response

Physical Regulation: _____

Immune: _____

_____

_____

_____

_____

_____

_____

Circulation: _____

_____

_____

_____

_____

_____

_____

_____

_____

_____

_____

_____

Oxygenation: _____

_____

_____

_____

_____

Hormonal/Metabolic Patterns: _____

_____

_____

_____

Nursing Diagnosis
(Altered/High Risk for/
Potential for Enhanced)

[Injury: Risk]
　Aspiration
　Disuse syndrome
　Poisoning
　Suffocation
　Trauma
[Physical regulation,
　　altered]
　Infection: risk
　Altered protection
　Thermoregulation,
　　ineffective
　　—Hypothermia
　　—Hyperthermia
Cardiac output,
　decreased
[Tissue perfusion,
　altered]
　Cardiopulmonary
　Cerebral
　Peripheral
[Fluid volume, altered]
　Deficit
　Deficit: risk
　Excess
　Imbalance
[Respiration, altered]
　Airway clearance,
　　ineffective
　Breathing pattern,
　　ineffective
　Gas exchange,
　　impaired
[Menstrual patterns]
[Premenstrual syndrome]

Energy Field Patterns

Nursing Diagnosis
(Altered/High Risk for/
Potential for Enhanced)

Energy field
disturbance

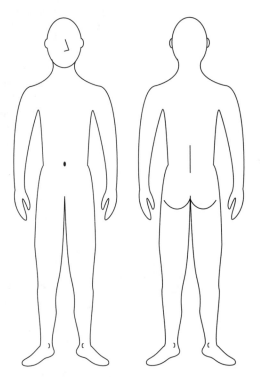

ADDITIONAL COMMENTS:

_____
_____
_____
_____
_____
_____
_____
_____
_____

Goals

1. _____
2. _____
3. _____
4. _____
5. _____

Prioritized Nursing Diagnosis/Problem
List/Theory-Based Plan of Care   **Date**

  1. _____   _____
  2. _____   _____
  3. _____   _____
  4. _____   _____
  5. _____   _____

Signature _____ Date _____

Holistic Nursing Care Plan

Name: _____   Client Goals:
Date: _____   1. _____
                                             2. _____
                                             3. _____
                                             4. _____

Nursing Diagnosis and Related Factors	*Client/Patient Outcomes Outcome Criteria*	*Therapeutic Intervention*	*Evaluation*

Client Signature_____

Date _____

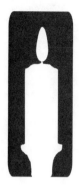

VISION OF HEALING
Actualization of Human Potentials

Each of us has the ability to achieve a balanced integration of human potentials: physical, mental, emotions, relationships, choices, and spirit. Effective self-care and self-healing depend on taking all these potentials into account. We are challenged to gain access to our inner wisdom and intuition and apply it in our daily lives. As we take responsibility for making effective choices and changes in our lives, we place ourselves in a better position to clarify our life patterns, purposes, and processes.

There are several ways to recognize and validate the healing work that we nurses do each day with our colleagues. After the beginning of shift report each day, for example, it may be possible to take a few minutes to share with each other different personal concerns that are in need of healing. One person may say, "When you think of me today, send me energy, because my sister is ill and I'm worried about her"; or "I'm grieving over Sarah's death last week, and my heart still aches." Another idea is to establish a certain time every other week to discuss healing moments that each person has experienced. Someone may have taught a patient a relaxation exercise that significantly reduced her anxiety; someone else may have learned a new technique to manage stress in the workplace. This time together can validate skills, as well as intuition, build trust, and develop a mutual appreciation that will facilitate the healing process in self and others.

An in-service education committee may develop a questionnaire to establish nurses' desires and needs to learn about specific skills necessary to promote healing. Some classes may be on self-nurturing, learning ways to increase skills of presence to serve and share with intention, therapeutic touch, or empowerment sessions.

Actualizing human potentials means first recognizing and then accepting all the potentials of our being, even those we wish to change. Developing our potentials requires a willingness to assess our position in life, to develop an action plan for change, and then to evaluate our new position in a lifelong process.

Chapter 15

Self-Assessments: Facilitating Healing in Self and Others

Barbara Montgomery Dossey and Lynn Keegan

NURSE HEALER OBJECTIVES

Theoretical

- List the six parts of the circle of human potential.
- Define biodance.

Clinical

- Identify specific areas in each potential that can increase and maximize a nurse's effectiveness in clinical practice.
- Seek ways to increase conscious attention to feelings, environment, relationships, life patterns, and processes in clinical practice.
- Use the self-assessment and the circle of human potential as interventions with clients.

Personal

- Tabulate your self-assessment score to determine if you are maximizing your human potential.
- Establish areas that you wish to focus on in order to create changes and choices that lead to new health behaviors.
- Increase your awareness of ways to gain access to your inner healing.

DEFINITIONS

Healing: a process of bringing all parts of one's self together at deep levels of inner knowing, leading toward an integration and balance, with each part having equal importance and value; also referred to as self-healing or wholeness.

Healing Awareness: the conscious recognition and focusing of attention on sensations, feelings, conditions, and facts dealing with needs of self or clients.

Nurse Healer: one who facilitates another person's growth and life process toward wholeness (body-mind-spirit connections) or who assists with recovery from illness or transition to peaceful death.

Process: the continual changing and evolution of one's self through life; the reflection of meaning and purpose in living.

Transpersonal Self: the self that transcends or goes beyond personal individual identity and meaning to include purpose, meaning, values, and unification with universal principles.

Transpersonal View: the state that occurs with a person's life maturity whereby the sense of self expands.

CIRCLE OF HUMAN POTENTIAL

The circle is an ancient symbol of wholeness. As seen in Figure 15-1, the circle of

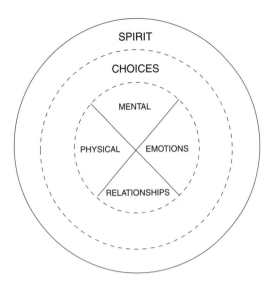

Figure 15-1 Circle of Human Potential

human potential has six areas: physical, mental, emotions, relationships, choices, and spirit. All are important parts of the self that are constantly interacting. When any one part becomes incomplete, the entire circle loses its completeness because all parts are necessary to maintain the whole. When people become aware of their strengths, as well as their weaknesses, they begin to move to their highest capabilities. The area of choices is surrounded by an inner and outer dotted circle to represent the idea that their continually evolving spiritual development guides what people consciously/unconsciously choose. Spirit is placed in the outer circle to show that it transcends all the other dimensions and helps to maximize our human potentials.

All people are complex feedback loops. As we learn about these feedback loops, we are able to understand our body-mind-spirit connections. Our bodies are in a constant state of change of which we are unaware. Life is a biodance, the endless exchange of all living things with the earth in which all living organisms participate. It exists not only as we live, but also as we die. We do not wait until death to make an

exchange with the earth, for we are constantly returning to the universe while alive. In every living moment, a portion of the 1,028 atoms in our body returns to the world outside. This is another idea of wholeness, which explains why the notion of "boundary" begins to seem an arbitrary idea rather than a physical reality.[1]

Assessing our human potential attunes us to our healing awareness; it is the innate quality with which all people are born. It must be developed in order to be actualized to the fullest. Healing is recognizing our feelings, attitudes, and emotions, which are not isolated, but are literally translated into body changes. Images cause internal events through mind modulation that simultaneously affects the autonomic, endocrine, immune, and neuropeptide systems (see Chapter 4). Everyone has the potential and choice to tap into this innate healing potential. When we acknowledge our body-mind-spirit relationships, true healing can occur. Times of stress and crisis in our daily routine can block self-healing. Therefore, it is necessary for us continually to assess and reassess our wholeness.

SELF-ASSESSMENTS

In order to maximize our human potentials, it is important to assess each aspect of our being: physical status, mental status, emotions, relationships, choices, and spirit. The self-assessments in Figures 15-2 through 15-7 help us more clearly identify our current positions in each of these areas.[2] Exhibit 15-1 explains the scoring.

The practice of self-assessment has mushroomed in the past several years as the number of assessment tools has increased and their use has become more common. There are now individualized tools for special interest groups. For example, a recent study provided evidence for the reliability and validity of a self-care instrument to measure the self-care component of the Abilities Assessment Instru-

PHYSICAL

Where I Am Now	Almost Always	Some-times	Almost Never	How I Want It To Be
Assess my general health daily	2	1	0	
Exercise 3 to 5 times a week for 20 minutes	2	1	0	
Eat nutritious foods daily	2	1	0	
Play without guilt	2	1	0	
Practice relaxation daily	2	1	0	
Energy level is effective for daily activities	2	1	0	
Do not smoke	2	1	0	
Drink in moderation	2	1	0	
Have regular physical and dental checkups	2	1	0	
Balance my work life with personal life	2	1	0	
Physical Score				

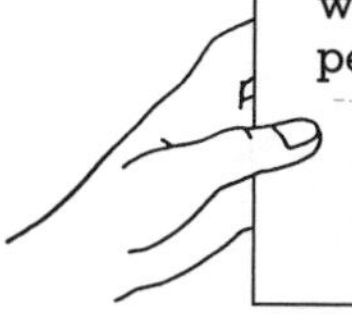

Figure 15–2 Physical Self-Assessment. *Source:* Reprinted with permission from L. Keegan and B. Dossey, *Self Care: A Program To Improve Your Life,* © 1987.

ment for elderly women.[3] Other new protocols are being offered as guidelines for clinicians to use in their assessment and management of the wellness spirituality of older adults.[4] Another new questionnaire has been used with college women to ascertain perceptions about body image, body self relations, and lifestyle behaviors.[5] Groups of people concerned with optimizing health are beginning to use self-

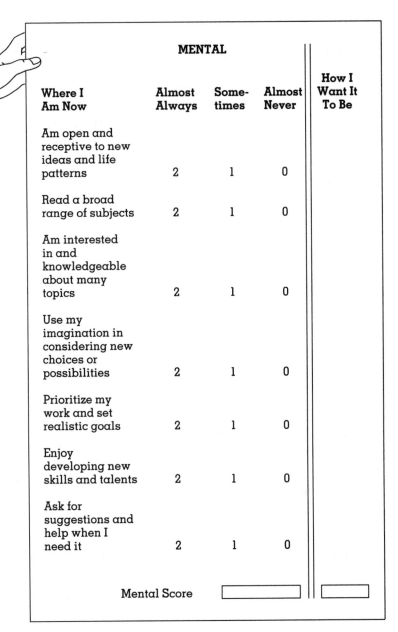

MENTAL				
Where I Am Now	Almost Always	Some-times	Almost Never	How I Want It To Be
Am open and receptive to new ideas and life patterns	2	1	0	
Read a broad range of subjects	2	1	0	
Am interested in and knowledgeable about many topics	2	1	0	
Use my imagination in considering new choices or possibilities	2	1	0	
Prioritize my work and set realistic goals	2	1	0	
Enjoy developing new skills and talents	2	1	0	
Ask for suggestions and help when I need it	2	1	0	
Mental Score				

Figure 15-3 Mental Self-Assessment. *Source:* Reprinted with permission from L. Keegan and B. Dossey, *Self Care: A Program To Improve Your Life,* © 1987.

assessment questionnaires. In Idaho at 1 of 25 annual statewide conferences for K–12 school personnel, self-assessment instruments are being used to monitor behavior change at 3 months, 6 months, and 1 year following conference participation.[6]

DEVELOPMENT OF HUMAN POTENTIALS

Physical Potential

All humans share the common biologic experiences of birth, gender, growth, ag-

EMOTIONS

Where I Am Now	Almost Always	Some-times	Almost Never	How I Want It To Be
Assess and recognize my own feelings	2	1	0	
Have a nonjudgmental attitude	2	1	0	
Express my feelings in appropriate ways	2	1	0	
Include my feelings when making decisions	2	1	0	
Can remember and acknowledge most events of my childhood including painful as well as happy ones	2	1	0	
Listen to and respect the feelings of others	2	1	0	
Recognize my intuition	2	1	0	
Listen to inner self-talk	2	1	0	
Emotions Score				

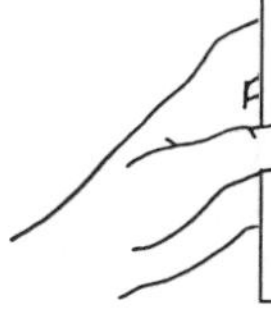

Figure 15–4 Self-Assessment of Emotions. *Source:* Reprinted with permission from L. Keegan and B. Dossey, *Self Care: A Program To Improve Your Life,* © 1987.

ing, and death. Once each person's basic biologic needs for food, shelter, and clothing have been met, there are many ways to seek wholeness of physical potential. Many elements influence physical potential; the major ones are physical awareness of proper nutrition, exercise, relaxation, and balance between work and play. Many people have become obsessed with these elements of the physical potential, but have failed to recognize that they are not separate from or more important than the

RELATIONSHIPS

Where I Am Now	Almost Always	Some-times	Almost Never	How I Want It To Be
I share my opinions and feelings without seeking the approval of others or fearing outcomes	2	1	0	
Create and participate in satisfying relationships	2	1	0	
Sexuality is part of my relationship	2	1	0	
Have a balance between my work and family life	2	1	0	
Am clear in expressing my needs and desires	2	1	0	
Am open and honest with people without fearing the consequences	2	1	0	
Do my part in establishing and maintaining relationships	2	1	0	
Focus on positive topics in relationships	2	1	0	
Relationships Score				

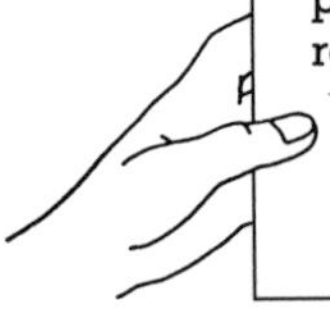

Figure 15–5 Self-Assessment of Relationships. *Source:* Reprinted with permission from L. Keegan and B. Dossey, *Self Care: A Program To Improve Your Life,* © 1987.

other potentials. Health is more than the absence of pain and symptoms; it is present when there is a balance. As we assess biologic needs, we must also take into consideration our perceptions of these areas. Many illnesses have been docu-mented as stress-related, because our consciousness plays a major role in health and physical potential.

Our body is a gift to nurture and respect. As we nurture ourselves, we increase our uniqueness in energy, sexuality, vitality,

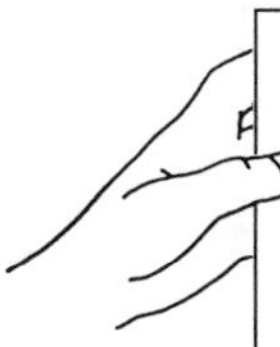

CHOICES				
Where I Am Now	**Almost Always**	**Some-times**	**Almost Never**	**How I Want It To Be**
Manage my time to meet my personal goals	2	1	0	
Am committed and disciplined whenever I take on new projects	2	1	0	
Follow through and work on decisions with clarity and action steps	2	1	0	
Am usually clear on decisions	2	1	0	
Take risks	2	1	0	
Can accept circumstances that are beyond my control	2	1	0	
Take on no more new tasks than I can successfully handle	2	1	0	
Recognize shortcomings of people and events for what they are	2	1	0	
Choices Score				

Figure 15-6 Self-Assessment of Choices. *Source:* Reprinted with permission from L. Keegan and B. Dossey, *Self Care: A Program To Improve Your Life,* © 1987.

and capacity for language and connection with our other potentials. This nurturance strengthens our self-image, which causes several things to happen. First, our body-mind-spirit responds in a positive and integrated fashion. Second, we become a role model with a positive influence on others. Finally, we actually enhance our general

SPIRIT

Where I Am Now	Almost Always	Some- times	Almost Never	How I Want It To Be
Operate from the perspective that life has value, meaning, and direction	2	1	0	
Know at some level a connection with the universe	2	1	0	
Know some Power greater than myself	2	1	0	
Feel a part of life and living frequently	2	1	0	
Recognize that the different roles of my life are expressions of my true self	2	1	0	
Know how to create balance and feel a sense of connectedness	2	1	0	
Know that life is important, and I make a difference	2	1	0	
Spirit Score	☐			☐

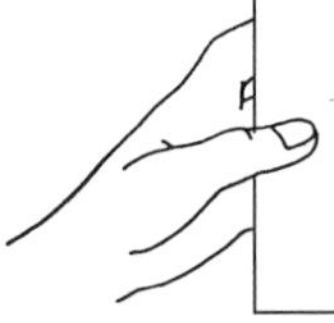

Figure 15–7 Spirit Self-Assessment. *Source:* Reprinted with permission from L. Keegan and B. Dossey, *Self Care: A Program To Improve Your Life,* © 1987.

feeling of well-being. It is impossible to gain such strengths or empowerment without these changes being manifest and influencing the lives of other people.

Mental Potential

Early in our lives, we have various role models who influence our thoughts, behav-

Exhibit 15–1 Meaning of the Tallied Scores

Scores of 14 to 20

Congratulations! Your score shows that you are aware of the important areas of your life. You are using your knowledge to work for you by practicing good life patterns that reflect health and balance. As long as you continue with high scores, you will be maximizing your human potential. You are a good model of health to family and friends. Since your score is high in this area, move to other areas where your scores are low and identify areas for improvement.

Scores of 10 to 13

Your life patterns in this area are good, but there is room for improvement. Reflect on the "Sometimes or Almost Never" answers. What could you do to change your score? Even the slightest change can make a difference to improve the quality of your life.

Scores of 6 to 9

Your life stressors are showing. You need more information about these important life areas and what changes you can make. Read on to obtain guidance.

Scores of 0 to 5

Your life is full of unnecessary stress. You are not taking good care of yourself. You need to take some time and learn the principles of self-care.

When you finish this exercise you have a composite picture not only of where you are now, but where you want to go. ENJOY THE JOURNEY!

Source: Copyright © L. Keegan and B. Dossey.

---

logical mental processes, we become interested in a broad range of subjects and expand our full appreciation of the many great pleasures in life. Not only should we increase our awareness of ways to use both logical and intuitive thought, but also we should increase our skills to create better simultaneous integration of both ways of knowing.

With such interventions as relaxation and imagery, we learn to be present in the moment. It is during these moments that we release our critical inner voice that is constantly judging in self-dialogue. These are the moments when we expand our mental knowing. As we increase our openness and receptivity to information and suggestions, mental growth can occur. Every aspect of our life is a learning experience and becomes part of a lesson in changing.

Emotions Potential

Involved in our emotions potential are our willingness to acknowledge the presence of feelings and value them as important, and the ability to express them. Emotional health implies that we have the choice and freedom to express love, joy, guilt, fear, and anger. The expression of these emotions can give us immediate feedback about our inner state, which may be crying out for a new way of being.[7]

Emotions are responses to the events in our lives. True healing occurs when we confront both positive and negative intense emotions. Various degrees of chronic anxiety, depression, worry, fear, guilt, anger, denial, or repression result from our failure to confront our emotions. One of the greatest challenges we have is to acknowledge, own, express, and understand our emotions. We are living systems who constantly make exchanges with our environment. All life events affect our emotions and general well-being.

As we become more balanced in living, we allow our humanness to develop. We

iors, and values. As we mature and gain life experience, shifts occur in our thinking, our behavior, and our values. Conflicts develop when we do not take the time to examine our new perceptions and discard old beliefs and values that no longer fit.

Our challenge is to create accurate perceptions of the world through our mental potential. Through both logical and non-reach out and ask for human dialogue that is meaningful. Increasing the emotions potential allows spontaneity and a positive, healthy zest for living to emerge. We must be aware of and take responsibility for expression that allows spirit and intuition to flower. It is important to have a consistent harmony between thought processes and emotions, as disharmony causes dissonance.

Emotions are gifts. Frequently, a first step toward releasing a burden in a relationship is to share deep feelings with another. There is no such thing as a good or bad emotion; each is part of the human condition. Emotions exist as the light and shadow of the self; thus, we must acknowledge all of them. They create the dance of life, the polarity of living. The only reason that we can identify the light is that we know its opposite, the shadow. When we see the value in both types of emotions, we are in a position of new insight and new understanding, and we can make more effective choices. As we increase our attention to body-mind-spirit interrelationships, we can focus on the emotions that move us toward wholeness and inner understanding.

Relationships Potential

Healthy people live in intricate networks of relationships and are always in search of new, unifying concepts of the universe and social order. Human beings need to explore and develop meaningful relationships. A healthy person simply cannot live in isolation. In a given day, we interact with many people—immediate family, extended family, colleagues at work, neighbors in the community, and numerous people in organizations. Because we spend at least half of our awake time with colleagues at work, we must support and nourish these relationships. We must also extend our networks to include our nation and planet Earth. Each of us must take an active role in developing local networks of

relationships that can have a ripple effect on global concerns.

Relationships have different levels of meaning, from the superficial to the deeply connected. The challenge in relationships is to extend ourselves and to learn to exchange feelings of honesty, trust, intimacy, compassion, openness, and harmony. Sharing life processes requires a true interchange between self and others. Only when we increase our awareness and intention can we promote such interchanges with our family, friends, work colleagues, clients, and community at large. As we increase our network from one person to another, the fact that one contact leads to many more extends our boundaries even further.

It is essential that we identify the cohesiveness in our relationships, as well as the disharmony. We must be aware of the impact that we have on clients, family, and friends. Something always happens when people come together, for life is never a neutral event. Our attitudes, healing awareness, and concern for self and others have a direct effect on the outcome of all our encounters.

Choices Potential

People have an enormous capacity for both conscious and unconscious choices in their lives. Conscious choices involve awareness and skills, such as discipline, persistence, goal setting, priorities, action steps, knowledge of options, and recognition of perceptions. We can enhance our awareness, knowledge, and new skills for living and be active participants in daily living, not passive observers who hope that life will be good to us.

The unconscious also plays a major role in our choices.[8] Jung conceived of the unconscious as a series of layers. Those closest to our awareness may become known; those farthest away are, in principle, inaccessible to our awareness and operate autonomously. Jung saw the unconscious as the home of timeless psychic forces that he called archetypes, which generally are invariant throughout all cultures and eras. He felt that every psychic force has its opposite in the unconsciousness—the force of light is always counterposed with that of darkness, good with evil, love with hate, life with death, etc. Jung believed that any psychic energy could become unbalanced and that life's greatest challenge was to achieve a dynamic balance of the innate opposites and to make this balancing process as conscious as possible.

Each of us is responsible for assessing our own values and desires. No one else can make decisions for us. When we do not exercise our ability to make choices, the values of others are imposed on us, and we never reach our highest potential. Choice involves taking risks. We may make some mistakes along the way, but we also gain experience.

Continuing to develop clarity in life enables us to meet goals. A simple process for changing behavior is to learn to change perception. Changing all the "shoulds" in our thoughts and actions to "I could, and I have a choice" is a good place to start. For example, "I should be more loving" can become "I could be more loving, and I have a choice." We create more effective choices when we take the time not to be judgmental and to release fears and guilt. We can all change, and it is a skill of awareness to acknowledge that we are worth the effort.

Spirit Potential

Throughout history, there has been a quest to understand the purpose of human life experience. Humankind is incomplete unless the human condition for transcendence evolves (see Chapters 1, 2, and 5). Spirit comes from our roots—the universal need to understand the human experience of life on earth. It is the vital element and the driving force in how we live our lives. It impacts every aspect of our life choices and the degree to which we develop our human potentials. Spirit involves the development of our higher self, also referred to as the transpersonal self. A transpersonal experience or transcendence is described as a feeling of oneness, inner peace, harmony, and wholeness and connection with the universe.[9-14] The meaning and joy that flow from developing this aspect of our human potential allow us to have a transpersonal view. Some of the ways we may come to know this transcendence are through prayer, meditation, organized religion, philosophy, science, poetry, music, inspired friends, and group work.

Like the other potentials, spirit potential does not develop without some attention. Every day, with each of our experiences, we need to acknowledge that our spirit potential is essential to the development of a healthy value system. We shape our perception of the world through our value system, and our perceptions will influence whether we have positive or negative experiences. Even through the pain of a negative experience, we have the ability to learn. Pain can be a great teacher. On the other side of the experience is new wisdom, self-discovery, and the chance for making new choices based on wisdom.

AFFIRMATIONS

As strong, positive statements acknowledging that something is already so, affirmations can help us change our perceptions and beliefs. If we believe an affirmation to be true, our perceptions selectively reinforce it because we change our self-talk. Our mind is constantly engaged in dialogue with ourselves; in fact, the person we talk to the most in a day is the self. Self-talk even operates in our unconscious through dreams while we sleep. Thus, an important way to influence our unconscious is to focus on positive images and affirmations before we drift to sleep and immediately on awakening. Positive images and affirmations also reinforce those things that have meaning and value. They help us in our spiritual development because they move into the deep layers of the unconscious, become part of our myths, and influence our daily lives.

If our thoughts are hopeful and optimistic, our body responds with confidence, energy, and hope. If negative thoughts dominate, however, our body responds with tightness, uneasiness, and an increase in breathing, blood pressure, and heart rate. Affirmations are statements we select to affirm our intentions and choices; they can help us

- identify what is true for us so that the truth can manifest itself in behavior and more options
- clarify goals, take actions, and conduct self-evaluations
- assume more responsibility for our actions, thoughts, beliefs, and values
- envision a new way of being

PHYSICAL

- I assess my general health daily.
- I exercise three to five times a week for 20 minutes.
- I eat nutritious food daily.
- I play without guilt.
- I practice relaxation daily.
- I have energy levels effective for daily activities.
- I do not smoke.
- I drink in moderation.
- I have regular physical and dental checkups.
- I balance my work life with my personal life.

EMOTIONS

- I assess and recognize my own feelings.
- I have a nonjudgmental attitude.
- I express my feelings in appropriate ways.
- I consider my feelings when making decisions.
- I acknowledge both happy and painful memories.
- I listen to and respect the feelings of others.
- I recognize my intuition.
- I listen to inner self-talk.

MENTAL

- I am open and receptive to new ideas and life patterns.
- I read a broad range of subjects.
- I am interested in and knowledgeable about many topics.
- I use my imagination in considering new choices or possibilities.
- I prioritize my work and set realistic goals.
- I enjoy developing new skills and talents.
- I ask for suggestions and help when I need it.

RELATIONSHIPS

- I share my opinions and feelings without seeking the approval of others or fearing outcomes.
- I create and participate in satisfying relationships.
- I allow sexuality to be a part of my relationships.
- I have a balance between my work and my family life.
- I am clear in expressing my needs and desires.
- I am open and honest with people without fearing the consequences.
- I do my part in establishing and maintaining relationships.
- I focus on positive topics in relationships.

CHOICES

- I manage time to meet my personal goals.
- I am committed and disciplined whenever I take on new projects.
- I follow through and work on decisions with clarity and action steps.
- I am usually clear on decisions.
- I take risks.
- I can accept circumstances beyond my control.
- I take on no more new tasks than I can successfully handle.

SPIRIT

- I operate from the perspective that life has value, meaning, and direction.
- I know, at some level, a connection with the universe.
- I know some power greater than myself.
- I feel a part of life and living frequently.
- I recognize that the different roles of my life are expressions of my true self.
- I know how to create balance and a sense of connectedness.

CONCLUSION

No matter where we are, each of our human potentials affects our whole being. Our challenge in all aspects of our personal and professional lives is to strive to integrate all our human potentials. When we assess our human potentials and decide how we want our lives to be, we evoke meaning and purpose in life. If one area of our human potential is left undeveloped, things do not seem to be as good as they could be. When one strives to develop all areas, however, a sense of wholeness emerges, one's self-worth increases, and life goals are actualized. Being alive becomes more exciting, rewarding, and fulfilling. Even when frustrations arise, the whole person is able to recognize choices and decrease the barriers to maximizing human potentials.

DIRECTIONS FOR FUTURE RESEARCH

1. Determine if the percentage of desired client outcomes increases when the nurse uses the circle of human potential as an assessment tool and a nursing intervention.

2. Determine if the nurse's self-esteem increases when the concepts of the circle of human potential and affirmations are integrated each day.
3. Determine if the client's self-esteem increases when the concepts of the circle of human potential and affirmations are taught.
4. Evaluate changes in behavior and perceived quality of life when clients learn awareness skills in regard to their human potentials.

NURSE HEALER REFLECTIONS

After reading this chapter, the nurse healer will be able to answer or begin a process of answering the following questions:

- What is my process when I assess my circle of human potentials?
- Am I consciously aware of the daily opportunity to manifest my own human potentials?
- What can I do to increase my conscious awareness of fully participating in living?
- How do I feel when I use the word healer to describe myself?
- What is my inner awareness when I acknowledge my healing potential?

NOTES

1. L. Dossey, *Space, Time and Medicine* (Boston: Shambhala, 1982).

2. L. Keegan and B. Dossey, *Self Care: A Program To Improve Your Life*, 1987.

3. C.M. Lyle and D.L. Wells, Description of a Self-Care Instrument for Elders, *Western Journal of Nursing Research* 19, no. 5 (1997):637–653.

4. M.C. Leetun, Wellness Spirituality in the Older Adult: Assessment and Intervention Protocol, *Nurse Practitioner* 21, no. 8 (1996):65–70.

5. E. Koff and C.L. Bauman, Effects of Wellness, Fitness, and Sport Skills Programs on Body Image and Lifestyle Behaviors, *Perceptual and Motor Skills* 82, no. 2 (1997):555–562.

6. L.L. Rankin and J.G. Mathews, Health Practices of Educators Participating in an Idaho Wellness Conference: One Year Follow-up, *Journal of School Health* 68, no. 1 (1998):18–21.

7. L. Keegan, *Nurse As Healer* (Albany, NY: Delmar Publishers, 1994).

8. L. Dossey, *Healing Words: The Power of Prayer and the Practice of Medicine* (San Francisco: Harper San Francisco, 1993).

9. J. Achterberg et al., *Rituals of Healing: Using Imagery for Health and Wellness* (New York: Bantam Books, 1994).

10. T. Moore, *Care of the Soul* (New York: Harper-Collins, 1992).

11. P. Burkhardt and M. Nagai-Jacobson, Reawakening Spirit in Clinical Practice, *Journal of Holistic Nursing* 12, no. 1 (1994):9–21.

12. J. Kornfield, *A Path with Heart* (New York: Bantam Books, 1993).

13. L. Dossey, *Recovering the Soul: A Scientific and Spiritual Search* (New York: Bantam Books, 1989).

14. L. Dossey, *Meaning and Medicine: Lessons from a Doctor's Tales of Breakthrough and Healing* (New York: Bantam Books, 1991).

VISION OF HEALING

Changing Outcomes

Whatever we focus on expands.

Glenda Lippman[1]

Because our thinking influences the way that we interpret our world, changing our thoughts can change our physical and emotional interaction with society. As clients share their inner dialogue and interpretation of events with nurses, we are allowed glimpses into their distinctive world view.

Our inner conversation forms a backdrop against which our lives unfold; if it is optimistic and affirmative, our actions and attitudes take on a positive tone. If, on the other hand, the inner conversation is negative and bleak, so follows our behavior, and in some cases, our mental and physical health. Gently helping clients identify discrepancies between their thoughts and reality allows them to bring the world into a clearer focus. By examining the silent dialogue that accompanies every interaction with the outer world, identifying false assumptions, distortions, and misinterpretations, clients can choose to make healthy changes. Sensitive questions, frequent restatement of clients' accounts of their perceptions, and requests for clarification will help guide the nurses and clients on the road to accurate interpretation of events, thoughts, and feelings.

Caregivers should proceed into the inner world of the clients' minds with reverence and respect. We are only guests in that world and must facilitate healthy redirection with regard for the multitude of unknown stories that contribute to the wholeness of our clients.

NOTE

1. Personal communication.

Chapter 16

Cognitive Therapy

Eileen M. Stuart-Shor and Carol L. Wells-Federman

NURSE HEALER OBJECTIVES

Theoretical

- Define cognitive therapy.
- Identify the three main principles of cognitive therapy.
- Discuss the connection between cognition(s), health, and illness.
- Identify four major contributors to the development of cognitive therapy.
- Compare and contrast potential bio-psycho-social-spiritual-behavioral responses to stress and their effects on health and illness.
- Discuss the roles of contracting and goal setting in cognitive restructuring.

Clinical

- Discuss the major diagnoses and health problems that respond favorably to cognitive therapy.
- Describe ways to facilitate cognitive restructuring.
- Identify stress warning signals.
- Describe and identify automatic thoughts.
- Describe and identify cognitive distortions and irrational beliefs.
- Describe a simple model for cognitive restructuring.
- Outline the guidelines for organizing a cognitive therapy session.

- Explore different practice settings in which cognitive restructuring can be used.
- Evaluate client progress toward goals by assessing both short-term and long-term goals of therapy.

Personal

- Identify stress warning signals.
- In response to stress: Stop, take a breath, reflect on the cause of the stress, and choose a more healthy response.
- Develop a list of meaningful personal rewards.
- Begin a healthy lifestyles/healthy pleasures journal.

DEFINITIONS

Cognition: the act or process of knowing.

Cognitive: of or relating to consciousness, or being conscious; pertaining to intellectual activities (such as as thinking, reasoning, imagining).

Cognitive Distortions: inaccurate, irrational thoughts; mistakes in thinking.

Cognitive Restructuring: examining and reframing one's interpretation of the meaning of an event.

Cognitive Therapy: a therapeutic approach that addresses the relationships among thoughts, feelings, behaviors, and physiology.

THEORY AND RESEARCH

Historically, cognitive therapy is rooted in the treatment of anxiety and depression; however, in the last 10 years its application has broadened greatly. This chapter explores the application of cognitive therapy in the context of nursing practice along the wellness–illness continuum and the bio-psycho-social-spiritual domains. Cognitive therapy is integrated into expert nursing practice in myriad ways, which are discussed throughout this chapter. In addition, the unique perspective that nurse healers bring to the application of cognitive therapy is addressed.

Cognitive therapy is based on the premise that stress and suffering are caused by *perception*, or the way people think, and postulates that the thoughts which create stress are often distorted. These negative thoughts can affect emotions, behaviors, and physiology and can influence the individual's beliefs. By changing negative thoughts, specifically those that trigger and perpetuate distress, the individual can change physical and emotional states.

In this chapter, understanding of the relationship between negative thoughts that trigger and perpetuate stress and changes in physical and emotional states is drawn from the biopsychosocial model.[1] The dimension of spirituality has been added to Engel's existing model.[2] In this eclectic bio-psycho-social-spiritual model, there is a tacit understanding that stress, or the perception of threat, can lead to changes in physical, emotional, behavioral, and spiritual states. If we accept that stress causes changes in physical and emotional states and is influenced by *perception*, and if we accept that *perception* is influenced by distorted thinking patterns (negative thoughts), then we have created a link between cognitive therapy, which restructures distorted, negative thinking patterns, and mind-body interactions, which influence health and illness. This link has implications for health promotion, symptom reduction, and disease management. Because understanding the dynamic interaction of cognitive therapy and the psychophysiology of mind-body connections is fundamental to the application of cognitive therapy in nursing, it is explored in greater detail later in this chapter.

Cognitive therapy was first used as a short-term treatment for depression and anxiety that focused on helping people to recognize automatic, distorted thoughts and to change those thoughts that trigger and perpetuate distress.[3] It is now being applied successfully to reduce health-risking behaviors, physical symptoms, and the emotional sequelae of a variety of illnesses to which stress is an important causative or contributing factor.[4] It is also useful in value clarification, which is the first step in establishing meaningful health goals.[5]

Cognitive therapy has ancient origins. A century ago, the Greek philosopher Epictetus described how people are most often disturbed not by the things that happen to them but by the opinions they have about those things. Theorists including Beck,[6] Ellis,[7] Meichenbaum,[8] and Burns[9] have advanced the modern interpretation of cognitive therapy. In the late 1960s, Beck conceptualized cognitive theory as a model to treat depression and anxiety and developed effective intervention strategies to restructure cognitive distortions and successfully mitigate the symptoms of depression and anxiety. Ellis developed the approach known as rational-emotive therapy to recognize and challenge distorted thinking. Ellis was particularly interested in uncovering those beliefs and assumptions that people hold as absolutes and that provide the lens (or filter of life experience) that causes distortions. Meichenbaum and Burns further enhanced the theory and practice of cognitive therapy through research and clinical experience.

Research on cognitive therapy continues to provide evidence of its broad application to both psychologic and physical health problems. In a 30-year retrospective, Beck provided a comprehensive overview of several important outcome studies.[10] He cited a meta-analysis of 27 studies that demonstrated the efficacy of cognitive therapy in treating unipolar depression and its superiority to other treatment methods, including antidepressant drug therapy. He also referenced five published studies that indicated that the use of cognitive therapy to treat depression is more effective in maintaining gains and preventing relapses than is antidepressant drug therapy. The review cited literature that demonstrates a nearly complete reduction of panic attacks after 12–16 weeks of treatment. Successful application of cognitive therapy to treat generalized anxiety disorder, eating disorders, heroin addiction, and inpatient depression has been reported.

Empirical evidence continues to grow in support of the application of cognitive therapy to treat a wide variety of physical symptoms. Emmelkamp and van Oppen[11] published an overview of the contribution of cognitive approaches to a reduction in physical symptoms and emotional sequelae of hypertension, bulimia, chronic pain, tension headache, acquired immunodeficiency syndrome (AIDS), cancer, and asthma. Other authors have reported its effective use to treat insomnia,[12] infertility,[13] and medically unexplained physical symptoms.[14] In addition to improving health outcomes, cognitive therapy has been shown to be cost effective as an intervention strategy in behavioral medicine.[15]

Effects of Cognition on Health and Illness

Stress (the *perception* of a threat to one's well-being, and the *perception* that one cannot cope) can cause physical, psychologic, behavioral, and spiritual changes.[16] Both cognition (the way one thinks) and perception (the way one views, interprets, or experiences someone or something) are important to an understanding of cognitive restructuring. If individuals change the way they think (cognition), they may change their perception of the situation. And if they change their perception of a situation so that they no longer view that situation as threatening, they will not experience stress. Thus, changing thoughts and perceptions can influence physiologic, psychologic, behavioral, and spiritual processes. The following paragraphs delineate the effects of stress on physical, psychologic, social/behavioral, and spiritual pathways.

Physiologic Effects of Stress

In response to a perceived threat (stress), the body gears up to meet the challenge. This perception of threat (stress) stimulates a cascade of biochemical events initiated by the central nervous system (Figure16–1).[17] Termed the *fight or flight response*[18] and later the *stress response*,[19] this heightened state of sympathetic arousal prepares the body for vigorous physical activity. Repeated exposure to daily hassles or prolonged stress activates the musculoskeletal system, increasing tension and rigidity. Concurrently, the autonomic nervous system, via the sympathetic branch, produces a generalized arousal that includes increased heart rate, blood pressure, and respiratory rate. In addition, there is a heightened awareness of the environment, shifting of blood from the visceral organs to the large muscle groups, altered lipid metabolism,[20] and increased platelet aggregability.[21] The neuroendocrine system, in response to stimulation of the hypothalamic-pituitary-adrenal axis and the secretion of corticosteroids and minerolocorticoids, increases glucose levels, influences sodium retention, and increases the anti-inflammatory response in the acute phase. Over time, however, immune function decreases.[22] In addition, levels of other hormones regulated by the neu-

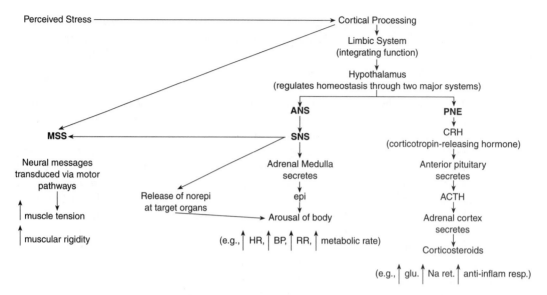

Figure 16-1 Stress Response. ACTH = adrenocorticotropic hormone; ANS = autonomic nervous system; BP = blood pressure; epi = epinephrine; glu. = blood glucose level; HR = heart rate; MSS = musculoskeletal system; Na ret. = sodium retention; norepi = norepinephrine; PNE = pituitary-neuroendocrine system; RR = respiratory rate; SNS = sympathetic nervous system. *Source:* Reprinted with permission from C.L. Wells-Federman, et al., *Clinical Nurse Specialist,* Vol. 9, No. 1, p. 60, © 1995, Williams & Wilkins.

roendocrine system, such as reproductive and growth hormones, endorphins, and encephalins, can be affected.

Prolonged or repeated exposure to stress has been shown to cause or exacerbate disease or symptoms of diseases such as angina, cardiac dysrhythmias, pain, tension headaches, insomnia, and gastrointestinal complaints. This influence is documented in extensive experimental and clinical literature.[23] Interestingly, but not surprisingly, Cohen and colleagues[24] found that, under stressful conditions, individuals are more likely to catch the common cold.

Psychologic Effects of Stress

The psychologic effects of stress are manifested by negative mood states such as anxiety, depression, hostility, and anger. These emotions (mood states) can in turn negatively influence a person's ability to concentrate and effectively problem solve. In addition, a growing body of evidence documents the correlation between prolonged negative mood states and increased morbidity and mortality in certain diseases. One such example is the relationship between anxiety and hypertension. The Framingham heart study found that, among middle-aged men, anxiety levels measured two decades earlier predicted the occurrence of hypertension.[25] Similarly, Williams and colleagues[26] found that increased measures of hostility at age 18 predicted hypertension at age 45. Depression has been shown to be associated with increased risk for morbidity and mortality, particularly from cardiovascular disease.[27]

Concurrently, a growing body of research supports the importance of controlling stress in the treatment of many diseases. Cancer and other diseases of the immune system have been shown to respond to interventions that reduce the stress response, as have arthritis, chronic pain, hypertension, cardiac dysrhythmias, insomnia, premenstrual syndrome, infertility, and the nausea and vomiting associated with chemotherapy.[28-32]

Kobasa[33] detailed the benefits of developing a positive attitude and approach to stress. Individuals with what they described as stress-hardy characteristics who also exercised and enjoyed social support were shown to be less vulnerable to stress-related symptoms and diseases. The characteristics of stress-hardiness are *control, challenge,* and *commitment.* For individuals with these characteristics, stress is seen as a *challenge* rather than a threat; they feel in *control* of situations in their lives and are *committed* to, rather than alienated from, work, home, and family.

Better health has also been associated with an optimistic explanatory style. The link between optimism and health was made by researchers tracking the lives of a group of Harvard graduates from the class of 1945.[34] They found that individuals who were optimistic in college were healthier in later life, whereas those who were pessimistic were less healthy. By middle age, pessimists experienced more health problems. It is theorized that a pessimistic explanatory style or attitude, in addition to adversely affecting behavior, may weaken the immune system through a prolonged increase in sympathetic arousal. For example, pessimists have more health-risking behaviors such as smoking, alcohol misuse, and sedentary lifestyle. Recognizing the influence of explanatory style on health and well-being furthers the understanding of how thoughts, feelings, behaviors, and physiology interact.

Social/Behavioral Effects of Stress

In response to stress, people often revert to less healthy behaviors. The *social/behavioral pathway* is best illustrated by appreciating the effect of behavior patterns on the incidence and progression of disease. How and what people eat, drink, and smoke, as well as how they take prescribed or illegal drugs, has important influence on health. For many, stressful events can increase behaviors such as overeating or excessive intake of alcohol. As stress increases, self-control decreases. Lapse to behaviors that provide immediate gratification is more likely when stress is high. This inability to control health-risking behaviors as a result of increased stress is called the *stress-disinhibition effect.*[35]

Behaviors such as social isolation that may be influenced by stress and negative thinking patterns have been shown to be associated with higher morbidity and mortality in the first year after myocardial infarction.[36] Conversely, social support has been found to have a positive effect on health outcome in medical settings. A report by Frasure-Smith and Prince[37] revealed that among patients hospitalized for myocardial infarction, those receiving social support through nurses' visits after discharge had a significantly lower risk of a second event compared with those in a control group. The authors theorized that positive changes in the emotional state of patients in the experimental group modulated the stress response.

Positive health outcomes in labor and delivery appear to be affected by emotional support as well. The most common surgical procedure performed in the United States is Caesarean section (C-section). Delivery by C-section increases the risk of complications for mother and child as well as extends hospital stay. The presence of a supportive woman during labor and delivery has been shown to reduce the need for C-section, shorten labor and delivery time, and reduce perinatal problems.[38,39] The benefits of social support to both patient's health and the health care system can easily be seen from these studies.

Recent research on programs that influence behavior change have shown positive modification of some of the most widespread diseases. Lifestyle behavior change has been demonstrated to cause regression of coronary atherosclerosis.[40–42] Fiatarone and colleagues[43] were able to counteract muscle weakness and physical frailty in very old individuals by adding high-intensity resistance exercise to their daily routines. These are only a few of the hundreds of studies that provide continuing evidence of the multidirectional relationships among thoughts, feelings, beliefs, behaviors, and physiology.

Spiritual Effects of Stress

In response to stress, people can become disconnected from life's meaning and purpose. Frankl,[44] in *Man's Search for Meaning*, draws a parallel between connection with life's meaning and survival. He describes the survivors of the World War II concentration camps as being those individuals who were able to retain their sense of meaning and purpose, and to draw meaning and purpose from this experience. A feeling of disconnection, however, in addition to being an effect of stress, can also be a precursor to stress. Several studies have examined the effects of spirituality, defined as connection with life's meaning and purpose, on health.[45–47] Increased scores on measures of spirituality correlated with increased incidence of health-promoting behaviors.[48] Other studies have explored the association between religious affiliation and health and have found a positive correlation.[49–52] This area of study is of considerable interest in the scientific literature today.

COGNITIVE THERAPY

In the preceding pages, a foundation has been established for how cognitions, which are exquisitely sensitive to perception, can influence physiologic, psychologic, social/behavioral, and spiritual processes. Because of this influence, cognitive therapy is an important intervention in optimizing the positive links between mind, body, and spirit and in minimizing the negative consequences of adverse interactions. Cognitive therapy helps individuals reappraise or reevaluate their thinking. It is often referred to as *cognitive restructuring* because the intent of the intervention is to change or restructure the distortions in thinking patterns that cause stress. The basic principles of cognitive therapy are the following:[53–55]

- Our thoughts, not external events, create our moods.
- The thoughts that cause stress are usually unrealistic, distorted, and negative.
- Distorted, illogical thoughts and self-defeating beliefs lead to physiologic changes and painful feelings, such as depression, anxiety, and anger.
- By changing maladaptive, unrealistic, distorted thoughts, individuals can change how they feel (physically and emotionally).

The goals[56] of cognitive therapy include training clients to

- Pinpoint the negative automatic thoughts and silent assumptions that trigger and perpetuate their emotional upsets.
- Identify the distortions, irrational beliefs, or *cognitive errors.*
- Substitute more realistic, self-enhancing thoughts, which will reduce the stress, symptoms, and/or painful feelings.
- Replace self-defeating *silent assumptions* with more reasonable belief systems.
- Develop improved social skills, as well as coping, communication, and empathic skills.

The Process of Cognitive Therapy

The nurse provider serves as a guide in the process of cognitive therapy. Unlike in biomedical interventions, the provider cannot perform this intervention to or for the client but guides the individual to do it for himself or herself. There is no way to predict what will surface during the therapy or what meaning it will have to the individual. The nurse must honor the premise that each individual can best interpret his or her own experience(s), belief(s), and/or distortion(s).

Step I: Awareness

Developing awareness is the first step in a systematic approach to guide clients to a restructuring of their cognitive distortions. Clients are asked to bring to their conscious awareness two things. First is an awareness of how negative thoughts and silent assumptions influence them physically, emotionally, behaviorally, and spiritually. Second is an awareness that a process (silent assumptions, irrational beliefs, and cognitive distortions) underlie these automatic negative thoughts. To facilitate development of this awareness, a four-step approach is used to explore a stressful situation systematically. Clients are asked to *stop* (break the cycle of "awfulizing," escalating thoughts—become aware that a stress has taken place); ***take a breath*** (release physical tension, promote relaxation—become aware of physical changes that have occurred in response to stress); ***reflect*** (realize what is going on—become aware of automatic thoughts, distortions, beliefs, assumptions); and ***choose*** (decide how to respond—become aware of choices in responding).[57]

Clients are first asked to identify their warning signals of stress. Exhibit 16–1 is a sample form for identifying and recording this information. These cues (or signals) can be physical, emotional, behavioral, or spiritual. When asked to monitor responses to a particular event, clients become more consciously aware of these cues. Exhibit 16–2 is an example of a format for recording this information. Although it may initially increase an individual's perception of physical pain or emotional discomfort, conscious awareness is a necessary first step in recognizing the relationship of thoughts, feelings, behavior, and biology to distorted thinking patterns.

Often, clients have long ignored the cues their minds or bodies give them. Consider the client with disabling headaches who often ignores the shoulder and neck tension that precede his headaches. Had he attended to his early stress warning signs (neck and shoulder tension), he might have avoided the headache. Becoming aware of these stress warning signs is the first step. Attending to the cues is the next. Once they make this connection, clients can much more easily develop skills to reduce negative mood states, unhealthy behaviors, and physical symptoms. To continue with the example above, it is easier to stop a tension headache when the client notices shoulder tension and stops, takes a few deep diaphragmatic breaths, and gently stretches the area than to wait for the headache to become incapacitating before acting.

> **Exercise:** Ask the client to identify his or her stress warning signals. Then, have the client identify a stressful experience and the physical or emotional reaction to this particular experience. For example, after being instructed to stop, take a breath, and notice the physical and emotional response to a stressful situation, one client related the following:
>
> *On my way home from work yesterday I sat in traffic. I noticed that my hands were gripping the steering wheel, my neck and shoulders were tight, and my jaw was clenched. I felt angry and frustrated because I wanted to be home.*

Becoming aware of stress warning signals is an important first step. Although this seems very straightforward, the average

Exhibit 16–1 Stress Warning Signals

Physical Symptoms
- ❏ Headaches
- ❏ Indigestion
- ❏ Stomachaches
- ❏ Sweaty palms
- ❏ Sleep difficulties
- ❏ Dizziness
- ❏ Back pain
- ❏ Tight neck, shoulders
- ❏ Racing heart
- ❏ Restlessness
- ❏ Tiredness
- ❏ Ringing in ears

Behavioral Symptoms
- ❏ Excess smoking
- ❏ Bossiness
- ❏ Compulsive gum chewing
- ❏ Attitude critical of others
- ❏ Grinding of teeth at night
- ❏ Overuse of alcohol
- ❏ Compulsive eating
- ❏ Inability to get things done

Emotional Symptoms
- ❏ Crying
- ❏ Nervousness, anxiety
- ❏ Boredom—no meaning to things
- ❏ Edginess—ready to explode
- ❏ Feeling powerless to change things
- ❏ Overwhelming sense of pressure
- ❏ Anger
- ❏ Loneliness
- ❏ Unhappiness for no reason
- ❏ Easily upset

Cognitive Symptoms
- ❏ Trouble thinking clearly
- ❏ Forgetfulness
- ❏ Lack of creativity
- ❏ Memory loss
- ❏ Inability to make decisions
- ❏ Thoughts of running away
- ❏ Constant worry
- ❏ Loss of sense of humor

Do any seem familiar to you?

Check the ones you experience when under stress. These are your stress warning signs.

Are there any additional stress warning signals that you experience that are not listed? If so, add them here.

_____

_____

_____

_____

_____

Source: Reprinted with permission from H. Benson and E.M. Stuart, *The Wellness Book*, p. 182, © 1992, Carol Publishing.

person is often quite unaware of the effects of stress on the bodymind. Once the client is aware of the effects of stress, he or she may be able to release tension more easily. Clients build on this awareness as they proceed through cognitive restructuring.

Step II: Automatic Thoughts

Once the client has been able to identify a stress or a stressful situation and identify the changes in bodymind that accompany this stress, the next step is to identify the automatic thoughts. These thoughts usu-ally occur automatically in response to a situation. Because these thoughts occur automatically and often are not in the conscious awareness of the individual, they are described as knee-jerk responses. Clients are taught a systematic approach to identifying these self-defeating automatic thoughts.

Automatic thoughts have certain characteristics in common. They are

- reflex or knee-jerk responses to a perceived stressor
- usually negative

Exhibit 16–2 Challenging Stress and Winning—Stop, Take a Breath, Reflect, Choose

Situation Briefly describe a situation that caused you stress this week.	**Physical Response** Describe how you felt physically in this situation.	**Automatic Thoughts** Write your automatic thoughts in this situation.	**Moods and Emotions** Describe how you felt emotionally in this situation.
Exaggerated Beliefs Write down the exaggerated beliefs behind your automatic thoughts.	**Behavior** Describe how you behaved during or immediately after the situation.	**More Effective Response** Describe how you might think or act differently that would help you cope more effectively.	**Potential Outcome** Describe how this might make you feel and behave.

Source: Reprinted with permission from H. Benson and E.M. Stuart, *The Wellness Book*, p. 182, © 1992, Carol Publishing.

- quick, fleeting, a kind of shorthand (e.g., should, ought, never, always)
- usually not in our conscious awareness
- frequently unrealistic, illogical, and distorted.

Because these thoughts form so quickly, it is often difficult to notice that they have occurred. Typically, people attribute the stress they experience or the feeling they have to the person or situation that is causing the stress. By stopping, taking a breath, and asking the question, "What is going on here?" clients gradually become aware that their stress does not always come from an outside event or situation but may come from the way they interpret these events.

Automatic thoughts can be viewed as inner dialogue or perceptions, which in turn create the experience and influence the individual's physiology, emotions, and behaviors.

> **Example:** A very popular and successful teacher was reviewing the evaluations at the end of the semester. He read 20 very positive reviews. Then he read one that contained some criticism of his teaching style. Instantly he felt a tense sensation in his stomach and chest.
>
> After stopping and taking a breath, he was able to identify the following automatic thoughts: *"there's **always** one in a crowd . . . **ought** to have done (whatever) . . . **never** could teach that concept well . . . **should** have included the new material I saw in the library . . . I **always** come up short."*

Notice that the teacher had an *instant* reaction to this stress (perception of threat) and that his automatic thoughts were quick, fleeting, negative, and probably not in his conscious awareness. (Does he *really* believe he *always* comes up short?) Identifying automatic thoughts is an important step in allowing clients to look realistically at their automatic reaction to a stressor and put it into perspective.

One of the most important and difficult tasks in cognitive restructuring is developing an awareness that these automatic thoughts occur. One reason that these reflex, knee-jerk responses are so pervasive is that the body does not know the difference between things that are imagined and things that are actually experienced. Another reason is that people are always talking to themselves, and after they say something to themselves often enough, they begin to believe it. A third reason is that people rarely stop to question their thoughts or emotions. For these reasons,

clients need to be taught a structured way of exploring stress and uncovering these automatic thoughts.

> **Exercise to uncover automatic thoughts, feelings, and physical response** (see Exhibit 16–2)
> - Stop (break the cycle of escalating, awfulizing thoughts).
> - Take a breath (release physical tension, promote relaxation).
> - Reflect:
>   — Physically how do I feel?
>   — Emotionally how do I feel?
>   — What are my automatic thoughts (e.g., should, always, ought, never, etc.)?

Step III: Cognitive Distortions

Once clients have learned to identify stressful situations, their physical, emotional, and behavioral responses to stress, and the automatic thoughts that precipitate the experience, the next step in the process is to teach clients to identify distortions in thinking. Cognitive distortions are illogical ways of thinking that lead to adverse body-mind-spirit states. The problem is not that these thoughts are wrong or bad, but that people hold the beliefs so strongly. Cognitive distortions are based on beliefs or underlying assumptions that are generally out of proportion to the situation. These beliefs or assumptions are usually long held, are based on life experience, and often are not in conscious awareness.

Through years of research and clinical experience, Burns[58] has identified 10 general categories of cognitive distortions that lead to negative emotional states:

- **All-or-nothing thinking:** Viewing things in black or white; considering oneself as a total failure when a performance falls short of perfection. (Think back to the example of the teacher. In the face of 20 excellent evaluations, and 1 constructive criticism, the teacher immediately focused all his attention on the imperfection and felt anxious and upset. *"I should have taught the course all differently." "I never get a good review.")*

- **Overgeneralization:** Viewing a single negative event as a never-ending pattern. *"Fixing my car cost twice what they said it would. All mechanics are dishonest and always will be."*
- **Mental filtering:** Picking out a negative detail and dwelling on it exclusively, "catastrophizing" or "awfulizing." *"I got a lousy grade on that test. I'll probably have to drop out of school. I won't be able to find a decent job and will have to move back in with my parents."*
- **Disqualifying the positive:** Rejecting positive experiences as if they don't count. *"It was nothing."* Being unable to accept praise. *"You're just saying that because you have to."*
- **Jumping to conclusions:** Reading the minds of others or predicting negative outcomes without sufficient evidence. *"He went off to bed without saying anything. He's angry with me for working late again."*
- **Magnification:** Exaggerating the importance of mistakes or inappropriately minimizing the significance of one's own assets. *"My performance tonight was horrible—I'll never get the lead part."*
- **Emotional reasoning:** Assuming that one's emotions reflect the way things are. *"I feel worthless—I must be worthless."*
- **"Should" statements:** Trying to motivate oneself with shoulds and shouldn'ts. *"Good employees should always get to the office early and be willing to stay late."*
- **Labeling:** Name calling; labeling oneself "a loser" if a mistake is made; making an illogical leap from one characteristic to a category. *"She's*

blond. What do you expect? She's an airhead."
- **Personalization:** Blaming oneself inappropriately as the cause of a negative event; seeing events only in relation to oneself. *"It's my fault that my child didn't do well in school, because I work."*

Exaggerated, unrealistic, illogical, and distorted automatic thoughts are a result of deeply held silent assumptions and beliefs that are usually not in conscious awareness. A client is more likely to experience stress in any given situation if he or she holds these beliefs as absolutes. Situations that are encountered are far more likely to precipitate stress if the world is viewed in terms of black or white (e.g., all good or all bad) than if there is room for shades of gray. An important understanding for the clinician is that it is not the belief that needs to be examined, it is the degree to which the belief is held. All clients are entitled to their individual sets of beliefs. Assigning any value, right or wrong, to their beliefs is not in the nurse's purview. The nurse is simply inviting clients to examine their beliefs in the context of their stress and to assess whether the degree to which they hold these beliefs serves them well or contributes to stress. Clients can very easily be alienated if they feel the nurse is making value judgments about their beliefs. The core concept here is not to examine beliefs to decide whether they are right or wrong, but to decide whether they are practical or impractical. Some commonly held assumptions and beliefs are:[59]

- If I treat others fairly, then I can expect them to treat me fairly.
- I must always be loved by family, friends, and peers to be worthwhile.
- I must be unfailingly competent and perfect in all that I do.
- My worth as a human being depends upon my achievements (or intelligence or status or attractiveness).

Everyone has a right to his or her beliefs and opinions. Problems develop only when these beliefs are held as absolutes and therefore provide no room for flexibility in an imperfect world.

Example: Reflect back on the previous example of the teacher reading course evaluations who had a strong reaction to criticism.

After taking a breath, interrupting his automatic response, and identifying his automatic thoughts, he was able to identify his cognitive distortions and irrational beliefs. They included *all-or-nothing thinking* (must be perfect all the time), *overgeneralization* (never will get it right), *disqualifying the positive* (20 excellent reviews wiped out by 1 negative review), and the *belief* that "I must be unfailingly competent and perfect in all I do in order to be loved and/or respected by family, friends, and peers."

Exercise to uncover cognitive distortions (see Exhibit 16-2)
- Stop (break the cycle of escalating, awfulizing thoughts).
- Take a breath (release physical tension, promote relaxation).
- Reflect:
  — Physically how do I feel?
  — Emotionally how do I feel?
  — What are my automatic thoughts (e.g., should, always, ought, never, etc.)?
  — What is going on here?
  — Is it really true?
  — Am I jumping to conclusions?
  — Am I catastrophizing, awfulizing, getting things out of perspective?
  — Is it really a crisis?
  — Is it as bad as it seems?
  — Is there another way to look at the situation?
  — What is the worst that can happen?

Because these strongly held assumptions and beliefs are mostly silent or not in people's conscious awareness, it is a challenge to discover their existence and, consequently, their influence on people's thoughts, emotions, and behaviors. In addition to the systematic approach described above to explore a stressful situation (stop, take a breath, reflect, and choose), another technique that is helpful in discovering underlying assumptions and beliefs is the Vertical Arrow Technique developed by Burns.[60]

Vertical Arrow exercise: Ask the client to identify a stressful situation and to challenge the underlying assumptions in this stress. The client can challenge the assumption by asking the question, "If that is true, why is it so upsetting?"

For example, a nursing school student had severe panic that kept her from speaking up in class. Class participation was 50 percent of the grade, so she wanted to change this behavior. When she was asked why it was stressful to ask a question, the following sequence of thoughts emerged.

"If I speak up, I may say something stupid."
↓
If this is true, why is it so upsetting?
↓
"They will think I'm stupid."
↓
If this is true, why is it so upsetting?
↓
"The smart students won't invite me to join their study group."
↓

If this is true, why is it so upsetting?

↓

"I won't pass unless I'm in a good study group."

↓

If this is true, why is it so upsetting?

↓

"I'll flunk out of school."

↓

If this is true, why is it so upsetting?

↓

"My family and friends will be embarrassed."

↓

If this is true, why is it so upsetting?

↓

"They won't love me."

↓

If this is true, why is it so upsetting?

↓

"I'm unlovable."

Viewing the stress in this manner allowed the student to see how out of perspective her thoughts were. She could clearly see that her stress was distorted by the rigid belief that to make a mistake would make her less than perfect and to be less than perfect was bad and would make people cease to love her. This awareness allowed her to put the stress in perspective and to get past her fear of asking a question.

Once a fear is recognized, it can be approached like any other stressor. If it is irrational, it can be challenged through cognitive restructuring. If it is rational, then appropriate problem-solving and coping strategies are required.

Identifying Emotions. The way people feel emotionally is an important part of health. Feelings of vigor, vitality, and general well-being are important correlates of health; conversely, feelings of anger, hostility, anxiety, or depression can contribute to ill health. Many people find their emotions troubling, either because they are out of touch with them or because they feel overwhelmed by them. Family and cultural influences have a great deal to do with the way emotions are experienced. Many families and cultures do not encourage the expression of emotions, and individuals learn to ignore this aspect of their lives. As individuals become aware of their body-mind-spirit responses to stress by identifying their emotional stress warning signals, they become aware of their feelings and emotions, and the connection between these feelings and emotions and stress.

Feelings of depression, anger, fear, and guilt are all part of the human experience; however, individuals may need to be encouraged to acknowledge and honor these emotions. Emotions are genuine, and people are entitled to the way they feel. On the other hand, emotions, particularly exaggerated emotions, can interfere with effective problem solving. Individuals need to be guided through the process of recognizing their emotions and the thoughts that underlie these feelings. For example, anger is often perpetuated by thoughts of unfair treatment. Frustration is often the result of unmet expectations. Thoughts related to loss contribute to the feeling of depression, and perception of a loss of control often causes anxiety. It is important to distinguish healthy fear from neurotic anxiety.[61] Thoughts underlying healthy fear are realistic, keep one alert, and warn one of dangers. Neurotic anxiety is related to thoughts that are distorted and unrealistic and often contain "what ifs": "What if I don't get the job?" "What if I don't find a partner?" A great deal of time and energy are wasted on events that may never take place. The nurse must guide the client in discovering the thoughts that are behind the emotion. In this way, the nurse can facilitate a process of challenging the thoughts and dealing with the emotions.

When feelings are ignored, denied, or suppressed, they often become intertwined with stress. In this case, clients sometimes have difficulty identifying either the emotion or the automatic thoughts related to the emotion. Cognitive restructuring allows individuals to become aware of the emotions, the automatic thoughts related to a particular emotion, and the connection with stress. Reflecting on these underlying themes often helps individuals to explain why they feel as they do and, in turn, to choose a more effective coping mechanism.

Another danger in denying feelings is that individuals can become trapped in one of these emotional states, so that the mind becomes a filter, letting into conscious awareness only material that confirms or reinforces their mood. For example, when people are depressed, they notice and experience only things that depress them more; nothing that would bring joy and pleasure is allowed into their awareness. Through cognitive restructuring, they can learn to reduce the frequency, length, and intensity of these feelings.

Exercise to uncover the relationship of thoughts and feelings (see Exhibit 16–2)

- Stop (break the cycle of escalating, awfulizing thoughts).
- Take a breath (release physical tension, promote relaxation).
- Reflect (What am I feeling? What am I thinking? Is there a theme that underlies my stress triggers?).

Feeling	Thoughts related to[62]
Anger	Being treated unfairly
Frustration	Unmet expectations
Depression	Loss
Anxiety	Loss of control, fear of the unknown

As an example, consider the situation of a person who is laid off from his or her job. An angry person often views situations through the lens of his or her standard of fairness. In response to being laid off, such a person might be angry and think, "Why me? I've worked hard all these years, never complaining, doing more than I was asked, and this is how they reward me?" A depressed individual often responds with distortions such as all-or-nothing thinking, personalization, and overgeneralization. In response to being laid off, such a person might become depressed and think, "This shows what a complete failure I am. I'll never amount to anything." In the same situation, an anxious person might experience an entirely different set of distortions. This person might predict dire consequences (jump to conclusions) and take them as facts. An anxious person who just got laid off might think, "I'll never get a job again. I'll be broke, on the street, and living on welfare in a matter of months."

The nurse helps the client become aware of the relationship of these emotional themes to stress triggers and cognitive distortions. When the nurse guides the client through a stress awareness exercise, if the client identifies his or her emotional response as anger, the nurse helps the client to make the connection with automatic thoughts related to being treated unfairly (e.g., "This shouldn't have happened to me"; "Why me?" "This is so unfair.").

Because clients have often spent so many years ignoring their emotional cues, they sometimes have difficulty recognizing either the thoughts or the emotions that are related to stressful situations. Keeping a dairy or journal reflecting thoughts and feelings about stressful events has been found to be a valuable tool clients can use to identify automatic thoughts and underlying emotions. This method will be explained further in the section on coping.[63] In addition to understanding stressors and common themes that trigger stress, acknowledging and honoring emotions is important to a healthy sense of self. Healthy self-esteem, in turn, is an important ingredient in stress-hardiness or the ability to greet stressful events as challenges to be met rather than as threats to be feared.

Step IV: Choosing Effective Coping

The final step in the process of cognitive therapy is to help the client restructure or reframe distortions and beliefs and choose a more effective way of responding or coping. To accomplish this, one must recognize that stressful situations have two components, which Ellis termed the *practical problem* and the *emotional hook*. The practical problem is the situation at hand, or the problem that needs to be addressed. The emotional hook is the client's opinion about the problem or the individual(s) who have caused the problem. Quite often people respond to situations as if they can solve the problem by addressing the emotional hook. In the following example, note the difference in these two elements of the stress.

> **Example:** John related that he became very upset when he was late for an appointment and, while he was in line at the grocery store, someone cut in front of him.
>
> To cope effectively with this situation, John needed to separate the *practical problem* (getting through the line) from the *emotional hook* (his opinion about people who cut in line and his "right" to be treated fairly). When asked to stop, take a breath, and reflect, he was able to uncover his physical response (tense, tight jaw), his emotional re-

sponse (anger), his automatic thoughts ("This *always* happens to me"; "People *ought* not to cut in line"; "Late"), and silent assumptions underlying the distorted thinking ("I treat others fairly, and I expect to be treated fairly").

This example shows clearly that the process of solving the practical problem is quite different from the process of addressing the emotional hook. If John were to expend his energy in convincing the person who cut in front of him of the error of his ways regarding behavior in line, John would be unlikely to solve his problem (he was late and needed to get through the line efficiently). Moreover, in practical terms, John had no control over this other person. How likely was it that John could influence this person's behavior in future situations? Automatic thoughts—shoulds, nevers, always, musts, and oughts—often interfere with finding practical solutions to the problem. The emotional hook robs individuals of their ability to see the options for responding. This failure can make it impossible for clients to recognize when they have no control over a situation and need to concentrate on the practical problem rather than the emotional hook.

In this example, once John recognized how his underlying beliefs and assumptions were influencing his choices, he could take steps to stop the escalation of emotional upset and choose the best solution for the problem. Doing so involved making a decision about how to respond from conscious awareness and without continued emotional arousal. He might see several options. For example, he might choose to change lines or to calmly ask the person who cut in front of him to go to the end of the line (direct action). Or, he might choose just to let it go because, although it is important to be treated fairly, in this instance he was in a hurry, he didn't have the time or desire to deal with this individual, and, since this didn't *always* happen to him, it wasn't worth getting upset about (acceptance, reframing). Whatever the decision, it could be made with awareness and choice, not in reaction to a deeply held belief about how people ought to behave, and without further escalating emotional distress.

Exercise for reframing and problem solving (see Exhibit 16–2)

- **Stop:** Train a client to stop each time a stress is encountered, before thoughts escalate into the worst possible scenario. The simple act of thinking "Stop" can help break a pattern of automatic response.
- **Breathe:** Teach the client to breathe deeply and release physical tension. Physically taking a deep, diaphragmatic breath can be important, because during times of stress, most people hold their breath. Taking a deep breath can elicit the physiologic changes of the relaxation response, the opposite of the stress response. This practice facilitates awareness of stress warning signals and the interaction between stress and body-mind-spirit changes.
- **Reflect:** Teach clients to ask themselves several questions about the automatic thoughts and underlying beliefs. Is this thought true? Is this thought helpful? (This is the process of developing awareness of automatic thoughts and cognitive distortions and challenging these distorted thoughts, beliefs, and assumptions.)
- **Choose:** Train clients to select the most effective way to cope with and/or solve the prob-

lem. Instruct the client to ask a series of questions:
- — What is the practical problem?
- — What is the emotional hook?
- — How can I substitute more realistic, self-enhancing thoughts to reduce the painful feelings?
- — How can I replace self-defeating silent assumptions (e.g., by substituting "I'm doing the best I can" for "I can't cope with this")?
- — What do I need?
- — What can I do?
- — What do I want?
- — What is possible?
- — Do I have the time, skills, and personal investment to achieve a practical solution? Is the practical problem within my control to solve?
- — Is it possible to deal with the *practical* problem? (i.e., Is it within my control?)
- — Do I need to temper my emotional response before I can act responsibly, practically, and appropriately?
- — Am I avoiding the best solution because it will be difficult for me?

Many techniques can be used to help clients effectively problem solve and cope with stressors. Effective coping requires that one attend to both the practical problem and the emotional hook. This sometimes requires two different approaches. Careful thought must be given to each stressful situation in order to choose the most effective coping strategy. The following list suggests a few ways to cope.[64]

Distraction. Worry about resolving a stress can be put off until the time is right.

(For example, the client receives a letter from the manager of the bank asking to speak with the client as soon as possible, but it is after closing hours. Distraction involves putting this worry aside until the bank opens the next day, at which time the client can deal directly with the situation. This is quite different from procrastination or denial because it is a necessary delay as opposed to avoidance.)

Direct action. The problem can be dealt with directly to resolve it.

Relaxation. Using relaxation techniques to reduce emotional arousal is a way of coping with a stress that cannot be changed or avoided. Techniques to elicit the relaxation response include meditation, yoga, mindfulness, T'ai Chi, as well as many others. Relaxation techniques are covered in Chapter 21.

Reframing. Looking at a situation differently can help individuals cope. A glass filled halfway can be labeled either half full or half empty. This label changes the experience greatly. Illness, for example, can be viewed as catastrophic and life shattering or as an opportunity for reconnection with what is meaningful in one's life.

Affirmations. Positive thoughts can be used to recondition one's thinking. For example, individuals frequently tell themselves they cannot do something, and the statement becomes a self-fulfilling prophecy. Affirmations are a way of countering self-defeating silent assumptions. An affirmation is simply a positive thought, a short phrase, or a saying that has meaning for the individual. Clients can be coached to create an affirmation as a way of reframing or choosing a more helpful, reasonable belief system.

Exercise for developing an affirmation. Ask the client to choose an aspect of life that is causing stress, such as work, family, or health. Have the client decide

what he or she would want to have happen or how he or she would want to feel in the situation. Formulate the goal as a first-person statement, in the present, and in the positive (e.g., "I am confident in my work"; "I can handle it"; "I am peaceful"; "I am becoming healthy and strong"). Have the client repeat the affirmation often during the day, perhaps before or after eliciting the relaxation response or as part of a breathing exercise.

In a short time, affirmations can become second nature and help to enhance self-esteem and reduce stress.

Spirituality. A sense of connection to the universe, God, or a higher power, or connecting with what is important and meaningful in our life, can aid in coping with stress. Connection with life's meaning and purpose is addressed in greater detail in Chapter 5.

Catharsis. Emotional catharsis, either laughing or crying, can be very effective in relieving emotional distress.

Journal writing. Using a journal to write about thoughts, feelings, and experiences is often helpful in processing emotions. Pennebaker and colleagues found that writing in order to get in touch with one's deepest thoughts and feelings can measurably improve physical and mental health.[65] Suggest to clients that they get a special notebook and colorful pens for their journal. Chapter 17 contains more detailed information on journal writing.

Social support. Having supportive family, friends, and co-workers is important to effective coping and has been shown to contribute to stress-hardiness.[66] Talking out problems is often helpful to obtain good advice or uncritical support. Social support has been found to reduce the incidence of heart disease as well as other health problems. In the social support literature, it has been noted that both the number of supporters and the quality of the relationships are important.[67]

Assertive communication. Communication is an important skill to help in solving problems and reducing conflicts and stress. Although communication is addressed in Chapter 11, it is considered in some detail below because it is an important coping and problem-solving skill that can be adversely affected by deeply held beliefs and silent assumptions. Cognitive restructuring can influence the ability to communicate effectively and, in turn, improve coping.

People who have problems with communication usually experience the following problems:[68]

- disparity between what they say (statement) and what they want (intent)
- confusion about or resistance to stating clearly how they feel, what they want, or what they need (assertiveness); there is either a tendency to deny their own feelings (passiveness) or to be indifferent toward the feelings of others (aggressiveness)
- inability to listen.

The importance of matching the statement with the intention is illustrated by the following.

Example: After spending a long day at work and stopping to pick up some groceries at the store, Jill arrives home to find her husband Jack at his desk in his office going over some bills. Coming in the door, she remarks, "Wow, busy day. I just picked up some groceries." She begins bringing the bags of groceries into the kitchen, walking past him. Following each trip to the garage, she shuts the door a little more forcefully and sets each

bag down a little more loudly as Jack continues to sit at his desk.

When he finally says, "Anything wrong?" Jill answers, "Nothing!" and storms out of the room, feeling that, if he loved her, he would know what she needed and wanted.

The first principle of effective communication is to be clear about what one wants and needs (intent) in statements to others. Although it would be wonderful if spouses, friends, and others were mind readers, assuming that they are does not help with communication. Matching statements with intentions is an art and a skill. It requires that individuals recognize their automatic thoughts, emotions, and cognitive distortions and take responsibility for their part of the conversation.

Consider the above example. If Jill's *intention* was for her husband to help bring the groceries into the house, then her *statement* should have reflected this. She might have said, "Wow, what a busy day. I just picked up some groceries. Could you help me bring them into the house?" Clients must understand that the other person is not obligated to respond as they would wish. However, what they are asking for will be a lot clearer to others if the statement reflects the intent.

The next principle of effective communication is to be assertive.[69] In most cases, assertive communication is the most effective way to communicate. An assertive statement expresses one's feelings and opinions and reaffirms one's identity and rights. It is not judgmental. The general format of an assertive statement is "I feel (label the emotion), when you (label the behavior) because (provide an explanation)." The formula requires that all three elements be included. Cognitive restructuring facilitates assertive communication because it requires clients to identify their thoughts and feelings. In the example above, Jill would

—stop (break the cycle of escalating, awfulizing thoughts)

—take a breath (release physical tension, promote relaxation)

—reflect:

1. Emotionally how do I feel? (frustrated)

2. What are my automatic thoughts? ("If he loved me, he would get up and help me! He never helps me with the house. He always expects me to do everything around here. He doesn't care about me. He's never going to change.")

Recognizing her thoughts and feelings would help Jill to formulate an assertive statement when her husband asks, "Anything wrong?" She could then say, "I feel *frustrated* (emotion) when you *don't help me bring in the groceries* (behavior) because *if you cared for me you would help me more with the chores around the house* (explanation)." In this way, she would both have made her feelings clear and have explained why she felt that way. This, in turn, would have provided a better opportunity to work on problem solving. If clients cannot articulate both their feelings and their needs, they leave it up to others to figure them out. When others fail to do so correctly, the clients feel let down and blame others for not understanding. The nurse can help clients to recognize that they have a right to speak up and a responsibility to do so in an assertive rather than passive or aggressive way. The nurse can guide clients in matching their emotions with the explanation (e.g., frustration = unmet expectation) by reviewing the exercise on matching thoughts and emotions as in the example above. Clients should be reminded that this technique will feel awkward and uncomfortable at first. They may have to practice it many times before communications improve. Other people need time to adjust to the changes they are trying to make. Effective communication takes practice as well as patience with oneself and with others.

Empathy. Empathy is the ability to take into consideration the other person's perspective. It is an effective coping technique because it facilitates communication. It helps clients become better listeners.

Exercise to promote empathy: Empathy can be facilitated through active listening. This technique requires conscious, nonjudging awareness. It helps to clarify the issues involved and can de-escalate many emotional exchanges. Consider a situation in which the mother announces, "I can't stand this room any more. It's a mess." The response to this statement may be critical to resolving the issues without contributing to further miscommunication and escalating the problem. Instead of becoming hooked by a defensive emotional reaction, clients can learn to operate from empathy using the four-step approach.

- **Stop** (break the cycle of escalating, awfulizing thoughts).
- **Take a breath** (release physical tension, promote relaxation).
- **Reflect:**
  — Emotionally how do I feel? (hurt, angry)
  — What are my automatic thoughts? ("How could she say that? I work hard too. I'm always being blamed for how things are around here. No one understands kids.")
  — What are the thoughts and emotions being expressed by the other person? (the simple practice of asking this question provides a very different perspective

as the client begins to formulate a response).

- **Choose:**
  — My feelings are hurt, but I
    choose not to react defen-
    sively.
  — I choose to listen actively to
    the other person's response
    and will try to understand
    that person's perspective,
    using this phrase: "You
    sound (emotion) about (situ-
    ation)."

Rogers suggested using this last phrase
as a way to facilitate communication and
gain awareness of another person's perspective.[70] In the above scenario, the teenage child might say, "You sound *upset*
about the *messy house.*" Possible responses might include: "It's not just the
room, everything seems to be in a mess,
here and at the office. I can't seem to get
anything done." Or she might say, "You're
right about that. I hate coming home to a
messy house after a busy day."

When a client uses the skill of active listening, the other person often feels heard,
which may help to defuse further emotional
arousal and defensive behavior. In addition,
he or she now has an opportunity to clarify
any misunderstanding. Also, active listening allows the client to buy time to obtain a
better perspective on what the other person
is thinking and feeling. Clients can then
choose how they want to respond. This may
be a time to use assertive communication or
problem solving, or a time to step away from
the interaction until emotions and defenses
have settled. Active listening allows reflective, empathic, objective, and nonjudgmental communication. Coaching clients to
use cognitive restructuring skills that include active listening techniques facilitates
effective communication, in turn reducing
conflict and stress.

Acceptance. Acceptance is facing the
fact that some situations or people cannot
be changed or avoided and letting go of re-

sentment. Forgiveness is often a part of acceptance. Coping successfully means
gaining the wisdom to achieve the delicate
balance between acceptance and action,
between letting go and taking control. It is
the art of choosing the right strategy at the
right time.[71]

When clients feel that they can cope effectively, the harmful effects of stress are
buffered. The situation is perceived not as
a threat but as a challenge. This subtle difference has profound physiologic, psychologic, behavioral, and spiritual effects. It is
what allows people facing great adversity
(such as illness) to see the opportunity the
situation presents. Above all, as noted
above, clients need to recognize that coping is the art of finding a balance between
acceptance and action, between letting go
and taking control. Cognitive restructuring
helps clients distinguish these differences
by providing a format for observing or objectifying their experiences. In so doing,
they gain a sense of control that minimizes
or buffers the harmful effects of stress.

Application of the General Principles of Cognitive Therapy

Cognitive therapy is most useful for individual mood problems, not for relationship
problems or interpersonal conflict.[72] The
nurse must be imaginative and tenacious.
Cognitive therapy requires constant shifting
between technique and process. The
therapy combines problem resolution using
cognitive and behavioral techniques with
empathic focus on the client's feelings. The
process requires the skills of presence, intention, and communication. Several attempts and several different ways of looking at a situation may be required before a
client recognizes the automatic thoughts
and underlying beliefs involved.

Cognitive therapy can be used in both
inpatient and outpatient settings, but the
goals and process are different in these settings. The goal of cognitive therapy in the

outpatient setting is generally to restructure cognitive distortions to enhance a variety of self-management skills and healthy lifestyle behaviors, which in turn help to promote health, reduce symptoms, or manage illness. Outpatient cognitive therapy can be provided either individually or in a group. The majority of this chapter has been written for this application.

The goal of cognitive therapy in the inpatient setting is typically confined to assisting the patient to cope more effectively with those stresses that arise during hospitalization for an acute illness. In this context, the nurse must remember that he or she is viewing the patient from a snapshot perspective (through one episode in the continuum of the patient's life). Patients bring to this hospital experience a reliance on long-standing coping styles—some adaptive, some maladaptive, and many influenced by cognitive distortions. In view of the short hospital stay and critical needs during this time, long-standing maladaptive coping patterns are best left to be addressed after discharge from the hospital.

In the hospital, cognitive therapy can be integrated effectively into the many nurse-patient communications that occur each day. Each interaction can be an occasion to assist patients in identifying the relationship of thoughts, feelings, and behaviors to biology as it applies to their current symptoms and illness. The nurse can utilize the structure of cognitive therapy to assist the patient in identifying distorted thinking patterns and realistically appraising the situation as well as in seeing opportunity in adversity. Thus, the patient can often choose a more realistic and less stressful way to view the situation. This, in turn, can decrease physical and emotional symptoms.

Hospitalization can be a time of opportunity despite its difficulties. Because hospitalization usually occurs when individuals are in need or crisis, they often feel vulnerable and may be more open to exploring different ways of thinking. In addition, they may be more open to discussing the role that negative thoughts, pessimism, and stress play in their illness, or the role that enhanced self-management skills would play in promoting wellness. For this reason, the inpatient stay offers multiple opportunities for the nurse to integrate cognitive therapy. Such integration can help establish a plan of care that is congruent with the patient's core values and beliefs. In one study, patients reported that the social support offered by nursing staff (organized around cognitive restructuring) was an important factor in their ability to successfully modify adverse lifestyle behaviors.[73]

HOLISTIC CARING PROCESS

Assessment

In preparing to use cognitive therapy interventions, the nurse assesses the following parameters:

- the client's ability to monitor and appraise inner dialogues and to communicate effectively
- the client's perception of the problem and the degree to which the client wishes to change a thought or behavior
- the client's ability to identify stress warning signals
- the client's readiness for and openness to changing thoughts or behaviors
- the client's level of experience with each of the interventions to be used.

Patterns/Problems/Needs

The following are the patterns/problems/needs compatible with cognitive therapy that are related to the nine human response patterns (see Chapter 14).

- *Communicating:* Altered verbal/nonverbal communications
- *Relating:* Altered, actual or potential Impaired social interaction

- *Choosing:*   Social isolation
                Altered parenting
                Altered coping,
                ineffective
                individual and
                family
- *Perceiving:* Altered self-
                concept:
                disturbance in
                self-esteem, body
                image, role
                performance,
                personal identity
- *Knowing:*   Altered thought
                processes
- *Feeling:*   Anxiety, fear

Outcomes

- Long-term goals (outcomes) are established prior to therapy, and short-term goals are set prior to each session.
- Goals are set with the client and must be mutually acceptable. A contract may be established to monitor progress and promote adherence.
- A general list of optimal cognitive therapy outcomes includes the following. The client will be able to:
  —recognize connections among cognition, emotions, behaviors, and physiology
  —identify physical, psychologic, and behavioral stress warning signals
  —demonstrate the ability to recognize cognitive distortions and examine the evidence for and against key beliefs
  —change the way that he or she thinks (views situations) and try alternative conceptualizations or more rational responses independently
  —report a decrease in arousal, anxiety, fear, depression, or somatic complaints and an elevation in self-esteem after correcting cognitive distortions.

Setting Goals

It is important to establish clearly defined desired outcomes that are mutually agreed upon by both client and nurse prior to beginning cognitive therapy. These mutually agreed upon outcomes form the basis for establishing long- and short-term goals. Clients are more likely to accomplish goals if they played an integral role in establishing these goals. As clients assume more responsibility for their health and become more active partners with health care providers, the nurse must respect their input to maximize successful outcomes. Goals should be specific, concrete, and measurable; in addition, they should be achievable.

The process of establishing outcomes should take into account the client's

1. beliefs about health and illness (i.e., health belief model)
2. experience with healthy behaviors (i.e., health behaviors)
3. self-awareness, self-monitoring (i.e., self-efficacy theory, self-regulation theory)
4. stage of change and readiness to change (i.e., change theory, the transtheoretical model)
5. motivation to change (i.e., the dynamics of motivation)
6. understanding of the relationship between illness/wellness and behavior (i.e., dynamics of health-wellness-disease-illness)
7. preferences (i.e., client rights)
8. attitudes, beliefs, and values.

Goal setting is a dynamic process that involves both the client and the nurse at each level. The nurse can facilitate this process by:

- Accumulating a complete bio-psycho-social-spiritual database that is appropriate to the setting and diagnosis.
- Identifying and prioritizing problems to be addressed.

- Setting mutually agreed upon long- and short-term goals.
- Helping clients clarify goals. This involves asking clients to determine what is important and meaningful to them. Suggest that they focus on those things that sustain meaning and purpose in their lives. Focus on goals that allow them to achieve rewards from health rather than from sickness. Encourage clients to challenge themselves when their behaviors are not congruent with what is important and meaningful to them. For example, when a client with a high cholesterol level eats high-fat foods, have them contrast that behavior with what is meaningful to them (e.g., family). The cost-benefit is usually clear and places the responsibility for the behavior with the client, not the provider. Asking the following questions may help clients clarify long-term goals.
  — What is most important and meaningful in your life?
  — What would you most like to change about your life right now?
  — How can you begin the first step in that change?
  — On what date would you like to achieve that goal?
  — How can you reward yourself for success?
  — How will your life be different when you succeed?
  — How can I help?
- Using the 2×50 rule when goal setting. Ask the client to state the goal, then double the amount of time set for accomplishing the goal or reduce its difficulty by 50 percent. For example, losing 10 pounds in the next month is probably an unrealistic goal; losing 10 pounds in 2 months or losing 5 pounds in the next month is probably a more realistic, attainable goal. Smaller, more attainable goals create a sense of achievement, build self-esteem,

and foster enthusiasm to set further goals.
- Establishing a health contract. A health contract is a formal way to enhance goal attainment. It is a way to increase the quality of communication between client and nurse and can also help a client become a more willing participant in self-care. The client's failure to achieve the goals of the contract opens the door to further discussion of the reasons for difficulties with compliance and ways of modifying behavior(s) to achieve a mutually agreed upon goal.

A successful contract includes more than simply a list of behavioral goals. Successful attainment of goals depends on skills the client learns during the process of developing the contract. This process provides the opportunity to analyze behaviors in relationship to the environment and to choose strategies that facilitate learning, changing, or maintaining a behavior.[74]

Contracts may be verbal, but all parties are likely to take written contracts more seriously. If a contract is written, both the client and the nurse should sign it. Contracts should always contain these key elements:
— a desirable, concrete, attainable, measurable goal
— a time for completion as well as identified times to evaluate progress toward goals
— the responsibilities of involved parties (e.g., client and nurse, client and spouse)
— an identified reward for achieving the stated goal

Some clients find the word *contract* threatening or uncomfortable. In this case, the contract may be referred to as an agreement or a statement of mutual goals. In establishing a contract, the nurse assumes the role of facilitator. The nurse introduces the concept of contracting and identifies the reasons that such an approach may be valid in the client's circumstances. After this, the nurse may limit his or her involvement to guidance and support. The greater the client input, the greater the likelihood that the client will achieve the goal of the contract. The contract should identify small, achievable steps to facilitate reaching the desired goals. In this way, the client is more likely to succeed.

- Assisting the client in identifying rewards for achieving a goal. Rewards can enhance goal attainment, but often clients find it difficult to identify appropriate rewards. Many people feel uncomfortable rewarding themselves and fail to realize that rewards are important in both learning and maintaining new behaviors. Rewards should be congruent with the difficulty of the goal set. The reward need not cost money or even be tangible. Ideally, as clients gain confidence and independence in self-management, they learn to self-reward.

Therapeutic Care Plan and Interventions

Before the Session

- Establish a therapeutic relationship by creating a space in which both you and the client feel physically and emotionally safe and comfortable.
- Provide materials for recording cognitive distortions and alternative rational thoughts and statements (e.g., paper and pen, blackboard, preprinted forms).
- Center yourself; clear your mind of personal or professional issues in order to be fully present.
- Establish the long-term goals (outcome) of therapy with the client.

At the Beginning of the Session

- Assess the client's level of mood, discomfort, or relaxation.
- Review homework from the previous session, if appropriate. Ask the client to describe any changes that have occurred since the previous session.

During the Session

- Determine, with the client, which issues need to be addressed and set short-term goals for the session.
- Listen and guide with focused intention. Provide appropriate feedback, clarification, support, or interpretation.

At the End of the Session

- Have the client identify and verbalize changes that have occurred during the session. Assess progress toward goals.
- Assign homework to be done for the next session.
- Schedule a follow-up session

Case Study

The same process that has been discussed throughout this chapter can also be used for inpatients, but the nurse would typically guide the patient through the process at the time of the stress. The following example considers the situation of a patient newly admitted to the coronary care unit who experiences chest pain. As the nurse responds to this potentially urgent clinical situation, he or she can gently guide the patient through the following exercise.

- **Stop:** Break the cycle of escalating, awfulizing, negative automatic thoughts. *"I need you to stop and focus on letting go of the worry cycle. If we work together, we will get the best outcome. We have things under control, and I want you to let me worry about the technical things that need to be done. I want you to . . ."*

- **Breathe:** Release physical tensions. *"Focus on your breathing and leave the rest to me. Take nice, slow breaths, in and out. Concentrate on letting go of tension in your hands, jaw, and feet. Put all of your effort into feeling your fingers and toes, and let the jaw be relaxed and easy. Do you still feel tension somewhere in your body? If so, begin to relax that area. With each breath in, breathe in relaxation; with each breath out, breathe out tension. Now, begin to think about a favorite place and, as you breathe in, feel the peace of that place fill you; as you breathe out, let the worries and tension of the moment flow out."*

The nurse guides the person through this relaxation/distraction exercise as he or she proceeds to treat the patient's chest pain. Obviously, it is not in the client's best interest for the nurse to stop what he or she is doing; rather, this skill needs to be such an integral part of the nurse's practice that it can be done while technologic tasks are performed. Empathic communication, presence, and touch enhance the process.

The next steps occur after the acute situation is over. "Tidying up" might be useful as a metaphor for dealing with the feelings that probably emerged in the patient. To continue with the chest pain example: the nurse guides the patient through the remainder of the cognitive restructuring steps.

- **Reflect:** Think back on what happened during the chest pain.
  - Physically how did you feel? Were there any areas you felt were particularly tense? Were you able to release physical tension? What works for you to release tension? The nurse discusses the effect of relaxation on ischemia and mental stress. The nurse empowers the patient with a specific skill that can be called upon to help treat their myocardial ischemia.

  - Emotionally how did you feel? The nurse invites the patient to talk about his or her feelings during this episode (e.g., worry, fear, anger, sadness). Using the concepts of awareness, automatic thoughts, and cognitive distortions, the nurse guides the patient through the process of realistic appraisal. Giving the patient permission to discuss his or her emotions and stress may help avoid all-or-nothing thinking, overgeneralization, jumping to conclusions, mental filtering, disqualification of the positive, and magnification. The patient is allowed to talk. The patient is gently encouraged to reveal any fears. The nurse helps the patient make an association between the emotional reaction to pain and the cycle of escalating pain this can create. Drawing a picture or writing in a journal can be useful if the person is reluctant to talk. The person's ability to identify his or her emotions needs to be accepted in a nonjudging way. Using a real-life, real-time, stressful experience provides a rich opportunity for dialogue and for teaching concrete self-management skills.

  - Is there another way to look at the situation? Are there opportunities here? An opportunity to reconnect with what is important in life? An opportunity to learn self-management skills that can treat the underlying pathophysiology? An opportunity to break the cycle of stress/ worry/chest pain/stress/worry/chest pain? This is also an opportunity for the nurse to praise the patient for doing the best he or she could in a very stressful situation.

- **Choose:** Replace maladaptive, unrealistic, distorted thinking patterns with a more effective and realistic response. At this stage of illness, it is most helpful to focus on a plan that replaces the anxiety/tension response to chest pain with focused relaxation and affirmation. Additional coping mechanisms can be addressed later in the hospital stay or in the outpatient setting.

Evaluation

Client outcomes that were established prior to initiating cognitive therapy and the client's subjective experiences are used to evaluate progress toward *long-term goals*. To evaluate progress toward *short-term goals*, client outcomes that were established prior to starting the session and the client's subjective experiences are used. Revising and updating goals are a part of each session.

Recognizing self-defeating automatic thoughts and silent assumptions in addition to changing long-standing health-risking behaviors is often challenging and frustrating to clients. With careful choice of interventions, honest and thoughtful feedback, and continuing support, the nurse can help clients gain significant health-affirming benefits. In turn, the nurse can realize the value of enhancing the client's autonomy and self-confidence in healthy behavior change and self-regulation.

DIRECTIONS FOR FUTURE RESEARCH

1. Evaluate the effectiveness of using the four-step approach of cognitive restructuring in helping clients change health-risking behaviors such as smoking, alcohol misuse, or overeating.

2. Evaluate whether there are differences in the application of cognitive therapy among different age groups?

3. Investigate cognitive distortions in children. Do the distortions change or intensify as children grow? Do children with similar distortions develop similar health issues as they mature?

NURSE HEALER REFLECTIONS

After reading this chapter, the nurse healer will be able to answer or begin the process of answering the following questions:

- What are my stress warning signals?
- What are the current stressors in my life?
- Can I pinpoint my negative automatic thoughts and silent assumptions that trigger and perpetuate my emotional upset?
- Can I use the four-step approach to help reduce my distress and effectively solve problems?
- Is there an affirmation I can create to help me counter self-defeating automatic thoughts and silent assumptions?
- When setting goals, have I made certain that:
  — they are desirable, concrete, attainable, and measurable?
  — I have set a time for completion, as well as identified times to evaluate progress?
  — I have identified steps or short-term goals that will help me achieve my desired long-term goal?
  — I have identified a reward for achieving the stated goal?

NOTES

1. G. Engel, The Clinical Application of the Biopsychosocial Model, *American Journal of Psychiatry* 137 (1980): 535–544.

2. E.M. Stuart et al., Spirituality in Health and Healing: A Clinical Program, *Holistic Nursing Practice* 3 (1989): 35–36.

3. A.T. Beck, A Systematic Investigation of Depression, *Comprehensive Psychiatry* 2 (1961): 163–170.

4. H. Benson and E. Stuart, *The Wellness Book: A Comprehensive Guide to Maintaining Health and Treating Stress-Related Illness* (New York: Fireside, Simon & Schuster, 1993).

5. Benson and Stuart, *Wellness Book*.

6. A.T. Beck, *Cognitive Therapy* (New York: New American Library, 1979).

7. A. Ellis, *Reason and Emotion in Psychotherapy* (New York: Lyle Stuart, 1962).

8. D. Meichenbaum, *Cognitive Behavior Modification: An Integrative Approach* (New York: Plenum Press, 1977).

9. D.D. Burns, *Ten Days to Self-Esteem* (New York: William Morrow, 1993).

10. A.T. Beck, Cognitive Therapy: A 30-year Retrospective, *American Psychologist* (1991): 368–375.

11. P.M. Emmelkamp and P. van Oppen, Cognitive Interventions in Behavioral Medicine [review], *Psychotherapy and Psychosomatics* 59 (1993): 116–130.

12. G.D. Jacobs et al., Home-Based Central Nervous System Assessment of a Multifactor Behavioral Intervention for Chronic Sleep-Onset Insomnia, *Behavior Therapy* 24 (1993): 159–174.

13. A.D. Domar et al., The Mind/Body Program for Infertility: A New Behavioral Treatment Approach for Women with Infertility, *Fertility and Sterility* 53 (1990): 246–249.

14. A.E. Speckens et al., Cognitive Behavioural Therapy for Medically Unexplained Physical Symptoms: A Randomised Controlled Trial, *British Medical Journal* 311, no. 7016 (1995): 1328–1332.

15. R. Friedman et al., Behavioral Medicine, Clinical Health Psychology, and Cost Offset, *Health Psychology* 14 (1995): 509–518.

16. E.M. Stuart et al., Managing Stress, in Benson and Stuart, *Wellness Book*, 177–188.

17. C.L. Wells-Federman et al., The Mind/Body Connection: The Psychophysiology of Many Traditional Nursing Interventions, *Clinical Nurse Specialist* 9, no. 1 (1995): 59–66.

18. W.B. Cannon, The Emergency Function of the Adrenal Medulla in Pain and the Major Emotions, *American Journal of Physiology* 33 (1914): 356–372.

19. H. Selye, History and Present Status of Stress Concept, in *Handbook of Stress: Theoretical and Clinical Aspects*, ed. L. Goldberger and S. Breznitz (New York: The Free Press, 1982), 7–20.

20. S.M. Grundy and A.C. Griffin, Relationship of Periodic Mental Stress to Serum Lipoprotein and Cholesterol Levels, *Journal of the American Medical Association*, 171 (1959): 1794–1796.

21. S.B. Malkoff et al., Blood Platelet Reactivity to Acute Mental Stress, *Psychosomatic Medicine* 55 (1993): 477–482.

22. J.K. Kiecolt-Glaser and R. Glaser, Psychological Influences on Immunity, *American Psychologist* 43 (1988): 892–898.

23. R.J. Gatchel et al., *Psychophysiological Disorders: Research and Clinical Applications* (Washington, DC: American Psychological Association, 1993).

24. S. Cohen et al., Psychological Stress and Susceptibility to the Common Cold, *New England Journal of Medicine* 325 (1991): 606–612.

25. J.H. Markovitz et al., Psychological Predictors of Hypertension in the Framingham Study. Is There Tension in Hypertension? *Journal of the American Medical Association* 270 (1993): 2439–2443.

26. R. Williams et al., Type A Behavior, Hostility and Coronary Artherosclerosis, *Psychosomatic Medicine* 42 (1980): 539–549.

27. N. Frasure-Smith et al., Depression Following Myocardial Infarction: Impact on 6 Month Survival, *Journal of the American Medical Association* 270 (1993): 1819–1825.

28. F.I. Fawzy et al., Malignant Melanoma: Effects of an Early Structured Psychiatric Intervention, Coping, and Affective State on Recurrence and Survival 6 Years Later, *Archives of General Psychiatry* 50 (1993): 681–689.

29. D. Spiegel et al., Effect of Psychosocial Treatment on Survival of Patients with Metastatic Breast Cancer, *Lancet* 2 (1989): 888–891.

30. K. Lorig et al., Evidence Suggesting that Health Education for Self-Management in Patients with Chronic Arthritis Has Sustained Health Benefits while Reducing Health Care Costs, *Arthritis and Rheumatism* 36 (1993): 439–446.

31. M.A. Caudill et al., Decreased Clinic Use by Chronic Pain Patients: Response to Behavioral Medicine Intervention, *Clinical Journal of Pain* 7 (1991): 305–310.

32. Benson and Stuart, *Wellness Book*.

33. S. Kobasa, Stressful Life Events, Personality and Health: An Inquiry into Hardiness, *Journal of Personality and Social Psychology* 37 (1979): 1–11.

34. R.C. Colligan et al., CAVEing the MMPI for an Optimum-Pessimism Scale: Seligman's Attributional Model and the Assessment of Explanatory Style, *Journal of Clinical Psychology* 50, no. 1 (1994): 71–95.

35. G.A. Marlatt, Relapse Prevention: Theoretical Rationale and Overview of the Model, in *Relapse Prevention*, ed. G. Marlatt and J. Gordon (New York: Guilford Press, 1985), 3–70.

36. N. Frasure-Smith and R. Prince, The Ischemic Heart Disease Life Stress Monitoring Program: Impact on Mortality, *Psychosomatic Medicine* 47 (1985): 431–445.

37. N. Frasure-Smith and R. Prince, Long-term Follow-up of the Ischemic Heart Disease Life Stress Monitoring Program, *Psychosomatic Medicine* 51 (1991): 485–512.

38. J. Kennell et al., Continuous Emotional Support During Labor in a U.S. Hospital: A Randomized Controlled Trial, *Journal of the American Medical Association* 265 (1992): 2197–2237.

39. M.K. Klaus et al., Maternal Assistance and Support in Labor: Father, Nurse, Midwife or Doula?, *Clinical Consultations in Obstetrics and Gynecology* 4 (1992): 211–217.

40. D. Ornish et al., Can Lifestyle Changes Reverse Coronary Heart Disease? The Lifestyle Heart Trial, *Lancet* 336, no. 8708 (1990): 129–133.

41. E.M. Stuart et al., An Integrated Multiple Risk Reduction Program: Psychosocial and Behavioral Outcomes, *Circulation* 96, no. 8 (1997): I–191.

42. E.M. Stuart et al., An Integrated Approach to Multiple Risk Reduction: Comparison of Outcomes from "Heart and Sole" and the Ornish Intensive Lifestyle Management Programs, *Circulation* 96, no. 8 (1997): I–350.

43. M.A. Fiatarone et al., Exercise Training and Nutritional Supplementation for Physical Frailty in Very Elderly People, *New England Journal of Medicine* 25 (1994): 1769–1775.

44. V. Frankl, *Man's Search for Meaning* (Boston: Beacon Press, 1963).

45. M. Schlitz, Intentionality and Intuition and Their Clinical Implications: A Challenge for Science and Medicine, *Advances: The Journal of Mind-Body Health* 12 (1996): 58–66.

46. D.B. Larson and M.A. Milano, Are Religion and Spirituality Clinically Relevant in Health Care? *Mind/Body Medicine* 1 (1995): 147–157.

47. A.H. Roberts et al., The Power of Nonspecific Effects in Healing: Implications for Psychosocial and Biological Treatments, *Clinical Psychology Review* 13 (1993): 375–391.

48. J.D. Kass et al., Health Outcomes and a New Index of Spiritual Experience, *Journal for the Scientific Study of Religion* 30 (1991): 203–211.

49. E.M. Adalf and R.G. Smart, Drug Use and Religious Affiliation, Feelings, and Behavior, *British Journal of Addiction* 80 (1985): 163–171.

50. J.J. Andreasen, The Role of Religion in Depression, *Journal of Religion and Health* 11 (1972): 153–166.

51. L.B. Bearon and H.G. Goenig, Religious Cognitions and Use of Prayer in Health and Illness, *The Gerontologist* 30 (1990): 249–253.

52. L. Dossey, Healing Words: *The Power of Prayer and the Practice of Medicine* (San Francisco: HarperCollins, 1993).

53. D.D. Burns, *The Feeling Good Handbook: Using the New Mood Therapy in Everyday Life* (New York: William Morrow, 1989).

54. A.R. Childress and D.D. Burns, The Basics of Cognitive Therapy, *Psychosomatics* 22, no. 12 (1981): 1017–1027.

55. A. Webster et al., How Thoughts Affect Health, in Benson and Stuart, *Wellness Book*, 189–208.

56. Childress and Burns, Basics of Cognitive Therapy.

57. E. Stuart et al., Coping and Problem Solving, in Benson and Stuart, *Wellness Book*, 230–248.

58. Burns, *Feeling Good Handbook*.

59. Ellis, *Reason and Emotion in Psychotherapy*.

60. Burns, *Feeling Good Handbook*.

61. Burns, *Feeling Good Handbook*.

62. Burns, *Feeling Good Handbook*.

63. J.W. Pennebaker, *Opening Up: The Healing Power of Confiding in Others* (New York: William Morrow, 1990).

64. Stuart et al., Coping and Problem Solving.

65. J.W. Pennebaker et al., Disclosure of Traumas and Immune Function: Health Implications for Psychotherapy, *Journal of Consulting and Clinical Psychology* 56 (1988): 239–245.

66. S.C. Kobasa et al., Hardiness and Health: A Prospective Study, *Journal of Personality and Social Psychology* 42 (1982): 168–177.

67. Frasure-Smith and Prince, Ischemic Heart Disease Life Stress Monitoring Program.

68. M.A. Caudill, *Managing Pain Before It Manages You* (New York: Guilford Press, 1995).

69. Burns, *Feeling Good Handbook*.

70. C. Rogers, *Client-Centered Therapy* (Boston: Houghton Mifflin, 1951).

71. Stuart et al., Coping and Problem Solving.

72. Burns, *Feeling Good Handbook*.

73. C. Medich et al., Healing Through Integration: Promoting Wellness in Cardiac Rehabilitation, *Journal of Cardiovascular Nursing* 11 (1997): 66–79.

74. S. Boehm, Patient Contracting, in *Nursing Interventions: Essential Nursing Treatments*, 2d ed., ed. G. Bulechek and J. McCloskey (Philadelphia: W.B. Saunders Co., 1992), 425–433.

VISION OF HEALING
Healthy Disclosure

Diaries, journals, logs, reviews, stories, and letters enable us to keep track of and enhance the patterns of our lives. Research shows that, in addition to helping us find meaning and depth in our life experiences, writing about occurrences such as trauma or illness improves our health.[1] Writing may also help us make the experience our own and explore its meaning for us, the way that we come to possess it, and, ultimately, the way that we can release it.[2]

As adolescents, we may have written in a diary, entering into it both the mundane and the deeply moving events of our days. With the transition into adulthood, we may well have reduced these diary entries to lists of things to do, appointments, chores, and dates. We find time only to jot short notes on a calendar or in a blank book, making longer entries in a loose-leaf notebook or perhaps putting into a box scraps of paper that contain ideas, thoughts, bits of poetry, and plans for a golden tomorrow. Even these abbreviated records provide a skeletal reflection of our lives, which can be filled out and given form by memories.

As nurses, we can refresh our own self-reflection techniques and perfect new ones to help us record and grow from our experiences, intuitions, and connections. We can learn to help ourselves and our clients tap into the spiritual and self-healing aspects of the complex and beautiful web of our existence. Self-reflection helps us evoke more trust and truth in daily living.

As the gods created the universe, they discussed where they should hide Truth so that human beings would not find it right away. They wanted to prolong the adventure of the search.

"Let's put Truth on top of the highest mountain," said one of the gods. "Certainly it will be hard to find there."

"Let's put it on the farthest star," said another. "Let's hide it in the darkest and deepest of abysses."

"Let's conceal it on the secret side of the moon."

At the end, the wisest and most ancient god said, "No, we will hide Truth inside the very heart of human beings. In this way they will look for it all over the Universe, without being aware of having it inside themselves all the time."[3]

NOTES

1. J. Pennebaker, *Opening Up: The Healing Power of Confiding in Others* (New York: Avon Books, 1990).

2. M. Crichton, *Travels* (New York: Ballantine Books, 1988), xi.

3. P. Ferrucci, *What We May Be* (Los Angeles: Jeremy P. Tarcher, 1982), 143.

Chapter 17

Self-Reflection: Consulting the Truth Within

Lynn Rew

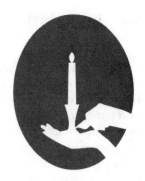

NURSE HEALER OBJECTIVES

Theoretical

- Define the concept of self-reflection.
- Discuss cognitive, intuitive, and transcendent awareness.
- Describe scientific evidence of the connections between mind, body, and spirit.
- Discuss theories of self-identity, awareness, and health as they relate to the concept of self-reflection.
- Describe self-reflection interventions.

Clinical

- Match each self-reflection intervention with a potential client.
- Keep a diary of self-reflection interventions used with clients for 1 month.
- Identify at least two positive outcomes for each client with whom you initiated a self-reflection intervention.

Personal

- Identify two ways in which your intuitive awareness has had a healing influence on your life.
- Keep a journal of self-reflection interventions that you use to enhance your own health or that of your family.

- Discuss with another nurse ways in which self-reflection has helped you improve your nursing practice.

DEFINITIONS

Awareness: alertness, watchfulness, and knowledgeability about oneself and the environment, including events that take place.

Health: harmony or unity of one's body-mind-spirit within an ever-changing environment.

Identity Status: one of four categories of adolescent identity formation processes.

Self: a principle underlying and organizing subjective experience.

Self-Identity: process of awareness of who one is and what one's place in the world is.

Self-Reflection: process of turning awareness inward, communicating with one's inner wisdom for the purpose of healing and well-being.

THEORY AND RESEARCH

Self-reflection is the process of turning one's attention or awareness internally to examine thoughts, feelings, beliefs, and behaviors. It is a deliberate process with the goal of discovery and learning.[1] Self-reflection means to look within oneself and to listen to the self-talk and associated feelings that guide behavior. Self-reflection activities are an essential component of expert nursing practice and may also be used as interventions for clients who would benefit from increased self-understanding.

Self-reflection nursing interventions have been developed in response to theories and research findings from a variety of disciplines. The concept of the self and theories of self-identity form the base for exploring the phenomenon of self-reflection. Similarly, theories of awareness that include cognitive, intuitive, and transcendent dimensions expand this basic framework and acknowledge the holistic nature of human beings. Recent research findings that validate the connections between body, mind, and spirit substantiate the theoretical understanding and support for these interventions.

Self

Questions about the reality of the self have been posed and answered historically through the disciplines of philosophy and psychology. The first American psychologist, William James, who was also a profound philosopher, provided one of the earliest explanations of the self and influenced the development of subsequent psychologic theories of the self. According to James, the self consists of the material Self (James used the upper case), the social Self, and the spiritual Self.[2] James identified the physical body and the clothes that a person wears as the innermost part of the material Self. In addition, the material Self includes a person's family, home, and material possessions. The social Self includes a person's fame, honor, and any image that another person carries of the person. The spiritual Self, according to James, is the inner or subjective being, which is the most intimate and enduring component of a person's self.

James noted that, to consider the spiritual self, one had to be reflective and to abandon one's outward point of view. This aspect of self is felt rather than seen. The spiritual self includes inner psychic qualities such as volition or will and emotions such as desire. Much debate has occurred in both philosophy and psychology since James's writings in the late 1800s. Primarily, the question of when the self is first recognizable in humans has not been easily answered. Some theorists believe that there is an innate "kernel of self" that gradually develops over time and through experience.[3] This innate self is the consciousness or awareness of self that emerges out of interactions with others and the ability to think about oneself.[4] Kagan, a developmental psychologist, argues convincingly that, until some time in the second year of life, there is little evidence that children are aware of themselves.[5] Kagan points out that two-year-olds smile when they master a task, even when playing alone, and they begin to attempt to direct the behaviors of others (e.g., by placing a toy telephone at the mother's mouth and gesturing for her to talk). Kagan concludes that the ability to reflect on one's experience, including one's feelings, thoughts, and behaviors, indicates that there is a unifying principle of the self.

Self-Identity

Human beings take their unique places in the world through a complex process of self-identification and differentiation. As infants grow and develop, they soon come to recognize what is oneself and what is the other. Their process of learning who they are and who they are not and what their place is in the world involves a dynamic interaction between the individual, the family, and the larger society. Erikson identified eight stages or crises through which each individual passes in the process of coming to know the self.[6] His theory is based on the assumption that within each person is a drive to overcome each developmental crisis and to form a solid sense of identity that then allows the individual to engage in intimate relationships with others, to be productive in life, and to feel that life has integrity. Self-identity is both a process and an outcome.[7]

According to Erikson's theory, infants face a crisis of trust versus mistrust as they learn to differentiate themselves from their mothers. An immature sense of the self and one's place in the world is nurtured through the relationship between the infant and the mother or other primary caregiver and other persons within the infant's larger family and community. This embryonic sense of identity is further developed in the second phase or crisis of development in which the toddler masters autonomy versus shame and doubt. With increasing awareness of themselves as different and independent from others, toddlers and young children gain confidence in their awareness and knowledge of who they are and what they are capable of doing. As young children develop further and expand their interaction with a larger society, as in the context of school and other social institutions, they face the third developmental crisis of developing initiative and industry versus guilt and inferiority. The development of initiative and industry occurs primarily in the performance of tasks that are shared with and/or evaluated by others. In the context of culture, older children spend increasingly longer periods of time away from the persons (parents) who nurtured them during their initial formation of a sense of identity and perceptions of the world at large. Children are exposed to further experiences that help them differentiate their sense of who they are and where they belong in the world through school and extracurricular activities. In each of these early stages of development, the individual becomes more and more capable of knowing about the self, about his or her intellectual, emotional, and spiritual capabilities. With each developmental success,

the child becomes more sure of the self and is capable of moving forward to resolve future developmental crises. With this development and maturity also comes the ability to think more deeply and seriously about the self.

The adolescent faces a new crisis of identity formation that calls into question how well the previous developmental crises have been mastered. Erikson called this the crisis of identity versus identity diffusion. Adolescence creates its own threats to identity related to the physiologic changes of puberty. This adolescent stage is often characterized by intense internal conflict and confusion about oneself. Rapid physical development and sexual maturity are accompanied by new and often more intense emotional experiences that can shake the foundation of one's sense of who one is and what one is to do in the world. Society also places increasingly greater demands on adolescents than on children, giving them both more freedom and more responsibilities. The purpose of the adolescent crisis of identity formation is to prepare the person for more intimate and responsible relationships with others and for feelings of being sound and whole. Much introspection occurs during adolescence, and this natural phenomenon informs much of what we know about self-reflection as a healing process.

Marcia studied the identity formation of adolescents and described four different outcomes of this process.[8] He referred to these resolutions of identity as *statuses* and conceptualized these as a type of path or continuum. In the ideal outcome, consistent with Erikson's conceptualization of identity formation, the person makes a commitment to a way of being in the world after first considering several possibilities. Persons with this ideal status are termed the *identity achievement group*; this group includes those who make a commitment to an identity after a period of exploring various possibilities. Another group of adolescents belong to the *foreclosure group*, those who make identity commitments without exploring possible alternatives. These individuals foreclose on an identity that may be more like their identity as a child and is often ascribed to them by those around them, such as teachers or other influential adults. A third set of youths belong to the *moratorium group*, which includes those who are actively in a state of crisis or exploration as they attempt to formulate an identity. A final category of adolescents are those in the *identity diffusion group*, who have made no identity commitments, have not explored possibilities, and have not foreclosed on an identity from childhood. The concept that one reflects on oneself and examines the possible alternatives of who one might become suggests that adolescence may be a time of profound self-reflection. It is this process of looking inward for a guiding wisdom that leads to a sense of purpose and generativity as well as feelings of wholeness and integrity that Erikson claims characterize the later stages of ideal adult development.

While there is little empirical research to support a relationship between an adolescent's position in one of the aforementioned groups and health, some evidence suggests that individuals who are in the moratorium group experience anxiety and guilt that can block further healthy exploration and development of a comfortable sense of self-identity. Similarly, many of those who are in the foreclosure group lack the practice of self-reflection and tend to engage in self-denial and excessive moralism that prevents them from being open to others and to new experiences.[9]

Self-Awareness

To optimize one's personal development as well as one's health and well-being, one must be fully aware of the self. To be aware is to be watchful, alert, and knowledgeable.[10] To be aware of oneself is to know one's own identity and one's relationship to others; to be aware of oneself is to know what one can do and where one fits within the social order of the world. The process of healing, which is never fully completed, requires an ongoing awareness of one's body-mind-spirit. Awareness of one's place within society and within the universe occurs in three dimensions: the cognitive, the intuitive, and the transcendent. This multidimensional awareness includes rational knowledge of facts and laws that govern the physical world. This is *cognitive awareness* and includes "consciously knowing facts and processing the constant flow of information coming in through the senses."[11(p.4)] This is the awareness that accompanies the first two stages of identity formation in Erikson's stages of development. Cognitive awareness is used throughout one's life to provide information about the physical world and one's behaviors in it.

Intuitive awareness is another way of knowing about oneself and the world. It is an affective sense of knowing by feeling some truth directly. Rather than following the rational and linear steps of empirical knowledge gained through the senses, intuitive awareness comes as an intense feeling of certainty that may be accompanied by a sense of mystery or confusion.[12] It is a direct way of knowing that is very personal and often poorly communicated to others. As individuals grow and develop, this sense of intuition may flourish or be stunted by those who do not trust its wisdom.[13]

A third kind of awareness is that of the spiritual dimension and is known as *transcendent awareness*. Transcendent awareness is not bound by time or matter. It is a way of knowing that represents an exchange of energy occurring without rational thought.[14] It may be evident to the individual through prayer or meditation. As depicted in Figure 17–1, these types of awareness vary in their degree of concreteness. On the most practical or concrete

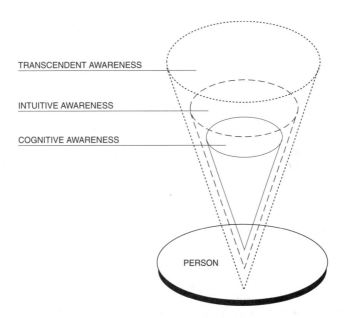

TRANSCENDENT AWARENESS

INTUITIVE AWARENESS

COGNITIVE AWARENESS

PERSON

Figure 17-1 Dimensions of Cognitive, Intuitive, and Transcendent Awareness. *Source:* From *Awareness in Healing, 1st edition,* by L. Rew, © 1995. Reprinted with permission of Delmar Publishers, a division of International Thomson Publishing. Fax 800-730-2215.

level is cognitive awareness, knowing about the physical world and one's own physical attributes. On the second, more abstract level is intuitve awareness, knowing by feeling or sensing something directly without having to think about it or without having direct evidence. Finally, on the most abstract level is transcendent awareness, knowing directly through one's soul or spirit. Within a person, each of these three types of awareness is synthesized into a resource of inner wisdom that may be tapped in self-reflection activities.

The idea of transcendent awareness is derived from the works of William James,[15] who identifed the spiritual Self, and Viktor Frankl,[16] who described self-transcendence as the tendency of human beings to reach beyond themselves and either to discover or to create purpose and meaning in their lives. Frankl's primary thesis was that the search for meaning is the primary motivation in human life. He identifed three major ways in which people find meaning or pur-

pose in life: (1) creating a work or doing a deed, (2) experiencing something or encountering another person, and (3) choosing an attitude in the face of circumstances that cannot be changed or that involve suffering. Others have studied self-transcendence as an aspect of the spiritual dimension of people. For example, Reed developed a mid-range nursing theory of self-transcendence based on life-span development theories.[17] She concluded that "in individuals who have an increased awareness of personal mortality through such experiences as terminal illness or advanced age, self-transcendence is a salient pattern and a correlate of well-being."[18(p.75)] She asserted that nurses can help clients expand their self-boundaries through meditation, visualization, peer counseling, journal keeping, self-reflection, and life review, thus enabling them to look both inwardly and outwardly. This view is similar to that of Newman, who theorized that health is expanding consciousness and that "unbroken wholeness is what is real—not the fragments we devise with our way of describing things."[19(p.37)]

Coward studied self-transcendence both in healthy populations and in people with acquired immune deficiency syndrome (AIDS) and advanced breast cancer. She found that self-transcendence was related to an increased sense of purpose and self-worth in patient populations, and that it was associated with emotional well-being, hope, sense of coherence, and self-esteem in the healthy population.[20] Transcendent awareness is the knowledge that one has a spiritual connection to something greater than the self. It may be experienced in quiet times of meditation and prayer or in situations of crisis. It is the type of awareness that may be experienced directly and suddenly, similar to intuitive awareness.[21] Each type of awareness—that is, cognitive, intuitive, and transcendent—contributes to the synthesis of the whole person and is manifest in self-awareness. Each is important in the development of a healthy person. Each of these types of awareness can be fostered through self-reflective strategies that focus on thoughts (cognitions), feelings and intuitions, and self-transcendent experiences or ideas.

Much research has shown that cognitive-perceptual factors are related to health-promoting behaviors and healthy outcomes.[22] Just as educational interventions can increase clients' knowledge about their bodies and physiologic processes, cognitive awareness can be improved and is related to better health outcomes. For example, in a meta-analysis of the effects of psychoeducational approaches in caring for adults with hypertension, nurse researchers found that education had statistically significant beneficial effects on blood pressure.[23] Little research exists, however, regarding the relation of intuitive and transcendent awareness in relation to health. Self-reflection skills combine the linear analysis of cognitive awareness with the intuitive, nonlinear, and more direct ways of knowing.[24] As these two aspects of knowing and perceiving are synthesized, changes in the bodymind, bodyspirit, and mindspirit occur.

Body-Mind-Spirit Connections

Recent research has provided much evidence of the connections between the mind, body, and spirit.[25,26] The burgeoning disciplines of psychoneuroimmunology and neuropsychology have shed much light on the holistic nature of human belief, thought, and behavior. Once the domain of philosophers and theologians, the realities of beliefs, conscious thought, and spiritual experience have now found their rightful places within new sciences that connect these abstract realities with chemistry and biology. For example, Pert's pioneering work in biochemistry revealed the presence of chemical messengers known as neuropeptides that, along with their corresponding receptors in cells, form a network for information processing between the body and the mind.[27,28] The presence of such a network literally allows various parts of the body to communicate with one another through a mind no longer limited to a space within the brain. Furthermore, there is increasing evidence that engaging in relaxation, guided imagery, and artistic endeavors changes physiology and results in altered immune function with consequent healing.[29]

Spiritual healing, which historically has been a part of many primitive medical systems, is now being explored seriously in scientific circles. Its effectiveness may be due in part to hypnosis, which mimics the focused attention and altered state of consciousness that is found in some ritualistic spiritual healing practices.[30] Scientific theoretical models are also being developed and tested to explain the healing effects of prayer.[31] These and other findings (see, e.g., the discussion of the psychophysiology of healing in Chapter 4) emphasize the interdependence of the mind-body-spirit dimensions of human beings and provide an important part of the framework for self-reflection interventions.

HOLISTIC CARING PROCESS

Assessment

In preparing to use self-reflection interventions, the nurse assesses the following parameters:[32]

- *the client's belief system:* Is it congruent with planned interventions?
- *the client's ability to read and write:* If the client cannot read or write, can family members or friends assist with audiotape recordings?
- *the client's experience with similar techniques:* Has the client ever kept a diary or discussed his or her dreams with others?
- *the client's personal goals and motivation for reaching them:* Are they clear to the nurse and can the nurse respect them if they are different from her own?
- *the client's understanding of the purpose of the intervention:* Does the client understand that the purpose is not to invade his or her privacy but to enhance self-understanding?

Patterns/Problems/Needs

The following are the patterns/problems/needs compatible with the interventions for self-reflection that are related to the nine human response patterns of the Unitary Person framework (see Chapter 14):

- *Communicating:* Altered communication: impaired verbal communication
- *Relating:* Impaired social interaction; Altered family processes; Social isolation
- *Valuing:* Spiritual distress; Disruption of person-environment pattern of the whole

- *Choosing:* Impaired adjustment; Ineffective family coping; Ineffective individual coping
- *Moving:* Activity intolerance: fatigue; Sleep pattern disturbance; Deficit in diversional activity
- *Perceiving:* Altered self-concept; Body image disturbance; Hopelessness; Powerlessness
- *Knowing:* Altered thought processes
- *Feeling:* Anxiety; Grieving: anticipatory and dysfunctional

Outcomes

Exhibit 17–1 guides the nurse in client outcomes, nursing prescriptions, and evaluation for the use of self-reflection as a nursing intervention.

Therapeutic Care Plan and Interventions

Following the client assessment and establishment of goals with the client, the nurse plans with the client to implement those self-reflection techniques that the client finds most appealing and eager to try, and that both nurse and client agree will have the highest likelihood in helping to reach the goals. Although most of these interventions require little technical skill on the part of the nurse, they do require a thorough assessment and a collaborative relationship with the client.

Before the Session

- To be fully present with the client and with the intention to facilitate healing, begin with centering. This is done by engaging in deep breathing and systematic relaxation, letting go of other issues and concerns, and allowing yourself to be fully present in the moment with the client.
- Complete other physical treatments for the client and ensure the client's physical comfort prior to beginning a

Exhibit 17–1 Nursing Interventions: Self-Reflection

Client Outcomes	Nursing Prescriptions	Evaluation
The client will demonstrate more effective coping skills as evident in weekly journal entries and clustering maps.	Guide the client in journal keeping and clustering to identify patterns of ineffective and effective coping skills.	The client demonstrates active problem solving and decreasing reliance on food and drugs.
The client will seek situations in which he or she interacts with others and will record feelings of belonging to a group through diary entries.	Guide the client to write daily about feelings and thoughts about the client and his or her relationships with others. Encourage the client to engage in lucid dreaming to imagine himself or herself interacting competently with others.	The client increases participation in social and family events and describes feelings of being more connected with others.
The client will reminisce about life through a life-review process and will verbalize a sense of meaning or purpose in life.	Facilitate six to eight sessions of reminiscence and life review in a support group setting. Encourage presentation of photographs and memorabilia.	The client states that, in addition to feeling sad about dying, he or she has come to realize that life has meaning and purpose and that he or she will be missed by family and friends.

self-reflection intervention so that the client may also be fully present in the moment and will not be distracted by physical sensations such as hunger or pain.

- Maintain privacy.
- Collect any special supplies required, such as paper, pencils, photograph albums, tape recorders, or music tapes, prior to initiating the intervention.[33]

At the Beginning of the Session

- Begin the intervention by describing what is to be done and what the client may expect to achieve as a result of participating in the activity.[34]
- Begin with a relaxation exercise, including deep breathing and systematic muscle relaxation (see Chapter 21 for details).
- Encourage the client to quiet the inner chatter or dialogue and to listen to his or her inner wisdom for guidance.

- If this is a second or subsequent session, review with the client events and situations that have transpired since the previous session before starting the relaxation exercise.

During the Session

- Support the client through physical presence and encouragement.
- If the client requests solitude, respect this need and encourage the client to indicate when he or she is ready for further interaction.
- Encourage the client to ask questions and clarify for the client the purpose and process involved in looking inward for wisdom and understanding.
- Monitor the environment to reduce stimuli in the form of noise, light, and odors that may distract the client from concentrating on the task at hand.
- Ensure that ample time and supplies are provided for the client to complete

the strategies and obtain the maximum benefit from them.

At the End of the Session

- Before leaving the client, bring the client's focus back to the present time and place, reorienting the client as needed.
- Review what has been done and what goals have been met.
- Encourage the client to continue with homework if needed and provide for a mutually convenient time to review this homework.
- Assess the client's ability to continue reflective work on his or her own and continue discussion if the client has difficulty in interpreting what has happened.

Specific Interventions: Self-Reflection

The purpose of self-reflection interventions is to help the client make sense of life events and circumstances that may be bewildering or discomforting. Many experiences in life lead to feelings of emptiness and disharmony because of the client's inability to connect the experience with thoughts, feelings, actions, and physiologic responses. Using the following strategies with clients empowers them and enables them to make new connections and to reframe and reinterpret their experiences in light of inner strengths and wisdom.

Keeping Diaries and Journals

Keeping diaries and journals is a simple way to begin the process of self-reflection. Notes may be kept in a variety of forms, but a notebook or journal that keeps notes together in a single-bound format facilitates the use of these documents for review and for discerning patterns of response to life's events. Diaries may be structured or un-structured. Structuring diaries often facilitates the recording of information such as eating patterns or patterns of pain and its management. Keeping a chart of symptoms such as those associated with headache pain may be useful in identifying interpersonal or environmental triggers for such symptoms.[35] Unstructured diaries or journals provide the space to record thoughts and feelings about those situations that create anxiety or symptoms of illness. There is no correct or incorrect way to make entries in such a diary or journal, and clients can be encouraged simply to allow themselves to follow the stream of consciousness and to play as they begin to write or draw in this format.[36] The purpose is to release feelings, to capture lessons learned in the past and apply those lessons to the present, and to connect feelings with thoughts, memories, beliefs, behaviors, and expectations about the future.

Diaries and journals may also be used as an arena in which to practice dialogues with personal body parts, other people, or groups. They may be used to log dreams and to record various interpretations of these dreams. These strategies may also be used with children, who may enjoy adding stickers to express feelings or to stimulate the imagination in helping them to deal with painful or frightening procedures or past events. Because the results of keeping a journal or a diary are very tangible, the selection of an appropriate style of documentation is important. Many fabric-covered blank books are available for this purpose, as are commercially produced daily diaries with dates. The importance of selecting writing or drawing instruments should be addressed, and the client should be assisted in choosing one or several that are pleasurable to use. Reviewing with the client the selection of the diary or journal and writing or drawing instruments may also enhance the experience of self-reflection as the client explains why these particular supplies are appealing.

Creating Works of Art

Creating works of art, including drawing, sketching, painting, sculpting, weaving, sewing, knitting, and so forth, may be used to explore beliefs and shape outcomes.[37] To use one of these strategies for self-reflection, the client, with the nurse's help, identifies the purpose of the activity in terms of process rather than product. The purpose is to examine values and beliefs that may be hidden from conscious awareness but that are influencing the client's experience of illness or disharmony. Images that emerge during the creative process are authentic and allow the individual to tap into wisdom that may lie beyond the client's usual ability to access. It is important to stress that this type of activity focuses on process, because the client may put up barriers to engaging in artwork because of a sense that the product or outcome will not be very good. A stimulating question to begin the activity might be, "What would you paint (draw, sculpt, etc.) if you were not trying to impress anybody with your result?"[38(p.19)]

Writing Letters

Writing letters is a way to express a variety of feelings. While clients may already be using such writing to express positive feelings to others (e.g., by writing a thank you note), they may be unaware of its usefulness as a strategy to express negative feelings such as anger and disappointment. The process of writing a letter is healing because it gives tangible expression to thoughts and feelings that are sometimes kept out of awareness. Letters that express negative emotions may be read aloud to another person such as the nurse, who acts as a sounding board, or may be read for audio recording. After listening to the letter, the nurse may provide objective feedback, or the client may wish to listen to himself or herself on a tape recording. The letter may then be rewritten to clarify an expression of feelings. The first draft of such a letter should be completed without editing and should be written as if it would not be sent to the person addressed. Later drafts may be edited and sent if the client determines that this would be helpful. The process of writing and rewriting a letter should continue until the strength of the emotion has diminished or the client feels at peace with the issue of concern. The letter may then be torn up, placed in a journal, burned, buried, or sent to the intended recipient.[39] If the letter is to be used for catharsis and not for direct communication between client and another person, this should be made clear prior to beginning the intervention. However, the goal may be changed as the client gains self-understanding.

Beginning an Intuition Log

Intuition is a way of direct knowing that is not based on the usual linear method or rational analysis of sensory data.[40] Sudden flashes of insight that are unexpected are common experiences, but few people have learned to trust them as sources of truth or wisdom. Learning to trust such truths, however, contributes to healing and spiritual growth.[41] Some clients may benefit from carrying a personal intuition log with them. Each time they hear a small inner voice, have a vague hunch, or experience a sudden "aha," they can record it in the log book.[42] These entries can then be reviewed with the nurse to begin to sort out the truths from the mere hunches. With validation, clients begin to trust their intuitions, and this intuitive awareness then empowers them with new solutions and deeper understandings that promote healing.

Using Metaphors

A metaphor is a word, phrase, or concept denoting one kind of idea that is used in place of another to suggest an analogy or similarity between the two.[43] This intervention helps clients deal with the questions

"Who am I?" and "What is my life all about?" The purpose is to examine the meaning of a problem situation or of one's life in general by using a metaphor to describe some aspect of one's past, present, or future. Using an object to represent their life or an illness, clients are instructed to write or talk about themselves; for example, a client may describe himself or herself as a banana that started out green but ended up mushy and sweet.[44] Clients may be instructed to complete the statement, "Right now my life feels like a ____." Once the metaphor is identified, clients are encouraged to describe it as fully as possible (e.g., size, color, weight, relation to other objects, etc.). After recording or relating the metaphor, clients may wish to change to a different metaphor to symbolize growth in the future.

Learning from Dreams

Most of the dreams people remember take place during the stage of sleep in which they experience rapid eye movements (REM). Periods of REM sleep occur approximately every 90 minutes after one first falls asleep and are essential for health. People deprived of this stage of sleep may experience memory loss, irritability, fatigue, and lack of concentration.[45] Dreams come from three different levels of consciousness: (1) the preconscious, which is the most readily accessible and contains material easily called into consciousness during the time one is awake; (2) the personal unconscious, which includes those memories that are generally hidden or repressed from waking consciousness, such as childhood traumas and fears; and (3) the collective unconscious, which includes the inherited aspects of mind that spawn the recurrent themes common in the mythology and legends of all cultures.

In his book entitled *Teach Yourself to Dream*, David Fontana offers a practical guide to harnessing the power of the mind and regaining wholeness.[46] He provides a variety of techniques based on Jungian psychology to help people discover the personal meanings of dreams, make dreams more vivid, use dreams to solve practical problems, and engage in lucid dreaming. For example, Fontana suggests that the client be directed to perform a brief ritual before falling asleep in which dreams are allowed full reign. Creating a framework based on music, drumming, gesturing, or chanting may facilitate dreaming. Thinking about one's dreams during the day and making imaginative connections between the dreams and actual events may help one to gain insights and facilitate meaningful interpretations of subsequent dreams. Reviewing the day's events prior to falling asleep will facilitate the recall of dreams and help one to build these meaningful connections.

The client may also be instructed to keep a dream diary and pen next to the bed in order to learn the most from dreams. As in writing any diary, the date should be noted and plenty of room should be left for interpretation of the dream. Fontana suggests always recording dreams in the present tense and making notes of the emotions that accompany the recording of the dream as well as drawing sketches, which may be either symbolic or real figures.[47] Recording the dream in the present tense brings the material directly into awareness, where the client can then deal with it.

Mind Maps and Clustering

Mind maps are a method for brainstorming by oneself. The purpose of this activity is to clarify one's thinking about a particular issue. As in group methods of brainstorming, four principles are involved: (1) Judgment or evaluation of ideas should be suspended. (2) Any idea or thought, no matter how illogical or absurd, is allowed. (3) The more ideas or thoughts generated, the better. (4) All combinations or modifications of existing ideas are allowed. The mapping of concepts, also known as clustering, begins with a key concept that comes to mind as one reflects on a problem or concern. This word, phrase, symbol, or sketch is placed in the center of a piece of paper and is circled. By connecting words or phrases to this central thought or idea, one can examine belief systems and integrate ideas. The process of writing down an idea, symbol, or picture and then circling it and connecting it to other words continues until an intuitive connection or insight is realized.[48] Using colors and following the natural shapes of plants, such as the roots, trunk, and branches of a tree, helps in expressing and exploring emotions and in examining the connections of these emotions with each other and with behaviors.[49] Figure 17–2 illustrates the use of clustering by a client in examining anxiety about an invasive diagnostic procedure. The concepts in the figure are numbered to demonstrate the sequence of

thinking and exploring done by the client; however, numbering is not necessary.

One type of mapping that is beneficial in self-reflection is to search the inner guides that Jung referred to as archetypes.[50] Jung conceptualized archetypes as patterns that are deeply imprinted in the human psyche and that exist in the "collective unconscious" of all people over all times. These are the patterns or themes that recur in dreams, myths, and legends. These archetypal patterns also serve as inner guides to the tasks or crises of growth and development. Some examples of archetypes and the corresponding tasks they help one to achieve are the Innocent, which assists in the attainment of happiness, and the Warrior, which assists in proving one's worth.[51] The Innocent archetype represents the natural state of dependency characteristic of infants and small children. Focusing on this aspect of oneself leads to fantasies of

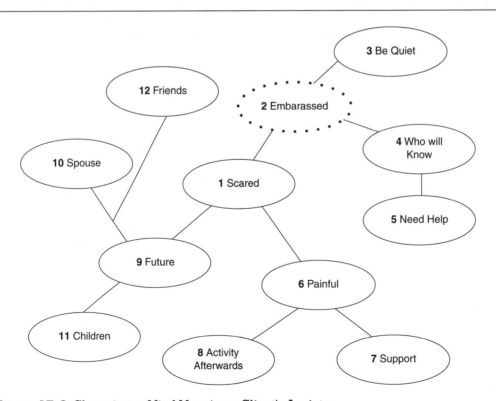

Figure 17–2 Clustering or Mind Mapping a Client's Anxiety.

paradise and living life somewhat passively, waiting to be cared for and rescued. One limitation of seeing oneself as an Innocent is that pain and suffering may be ignored. A strength of the Innocent archetype, however, is that it can attract and activate positive energy in social relationships so that change and growth can occur. The nurse who elects to use archetypes to help clients explore personal growth must be well-acquainted with Jung's work and the collective meaning of these archetypes.

Using the Mandala and Focusing

The mandala, from the Sanskrit word meaning *circle,* is a ritualistic device used in Buddhism as a focus for meditation. Any circular geometric design can be used to focus the attention and quiet the inner dialogue. Focusing on such a harmonic symbol may serve as preparation for listening to the wisdom within.[52] Focusing may then be used to stimulate self-awareness and emotional healing by drawing attention to physical symptoms of illness or other bodily sensations. Focusing may begin by using a physical symbol such as the mandala or by using directed imagery. The purpose is to direct the awareness of the client so that the body is sensed in a systematic manner.[53] In this technique, the internal dialogue that is constantly part of one's inner experience is first quieted, and then awareness is allowed to turn directly to the meaning of a problem or symptom.

Sharing Stories

Each person's life is composed of stories. By telling stories about themselves, people can re-create who they are and who they will become. By sharing and hearing stories, people may develop a deeper understanding of themselves and the meaning of their lived experiences.[54] To make sense of the world, humans create internal models or frames of reference based on a story line that connects experiences with thoughts, feelings, and beliefs. Telling one's personal story is empowering, but writing it is stronger and more permanent than simply speaking it.[55] Stories that are based on the facts of a client's life or that represent dreams and goals for the future may be shared between client and nurse or among a group of clients. Telling his or her story in a variety of settings to various audiences allows the client to incorporate the details of events that may otherwise be emotionally draining. Children, in particular, benefit from telling about their traumatic or frightening experiences. Writing a story allows the client the opportunity to revisit and revise the story as new insights are gained. The powerful impact of gaining insight from storytelling may be enhanced by encouraging the client to use the present tense. Visual images that arise during the telling or writing of the story can also be used to enhance the healing process associated with this intervention.[56]

Fictional story writing may be used in conjunction with the keeping of a diary or journal. Summarizing the theme of a series of events may help the client bring closure to circumstances that have challenged the sense of self. For example, after keeping a journal about the daily feelings and sensations associated with having a mastectomy, a client may write a story that identifies the fears and strengths of an imaginary woman with the same diagnosis. The story, which may incorporate elements of truth and fantasy, may then be read aloud into a tape recorder or to a support group.

Reminiscing and Embarking on a Life Review

Life review is the process of consciously returning to past experiences, often including traumatic life events, that can be surveyed, resolved, and reintegrated into the self.[57] The goal of this integration is the personal realization that life has been unique and has some kind of meaning.[58]

McDougall and colleagues studied this process in 80 adults over the age of 65 who had been diagnosed with depression.[59]

Subjects received follow-up care in their homes from an advanced-practice geronto-psychiatric nurse. During each of three sessions per week for 60 days, the nurse used life review to elicit issues about past experiences from the clients, who were formerly hospitalized for their symptoms of depression. These issues included negative life events, unresolved conflicts, and feelings of guilt. The researchers concluded that being in familiar surroundings within their homes enabled these older adults to discuss topics that might otherwise have remained unexplored and unresolved in this population. As a result of this intervention, the subjects showed a decrease in feelings of anxiety, denial, isolation, and despair.

Various self-help books are available commerically to use with clients who are self-directed or who might benefit from additional homework exercises. Many of these are in workbook format with inviting prompts to encourage completion of the activities. Some are meant specifically for women and others specifically for adolescents. A sampling of such books can be found at the end of the chapter under "Suggested Readings."

Case Studies

The two case studies that follow demonstrate the use of self-reflection strategies to aid a man who is dying and an adolescent who has an eating disorder.

Case Study No. 1

Setting:	Community-based AIDS support group
Client:	K.H., a 47-year-old man
Nursing Diagnoses:	1. Anticipatory grieving
	2. Altered comfort
	3. Powerlessness
	4. Social isolation, related to family's response to his diagnosis

Ten years ago, K.H. divorced his wife of 15 years when he decided to acknowledge his homosexuality. At the time, K.H. and his wife had three children ranging in age from 5 to 10 years. They had been a close-knit family and had been active in their community. K.H.'s wife won custody of the children but agreed that K.H. could retain weekly visitation rights. Shortly after the divorce, K.H. moved into an apartment with another man in the same city where his ex-wife and children lived. Over the next year, relations among the family members were strained, but K.H. was determined to be involved in raising his children. Approximately 5 years ago, K.H. learned that he and his partner were both positive for human immunodeficiency virus (HIV) although asymptomatic.

Now K.H. has full-blown AIDS and, although he is receiving treatment, he understands that his condition is fatal. His children are now 15, 18, and 20 years old. In the support group, which he attends with his partner (who remains asymptomatic), K.H. engages in reminiscing and life review. He also begins keeping a daily journal in which he records his physical sensations as the symptoms of his disease progress, his emotional feelings of sadness and regret, and his spiritual development as he becomes aware that life includes more than just the physical-emotional dimensions. With the guidance of the holistic nurse, and by sharing stories with other group members, he works through issues of conflict and guilt, particularly those related to raising his children. As a result of this process of self-reflection and increased understanding, K.H. writes a personal letter to each of his children. In each letter he reveals his deepest feelings of love and concern about the child's welfare and shares his experiences of growth and development as a whole person who is willing and ready to die in peace and harmony.

Case Study No. 2

Setting:	Outpatient psychiatric unit
Client:	R.D., an 18-year-old female with anorexia nervosa

Nursing Diagnoses:
1. Altered nutrition: less than body requirements
2. Altered family process
3. Ineffective individual coping
4. Disturbance in self-concept

R.D. is in her final year of high school and is making plans to attend an out-of-state college in less than a year. Her senior year is marked by an increasing withdrawal from her parents and younger brother. During family celebrations she refuses to participate in special meals and frequently retires to her room before dessert is served. She admits that she is engaging in an intense diet and exercise program to control her weight so that she will not be teased about being fat when she goes away to college.

R.D. finally agrees to visit her family physician when she begins to experience a persistent cough and finds it difficult to concentrate on her schoolwork. Her disordered eating is diagnosed and treated aggressively. Following a period of hospitalization in which she gains 15 pounds, she begins to attend outpatient group meetings for young women with various eating disorders. In this setting, she learns about techniques for self-reflection and begins to understand her own behavior and its connections to her deepest fears and needs. She finds that clustering is helpful in sorting out her fears about being out of control. Through this process she begins to understand that her eating behaviors have been ineffective in solving her problems with family members. R.D. also keeps a dream diary and is surprised to find some recurrent themes that enable her to confront her anxiety about growing up and leaving home.

Evaluation

With the client, the nurse determines whether the client outcomes for self-reflection (see Exhibit 17–1) were successfully

achieved. To evaluate the session further, the nurse may again explore the subjective effects of the experience with the client using the evaluation questions in Exhibit 17–2. Periodically, the nurse and the client review the progress made toward achieving the goals or outcomes identified before beginning the self-reflection interventions. Many of the interventions described here take place over relatively long periods of times. Throughout the process, the nurse must monitor the client's progress and provide both presence and encouragement to continue the process of self-understanding and acceptance. If specific techniques are used in a formal session, the nurse should encourage the client to evaluate each session as it ends.

DIRECTIONS FOR FUTURE RESEARCH

1. Evaluate the effectiveness of self-reflection interventions in achieving the desired client outcomes.

Exhibit 17–2 Evaluation of the Client's Subjective Experience of Self-Reflection

1. Was this a new experience for you? Can you describe it?
2. Did you have any physical or emotional responses to the experience? Can you describe them?
3. Were there any distractions?
4. Did this exercise change the way you see yourself or your experiences?
5. Did the experience help you recall any memories or details of your life?
6. What are your thoughts and feelings when you review your journal, diary, log, or other self-reflection tool?
7. Would you like to try this again?
8. What would make this experience more meaningful for you?
9. Do you see yourself using this exercise on a regular basis in your life?

2. Use qualitative methods to facilitate an understanding of how these interventions affect clients' experiences of healing.
3. Use qualitative methods to develop grounded theory to support the use of these strategies in achieving specific outcomes.
4. Conduct quantitative research to document relationships between the use of specific techniques and a variety of physiologic, behavioral, emotional, and spiritual outcomes for clients and for nurses themselves.
5. Develop appropriate instruments to provide objective evidence that self-awareness and self-understanding have taken place.

NURSE HEALER REFLECTIONS

After reading this chapter, the nurse healer will be able to answer or begin the process of answering the following questions:

- What inner knowledge and awareness can be created by keeping a personal journal or dream diary?
- How can personal creativity and problem solving be enhanced by self-reflective techniques such as lucid dreaming or meditation?
- How can the life review process be used to ease the pain of death in clients?
- How can I learn to trust intuition in working with clients?

NOTES

1. E.B. Clarke and J.A. Spross, Expert Coaching and Guidance, in *Advanced Nursing Practice: An Integrative Approach*, ed. A.B. Hamric, J.A. Spross, and C.M. Hanson (Philadelphia: W.B. Saunders Co., 1996), 148–153.
2. W. James, *The Principles of Psychology*, vol. 1 (New York: Dover Publications, 1890, 1950).
3. R.A. Wicklund and M. Eckert, *The Self-Knower: A Hero under Control* (New York: Plenum Press, 1992).
4. A.H. Modell, *The Private Self* (Cambridge, MA: Harvard University Press, 1993).
5. J. Kagan, Is There a Self in Infancy? in *Self-Awareness: Its Nature and Development*, ed. M. Ferrari and R.J. Sternberg (New York: Guilford Press, 1998), 137–147.
6. E. Erikson, *Identity: Youth and Crisis* (New York: W.W. Norton & Co., 1968).
7. R. Josselson, The Theory of Identity Development and the Question of Intervention, in *Interventions for Adolescent Identity Development*, ed. S.L. Archer (Thousand Oaks, CA: Sage Publications, 1994), 12–25.
8. J.E. Marcia, Identity in Adolescence, in *Handbook of Adolescent Psychology*, ed. J. Adelson (New York: John Wiley & Sons, 1980), 159–187.
9. Josselson, Theory of Identity Development.
10. L. Rew, *Awareness in Healing* (Albany, NY: Delmar Publishers, 1996).
11. Rew, *Awareness in Healing*.

12. Rew, *Awareness in Healing*.
13. N. Noddings and P.J. Shore, *Awakening the Inner Eye: Intuition in Education* (New York: Teachers College Press, 1984).
14. Rew, *Awareness in Healing*.
15. James, *Principles of Psychology*.
16. V. Frankl, *Man's Search for Meaning* (New York: Pocket Books, 1963).
17. P.G. Reed, Toward a Nursing Theory of Self-Transcendence: Deductive Reformulation Using Developmental Theories.
18. Reed, Toward a Nursing Theory of Self-Transcendence.
19. M.A. Newman, Experiencing the Whole, *Advances in Nursing Science* 20, no. 1 (1997): 34–39.
20. D.D. Coward, Self-Transcendence and Correlates in a Healthy Population, *Nursing Research* 45, no. 2 (1996): 116–121.
21. Rew, *Awareness in Healing*.
22. J.L. Bottorff et al., The Effects of Cognitive-Perceptual Factors on Health Promotion Behavior Maintenance, *Nursing Research* 45, no. 1 (1996): 30–36.
23. E.C. Devine and E. Reifschneider, A Meta-Analysis of the Effects of Psychoeducational Care in Adults with Hypertension, *Nursing Research* 44, no. 4 (1995): 237–245.
24. L.G. Kolkmeier, Self-Reflection: Consulting the Truth within, in *Holistic Nursing: A Handbook*

for Practice, 2d ed., eds. B.M. Dossey et al. (Rockville, MD: Aspen Publishers, 1988).

25. L. Dossey, Who Gets Sick and Who Gets Well? *Alternative Therapies* 1, no. 4 (1995): 6–11.

26. E. Rossi, *The Psychobiology of Mind-Body Healing* (New York: W.W. Norton & Co., 1993).

27. C. Pert, Neuropeptides: The Emotions and Body-Mind, *Noetic Sciences Review* Spring 1987, 13–18.

28. C. Pert, The Wisdom of the Receptors: Neuropeptides, the Emotions, and Body-Mind, in *The Healing Brain: A Scientific Reader*, ed. R. Ornstein and C. Swencionis (New York: Guilford Press, 1990), 147–158.

29. M. Samuels, Art as a Healing Force, *Alternative Therapies* 1, no. 4 (1995): 38–40.

30. J. McClenon, Spiritual Healing and Folklore Research: Evaluating the Hypnosis/Placebo Theory, *Alternative Therapies* 3, no. 1 (1997): 61–66.

31. J.S. Levin, How Prayer Heals: A Theoretical Model, *Alternative Therapies* 2, no. 1 (1996): 66–73.

32. Kolkmeier, Self-Reflection.

33. Kolkmeier, Self-Reflection.

34. Kolkmeier, Self-Reflection.

35. Kolkmeier, Self-Reflection.

36. Kolkmeier, Self-Reflection.

37. P.B. Allen, *Art Is a Way of Knowing* (Boston: Shambhala, 1995).

38. M. Cassou and S. Cubley, *Life, Paint and Passion: Reclaiming the Magic of Spontaneous Expression* (New York: G.P. Putnam's Sons, 1995).

39. Kolkmeier, Self-Reflection.

40. L. Rew, Intuition: Concept Analysis of a Group Phenomenon, *Advances in Nursing Science* 8, no. 2 (1986): 21–28.

41. L. Rew, Intuition: Nursing Knowledge and the Spiritual Dimension of Persons, *Holistic Nursing Practice* 3, no. 3 (1989): 56–68.

42. Kolkmeier, Self-Reflection.

43. F.C. Mish, *Merriam Webster's Collegiate Dictionary*, 5th ed. (Springfield, MA: Merriam-Webster, 1993).

44. R. von Oech, *A Whack on the Side of the Head: How You Can Be More Creative* (New York: Warner Books, 1990).

45. D. Fontana, *Teach Yourself to Dream* (San Francisco: Chronicle Books, 1997).

46. Fontana, *Teach Yourself to Dream.*

47. Fontana, *Teach Yourself to Dream.*

48. Rew, Intuition.

49. T. Buzan and B. Buzan, *The Mind Map Book* (New York: Penguin USA, 1993).

50. C.G. Jung, *Man and His Symbols* (New York: Dell Publishing, 1964).

51. C.S. Pearson, *The Hero Within* (San Francisco: HarperSanFrancisco, 1998).

52. Rew, *Awareness in Healing.*

53. A.W. Cornell, *The Power of Focusing: A Practical Guide to Emotional Self-Healing* (Oakland, CA: New Harbinger Publications, 1996).

54. M.G. Nagai-Jacobson and M.A. Burkhardt, Viewing Persons as Stories: A Perspective for Holistic Care, *Alternative Therapies* 2, no. 4 (1996): 54–58.

55. S.W. Albert, *Writing from Life: Telling Your Soul's Story* (New York: Jeremy P. Tarcher/Putnam, 1996).

56. R. Stone, *The Healing Art of Storytelling* (New York: Hyperion, 1996).

57. G.J. McDougall et al., The Process and Outcome of Life Review Psychotherapy with Depressed Homebound Older Adults, *Nursing Research* 46 (1997): 277–283.

58. Nagai-Jacobson and Burkhardt, Viewing Persons as Stories.

59. McDougall et al., Process and Outcome of Life Review Psychotherapy.

SUGGESTED READING

Albert, S.W., *Writing from Life: Telling Your Soul's Story* (New York: Jeremy P. Tarcher/Putnam, 1996).

Allen, P.B., *Art Is a Way of Knowing* (Boston: Shambhala, 1995).

Bingham, M., et al., *Choices: A Teen Woman's Journal for Self-Awareness and Personal Planning* (Santa Barbara, CA: Advocacy Press, 1993).

Cassou, M. and Cubley, S., *Life, Paint and Passion: Reclaiming the Magic of Spontaneous Expres-sion* (New York: G.P. Putnam's Sons, 1995).

Chapman, J., *Journaling for Joy: The Workbook* (Van Nuys, CA: Newcastle Publishing Co., 1995).

Fontana, D., *Teach Yourself to Dream* (San Francisco: Chronicle Books, 1997).

Murdock, M., *The Heroine's Journey Workbook* (Boston: Shambhala, 1998).

Olson, M., Death and Grief, in *Core Curriculum for Holistic Nursing*, ed. B.M. Dossey (Gaithersburg, MD: Aspen Publishers, 1997), 126–133.

VISION OF HEALING

Nourishing the Bodymind

In large measure, joy and vitality can come from eating well. A wise nurse endeavors to maximize and develop the best nutrition habits and skills both for the self and for the client. As we approach the 21st century, the ancient Greek ideal of a sound mind in a strong, able body is once again in fashion. A healthy physical body can indeed be the temple for the mind-spirit. The way in which we care for and nourish our bodies not only affects our general physical well-being but also increases our mental and spiritual capacities.

When planned with knowledge and commitment, nutritional intake promotes high-level wellness behavior. Foods have power. Foods transfer their power to human beings when we digest and assimilate them. One of the basic premises behind the view that foods heal is that food is comprised of organic chemicals just as we are. As physical organisms, we are composed of millions of biochemicals. Their daily replacement through the ingestion of healthy nutrients is critical to our optimal functioning. Food consumption and physical activity have a direct effect on the body-mind-spirit. Unlike taking medicines, healthy eating enables us to build up or tear down the actual tissues of our bodies. When

we eat well, we build strong, healthy bodies, but when our diets are defective, we deprive our bodies. In general, the feeling of well-being that comes from physical health permeates every individual activity, enabling the quickest thinking, permitting a better night's sleep, and perhaps facilitating spirituality.

The lack of proper nutrition is a major risk factor for diseases, such as hypertension, hypercholesterolemia, and obesity. Eating habits affect exercise abilities and vice versa. However, nutrition patterns can be modified when individuals make the decision to move toward wellness. For those who are nutritionally compromised or physically weakened because of illness and disease or because of mental, emotional, or spiritual ennui, the good news is that anyone with motivation can use the principles of healing nutrition to activate and nourish the bodymind.

As we embark on the 21st century, each of us has the capacity to acquire information, not only to prevent disease, but also to achieve a vital, productive life. Nurses can increase their own vigor and vitality and then use the same methods to assist their clients. As a collective whole, nurses can join with other professionals to meet the objective of increased health and vitality for all people.

Chapter 18

Nutrition

Susan Luck

NURSE HEALER OBJECTIVES

Theoretical

- Learn the definitions of terms in this chapter.
- Differentiate between the recommended daily allowance (RDA) and the optimal daily allowance (ODA).
- Develop a plan that combines good nutrition with exercise and body awareness.
- Learn the benefits of healthy eating for health maintenance and disease prevention.

Clinical

- Assess the quality of your food intake and note how it increases or decreases your energy level at work.
- Observe the meaning of foods in different cultural traditions.
- Identify nutritional foods that support your client's healing process.
- Employ strategies to improve nutrition in your workplace environment.

Personal

- Heighten your awareness of the way in which what you eat affects how you feel.
- Examine your eating patterns and the meaning of food in your life.

- Explore new foods and food preparation that support your health.
- Plan a day's menu, asking yourself, "What does my body need to enhance my wellness?"

DEFINITIONS

Antioxidants: substances that limit free radical formation and damage by stabilizing or deactivating free radicals before they attack cells.

Free Radicals: electrically charged molecules with an unpaired electron capable of attacking healthy cells in the body, causing them to lose their structure and function.

Glycemic Index: an index that classifies carbohydrate foods according to their glycemic response (effect on blood glucose levels), which varies with fiber content, starch structure, food processing, and presence of proteins and fats.

HDL: high-density lipoprotein form of cholesterol associated with reduced risk of artherosclerosis.

Homocysteine: an intermediate product of methionine metabolism and a marker for many clinical conditions, including cardiovascular disease.

LDL: low-density lipoprotein form of cholesterol strongly associated with increased risk of artherosclerosis.

Mineral: an inorganic trace element or compound that works in synergy with other compounds and is essential for human life.

Optimal Nutrition: adequate intake of nutrients for health promotion and disease prevention.

Phytochemicals: biologically active compounds found in foods.

Phytoestrogens: family of compounds found in plants that have some estrogenic and/or antiestrogenic activity in humans.

Probiotic: formulation containing beneficial living microorganisms that maintain health as part of the internal ecology of the digestive tract.

Vitamin: an organic substance necessary for normal growth, metabolism, and development of the body; acts as a catalyst and coenzyme, assisting in many chemical reactions while nourishing the body.

Xenoestrogens: synthetic, hormone-mimicking compounds found in certain pesticides, drugs, and plastics.

THEORY AND RESEARCH

Over the last few decades, nutrition has moved into the forefront as a major component in health promotion and disease prevention. The scientific knowledge of nutrition is expanding rapidly. As nutritional science has developed, so have its clinical implications and applications. Understanding of clinical nutrition has broadened, so that it is now included as part of an integrated, comprehensive approach to health care. Today, nutritional assessment and interventions are often prescribed along with conventional medical protocols in the treatment of many health conditions, including heart disease, arthritis, diabetes, obesity, cancer, immune dysfunction, and a variety of women's health problems.

In the past decade, science has vigorously researched the impact of nutrition on health and disease. Food is no longer viewed merely as providing substances whose absence would produce disease but as having a positive impact on the individual's health, physical performance, and state of mind. Foods, and the nutrients derived from them, are considered to promote health, assist healthy aging, and support complete physical, mental, and social well-being. Modern society makes available an increasingly wide variety of processed, denatured foods that are depleted of nutrients and often contain toxic chemicals. Research implicates these changes in the food supply as contributing to a number of health problems, including atherosclerosis, heart disease, hypertension, diabetes, and various cancers. These diseases were virtually unknown a hundred years ago. Therefore, nutritional requirements are being reevaluated to meet the demands of today's world and the needs of people throughout the various stages of life, beginning with prenatal development and continuing into old age. The individual's metabolism, environment, genetics, emotional health, and life stressors must be considered in evaluating nutritional needs and nutritional goals. Nutrition is becoming an important component of early intervention strategies to improve physiologic, cognitive, emotional, and physical functioning of the individual.

For more than 40 years, the recommended daily allowances (RDAs) for various nutrients established by the U.S. Food and Nutrition Board have been the standard guidelines for defining nutritional needs. RDAs specify the levels of nutrients required to prevent overt symptoms of deficiency.[1] Since their inception, the RDA guidelines have been periodically reevaluated and updated based on continuing analysis of science advances in the field. The RDA guidelines have generated controversy, with many governmental and private groups asking questions such as the following:

- Can one get all of the nutrients one needs from the foods available in today's food supply?
- Do the RDAs take into account individual lifestyle, food availability, individual health needs, and so on?
- Do the RDAs consider optimal health and well-being?

Many researchers and practitioners advocate nutrient supplementation in addition to consumption of healthy foods that conform to nutritional guidelines to help people meet the growing health challenges confronting our world today. They recommend new standards known as optimal daily requirements (ODAs).

Overt symptoms of nutrient deficiency are merely the last event in a long chain of reactions in the body. When a person does not receive adequate nutrients, the initial reactions occur on a molecular level. First, essential enzymes that are dependent on the deficient nutrients become depleted. This depletion then brings about changes in cells themselves. These deficiencies can continue for many years until the body can no longer carry out its normal functions. Eventually, overt signs and symptoms appear, even though the deficiency may still be considered subclinical since routine laboratory tests do not necessarily uncover nutritional deficiencies. Nevertheless, these subclinical deficiencies can lead to a broad range of nonspecific conditions that can diminish an individual's overall quality of life. Undiagnosed, these deficiencies, over many years, leave the body more vulnerable to illnesses to which the individual may be genetically predisposed and to immune system compromise. Only recently, high levels of homocysteine have been recognized to be associated with increased risk for cardiovascular disease and stroke. Homocysteine is found in low amounts in healthy individuals. Research has shown repeatedly that elevated homocysteine levels result from subclinical deficiencies of B

vitamins, including folic acid, vitamin B_6, and vitamin B_{12}.[2] Vigilance for nutrient deficiencies and their potentially life-threatening consequences is slow to become part of routine physical examinations and health assessments.[3] Two articles in a recent issue of the *New England Journal of Medicine* report, "High plasma homocysteine concentrations and low concentrations of folate and Vitamin B_6 through their role in homocysteine metabolism, are associated with an increased risk of extracranial carotid-artery stenosis in the elderly."[4] Attention to the role of nutrients in maintaining health and preventing disease is gradually becoming a recognized component in the provision of comprehensive care.

Nutrient deficiencies can result from a high intake of refined foods. Americans consume approximately 18 percent of their calories as refined sugar, devoid of the vitamins or minerals necessary for its metabolism. It is estimated that an additional 18 percent of a typical American diet consists of refined products. These include white bread, which is deficient in 28 essential nutrients that were contained in the whole grain prior to its processing. Deficiencies in many of these nutrients—especially vitamin B_6, the most commonly deficient B vitamin in the diet—are associated with diabetes, heart disease, depression, and premenstrual syndrome. Many epidemiological studies report strong correlations between Western diseases and dietary habits.[5] Mortality rates for certain cancers as well as the incidence of cardiovascular disease are higher among those consuming an American diet than among those consuming Asian, Scandinavian, or Mediterranean diets.[6] (The Mediterranean diet pyramid is shown in Figure 18–1.)

Nutrient Sources

Carbohydrates

Carbohydrates provide the main source of energy for all body functions, aiding in

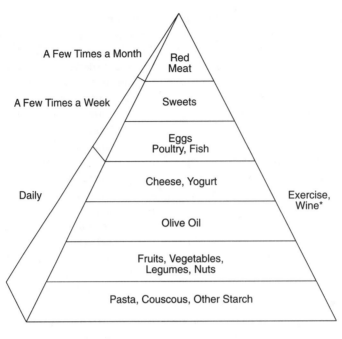

A Few Times a Month — Red Meat

A Few Times a Week — Sweets

Eggs Poultry, Fish

Cheese, Yogurt

Daily

Olive Oil

Exercise, Wine*

Fruits, Vegetables, Legumes, Nuts

Pasta, Couscous, Other Starch

*Daily, wine in moderation

Figure 18-1 Mediterranean Diet Pyramid. *Source:* Oldways Preservation & Exchange Trust. *Source:* Reprinted by permission of Dow Jones, Inc. via Copyright Clearance Center, Inc., © 1999, Dow Jones and Company, Inc. All Rights Reserved Worldwide.

digestion, assimilation, and metabolism of proteins and fats. Carbohydrates are classified as simple and complex. Simple carbohydrates include refined white flour products, white rice, white table sugar (dextrose), honey, fruit sugars (fructose), and milk sugars (lactose). Complex carbohydrates are found in whole grains, legumes, and vegetables and contain protein, vitamins, minerals, and fiber. They have been an important staple of the diet in diverse cultures throughout human history. Complex carbohydrates supply the body with essential nutrients and provide longer lasting energy than simple carbohydrates.

Fiber

Fiber contains polysaccharides and can be subdivided into insoluble fiber and soluble fiber, each with a different mixture of compounds. Insoluble fiber includes pectin and cellulose, hemicellulose, and lignins. Insoluble fiber is present in fruits, vegetables, whole grains, and beans. *Insoluble fiber* is found in apples, leafy vegetables, and brans. *Soluble fiber* is identified as gelatinlike substances including the mucilage qualities found in oatmeal and legumes. Research clearly documents that the modern Western diet, with its low fiber content, has led to an increase in digestive problems, including diverticulitis, constipation, colon cancer, gallstone formation, and other gastrointestinal disturbances. Although dietary fiber is not digested and provides no caloric contribution, it increases fecal bulk and weight, making the passage of waste products more efficient so that toxins and cancer-causing substances are eliminated quickly from the system. Fiber also is important in modulating insulin response and thereby stabilizing blood sugar levels. In recent years, research into the benefits of dietary fiber has led many practitioners to recommend a low-fat, high-fiber diet for prevention of heart disease, diabetes, obesity, digestive disorders, and cancer.[7] According to Seymour Handler, of the North Memorial Medical Center in Minneapolis, most of the serious diseases of the colon, including appendicitis and diverticular disease, are linked etiologically to the high–saturated-fat, low-fiber Western diet. Colon cancer may be caused in part by carcinogens created in the colon. A diet high in saturated animal fat and low in fiber increases the risk. Guidelines for minimizing risk include reducing consumption of saturated fats and increasing consumption of complex carbohydrate foods offering protein, vitamins, minerals, and fiber.[8]

Protein

Protein is the second most plentiful substance in the body (after water) and constitutes approximately one-fifth of body weight. Protein is the basic building block of the body and makes up the rigid structures such as bone, solid organs, and blood vessels. It is essential for the growth and maintenance of all body tissues, including muscle, skin, hair, nails, and eyes. Hormones, chemicals such as antibodies, and enzymes are comprised of protein. Protein molecules, comprised essentially of amino acids, form long chains and branched structures. Amino acids contain nitrogen, carbon, hydrogen, and sometimes sulfur. Twenty-two amino acids are required to build protein; half of these are produced in the body when adequate nutrients are available; eight are considered essential. Excessive protein consumption taxes the kidneys and digestive system. Since the majority of Americans consume most of their protein through animal products—a source of saturated fat as well—consump-

tion of a large quantity of animal protein is associated with increased risk of cardiovascular disease and breast, colon, and prostate cancers. Plant foods such as whole grains, legumes, seeds, and nuts provide excellent protein, but this protein is incomplete, and these foods must be combined to provide all of the essential amino acids. Protein requirements depend on the individual's activity level, energy requirements, age, and digestive health. The recommended protein allowance for health maintenance in the United States is 0.8 gram per kilogram of body weight per day. Men and women who body-build require up to 1.2 grams per kilogram of body weight.[9]

Lipids

Lipids are a group of fats and fatlike substances, including essential fatty acids, that account for more than 10 percent of body weight in most adults. The principal function of fats is to serve as a source of energy. Stored fats also act as a thermal blanket, insulating the body and providing a protective cushion for many tissues and organs. According to the third National Health and Nutrition Examination Survey, Americans are eating less fat than they were 10 years ago. Americans now average 34 percent of their total daily calories (82 grams) from fat with approximately 12 percent (29 grams) from saturated fats. Current dietary recommendations call for 20 percent of total calories from fat and less than 10 percent from saturated fats. The RDA for dietary fat suggested by the National Academy of Sciences to ensure the intake of essential fatty acids is 25 grams.[10] Unsaturated fats are usually liquid at room temperature and are derived from vegetables, nuts and seeds, soybeans, and olives. Saturated fats—found in animal products, including meat and dairy products—are generally associated with increased risk of cancer and cardiovascular disease. Foods often contain a mixture of saturated and unsaturated fatty acids. Fats are calorie rich and contain approximately 9 calories per gram, almost twice the calories of carbohydrates and proteins.

Essential fatty acids are found in both monosaturated and polyunsaturated fats. Monosaturated fats include olive oil, peanut oil, avocado oil, and canola oil. Polyunsaturated fats (PUFAs) are found in safflower, sunflower, corn, sesame, and soy oils. Fats can be further divided into two main classes: Omega-3 fatty acids and omega-6 fatty acids. Essential fatty acids form a structural part of all cell membranes. They hold proteins in the membrane, maintain fluidity of the membrane, and create electrical potentials across the membrane, facilitating the generation of bioelectrical currents that transmit messages. Certain essential fatty acids substantially shorten the time required for the recovery of fatigued muscles after exercise by facilitating the conversion of lactic acid to water and carbon dioxide. Essential fatty acids act as precursors for a family of hormonelike substances called prostaglandins, which regulate many functions in the body, including inflammatory processes and immune responses. Essential fatty acids contain no cholesterol. They must be supplied through the diet because they cannot be synthesized by the body, although they are essential to health. Omega-3 essential fatty acids are immune enhancing and are generally deficient in the modern diet. They contain high concentrations of linoleic acid and are necessary for normal growth and development throughout the life cycle. Omega-3 essential fatty acids are found in high concentrations in fish, fish oils, flax seeds, and pumpkin seeds. Research has shown that these essential fatty acids can lower blood pressure, lower cholesterol levels, and reduce the risk of heart disease, stroke, and immune system disorders. These essential fatty acids are found in high concentrations in the brain. Japanese researchers concur that a deficiency of these essential fatty acids can lead to im-paired ability to learn and decreased cognitive function.[11] Researchers believe that many of the health problems seen today are the manifestations of essential fatty acid deficiency. Deficiency symptoms include poor immune response, dry skin and hair, behavioral changes, menstrual irregularities, arthritislike conditions, and cognitive difficulties. Table 18–1 serves as a guide for general dietary goals and recommendations.

Vitamins

Vitamins are nutrients essential to life. They contribute to good health by regulating the metabolism and assisting in biochemical processes that release energy from digested food. Vitamins function mostly as coenzymes that activate the chemical reactions continually occurring in the body. Vitamins are the foundation for all aspects of body function, from nervous system transmission to proper composition of bodily fluids. Vitamins are divided into two major groups: water soluble and fat soluble. Water-soluble vitamins must be taken into the body daily and are excreted within 1 to 4 days. These include vitamin C and the B-complex vitamins. Because excessive quantities are excreted rather than stored, water-soluble vitamins are seldom associated with toxicity problems. Fat-soluble vitamins are absorbed into the blood along with dietary fats. Since they are insoluble in water, they are transported via the lymphatic vessels of the blood and are stored in the body's adipose tissue and in the liver. Fat-soluble vitamins include vitamins A, D, E, and K.

Table 18–2 provides more information about vitamins and their food sources.

Minerals

Minerals are naturally occurring elements or compounds found in the earth. They are passed from soil to plants and are then consumed by animals and humans. Minerals are essential components of all

Table 18-1 Dietary Goals and Recommendations

Dietary Goal	Food Group	Recommendation
Reduce fat	Meat (beef, chicken, pork, turkey, lamb)	Avoid high-fat meats Lean meat—trim fat Bake, broil, seam Increase fish intake Remove skin from poultry
	Dairy	Skim milk, low fat yogurt, goat (feta), low fat cheeses (mozzerella, cottage), low fat sorbet or sherbet
	Fats/oils	Avoid fried foods Avoid margarine, hydrogenated fats Use Olive, Flaxseed, Canola oil (cold pressed)
	Eggs	2–3 whole eggs/week (boil, poach) Eggs whites—as desired
Reduce refined sugar	Soft drinks, pastries, white sugar	Avoid sodas, cookies, pastries, table sugar Increase fruits
Increase complex carbohydrates	Whole Grains, Beans, Seeds, Nuts	Increase beans, whole grains: lentils, tofu, brown rice, oats, whole grain breads, fiber cereals, almonds, sunflower seeds
Reduce sodium	Salt	Eliminate processed foods high in salt Substitute condiments for flavoring (garlic, onions, spices)
Reduce caffeine	Coffee, Soda, Chocolate	Coffee substitutes—caffix, postum, decaffeinated coffee Eliminate soda and diet soda, fruit juices, iced herbal teas
Reduce alcohol	Alcohol	Limit (reduce) intake

*Read ingredients on labels

cells and function as coenzymes. They are necessary for proper composition of body fluids, formation of blood and bone, and maintenance of healthy nerve function. Once a mineral is absorbed, it must be carried from the blood to the cells and must then be transported across the cell membrane in a form that can be utilized by the cell. Minerals, like vitamins, work in combination with other nutrients and have both synergistic and antagonistic effects. Some minerals compete with one another for absorption, while others enhance the absorption of other minerals.[12] For example, too much calcium can decrease the absorption of magnesium, and therefore these minerals should be consumed in the proper ratio to maintain balance.[13]

Minerals are classified as either major minerals or trace minerals; however, this classification does not reflect their importance. A deficiency of either type of mineral can have a deleterious impact on health. To be classified as a major mineral, the mineral must make up no less than 0.01 percent of body weight. Major minerals include calcium, magnesium, phosphorus, potassium, sodium, and chloride. Trace minerals include arsenic, boron, chromium, cobalt, copper, fluoride, iodine, iron, manganese, molybdenum, nickel, selenium, silicon, tin, vanadium, and zinc.

Table 18–2 Fat-Soluble and Water-Soluble Vitamins

Vitamin	Function	Food Source
Fat-Soluble Vitamins		
Vitamin A (retinol)	Antioxidant. Aids in maintenance and repair of mucous membranes and epithelial tissue. Assists in growth and development of bones.	All orange and yellow fruits and vegetables: sweet potatoes, squash, yams, carrots, pumpkin, parsley, mango, apricots. Dark leafy greens: kale, spinach, broccoli, salmon, fish oils
Carotenoids (carotenes, lycopenes)	Antioxidant. Enhance cell communication and immune competence.	Orange, yellow, and dark green fruits and vegetables.
Vitamin D	Aids in transport of calcium. Promotes intestinal and renal absorption of phosphorus. Aids in growth of bones and teeth.	Liver, oils, egg yolk, alfalfa, dairy products, fish, especially fatty fish such as halibut, salmon, sardines.
Vitamin E	Antioxidant. Promotes wound healing. Protects cell membranes against lipid perioxidation and destruction. Improves circulation.	Cold-pressed vegetable oils, whole grains, dark leafy green vegetables, nuts, seeds, legumes, wheat germ, oatmeal.
Vitamin K	Aids in blood clotting. Promotes formation and maintenance of healthy bone.	Green leafy vegetables, egg yolks.
Water-Soluble Vitamins		
Vitamin B$_1$ (thiamine)	Coenzyme in oxidation of glucose. Assists in production of hydrochloric acid.	Dried beans, brown rice, egg yolks, fish, chicken, peanuts.
Vitamin B$_2$ (riboflavin)	Assists in red blood cell formation. Aids in metabolism of carbohydrates, fats, and proteins.	Beans, eggs, fish, poultry, meat, spinach, yogurt, asparagus, avocado.
Vitmain B$_3$ (niacin)	Promotes healthy skin and nervous system. Lowers cholesterol, improves circulation.	Fish, eggs, beef, cheese, potatoes, whole wheat.
Vitamin B$_5$ (pantothenic acid)	"Antistress" vitamin. Aids in production of adrenal hormones. Assists in formation of antibodies and protein metabolism.	Beans, beef, eggs, mother's milk, fresh vegetables, whole wheat, pork, saltwater fish.
Vitamin B$_6$ (pyridoxine)	Acts as coenzyme in metabolism of amino acids and essential fatty acids necessary for production of serotonin and other neurotransmitters. Essential for healthy nervous system. Assists in converting iron to hemoglobin.	Eggs, fish, spinach, peas, meat, nuts, carrots, poultry, soybeans, bananas, avocado, whole grain cereals, prunes.
Vitamin B$_{12}$ (cobalamin)	Aids in synthesis of red blood cells. Required for proper digestion and absorption of foods. Prevents nerve damage.	Beef, herring, cheese, sardines, salmon, shellfish, tofu, eggs, dairy products.
Vitamin C (ascorbic acid)	Antioxidant. Aids in collagen formation, absorption of iron, interferon production. Promotes capillary integrity. Aids in release of stress hormones.	Citrus fruits, papaya, parsley, watercress, berries, tomatoes, broccoli, brussels sprouts.
Folic acid	Participates in amino acid conversion, manufacture of neurotransmitters.	Dark green vegetables, kidney beans, asparagus, broccoli, whole grains, cereals.

Although normal dietary intake of trace nutrients poses no threat to human health, long-term therapeutic doses of one or more minerals at the expense of other minerals might result in secondary deficiencies that could impair immunological or antioxidant processes. Reduced bioavailability is aggravated by marginal dietary intake of the unsupplemented mineral. Even borderline levels of certain minerals can suppress a variety of immune functions. Cell-mediated immunity, antibody response, and other immune responses may be impaired by marginal deficiencies in trace minerals.[14] For example, borderline zinc deficiency is associated with depletion of lymphocytes and lymphoid tissue atrophy. Excessive long-term consumption of competing minerals, such as iron, might suppress immune response by producing a secondary deficiency of zinc.[15]

Bioavailability and supplementation are some of the most controversial areas in nutrition research and practice. Nutrient intake through food consumption depends on many factors, including the quality of the soil in which the foods were grown, use of fertilizers, and genetic engineering of foods, to name a few. Consumption of a wide variety of fresh fruits and vegetables and unprocessed whole foods is recommended.

Table 18–3 provides further information on minerals and their food sources.

Antioxidants

Some vitamins and minerals function as antioxidants. These include vitamins C and E, beta-carotene (a precursor of vitamin A), and the trace mineral selenium.[16] *Antioxidants* protect the body from the formation of free radicals. Free radicals are electrically charged molecules that have an unpaired electron. Free radicals can cause damage to healthy cells. They can also stress the immune system and suppress its ability to defend the host adequately against organisms, toxins, and metabolic by-products, all of which can lead to degenerative or infectious disease states.[17] Antioxidants can stabilize or deactivate free radicals before the latter attack cells. Antioxidants are absolutely critical for maintaining optimal cellular and systemic health and well-being.[18]

The body can also manufacture its own antioxidant, glutathione. Glutathione is a powerful antioxidant comprised of the amino acids cysteine, glycine, and glutamic acid. It is potentized and recycled by other antioxidants, including vitamin C, selenium, and coenzyme Q10. It is produced by and is most concentrated in the liver, where it is involved in detoxification pathways and protects against free-radical damage. Glutathione helps to recycle other antioxidants. Liver stores of glutathione can be depleted by disease processes, malnutrition, or poor-quality nutrient intake. Dietary amino acids are essential to glutathione synthesis. Lifestyle factors that affect efficient utilization of glutathione include stress, alcohol, cigarette smoking, and drug use.[19]

Digestion

Diet is the food we eat. Nutrition is the study of what happens after we eat it. Optimal absorption of nutrients depends on the integrity of the digestive system. The process of digestion begins in the mouth with chewing. Food is ground up into small particles and mixes with salivary enzymes. The entire gastrointestinal tract is lined with mucosal tissue that secretes enzymes and protective antibodies known as IgA molecules, an important part of our immune defense. The gastrointestinal tract also contains billions of friendly microflora. These microorganisms assist in metabolic processes while maintaining the integrity of the mucosal lining.

Digestion in the stomach occurs as food is churned and mixed with hydrochloric acid and various enzymes, which prepare it

Table 18–3 Major Minerals and Trace Elements

Mineral	Function	Food Source
Calcium	Formation of strong bones, transmission of nerve impulses, muscle growth and movement. Blood clotting. Prevention of hypertension.	Dairy products, salmon, sardines, green leafy vegetables, seeds and nuts, tofu, blackstrap molasses, seaweed.
Chromium	Metabolism of glucose. Stabilization of blood sugar levels. Synthesis of cholesterol, fats, and proteins.	Brewer's yeast, brown rice, cheese, whole grains, beans, mushrooms, potatoes.
Copper	Formation of bone, hemoglobin, red blood cells. Healing process.	Whole grains, avocado, oyster, lobster, dandelion greens, mushrooms, blackstrap molasses, nuts, seeds, soybeans.
Iodine	Energy production. Body temperature regulation, thyroid gland health.	Seaweed, iodized salt, dairy products, seafood, saltwater fish, garlic, swiss chard, summer squash.
Iron	Hemoglobin production. Stress and disease resistance. Energy production. Immune system health.	Eggs, fish, poultry, dark leafy greens, blackstrap molasses, almonds, seaweed.
Magnesium	Formation of bone. Carbohydrate and mineral metabolism. Maintenance of proper pH balance. Immune function.	Dairy products, fish, seafood, blackstrap molasses, garlic, whole grains, seeds, tofu, green leafy vegetables, nuts.
Manganese	Enzyme activation. Sex hormone production. Nerve health. Energy production.	Avocados, nuts, seeds, seaweed, whole grains.
Phosphorus	Bone and teeth formation. Cell growth. Contraction of heart muscle. Kidney function.	Asparagus, brewer's yeast, fish, dried fruits, garlic, legumes, seeds and nuts.
Potassium	Healthy nervous system. Regulation of body fluids with sodium. pH balance.	Apricots, bananas, potatoes, sunflower seeds, blackstrap molasses, sprouts, broccoli.
Selenium	Antioxidant function. Immune system protection, cancer prevention.	Brazil nuts, brewer's yeast, brown rice, dairy products, garlic, onions, whole grains.
Sodium	With potassium, regulation of body fluids necessary for nerve and muscle function.	Table salt, seaweed.
Zinc	Burn and wound healing. Carbohydrate digestion. Prostate gland function, reproductive organ growth and development. Immune system health, production of antibodies.	Sardines and other fish, legumes, poultry, meat, egg yolks, beans, pumpkin seeds, sunflower seeds.

for entry into the small intestine via the duodenum. In the small intestine, digestive enzymes from the liver, gallbladder, and pancreas are added to the still partially digested food. The pancreas secretes amylase, lipase, and chymotrypsin, while the liver and gallbladder secrete bile to aid in the digestion of fats and the absorption of essential fatty acids and fat-soluble vitamins. Food spends 1 to 4 hours in the small intestine, which is approximately 25 feet long. As food is digested, it is absorbed into small blood vessels in the lining of the intestine. Toxins and waste products enter the large intestine and are excreted as fecal matter. The large intestine processes primarily fiber and water. The proper absorption and utilization of nutrients depends on a complex orchestration of processes in the digestive tract, and therefore it is essential to maintain the health and balance of this system.

The friendly bacteria that live in the gastrointestinal tract, including strains of *Lactobacillus* and *Acidophilus*, have many beneficial effects on health. They assist in synthesizing B vitamins, digesting proteins, balancing intestinal pH, reducing serum cholesterol, strengthening the immune system in the gut, eliminating parasites and preventing overgrowth of yeast, and maintaining regularity. The most common reason for the destruction of friendly bacteria is the use of antibiotics. Studies indicate that beneficial bacteria must be replaced (by probiotic supplementation) when antibiotic therapy is administered. Symptoms of dysbiosis include fatigue, bloating, gas, diarrhea, constipation, food allergies, inflammatory disorders, migraine headache, and weight gain.[20]

Dietary modification, including elimination of fried foods, sugars, and foods that stress an individual's digestive system, can also aid in the treatment of gastrointestinal problems. Keeping a food journal and then following an elimination diet is helpful. Identifying foods that may trigger digestive disorders, food allergies, and autoimmune responses, and then removing them from the diet for a minimum of 21 days can be an important dietary intervention for those with food sensitivities.[21] The individual can slowly reintroduce the food item and observe if symptoms return. Each person has a unique relationship with food and its chemical properties, and therefore nutritional assessment and dietary recommendations are based on individual biochemistry.

EATING TO PROMOTE HEALTH

Increasing awareness of how one's diet can effect one's health and well-being is essential to nutrition education. The following questions may be used as a guideline. Sit down in a quiet place and plan a day's menu by asking yourself:

- What does my body need to enhance wellness?
- What are my past eating patterns? Which do I want to keep? Which do I want to change?
- What are my activity levels and how should I include foods that meet my needs?
- How do I need to plan for psychologic factors?
- What factors, unique to me, influence my food planning?

As nutrition is integrated into clinical care, assessing the unique needs of each individual while offering health education and self-care tools can impact the health and well-being of the individual over time. Nutrition offers a holistic approach and takes into account the individual's physiologic, psychologic, social, genetic, cultural, religious, economic, and environmental needs. The individual's eating patterns, food preferences, motivation, attitudes, and beliefs are all part of nutrition counseling and education .

Cardiovascular Disease and Cancer

Cardiovascular disease and cancer are the two leading causes of death among women in the United States. Heart disease is responsible for 45 percent of all deaths among women, and nearly 40 percent of all females are expected to develop cancer at some point in their lifetime. A substantial body of research suggests that both heart disease and cancer are strongly related to dietary habits and nutrient status. Helping women to maintain optimal health with diet and healthy lifestyle choices can have a great impact on the prevalence of disease among women. Recent research demonstrates the cardioprotective effects of several dietary nutrients, including fiber (both soluble and insoluble), antioxidants (vitamins C and E, beta-carotene, selenium, coenzyme Q10), folic acid (homocysteine levels are highest among those with low folic acid levels), and essential fatty acids (omega-3 fish oil).[22]

Breast cancer is the second most common cause of cancer-related deaths in women in the United States. Two important environmental risk factors for breast cancer are diet and exposure to xenotoxins.[23] An estimated 80 percent of cancers are thought to be related to environmental factors; diet alone is estimated to play a role in at least 35 percent of all cancers. It has been estimated that as much as 50 percent of breast cancer might be prevented by dietary changes.[24]

Environmental xenoestrogens—synthetic hormone-mimicking compounds found in certain pesticides, drugs, and plastics—may play a role in the etiology of breast cancer. Women with breast cancer often have higher concentrations of pesticides in their blood and fatty tissue.[25] Xenoestrogens accumulate in the fatty tissues of the body and may interact with estrogen receptor sites in the breast, enhancing breast cell proliferation.[26]

Many epidemiological studies have associated a high-fat, low-fiber diet with an increased risk of developing cancer of the colon, prostate, and breast. A review of the literature also suggests an inverse relationship between the quantity of fresh fruits and vegetables consumed and the incidence of cancer. Fruits and vegetables are rich in fiber, antioxidants, and other plant-derived substances, or phytonutrients, that are believed to have cancer-protective properties.[27] Fiber is thought to influence hormone levels by facilitating the fecal excretion of estrogen metabolites, which at high levels can pose a risk for many women.[28]

Fat intake and obesity appear to be primary risk factors associated with cardiovascular disease, diabetes, and endometrial and ovarian cancers. Weight loss plans that support a low-fat, high-fiber diet, stress reduction, and exercise are part of a comprehensive health approach for the prevention of cardiovascular disease and breast cancer in women.[29]

Other dietary ingredients shown by research to have anticancer properties include soy-based products (tofu, miso, tempeh, soybeans) and cruciferous vegetables (broccoli, cauliflower, brussels sprouts). Soy products contain natural plant phytoestrogens (genistein and daidzen) called isoflavones that play a significant role in the prevention, and possibly treatment, of some hormone-related diseases. These phytonutrients appear to be protective against both breast cancer and prostate cancer.[30] Asian women, who consume approximately 30 to 50 times as much soy as American women, have low rates of breast cancer.[31] Cruciferous vegetables are rich in indoles and isothiocyanates. These substances may help in liver detoxification and aid in the removal of carcinogens, and appear to play a role in the prevention of cancer.

According to a report released in September 1998 through the Harvard School of Public Health, 40 percent of all cancers could be avoided by changes in lifestyle and diet. Walter C. Willett, a Harvard researcher, spent 14 years reviewing 4,500 studies from around the world on nutrition and cancer and compiled a 650-page report sponsored by the American Institute for Cancer Research.[32] The recommendations in this report are as follows:

- Choose a predominantly plant-based diet rich in a variety of vegetables and fruits.
- Avoid being underweight or overweight, and limit weight gain in adulthood to less than 11 pounds.
- Eat 8 or more servings per day of cereals and grains (e.g., brown rice, whole grain breads), legumes (e.g., lentils, soy), tubers (e.g., potatoes), and roots (e.g., beets).
- Eat five or more servings per day of other fruits and vegetables.
- Limit consumption of white sugar.
- Limit alcoholic drinks.
- Limit intake of red meat to less than 3 ounces a day, if it is eaten at all. In

place of red meat, eat fish, poultry, or soy products.

- Limit consumption of fatty foods, particularly those of animal origin.
- Limit consumption of salted foods. Use herbs and spices to season foods.
- Do not eat charred foods.
- Do not smoke or chew tobacco.

Osteoporosis

Many older adults are concerned about osteoporosis, a metabolic bone disorder characterized by a reduction in the amount of bone mass, which leads to bone fragility. Decrease in bone density results in loss of bone strength and increased risk of fractures of the spine, hip, and wrist. Osteoporosis has become a major health problem in the United States, although it often goes undetected until an accident or a fall results in a fracture. Osteoporosis primarily affects women. It is responsible for 1.5 million fractures annually, including more than 300,000 hip fractures. Peak bone mass is achieved at about 35 years of age; as estrogen levels decrease with age, the risk of decreased bone density rises. Women who have a strong family history of osteoporosis, have a small body frame, and are of Caucasian or Asian descent have a high risk for the disease.[33] Research suggests that, in those at risk, age-related bone loss may be reduced or even reversed through a comprehensive approach that combines nutrient supplementation, dietary adjustments, and lifestyle changes, including participation in a regular exercise program. The earlier in life a woman began to integrate an osteoporosis prevention program, the more she will reduce the risk of bone loss later in life. Bone is a dynamic tissue, and adequate nutrition is required for its maintenance and growth.

In the body's essential metabolic processes, there is a continuous exchange of calcium between bone and plasma. Plasma levels are given priority over bone density. If the body needs additional calcium for essential functions and it is not readily available, calcium is taken from the bones to meet these metabolic needs. When this occurs, bone strength is compromised and bones are weakened. A recurrent theme in nutritional medicine is that degenerative diseases are the result of our modern diet. Considering that bone is living tissue, it is susceptible to both dietary excess and deficiencies. One study found that two-thirds of women in the United States between the ages of 18 and 30 ingest less calcium than the RDA. Several studies have also linked high animal protein diets to loss of calcium from bone, concluding that individuals who consume a balanced vegetarian diet have stronger bones later in life than those who eat high amounts of animal flesh.[34]

Osteoporosis is often the result of deficiencies of several key nutrients of which calcium is but one. Statistics show that only 25 percent of women with osteoporosis are calcium deficient. Research has demonstrated that other essential nutrients, including magnesium, boron, vitamin D_3, and other trace minerals, must be available in the proper balance to facilitate calcium resorption and uptake into the bone. Studies have correlated long-term low-calcium diets with the development of osteoporosis later in life.[35] The best treatment for osteoporosis is prevention.

Common Risk Factors for Osteoporosis
- low intake of calcium, magnesium, vitamin D, and trace minerals
- high intake of animal protein
- high caffeine intake
- excessive intake of carbonated beverages
- high sodium intake
- high refined sugar intake
- lack of exercise
- lack of sunlight exposure
- excessive alcohol intake
- smoking

- use of certain medications, including antacids steroids, thyroid replacement drugs, chemotherapy agents
- hypochlorhydria (low HCI)

Guidelines for Healthy Bones
- Increase consumption of calcium-rich foods, including green leafy vegetables, whole grains, beans, tofu, dairy products, nuts and seeds.
- Increase weight-bearing exercise, such as walking.
- Decrease consumption of soda, caffeine, and alcohol.
- Spend 15 minutes a day exposed to direct sunlight.

Supplement Recommendations for Healthy Bones. The current RDA for calcium is 800–1200 milligrams per day of elemental calcium. Magnesium and calcium function in balance. The recommended ratio of calcium to magnesium is 2:1, thus, the recommended dosage of magnesium is 400–600 milligrams per day. Vitamin D reduces bone loss. Daily dose should not exceed 800 international units (IU) (RDA 400 to 600 IU). These nutrients work together to enhance each other's absorption and utilization in the body. Other nutrients that help maintain bone mass include vitamin K, boron, vitamin B_6, manganese, folic acid, vitamin C, and zinc.[36]

Regardless of a person's age, calcium and trace nutrients are essential for maintaining bone mass and overall good health.

Obesity

One of the most common nutritional problems is obesity. Obesity has been defined as weighing in excess of forty pounds above ideal body weight. Being overweight predisposes an individual to high blood pressure, elevated blood cholesterol levels, diabetes, stroke, heart attack, gallbladder disease, cancer, and musculoskeletal problems. Contributing factors include excessive intake of calories (especially from fat), excessive consumptions of refined sugar, vitamin and mineral deficiencies, maldigestion, insufficient exercise, hypothyroidism, and hereditary factors.

Individual diet-nutrition counseling includes exercise planning and behavior modification education. Decreasing caloric intake, increasing exercise, and developing a healthy relationship with food are essential to long-term weight-loss strategies. Successful weight loss is gradual and highly individualized.

The following are some general guidelines for weight management:

- Recognize management of obesity as a life-long commitment that requires lifestyle changes.
- Set realistic goals for weight loss.
- Do meal planning with daily menus.
- Serve smaller portions (use smaller plates).
- Avoid keeping ready-to-eat snack food around the house.
- Do grocery shopping from a list and not on an empty stomach.
- Do all eating in one room and focus on eating without distractions.
- Increase intake of vegetables ("free" foods).
- Leave a small amount of food on the plate.
- Increase activity level.
- Avoiding skipping meals.
- Avoid late-night eating.
- Drink at least six glasses of water daily.
- Try a food allergy elimination diet.
- Eliminate all junk foods (processed, refined foods) from the diet.

Weight loss is achieved and maintained with a regular exercise program, psychologic support, and a personal commitment to wellness.

Nutrition and Aging

Lifestyle and nutrition practices are recognized to play a fundamental role in healthy aging. Health benefits from optimal nutrition in the older years can prevent much of the decline seen with aging. The National Health and Nutrition Surveys conducted by the Department of Health and Human Services reveal that the nation's older citizens remain at high risk of macronutrient and micronutrient deficiencies. Untreated and often undiagnosed deficiencies have taken a heavy toll among older people, resulting in an accelerated aging process.[37] Research studies over the past decade clearly show that many of the ailments previously thought to be an inevitable result of old age can be prevented by aggressive detection and treatment of subclinical nutrient deficits. Cognitive impairment, depression, lethargy, anemia, and poor response to medical and surgical interventions may be the expression of nutrient deficiencies.[38]

While patients must be evaluated individually, many psychosocial factors should be considered when addressing nutrition needs and goals, including economics, the person's ability to shop and prepare meals, and social support. As many as 50 percent of elderly people suffer from atrophic gastritis, a condition that impairs absorption of micronutrients, especially of vitamin B_{12}.[39] Often elderly people have undetected hypochlorhydria, a deficiency of hydrochloric acid in the stomach that leads to bacterial overgrowth in the stomach and small bowel and results in impaired digestion and absorption of essential nutrients, including vitamins B_6 and B_{12}. Americans over the age of 65 consume 30 percent of the over-the-counter and prescription drugs sold in the United States. Many of these medications are known to impair food intake, absorption, and metabolism of nutrients. Some drugs such as phenobarbital are specific nutrient antagonists. The most commonly used over-the-counter drugs among elderly people are laxatives, which can impair the status of the fat-soluble vitamins A, E, D, and K. Other problems that interfere with nutrient intake include chewing difficulties, impaired cognitive function and forgetting to eat, social isolation and apathy in food preparation, and inability to shop or carry packages. Impaired memory in elderly people is often related to the effect of B-vitamin, antioxident, and essential fatty acid deficiencies.

One of the hallmarks of biologic aging is decreased ability to manage glucose metabolism. This imbalance is a contributing factor in many age-related diseases, including heart disease, inflammatory disorders, dementia, and diabetes. The physiologic control of glucose metabolism is one of the central regulatory activities, along with control of electrolyte levels, intracellular pH, oxygen and carbon dioxide concentrations, and membrane polarity.[40]

Many substances affect glucose metabolism, including insulin, hormones, and specific nutrients. Nutrients such as amino acids, fatty acids, trace minerals, and vitamins potentiate the effects of glucose by modifying insulin production and secretion. Increased levels of glucose activate inflammatory immune responses, increase oxidative stress, and accelerate biologic aging. Recent research has indicated that many nutritional substances can help modulate glucose regulation, including selenium, chromium, other trace minerals, alpha lipoic acid, vitamin B complex, vitamin C, and essential fatty acids.

Hypoglycemia and carbohydrate cravings are common syndromes that affect a large portion of the population. A refined-food diet high in simple sugars and low in fiber and nutrients often manifests as glycemic dysregulation and can lead to hyperglycemia and diabetes with aging. Recommendations for stabilizing blood sugar level at any age include eating several smaller meals daily that consist of protein and complex carbohydrates, and avoiding soda, caffeine, and refined or processed foods devoid of nutrients and fiber (see Exhibit 18–1 for a hypoglycemic diet plan).[41]

Exhibit 18-1 Hypoglycemic Diet Plan

GUIDELINES—LOW FAT/LOW REFINED CARBOHYDRATES/HIGH PROTEIN DIET

- Eliminate caffeine, soda, fruit juice white sugar, white flour, white rice, white bread.
- Limit fruits—2 per day and divide into 4 portions. Avoid grapes and bananas (high in sugar).
- Throughout the day, consume several small meals consisting of protein with complex carbohydrate if needed.
- Vegetables—*Unlimited*—raw or cooked depending on your preference (and digestion); limit beets and carrots

SAMPLE MENU CHOICES

Protein

Fish	canned tuna, sardines, broiled, baked, steamed fish
Chicken	baked, broiled, remove skin
Turkey	fresh turkey, white meat
Beans	soy (tofu), black, lentil, red, garbanzo, etc.
Whole Grains	brown rice, oatmeal, quinoa, millet, buckwheat (kasha), barley, whole wheat
Eggs	boiled, poached
Dairy	low fat cheese—mozzarella, goat, yogurt (plain)
Vegetables	salads, steamed vegetables; fresh or frozen; avoid canned.

- **Whole Grains + Beans (Complex Carbohydrates) = Complete Protein**

SAMPLE MENU SERVINGS

Breakfast

- 1 boiled egg with whole wheat bread; **or**
- 1 cup cooked old fashioned oatmeal, **or**
- Cold cereal with low fat milk, plain low fat yogurt, or milk substitute (soy, rice, or almond milk)

Lunch/Dinner

- Salad with grilled chicken or fish
- Tuna in whole wheat pita
- Lentil soup with whole wheat crackers
- Grilled chicken breast with ½ cup brown rice and steamed vegetables
- Tofu or black beans with brown rice and steamed vegetables
- Grilled fish with ½ baked potato and salad

Snacks (small meals)

Low fat plain yogurt with ½ fresh fruit, whole wheat cracker with tuna salad, hummus with whole wheat pita, 1 tablespoon almonds or sunflower seeds, or nut butter; almond or sesame tahini on whole wheat cracker, left over lunch portion.

Helpful Hints: Exercise, and Physical activity can be an important part of weight loss and blood sugar control. Check with your physician or physical therapist.

Vitamin deficiencies remain subclinical in elderly people and are the result of inadequate nutrient stores over many years. Establishing a reservoir of nutrients beginning in the younger years is an essential component of disease prevention and health maintenance for healthy aging. All guidelines for a healthy diet are essential to follow throughout life and are beneficial as one transitions into the senior years.[42]

HEALTHY CHOICES IN NUTRITION

High-Fiber Diet

- whole grains: oatmeal, brown rice, millet, whole wheat, enriched pasta
- beans: lentils, tofu, split peas, garbanzo beans, black beans, tempeh
- vegetables: green, yellow, orange—steamed, raw, or stir-fried
- nuts and seeds: sunflower seeds, Brazil nuts, almonds, sesame seeds, pumpkin seeds, nut butters
- fruits: local and in season, such as papaya, melon, mango, grapefruit, berries

Note: Grains + beans = complete protein.

Low-Fat Diet

- Limit meats.
- Eliminate sandwich meats (ham, salami, bacon, sausage).
- Increase fish, chicken, turkey.
- Use cold-pressed, unprocessed oils—olive, canola, sesame.
- Use butter instead of margarine.
- Use low-fat dairy products.
- Bake, broil, steam, or poach food.

Foods To Avoid

- sugars—cookies, soda, candy, jelly, syrup
- processed foods—additives, preservatives, artificial colorings and flavorings
- canned foods—fresh is best, frozen is next best
- refined hydrogenated oils (Crisco, palm oil, cottonseed oil)
- fast foods and junk foods

Other Important Health Factors

- Drink four to six glasses of liquid daily—spring or filtered water, herbal teas.
- Cook and prepare food in cast-iron or stainless steel cookware (avoid aluminum).
- Chew foods slowly and thoroughly.
- Eat smaller, simpler meals.
- Include fiber with each meal.
- Exercise daily—walk, bicycle, jog, dance, swim, stretch.
- Reduce stress through yoga, meditation, deep breathing, relaxation practice, visualization.
- Avoid alcohol, caffeine, smoking, recreational drugs, over-the-counter drugs.
- Get sufficient rest and sleep.

HOLISTIC CARING PROCESS

Assessment

In preparing to use nutrition interventions, the nurses assesses the following parameters:

- the client's relationship to nutrition and diet: biochemical, genetic, cultural, social, emotional, religious, economic, environmental, and physiologic components
- the client's eating habits, food preferences, and nutritional needs
- the client's motivation and ability to make the necessary dietary and lifestyle changes
- the client's understanding that changing food and eating patterns is part of a wellness process

Patterns/Problems/Needs

The following are the patterns/problems/needs compatible with nutrition interventions that are related to the nine human response patterns of the Unitary Person framework (see Chapter 14):

- *Exchanging:* Altered nutrition
  Altered circulation
  Altered oxygenation
- *Choosing:* Altered coping
- *Moving:* Altered physical mobility
  Sleep pattern disturbances

Altered patterns of
daily living
- *Perceiving:* Disturbance in body
image
Disturbance in self-
esteem
Potential hopelessness
Potential
powerlessness
- *Knowing:* Knowledge deficit
- *Feeling:* Pain
Anxiety
Grieving
Depression
Fear

Outcomes

Exhibit 18–2 guides the nurse in client
outcomes, nursing prescriptions, and
evaluation for the use of nutrition as a
nursing intervention.

Therapeutic Care Plan and Interventions

Before the Session

- Create an environment in which the
client feels comfortable discussing
physical and nutritional needs.
- Prepare assessment tools and educational materials.
- Focus on the client's nutritional and
physical needs.
- Use relaxation techniques to assist client before session begins.

At the Beginning of the Session

- Take and record the necessary physical assessment data (e.g., weight, skin
fold and thickness measurements).
- Guide the client to disclose past habit
patterns that affect eating behavior.

Exhibit 18–2 Nursing Interventions: Nutrition

Client Outcomes	Nursing Prescriptions	Evaluation
The client will be motivated to improve nutrition.	Assist the client in a personal self-assessment. Encourage the client to participate with the nurse to develop goals and action plans. Prepare the client to follow through with the nurse on evaluation and formulation of new goals.	The client completed a self-assessment form. The client participated with the nurse to develop a personalized program. The client met with the nurse for program evaluation.
The client will demonstrate knowledge of healthful nutrition.	Motivate the client to contribute to discussions about his or her program. Encourage the client to learn more about healthful behaviors as he or she works with the nurse.	The client participated in the session discussion. The client demonstrated new knowledge.

- Have the client document food intake and association between food and feelings of well-being or distress.
- Assist the client in creating a sample menu.
- Encourage the client to participate in setting nutritional goals and action plans.
- Present specific nutritional guidelines for the client to follow.
- Direct the client to keep a food journal to present at follow-up session.

During the Session

- Have the nurse serve as guide.
- Emphasize the connection between nutrition and whole person health.
- With the nurse's guidance, have the client develop strategies for changing nutrition habits, nutrient intake, and eating patterns.
- Have the nurse assist the client in optimizing diet and nutrition by:
  — Creating an image for food as a healing medicine
  — Reframing the nutrition process into a positive action
  — Reframing nutrition and food as an empowerment tool
  — Illustrating how external nutrition changes promote internal healing responses
  — Reinforcing the client's positive changes in nutrition as part of the healing process
  — Ending sessions with images of desired state of well-being.

At the End of the Session

- Have the client identify the options presented that best fit with his or her own lifestyle.
- Work together with the client to write down goals and target dates.
- Give the client specific affirmations to use to support these goals.

- Give the client handout material to reinforce the teaching.
- Use the client outcomes that were established before the session (see Exhibit 18–2) and the client's subjective experiences (Exhibit 18–3) to evaluate the session.
- Schedule a follow-up session.

Specific Interventions: Ensuring Optimal Nutrition

To optimize nutrient intake, the nurse may advise the client to

- adhere to recommended healthy diet
- practice relaxation techniques
- increase exercise following evaluation by a trained professional

The nurse can share information and research data on health benefits of antioxidants and other nutrients known to assist in the health and healing process.

A daily menu plan can be created to fit the client's particular needs. The following should be considered:

- daily activity status
- current health status
- any physical limitations
- economic considerations
- social and cultural influences
- emotion state of being
- individual differences, including food preferences and religious dietary customs

To motivate and assist the client, the nurse can

- encourage the client to write a food journal daily
- demonstrate the daily practice of asking the body what it needs to be healthy
- create daily menus using healthy choices that are mutually agreed upon
- teach the client to self-assess health changes that occur with dietary interventions

- encourage the client who is currently using nutritional supplementation to organize a routine to optimize compliance and benefits

Open-ended questions, images, journal writing, drawing, and other creative strategies to integrate nutrition into the client's daily life can be used to close the session.

Case Study

Setting:	A nurse-based wellness center
Client:	B.V., a 40-year-old married woman who seeks counseling for weight loss
Nursing Diagnoses:	1. Altered nutrition (more than body requirements) related to improper eating and lack of exercise
	2. Altered self-esteem related to obesity
	3. Ineffective reversal/prevention of coronary artery disease risk factors (hypertension, hypercholesterolemia, obesity) related to stress and low self-esteem

B.V. came to the wellness center after having a physical examination by a physician and being told for the sixth straight year that she needs to lose weight. Her total cholesterol is 340 milligrams per deciliter, blood pressure is 180/100, height is 5 feet, 7 inches, and weight is 220 pounds. She is a nurse and seeks help from a nurse colleague at the wellness center because her elevated cholesterol level has finally motivated her to lose weight. Her husband has been encouraging this for years, but she just cannot seem to make it happen.

During the initial session, the nurse takes an eating and diet history. Like most self-referrals for weight loss, B.V. is knowledgeable about various diet programs and has tried different plans for several years. She has a pattern of losing and then regaining up to 50 pounds on each attempt. At this point, she is willing to try anything.

The nurse discovers during the interview that B.V. has been on numerous antihypertensive drugs for 10 years without attaining consistent control. The assessment shows that, in general, B.V. is physically out of shape and emotionally depressed and discouraged. She is a fellow health care professional who has reached burnout.

After establishing 6-week and 6-month goals, B.V. and the nurse schedule weekly sessions. B.V. is given a standard form of a weekly diet, exercise, and emotion and attitude recording sheet. She is instructed to write down everything she eats, as well as the feeling that she has before, during, and after the eating periods during the next week.

In the second session, B.V. and the nurse review the eating/feeling diary and discuss where significant relationships between feelings and eating are observed. During this and subsequent sessions, it is important to examine and try to understand the client's feelings, for they are closely tied to the eating behavior. In addition, the physical parameters of weight and body fat calibration measurements are recorded.

Goals that are too difficult to achieve can discourage the client altogether. Therefore, during each session, several small attainable goals are set for the following week. Both exercise and eating patterns gradually improve.

B.V. meets with the nurse on a regular basis for 6 months. During that time, she reduces her weight to 160 pounds, works out in a regular aerobic exercise program four times a week, and increases her knowledge and interest in healthful food consumption. At the end of this period, B.V. and the nurse agree to move to monthly visits for the next three sessions and plan for termination of the appointments at that time.

Evaluation

With the client, the nurse determines whether the client outcomes for nutrition

Exhibit 18–3 Evaluation of the Client's
Subjective Experience with Nutrition

1. Is this the first time you have considered the effects of healing nutrition from a holistic perspective?
2. Have you discovered ways you can eat for increased vitality and vibrant living?
3. Do you think there are any links between your food intake and the potential for development of a chronic disease in your life?
4. Is your life filled with healing foods? Do you want it to be?
5. What support systems would help you develop and adhere to a lifestyle that includes healing foods?
6. Can you think of anything else that would help you to maintain a routine that includes healing nutrition?
7. What is your next step (or your plan) to integrate these experiences on a daily basis?

(Exhibit 18–2) were successfully achieved. To evaluate the session further, the nurse may again explore the subjective effects of the experience with the client using the evaluation questions in Exhibit 18–3.

Nurses should chart all information they impart to the client, as well as evaluation of the session. When the nurse works in an inpatient facility, other staff need to be appraised of the program and its progress. Nurses who work in wellness centers, in centers using integrated models, and in private practice should also keep records for each client and should state nursing di-

agnosis, type of counseling employed, and the effectiveness of each session.

The nurse is in a prime position to model the effects of healthy nutrition and lifestyle by integrating these elements into daily life and practicing self-care.

DIRECTIONS FOR FUTURE RESEARCH

1. Investigate the hypothesis that those who eat a nutritionally balanced diet live longer.
2. Continue the investigation on how healthy behaviors in nutrition affect a person's general sense of well-being.
3. Study the relationship of vitamin and mineral supplementation to disease prevention and high-level wellness.
4. Study the specific factors for tailoring a nutrition program to different cultural and ethnic groups.

NURSE HEALER REFLECTIONS

After reading this chapter, the nurse healer will be able to answer or begin the process of answering the following questions:

- What sensations accompany physical well-being because of my improved nutrition?
- What comprises healthy eating for both myself and my clients?
- How can I model healthy nutrition practices?

NOTES

1. National Research Council, *Recommended Daily Allowance*, 10th ed. (Washington, DC: National Academy Press, 1989).
2. A.G. Motulsky, Nutrition and Genetic Susceptibility with Common Diseases, *American Journal of Clinical Nutrition* 5, supplement (1992): 1244S–1245S.
3. K.A. Math, Homocysteine Athrothrombosis, *New England Journal of Medicine*, 399, no. 7 (1998): 478–479.
4. J.C. Deutch, et al., Plasma Homocysteine Levels and Folic Acid Supplementation, *New England Journal of Medicine*, 339, no. 7 (1998): 475.
5. B. Posner, et al., Diet and Heart Risk Factors in

Adult American Men and Women, *International Journal of Epidemiology*, 22 (1993): 1014–1025.

6. K.H. Thompson and D.V. Goodin, Micro Nutrients and Antioxidants in the Progression of Diabetes, *Nutrition Research* 15, no. 9 (1995): 1377–1410.

7. D. Jenkins, and T. Wolever, Slow Release Carbohydrate and the Treatment of Diabetes, *Nutrition Soc*, 40 (1981): 227–234.

8. S. Handler, Dietary Fiber: Can It Prevent Certain Colon Diseases? *Postgraduate Medicine* 73 (1983): 301–307.

9. J. Budwig, *Flax Oil as a True Aid Against Arthritis, Heart Infarction, Cancer, and Other Diseases* (Vancouver, BC: Apple Publishing, 1992).

10. C. Lafante and N. Ernst, Daily Dietary Fat and Total Food Energy Intakes—NHANES 111. Phase 1, *Journal of the American Medical Association* 217 (1994): 1309.

11. W. Connor et al., Essential Fatty Acids: The Importance of n-3 Fatty Acids in the Retina and Brain, *Nutrition Reviews* 50 (1992): 21–29.

12. M. Werbach, *Nutritional Influences on Illness* (New Canaan, CT: Keats Publishing, 1988).

13. Werbach, *Nutritional Influences on Illness*.

14. R. Chandra, Trace Element Regulation of Immunity and Infection, *Journal of the American College of Nutrition* 4 (1985): 5–16.

15. S. Solomon and R. Jacob, Studies on the Bioavailability of Zinc in Humans: Effects of Heme and Non Heme Iron on the Absorption of Zinc, *American Journal of Clinical Nutrition* 4 (1985): 5–16.

16. H. Sies et al., Antioxidant Function of Vitamins, *Annals of the New York Academy of Sciences* 669 (1992): 7–20.

17. O.I. Arumoa et al., Free Radicals, *Bio Ned* 6 (1989): 593–597.

18. B. Halliwell, Free Radicals, Antioxidants, and Human Disease: Curiosity, Cause or Consequence? *Lancet* 344 (1994): 721–724.

19. J. Bland, Antioxidants in Nutritional Medicine: Tocopherol, Selenium, and Glutathione, in *Yearbook of Nutrition Medicine 1984–1985* (New Canaan, CT: Keats Publishing), 213–237.

20. R. Fuller, Probiotics in Human Medicine, *Gut* 32 (1991): 439–473.

21. H. Sampson et al., Food Allergy, *Journal of the American Medical Association*, 258, no. 20 (1987): 2886–2890.

22. D. Hunter et al., A Prospective Study of the Intake of Vitamins C, E, A and the Risk of Breast Cancer, *New England Journal of Medicine* 3399 (1993): 234–240.

23. E. Dewailly et al., High Organochlorine Body Burden in Women with Estrogen Receptor Positive Cancer, *Journal of the National Cancer Institute* 85, no. 8 (1993): 598–599.

24. A. Diplock, Antioxidant Nutrients and Disease Prevention: An Overview, *American Journal of Clinical Nutrition* 53 (1991): 189S–193S.

25. P. Martin et al., Phytoestrogen Interaction with Estrogen Receptors in Human Breast Cancer Cells, *Endocrinology* 100, no. 5 (1978): 1860–1867.

26. D. Hunter and T. Kelseyk, Pesticide Residues and Breast Cancer: The Harvest or the Silent Spring? *Journal of the National Cancer Institute* 85, no. 8 (1993): 598–599.

27. G. Block, The Data Supports a Role for Antioxidants Reducing Cancer Risk, *Nutrition Reviews* 50 (1992): 207–21326.

28. D. Rose et al., High Fiber Diet Reduces Serum Estrogen Concentrations in Premenopausal Women, *American Journal of Nutrition* 54 (1991): 520–527.

29. R.J. Herscopf, Obesity, Diet, Endogenous Estrogens, and the Risk of Hormone-Sensitive Cancer, *Journal of Clinical Nutrition* 45 (1987): 283–289.

30. T.B. Clarkson et al., Estrogenic Soybean Isoflavones and Chronic Disease Risk Factors and Benefits, *Trends in Endrocrinology and Metabolism* 6 (1995): 11–16.

31. D. Ingram et al., Case Study of Phytoestrogens and Breast Cancer, *Lancet* 350 (1997): 990–994.

32. Willett Report

33. B.R. Goldin et al., The Relationship between Estrogen Levels and Diets in Caucasian and Oriental Immigrant Women, *American Journal of Nutrition* 44 (1986): 945–953.

34. V.W. Bunker, The Role of Nutrition in Osteoporosis, *British Journal of Biomedical Science* 51, no. 3 (1994): 228–240.

35. E.L. Smith et al., Calcium Supplementation and Bone Loss in Middle Aged Women, *American Journal of Clinical Nutrition* 50, (1989): 833–842.

36. J. Wright and J. Gaby, *Preventing and Reversing Osteoporosis* (Rocklin, CA: Prima Publishing, 1994), 21–93.

37. J. Morley, Nutrition and the Older Female: A Review, *Journal of the American College of Nutrition* 12 (1993): 337–343.

38. C. Jeandel et al., Antioxidant Status in Alzheimer's Patients, *Gerontology* 35 (1989): 275–282.

39. J. Prendergast, Nutritional Intervention in the Aging Process (New York: Springer Publishing Co., 1984), 265–280.

40. G. Reaven, Pathophysiology of Insulin Resistance in Human Disease, *Physiological Reviews* 75, no. 3 (1995): 473–485.

41. Reaven, Pathophysiology of Insulin Resistance.

42. A.H. Schapira, Oxidative Stress and Mitochondrial Dysfunction in Neurodegeneration, *Current Opinions in Neurology* 9 (1996): 260–264.

SUGGESTED READING

A. Adlercreutz, et al., Dietary Phyto-estrogens and the Menopause in Japan, *Lancet* 339 (1992): 1233.

T. Amimoto et al., Acetaminophen-Induced Hepatic Injury in Mice: The Role of Lipid Peroxidation and Effects of Pre-treatment with Coenzyme Q 10 α-Tocopherol, *Free Radical Biology and Medicine* 19 (1995): 169–176.

K. Anderson and K. Arrallah, Dietary Regulation of Cytochrome P450, *Annual Review of Nutrition* 11 (1991): 141–167.

E.E. Balieu, Dehydroepiandrosterone (DHEA): A Fountain of Youth? *Journal of Clinical Endocrinology and Metabolism* 81 (1996): 3147–3151.

M.K. Baum, et al., Micronutrients and HIV-1 disease progression, *AIDS* 9 (1995): 1051–1056.

E.G. Bliznakov, Coenzyme Q, in the Immune System and Aging, in *Biochemical and Clinical Aspects of Coenzyme Q10*, vol. 3, ed. K. Folkers and Y. Yamamura (New York: Elsevier Science, 1991), 331–336.

M. Boris and F.S. Mandel, Foods and Additives Are Common Causes of the Attention Deficit Hyperactive Disorder in Children. *Annals of Allergy* 72 (1994): 462–468.

V.W. Bunker, The Role of Nutrition in Osteoporosis, *British Journal of Biomedical Science* 51 (1994): 228–240.

H. Chen and A.L. Tappol, Vitamin E, Selenium, Trilox C, Ascorbic Acid Palmitate, Acetylcysteine, Coenzyme Q, B-Carotene, Canthaxanthin and (+)-Catechin Protect against Oxidative Damage to Kidney, Heart, Lung and Spleen, *Free Radical Research* 22 (1995): 177–186.

M.H. Coconnier et al., Inhibition of Adhesion of Enteroinvasive Pathogens to Human Intestinal Caco-2 Cells by Lactobacillus acidophilus Strain LB Decreases Bacterial Invasion, *FEMS Microbiology Letters* 110 (1993): 299–306.

G.B. Corcoran and B.K. Wong, Role of Glutathione in Prevention of Acetaminophen-Induced Hepatotoxicity by N-acetyl-l-cysteine in Vivo. *Journal of Pharmacology and Experimental Therapeutics* 238 (1986): 54–61.

L.G. Darlington, Dietary Therapy for Arthritis, *Rheumatic Diseases Clinics of North America* 17 (1991): 273–285.

K. Dubena and D.N. McMurray, Nutrition and the Immune System: A Review of Nutrient-Nutrient Interactions, *Journal of the American Dietetics Association* 96 (1996): 1156–1164.

L. Ernster and G. Dallner, Biochemical, Physiological and Medical Aspects of Ubiquinone Function, *Biochimica et Biophysica Acta* 1271 (1995): 195–204.

K. Folkers et al., The Activities of Coenzyme and Vitamin B6 for Immune Responses, *Biochemical and Biophysical Research Communications* 193 (1993): 88–92.

K. Folkers and R. Simonsen, Two Successful Double-Blind Trials with Coenzyme Q10 (Vitamin Q10) on Muscular Dystrophies and Neurogenic Atrophies, *Biochim Biophys Acta Mol Basis Dis* 1271 (1995): 281–286.

R. Fuller, Probiotics in Human Medicine, *Gut* 32 (1991): 439–473.

R. Fuller and G.R. Gibson, Modification of the Intestinal Microflora using Probiotics and Prebiotics, *Scandinavian Journal of Gastroenterology* 222, supplement (1997): 28-31.

G.B.J. Glass and B.L. Slomiary, Derangements of Biosynthesis, Production and Secretion of Mucus in Gastro Intestinal Injury and Disease, *Advances in Experimental Medicine and Biology* 189 (1976): 311–347.

S. Greenberg and W.H. Frisshman, Coenzyme Q10: A New Drug for Cardiovascular Disease, *Journal of Clinical Pharmacology* 30 (1990): 596–608.

L.S. Harbige, Nutrition and Immunity and Emphasis on Infection and Autoimmune Disease, *Nutrition and Health* 10, no. 4 (1996): 285–312.

A. Herp et al., Biochemistry and Lectin Binding Properties of Mammalian Salivary Mucous Glycoproteins, *Advances in Experimental Medicine and Biology* 33, no. 11 (1988): 1359–1363.

M.G. Hertog et al., Dietary Antioxidant Flavinoids and Risk of Coronary Heart Disease: The Zutphen Elderly Study, *Lancet* 342 (1993): 1007–1011.

A.M. Hoyumpa and S. Schenker, Drugs and the Liver, in *Gastroenterology and Hepatology: The Comprehensive Visual Reference*, ed. W.C. Maddrey (Philadelphia: Current Medicine, 1996): 6.1–6.22.

D. Ingram et al., Case-Control Study of Phyto-estrogens and Breast Cancer, *Lancet* 350 (1997): 990–994.

P. Jennerr, Oxidative Damage in Neurodegenerative Disease, *Lancet* (September 17, 1994), 796–798.

V.A. Jones et al., Crohn's Disease: Maintenance of Remission by Diet, *Lancet* 2 (1985): 177–180.

M. Kaminski, Jr., et al., Aids Wasting Syndrome as an Entero-Metabolic Disorder: The Gut Hypothesis, *Alternative Medicine Review* 3, no. 1 (1998): 40–53.

T.N. Kaul et al., Antiviral Effect of Flavinoids on Human Viruses, *Journal of Medical Virology* 15 (1985): 71–79.

J. Kjeldsen-Dragh et al., Controlled Trial of Fasting and One Year Vegetarian Diet in Rheumatoid Arthritis, *Lancet* 338 (1991): 899–902.

C.A. Lang et al., Low Blood Glutathione in Healthy Aging Adults, *Journal of Laboratory and Clinical Medicine* 120 (1992): 720–725.

C.W. Lo and W.A. Walker, Changes in the Gastrointestinal Tract During Enteral or Parental Feeding, *Nutrition Reviews* 47, no. 7 (1989): 193–198.

F. Lockwood et al., Progress on Therapy of Breast Cancer with Vitamin Q 10 and the Regression of Metastases, *Biochemical and Biophysical Research Communications* 212 (1995): 172–177.

B.M. Lomaestro and M. Malone, Glutathione in Health and Disease: Pharmacotherapeutic Issues, *Annals of Pharmacotherapy* 29 (1995): 1263–1273.

H. McCoy and M.A. Kenney, Magnesium and Immune Function: Recent Findings. *Magnesium Research* 5, no. 4 (1992): 281–293.

M. Messina et al., Photoestrogens and Breast Cancer. *The Lancet* 350, no. 9083 (1997): 990–994, 971–972.

A.J. Morales et al., Effects of Replacement Dose of Dehydroepiandrosterone in Men and Women of Advancing Age, *Journal of Clinical Endocrinology and Metabolism* 78 (1994): 1360–1367.

R. Nanda et al., Food Intolerance and the Irritable Bowel Syndrome, *Gut* 30 (1989): 1099–1104.

W.R. Phipps et al., Effect of Flax Seed Ingestion on the Menstrual Cycle, *Journal of Clinical Endocrinology and Metabolism* 77 (1993): 1215–1219.

A.H. Rowe and E.J. Young, Bronchial Asthma due to Food Allergy Alone in Ninety-Five Patients, *Journal of the American Medical Association* 169 (1959): 1158–1162.

E. Smith et al., Deterring Bone Loss by Exercise Intervention in Premenopausal and Postmenopausal Women, *Calcified Tissue International* 44 (1998): 312–321.

B.A. Stoll, Essential Fatty Acids, Insulin Resistance, and Breast Cancer Risk, *Nutrition and Cancer* 31, no. 1 (1998): 72–77.

A.M. Tang et al., Low Serum Vitamin B12 Concentrations Are Associated with Faster Human Immunodeficiency Virus Type 1 (HIV-1) Disease Progression, *American Journal of Clinical Nutrition* 127, no. 2 (1997): 345–351.

VISION OF HEALING
Moving Through Strength

It is remarkable how much better we can feel from the simple acts of exercising regularly and moving creatively to the rhythm of life. Holistic nurses endeavor to maximize and develop the best of exercise and movement skills, both for the self, for the individual client, and for groups. It is through various kinds of movement that we begin to strengthen and maximize the abilities of the physical body.

As we begin the new millennium, the ancient Greek ideal of a sound mind in a strong, able body is once again in fashion. A healthy physical body is indeed the temple for the mind-spirit. The way in which we care for our body permeates all aspects of our being including such things as our self-esteem and self-care practices. It even affects longevity and the ability to care for and be of service to others.

Holistic nurses will want to learn about various movements in order to personally and professionally use them with knowledge. A program of conscious, controlled, regular body movement promotes physical power. Unlike medicines, active movement enables us to build up the actual tissues and muscle mass of our bodies. When we exercise, we build strong healthy bodies, but when we are sedentary and slothful, we deprive ourselves and set up an internal environment for physical deterioration.

The feeling of well-being that comes from physical health permeates every individual activity, enabling the quickest thinking, permitting a better night's sleep, and perhaps facilitating spirituality. The lack of proper exercise and movement can even contribute to the risk of contracting major diseases, such as hypertension, hypercholesterolemia, and obesity. However, both movement and exercise patterns are modifiable when individuals make the decision to move toward wellness. For those who are physically weakened because of illness and disease or because of emotional, mental, or spiritual ennui, the good news is that anyone with motivation can begin a personally tailored exercise program to activate healing of the bodymind.

Now is the ideal time for making new personal beginnings. Think about why you want to make a new commitment to acquiring the knowledge and skills necessary for an effective movement program and how you will go about achieving your goals. Choose a program of strengthening exercise or movement routines then join with others for the support and motivation it takes to successfully carry through on your new program. It is when we become individually strong that we can best join with other like-minded nurses to demonstrate ways of moving through strength. When we believe and model the fact that physical strength is an important ingredient in optimum health we are in the best position to help our clients achieve their goals.

Chapter 19

Exercise and Movement

Beryl H. Cricket Rose and Lynn Keegan

NURSE HEALER OBJECTIVES

Theoretical

- Learn the definitions of terms in this chapter.
- Differentiate among exercise, fitness, and movement.
- Develop a fitness plan that combines movement and exercise.
- Learn the benefits of exercise and movement both in illness and in health.

Clinical

- Develop an awareness of body mechanics (movement and posture) during both clinical and physical activity and stationary desk or phone work.
- Employ strategies to improve exercise and movement in the workplace.
- Involve clients in self-assessment of their movement and exercise patterns as a routine part of health promotion and a strategy for management and recovery in illness.
- Include exercise and movement assessments of children in health care of a family.
- Seek current clinical research regarding special health concerns and the recommendations for therapeutic exercise and movement and make the information available to clients.

- Consider ways in which the nurse can initiate or promote community-based health programs supporting exercise and movement.
- Consider ways in which the nurse serves as a role model during the workday.
- Learn the value of kinetic energy at work and become an exercise leader in the clinical setting.

Personal

- Spend time becoming aware of your current activities of exercise and your patterns of movement.
- Assess your physical habits related to both exercise and movement .
- Begin to experiment with new patterns of exercise and movements.
- Become increasingly sensitive to nuances of feeling as you gradually refine your skills in these physical activities, increasing kinesthesia.
- Attend to the mind/body/spirit responses you feel and evaluate the results.

DEFINITIONS

Aerobic Exercise: sustained muscle activity within the target heart range that challenges the cardiovascular system to meet the muscles' needs for oxygen.

Anaerobic Exercise: exercise that is fueled by the energy within the muscles used.

Endurance: the period of time the body can sustain exercise or movement.

Fitness: the ability to carry out daily tasks with vigor and alertness, without undue fatigue, and with ample reserve to enjoy leisure pursuits; the ability to respond to physical and emotional stress without an excessive increase in heart rate and blood pressure. Fitness is increased with endurance exercises.

Flexibility: the ability to use a joint throughout its full range of motion and to maintain some degree of elasticity of major muscle groups.

Kinetic energy: energy associated with motion, energizing, or dynamic energy.

Maximal Heart Rate: the rate of the heart when the body is engaged in intense physical activity.

Movement: changes in the spatial configuration of the body and its parts, such as in breathing, eating, speaking, gesturing, and exercising; motion away from mental, physical, emotional, or spiritual stasis.

Nonaerobic Exercise: sustained physical activity above the normal resting state that uses one or more major muscle groups but is not intense enough to cause an increased muscle oxygen uptake.

Posture: pose, or placement of parts of the body in spatial relationships.

Resistance Training: the use of weights or opposing forces to exercise (strengthen) muscle groups.

Resting Heart Rate: the rate of the heart when the body is in deep rest.

Strength: the power of muscle groups.

Target Heart Rate: the safe rate for the heart during exercise.

Training: repetitive bouts of exercise over a period of time with the intention of developing fitness.

THEORY AND RESEARCH

Exercise

Traditionally, regular exercise programs were thought to be necessary only for athletes in training. We now know that vigorous aerobic exercise is good for everyone. The new guidelines issued by the American College of Sports Medicine (ACSM) note that body composition, strength, endurance, and flexibility are joined with cardiorespiratory vigor in supporting fitness.[1] Today, less than 1 percent of all the energy used in factories, workshops, and farms comes from human muscles. During the next few years, continued growth will be seen in information and technology occupations, which are increasingly sedentary and, hence, potentially unhealthy, reducing the fitness of many people.

Exercise is any form of movement in a continuum from active physical exertion to subtle motions that are only slightly perceptible. In a review of national surveys, one study found that approximately 20 percent of adults exercise with the intensity and frequency necessary for cardiovascular benefit, 40 percent are moderately active, and 40 percent are basically sedentary.[2] Thus, even though the number of adults who exercise regularly is increasing, most are not exercising at the intensity or frequency necessary to obtain maximal health benefits.

Physical activity is positively associated with a vigorous life and fitness. According to the 1998 guidelines from the ACSM, walking briskly every day substantially increases stamina, prevents obesity, and improves general fitness. A variety of clinical trials support the contention that regular participation in physical activity either delays the onset or reduces the severity of several chronic diseases, including obesity and coronary heart disease.[3–5]

Eastern approaches to exercise and movement, such as Ayurveda and yoga practices, are distinctly different from Western medical approaches; these Eastern practices advise movements and exercises for health promotion and restoration. Ayurvedic medicine prescribes daily exercises that, although specific to the individual, are generally designed to be performed at 50 percent of maximum heart rate and are balanced with breathing exercises and yoga postures and stretching. In ayurvedic practice, daily physical exercise balanced with mental and spiritual exercises is essential, but exercise is performed at submaximal levels designed to slowly increase capacity and endurance and provide positive self-reinforcement for the behavior. Thus, ayurvedic exercises are achievable by persons whose goal is not to develop athletic ability but rather to gain a healthy vitality.[6,7]

Exercise Needs in Special Situations

Acquired Immunodeficiency Syndrome. In a study to determine if progressive resistance exercise could improve muscle function in patients with acquired immune deficiency syndrome (AIDS), the experimental group who engaged in such exercise three times a week for 6 weeks improved significantly in 13 of 15 study variables. Thus, when patients are in the nonacute stage of AIDS, exercise can produce physiologic adaptation that improves muscle function and increases body dimensions and body mass.[8,9]

Cardiovascular Disease. In acute heart failure, rest is a useful adjunct to pharmacologic treatment. In chronic heart failure, however, avoidance of exercise can lead to deconditioning changes in skeletal muscle and in the peripheral circulation that may actually impair exercise tolerance. Although some controversy still exists as to whether training improves the prognosis

for patients with chronic heart failure and how soon after myocardial infarction they can safely commence training, exercise is likely to become an increasingly popular and useful adjunct in the care of patients with chronic heart disease.[10,11]

The cardiovascular effects of aerobic exercise include a decrease in the resting heart rate and the heart rate response to submaximal exercise, an increase in resting and exercise stroke volume, an increase in maximal cardiac output, an increase in maximum oxygen consumption, and an increase in arteriovenous oxygen difference. These effects of cardiovascular fitness have a beneficial effect on the coronary artery disease risk profile. An inverse relationship exists between physical fitness and resting heart rate, body weight, percentage of body fat, systolic blood pressure, and serum levels of cholesterol, triglycerides, and glucose. In addition, exercise increases the high-density lipoprotein fraction of total cholesterol.[12] To develop and maintain cardiovascular fitness, an individual should engage in aerobic exercise 3 to 5 days per week at an intensity of 55 to 90 percent of heart rate maximum or 40 to 85 percent of heart rate maximum reserve for 20 to 60 minutes (or a minimum of three 10-minute bouts accumulated throughout the day).[13] In addition, stretching and resistance training for the major muscle groups should be carried out 2 or 3 days a week. For resistance training, using one set of 8 to 10 exercises with 8 to 12 repetitions per exercise is recommended. Studies of stretching routines suggest that any of several techniques is beneficial. Four repetitions should be performed with each major muscle/tendon group. Therapists generally recommend stretching exercises for warm-ups and cool-downs during aerobic exercise, but isolated stretching or nonaerobic exercises such as yoga and T'ai Chi exercises are beneficial in themselves.[14-16]

Studies suggest that clinically stable, aerobically trained cardiac patients may perform resistance exercises like circuit training comfortably.[17] A carefully supervised, long-term program of low-resistance training appears to be safe with regard to blood pressure and beneficial in terms of strength gain.[18,19]

Age does not seem to influence the results in cardiac rehabilitation programs. One study found that improvements in exercise capacity, obesity indexes, and lipid levels were very similar in older and younger patients enrolled in cardiac rehabilitation and exercise programs.[20] Because nurses play a key role in the development and implementation of these programs, they should be aware of research findings in this area so that they can personalize programs to meet the needs of different types of patients.[21]

Diabetes. Control of diabetes is enhanced with control of stress (related to the fact that catecholamine or adrenalin production causes elevations in blood sugar). Yoga and therapeutic movement (dance) are recommended for stress management in diabetic individuals. Regular aerobic exercise, particularly bicycling and swimming, are beneficial for the diabetic individual in order to control weight, increase tissue oxygenation, and maintain energy levels. General health, other risk factors, and glucose control must be assessed before specific exercise prescriptions can be advised.[22,23]

Neuromuscular Conditions. In several small studies, patients with slowly progressive neuromuscular diseases (muscular dystrophy) were trained with moderate resistance exercise programs to study the safety and efficacy of strength training programs. Results provide evidence that a supervised submaximal strength training program is practical and safe for these individuals and can produce moderate improvement in measured strength.[24]

Low Back Pain. To determine whether graded physical exercise could restore occupational function in industrial blue-collar workers who were sick-listed for 8 weeks because of subacute, nonspecified, mechanical low back pain, 103 subjects were randomly assigned to either an activity group or a control group. Subjects in the graded activity group became occupationally functional again, as measured by their earlier return to work, and their time on long-term sick leave was significantly reduced.[25] Another group of researchers explored the effect of a weekly exercise program on the amount of short-term sick leave (50 days or less) attributable to back pain and the possible correlation between changes in absenteeism and changes in cardiovascular fitness. They found that, during the intervention period, the number of episodes of back pain and the number of sick leave days attributable to back pain decreased by more than 50 percent in the exercise group.[26] Spinal flexion exercises have been found to increase sagittal mobility more than do extension exercises.[27,28]

Osteoporosis. Weight-bearing, bone-jarring exercise and resistance training builds bones. For this purpose, dancing is better than swimming. One study reported that 30 women increased their spinal bone mass by 0.5 percent in 1 year by performing 50 minutes of vigorous walking four times per week, irrespective of calcium consumption, while nonexercisers lost 7 percent of spinal bone mass.[29] Epidemiological studies show that women who are able to maintain a high level of physical activity have a lower incidence of hip fractures, which may be an indirect result of postural stabilization, improved coordination, strength, and flexibility enabled by regular exercise.[30]

Asthma. Sixty-seven asthmatic adults participated in a 16-week program and were randomly assigned to a deep diaphragmatic breathing training group, a physical exercise training group, or a waiting list control group. Deep diaphragmatic training produced significant reductions both in medication use and in the intensity of asthmatic symptoms. Importantly, diaphragmatic training also made possible a nearly 300 percent increase in time spent in physical activities.[31]

Cystic Fibrosis. One study sought to determine whether substituting regular exercise, which also promotes coughing, for two of three daily bronchial hygiene treatments could improve pulmonary function and exercise response in patients hospitalized with cystic fibrosis. Results indicate that, in some cystic fibrosis patients, exercise therapy is an effective substitute for at least part of the standard protocol of bronchial hygiene therapy.[32]

Fibromyalgia. Strenuous exertion may exacerbate the disease of fibromyalgia, but specific low-intensity exercises such as walking, biking, and swimming with a kick board have been observed to aid in their physical fitness achievements. Aerobic exercise is contraindicated according to anecdotal evidence from therapists working with fibromyalgia patients.[33]

Rheumatoid Arthritis. Although patients with rheumatoid arthritis are not expected to maintain high levels of physical fitness, a 1975 study evaluated 34 patients who participated in a 6-week training program of physical therapy. Patients in the control group ($n = 11$) were given only physical therapy. Patients in the experimental group ($n = 23$) were also given cycle ergometer workouts five times a week. The training group showed significant improvement in a walk test and an oxygen uptake test with no change in joint status as judged by pain and swelling. A 6-month follow-up showed that 18 of the 23 patients continued exercising at least twice a week. After 8 years, those in the training group were three times more physically active, experienced less stiffness, and had fewer sick days and fewer hospitalizations than the control group. Several other studies support the prescription of moderate exercise (at 50–70 percent of maximal heart rate) and some resistance training for patients in a moderate phase of rheumatoid arthritis.[34]

Psychiatric Conditions. The effects of exercise on clients in a psychiatric rehabilitation program were investigated in three studies. Results indicate that, the higher the level of aerobic fitness, the lower the level of self-reported depression.[35,36] Nurses may want to act on such data by establishing exercise programs in psychiatric settings.

Aging Adults and Exercise

Loss of lower-extremity strength increases the risk of falls in older persons.[37] One exercise program study involving elderly male nursing home residents demonstrated that an appropriately designed high-intensity exercise program can result in significant, although limited, improvements in clinical mobility scores, strength, muscular endurance, and certain gait parameters.[38] In another study, a 12-week randomized clinical trial used an exercise program that focused on strength and balance to achieve a clinically significant improvement in gait velocity.[39] Exercise was also found to improve balance in elderly women.[40] Postural stability, cardiovascular toning, increased muscle mass and strength, added bone density, and psychological boost are all advantages of physical activity in the aging person. Running, walking, swimming, cycling, dancing, stretching, or other movement programs can add vigor to the life of an elderly person.[41]

Movement

Various aspects of movement, such as dance, theater, and sport, have been used in ritual, celebration, and healing rites since humans first organized into collective tribes and families. For thousands of years, Eastern cultures and philosophies have considered symbolic physical motion to be essential for physical and mental well-being. Yoga and T'ai Chi, for example, are two ancient physical movement forms that are still practiced today to enhance overall health. T'ai Chi, a traditional Chinese exercise, is a series of individual dancelike movements linked together in a continuous, smooth-flowing sequence. Movements within such disciplines are based on concepts of total concentration, strength, relaxation, and symbolic motion.

Movement ranges from the rapid motions of active dance or acrobatics to the subtle rhythm characterized by breathing and choral singing, to the slow, careful movements of T'ai Chi. It includes the way that individuals hold and carry their bodies (i.e., posture) and the way that groups communicate nonverbally (i.e., body language). Movement also includes dancing, swimming, and other leisure sports. Exercise is the form of movement to which we give most attention because of its known benefits to health maintenance. In health care, movement is used for a number of therapeutic purposes; range-of-motion exercises, water exercises, and specific physical therapy movements are incorporated into a variety of rehabilitative programs.[42]

The use of bodywork and movement to influence physiologic functioning is evident in several therapies emerging in alternative medicine: the Alexander technique, Feldenkrais method, rolfing movement integration, Aston-patterning, Hellerwork, and Trager approach. Most of these therapies are holistic approaches to reeducating body mechanics, balance, and postural alignments that are used by many nontraditional physical therapists and healers. The Alexander technique was developed by an actor who kept losing his voice and found his body movements and postures to be at fault.[43] In the Trager approach, the mindfulness of patterns of movement assists in improving balance in the frail elderly, easing tension in myofascial pain syndrome, and promoting recovery from surgeries in which movement is restricted for a time (mastectomy, surgery of the back, knee, or shoulder).[44]

In one study to determine the potential value of T'ai Chi in promoting postural control in well elderly people, the performance of nine T'ai Chi practitioners on five balance tests was compared to the performance of nine nonpractitioners. Statistical analysis demonstrated that, in three of the tests, the T'ai Chi practitioners had significantly better postural control than did the sedentary nonpractitioners. Men performed significantly better on the same three tests than did women in both the practitioner and nonpractitioner groups.[45] T'ai Chi has also been found to be a safe movement therapy for clients with rheumatoid arthritis.[46,47]

Because we all use movement continually, we usually take it for granted. For many who have disabilities, or are in rehabilitative programs, however, the design of creative movement plans can make the difference between partial and full development of their physical potential. Others can use movement therapies to improve body mechanics and help cope with the sedentary workplaces of our era. Although occupational or physical therapists often design and teach movement programs, new types of therapists have emerged with the increased emphasis on wellness programs. Dance therapists and T'ai Chi instructors are now more widely consulted, particularly by those seeking high-level wellness. Creative movement programs are taught in group sessions, at wellness centers, or in continuing education classes, and may be led by nurses.

Creative movement, including dance, T'ai Chi, and other expressive movements, is a health-promoting behavior that is appropriate for a variety of populations and age groups. Movement can be a nursing intervention with independent, active people, as well as with those who have mobility deficits.[48] Dance, which is one of the major movement therapies, emphasizes the holism of human beings. In dance, one can externalize concepts created in the mind, thus making possible another bodymind experience.

HOLISTIC CARING PROCESS

Assessment

In preparing to use exercise and movement interventions, the nurse assesses the following parameters:

- the client's financial and religious restrictions, as well as habit patterns formed during childhood and cultural approaches to exercise and movement
- the client's nonverbal movement patterns and known movement limitations
- the client's motivation, desire, and ability to make the necessary lifestyle changes in the areas of exercise and movement

Patterns/Problems/Needs

The following are the patterns/problems/needs compatible with the interventions for exercise and movement that are related to the nine human response patterns of the Unitary Person framework (see Chapter 14):

- *Exchanging:* Altered nutrition
  Altered circulation
  Altered oxygenation
- *Choosing:* Altered coping
- *Moving:* Altered physical mobility
  Sleep pattern disturbance
  Altered activities of daily living
- *Perceiving:* Disturbance in body image

Disturbance in self-esteem
Potential hopelessness
Potential powerlessness
- *Knowing* Knowledge deficit
- *Feeling* Pain
  Anxiety
  Grieving

Outcomes

Exhibit 19–1 guides the nurse in client outcomes, nursing prescriptions, and evaluation for the use of exercise and movement as nursing interventions.

Therapeutic Care Plan and Interventions

Before the Session

- Create an environment in which the client feels comfortable discussing the needs of his or her physical body from a physical movement perspective.
- Clear your mind of other client or personal encounters in order to be fully present when meeting with the client.
- Gather input data forms and teaching charts.
- Prepare all necessary assessment equipment.
- Prepare handouts or between-session worksheets to give to the client during the session.

At the Beginning of the Session

- Take and record the necessary physical assessment data (e.g., height, weight, skin-fold thickness measurements, body contour measurements, blood pressure, data on range of motion and mobility limitations).
- Guide the client as he or she discloses past habit patterns that affect exercise behavior.

Exhibit 19-1 Nursing Interventions: Exercise and Movement

Client Outcomes	Nursing Prescriptions	Evaluation
The client will be motivated to improve exercise and movement practice.	Assist the client in a personal self-assessment. Encourage the client to participate with the nurse to develop goals and action plans. Prepare the client to follow through with the nurse on evaluation and formulation of new goals.	The client completed a self-assessment form. The client participated with the nurse to develop a personalized program of exercise and movement. The client met with the nurse to evaluate program results.
The client will demonstrate knowledge of healthful exercise and movement programs and resources.	Motivate the client to contribute to discussions about his or her program. Encourage the client to learn more about healthful behaviors as he or she works with the nurse.	The client participated in the session discussions. The client demonstrated content knowledge and resource acquisition for using new behaviors in exercise and movement programs.

During the Session

- Review with the client current weekly exercise patterns.
- Be alert to psychologic clues that may relate to exercise behavior or extremes (exhaustion versus training versus sedentariness).
- Following data collection, work with the client to develop an individualized exercise and movement program.
- Make certain that teaching is at the client's intellectual and emotional level.

At the End of the Session

- Have the client identify the options presented that best fit with his or her own lifestyle.
- Work with the client to write down goals and target dates.
- Give the client specific affirmations to use to support these goals.
- Give the client handout material to reinforce the teaching.

- Use the client outcomes that were established before the session (see Exhibit 19–1) and the client's subjective experiences (Exhibit 19–2) to evaluate the session.
- Schedule a follow-up session.

Specific Interventions: Exercise and Movement

Exercise (Basic)

A new paradigm of fitness is emerging. Its orientation is broader and it focuses more on enjoyment. As the new paradigm gains strength, both the number of people exercising and those exercising at the level of vigor necessary to achieve improved vitality and health promotion will probably increase. Table 19–1 depicts the old and new fitness paradigms.

The primary purpose of exercise is to produce fitness. The basic components of fitness are

Table 19-1 Old and New Fitness Paradigms

Old Fitness Paradigm	*New Fitness Paradigm*
Physical education, athletics programs	Bodymind integration, kinetic energy
Competition and comparison with others	Noncompetition, self-comparison only
Regulated calisthenics, aerobics, sports	Technology, feedback, and mechanical advantages to motivate and inspire action
Rigorous and punitive	Exhilirating and fun
Muscle building, body building, shape orientation	Integration of body-mind-spirit in temporal physicality

1. flexibility: the ability to use a joint throughout its full range of motion and to maintain some degree of elasticity of major muscle groups. It is important because
   - it provides increased resistance to muscle and joint injury
   - it helps prevent mild muscle soreness if flexibility exercises are done before and after vigorous activity
2. muscle strength: the contracting power of a muscle. It is important because
   - daily activities become less strenuous as muscles become stronger
   - strong abdominal and lower back muscles help prevent lower back problems
   - appearance improves as muscles become firmer
3. cardiorespiratory endurance: the ability of the circulatory and respiratory systems to maintain blood and oxygen delivery to the exercising muscles. It is important because
   - it increases resistance to cardiovascular diseases
   - it improves the ability to maintain activity levels
   - it allows for a high energy return for daily activities
4. postural stability: the body's ability to balance and stay balanced during dynamic action; declines naturally with age; exercise continuation assists with preventing falls through integration of neuromuscular and sensory responses.

Beginning the regimen in a disciplined manner increases the chances of maintaining the program. Thus, before beginning an exercise program, an individual should be encouraged to follow these basic guidelines:

- Learn about the different types of exercise programs available in your area.
- Consult your physician or exercise authority. If you are over 35, have never seriously exercised, or have a disability or chronic illness, obtain guidance to avoid injuries or complications.
- Establish an exercise routine. Choose exercises or sports you will enjoy. Decide on a place and time of day to exercise. Ask a friend to join you or meet some new people at the jogging trail or health club. Create or join an exercise class before, during, or after work. There are endless possibilities.
- Warm up and cool down. Stretching exercises are essential before and after each aerobic or nonaerobic exercise period.
- Set realistic goals and work toward them. Some benefits of exercise may not be quickly apparent. Be patient.

Build up slowly to your long-term goals.

• Evaluate the program periodically. Determine if you are making progress. If you want to go further, set new goals.
• Create competition for yourself only if it benefits you. If you have allowed too much competition, exercise may become more of a burden than a joy.

Many rewards of exercise and physical activity begin immediately. Mental and spiritual improvements include beneficial changes in

• mental attitude toward your work, yourself, and life in general
• ability to cope with stress
• ability to avoid or control mild depression
• sleep patterns
• strength and endurance
• eating habits
• appearance and vitality
• posture
• physical stamina as you age

To reduce risks associated with exercise, one must know not only how often and how long to exercise but also how vigorously to exercise. Although the target pulse range allows for a heart rate within 60 to 80 percent of maximal capacity, the American Heart Association guidelines state that regular exercise of a moderate level, or from 50 to 75 percent of maximal capacity, appears to be sufficient. Maintaining the target pulse rate during physical exercise for 15 to 30 minutes three to five times per week reduces the risk of overexertion, enhances enjoyment, and results in cardiovascular fitness. Because uncontrolled exercising may result in injury, it is wise to follow these guidelines:

• Always warm up for a minimum of 10 minutes.
• If you are tired, stop.

• If something hurts, stop.
• If you feel dizzy or nauseated, stop.
• Take your pulse at regular intervals.
• Cool down after exercising.

To ease your heart rate into the training range, begin with 10 minutes of low-intensity warm-up exercise. To cool down, do 10 minutes of the same slow activity.

Adherence rates for nurse-led exercise programs are considerably higher than are those for other programs. Women tested at 3- and 6-month intervals after exercise intervention stated that they tried many fitness clubs and spas in the area but could find no exercise programs that were tailored to their age and fitness level or that took into consideration their individual health needs. Nurses interested in and knowledgeable about the changes associated with aging are in an ideal position to develop and lead exercise programs for older individuals, particularly those with chronic, nondisabling physical problems.[49] Technological advances that may help in the provision of educational services include videocassettes and interactive computer programs.[50]

Movement (Basic)

There are four components of creative movement: centering, warm-up, exploration of surrounding space, and stretching.[51]

1. Centering is the inward focusing on one's own physical reality. The duration of this process varies, but it usually lasts 3 to 10 minutes.
2. The stretching, breathing warm-up exercises follow the centering exercise and are designed to "wake up" the muscles while maintaining the harmonious integration of psyche and soma that was begun through centering.
   • Musical accompaniment has a positive effect on one's ability to perform. Music seems to bypass the psychological feedback of the sen-

sations of exertion and fatigue and instead produces feelings of exuberance and strength.

- Exercises are done to synchronize breathing and symbolic imagery slowly and rhythmically. The individual uses images in concert with motion.
- Social involvement during warm-up adds another dimension to creative movement. Initially, people may be shy with one another, but relaxation and enjoyment increase as the movement accelerates.
- Additional warm-up techniques allow people to delve deeper into their own personal inward life before proceeding further into group activities, if they wish.

3. Exploration of surrounding space occurs as movement proceeds and there is an awakened sense of self-awareness. With this discovery of new physical capacities comes increased kinetic and spatial awareness. During this time, there may be swinging, swaying, and laughter.

4. Stretching concludes a dance movement, allowing for relaxation as it brings one to a resting state. At the conclusion, one should savor the feeling of energetic relaxation.

Case Study

Setting:	Public health clinic
Client:	E.J., a 55-year-old Hispanic widow with diabetes, living with a partially blind adult son.
Nursing	1. Altered nutrition (more than body requirements) related to excessive intake, improper eating patterns, and lack of exercise
	2. Alteration in tissue perfusion related to decreased cellular exchange

3. Ineffective management of therapeutic regimen related to health beliefs

E.J. came for a routine checkup after years of uncontrolled diabetes mellitus. Oral hypoglycemic drugs had been prescribed for her several years earlier, but due to financial circumstances she did not continue to obtain health care and neglected her prescription for over 6 months. Worried because of increasing symptoms, she found the health department services and made an appointment with the family practice clinic. Her blood glucose level (fasting) was 240 mg/dl; her blood pressure was 150/88; she weighed 168 pounds and was 5 feet tall. She had not worked for the past 6 months. Her son lives with her and helps her financially as much as he can, working at nonskilled jobs. She has some friends and relatives that are nearby and who encouraged her to obtain treatment at a clinic.

Through the intake interview and history, the nurse learned that E.J. used to dance every weekend when her husband was alive and that she lives in a beautiful country setting in a trailer park. E.J. reported no meaningful activities outside of her church, for which she sometimes cleans and cooks. She had become more sedentary over the past 6 months, watching TV most of the day.

Willing to gain some control over her diabetes, E.J. agreed to follow a diet and exercise plan along with taking her prescriptions. She arranged to record her activities every day, to include daily walks in her neighborhood, and to begin using her record player at home to dance for 20 to 30 minutes three or four times a week. Together with the nurse, she designed an exercise program for a trial period of 6 weeks. She was given follow-up appointments with the nutritionist, the nurse, the physician, the laboratory, and a social worker.

Since her plan for exercise and movement included keeping a daily journal of her activities, she was instructed to bring this journal back to review with the nurse in 2 weeks during a short visit.

After 6 weeks, the nurse and the social worker had introduced E.J. to a senior citizen group that holds regular dances each month and an exercise class located in a church basement. E.J. met several other middle-aged women who walk in her neighborhood and formed a loose group of walkers. She reported only occasional lapses in exercise, usually due to her son's health or the weather. Together E.J. and the nurse discussed strategies for dealing with the changing weather and her daily walks. Overall, E.J. felt successful and energetic, and appeared to have recovered from the gloomy withdrawal she felt earlier.

Ongoing assessments of her activity level were to be scheduled according to her needs, but at least annually. E.J. revealed great joy in the experience of keeping a journal, as she felt she could show her son what she was doing and be proud of her smallest accomplishments regarding exercise and movement. Her ability to control this element in her self-care contributed both to her self-esteem and to the management of her diabetes. She also lost 8 pounds. In general, she experienced many benefits from establishing an exercise and movement program.

Evaluation

The nurse determines with the client whether the client outcomes for exercise and movement (Exhibit 19–1) were successfully achieved. To evaluate the session further, the nurse may again explore the subjective effects of the experience with the client using the evaluation questions in Exhibit 19–2.

Exhibit 19–2 Evaluation of the Client's Subjective Experience with Exercise and Movement Interventions

1. Is this the first time you have experimented with your exercise routine?
2. Have you experienced any sense of release during the changed physical activity?
3. Has your vitality increased since beginning regular exercise?
4. Does exercise give you a sense of reduced stress in your life?
5. Do you find time during your normal day to integrate special movement techniques?
6. If not, would you like to learn more ways to improve your movement periods at work?
7. What support systems have you discovered that assist you with maintaining and developing your exercise regimen?
8. Is there some other support that you need to assist you in adhering to your new exercise regimen?
9. What is your next step for integrating exercise and therapeutic movement into your daily life?
10. Do you need help in obtaining more resources for this final step?

Nurses should chart the information they impart to the client as well as the evaluation of the session. When the nurse works in an inpatient facility, other staff must be apprised of the program and the client's progress. Nurses who work in wellness centers, independent practice, or other areas in which counseling sessions are the primary care modality should keep records for each client that state the nursing diagnosis, type of counseling employed, and effectiveness of each session.

Attention to exercise and movement can lead to a general improvement of health and decrease the risk factors of major diseases. The nurse is in a prime position to model the effects of healthy exercise and movement behaviors.

DIRECTIONS FOR FUTURE RESEARCH

1. Investigate the hypothesis that those who exercise feel better and live longer.
2. Continue the investigations into the ways in which the lifestyle behaviors of exercise and movement affect a person's general sense of well-being.
3. Investigate the determinants that allow or encourage exercise in unstructured or spontaneous situations.
4. Study the specific factors that are important in tailoring exercise programs to ethnic and cultural groups.

NURSE HEALER REFLECTIONS

After reading this chapter, the nurse healer will be able to answer or begin the process of answering the following questions:

- How would I describe the place of movement and exercise in my life today?
- What mental or spiritual sensations accompany my physical sensations because of my improved exercise and movement status?
- How should I feel when I am physically fit?
- What exercise and movement changes can I incorporate in my daily life to improve my fitness?
- How can I learn, practice, and model healthy exercise and movement?

NOTES

1. American College of Sports Medicine, Position Stand, The Recommended Quantity and Quality of Exercise for Developing and Maintaining Cardiorespiratory and Muscular Fitness, and Flexibility in Healthy Adults, *Medicine and Science in Sports and Exercise* 30, no. 6 (1998): 975–991.
2. T. Stephens et al., A Description of Leisure Time Physical Activity, *Public Health Reports* 100 (1985): 147–157.
3. Burton Goldberg Group, *Alternative Medicine: The Definitive Guide* (Puyallup, WA: Future Medicine Publishing, 1994), 721, 729.
4. American College of Sports Medicine, Position Stand, Recommended Quantity and Quality of Exercise.
5. W.L. Haskett, Overview: Health Benefits of Exercise, in *Behavioral Health: A Handbook of Health Enhancement and Disease Prevention*, ed. J.D. Matarazzo et al. (New York: John Wiley & Sons, 1984).
6. H. Sharma and C. Clark, *Exercise in Contemporary Ayurveda: Medicine and Research in Maharishi Ayur-Veda* (New York: Churchill Livingstone, 1998), 117–126.

7. Burton Goldberg Group, *Alternative Medicine*, 69.
8. D.W. Spence et al., Progressive Resistance Exercise: Effect on Muscle Function and Anthropometry of Select AIDS Population, *Archives of Physical Medicine and Rehabilitation* 71, no. 9 (1990): 644–648.
9. L. Goldberg and D.L. Elliot, *Exercise for Prevention and Treatment of Illness* (Philadelphia: F.A. Davis Co., 1994), 301, 308.
10. Goldberg and Elliot, *Exercise for Prevention and Treatment of Illness*, 49.
11. A.J. Coats, Exercise Rehabilitation in Chronic Heart Failure, *Journal of the American College of Cardiology* 22, no. 4 (1993): 172A–177A.
12. L.T. Braun, Exercise Physiology and Cardiovascular Fitness, *Nursing Clinics of North America* 26, no. 1 (1991):135–147.
13. American College of Sports Medicine, Position Stand, Recommended Quantity and Quality of Exercise.
14. J. Lasater, Untying the Knot: Yoga as Physical Therapy, in *Complementary Therapies in Rehabilitation: Holistic Approaches for Prevention*

and *Wellness,* ed. C.M. Davis (Thorofare, NJ: Slack, 1997): 125–131.

15. R.K. Ng, Cardiopulmonary Exercise: A Recently Discovered Secret of T'ai Chi, *Hawaii Medical Journal* 51 (1992): 216–217.

16. J.S. Lai et al., Two-Year Trends in Cardiorespiratory Function among Older T'ai Chi Chuan Practitioners and Sedentary Subjects. *Journal of American Geriatric Society* 43 (1995): 1222–1227.

17. American College of Sports Medicine, Position Stand, Exercise for Patients with Coronary Artery Disease. *Medicine and Science in Sports and Exercise* 26, no. 3 (1994): i–v.

18. American College of Sports Medicine, Position Stand, Exercise and Physical Activity for Older Adults, 992–1008.

19. P.B. Sparling et al., Strength Training in a Cardiac Rehabilitation Program: A Six-Month Follow-up, *Archives of Physical Medicine and Rehabilitation* 71, no. 2 (1990): 148–152.

20. C.J. Lavie et al., Benefits of Cardiac Rehabilitation and Exercise Training in Secondary Coronary Prevention in the Elderly, *Journal of the American College of Cardiology* 22, no. 3 (1993): 678–683.

21. M.A. Parchert and J.M. Simon, The Role of Exercise in Cardiac Rehabilitation: A Nursing Perspective, *Rehabilitation Nursing* 13, no. 1 (1988): 11–14.

22. Goldberg and Elliot, *Exercise for Prevention and Treatment of Illness,* 181.

23. Burton Goldberg Group, *Alternative Medicine,* 652–653.

24. Goldberg and Elliot, *Exercise for Prevention and Treatment of Illness,* 121.

25. I. Lindstrom et al., The Effect of Graded Activity on Patients with Subacute Low Back Pain: A Randomized Prospective Clinical Study with an Operant-Conditioning Behavioral Approach, *Physical Therapy* 72, no. 4 (1992): 279–293.

26. K.M. Kellett et al., Effects of an Exercise Program on Sick Leave due to Back Pain, *Physical Therapy* 71, no. 4 (1991): 283–291.

27. I.M. Elnaggar, The Effects of Spinal Flexion and Extension Exercises on Low Back Pain Severity and Spinal Mobility in Chronic Mechanical Low Back Pain (PhD diss., New York University, New York, 1988).

28. Goldberg and Elliot, *Exercise for Prevention and Treatment of Illness,* 165–167.

29. L.A. Pruitt, et al., Weight-Training Effects on Bone Mineral Density in Early Postmenopausal Women, *Journal of Bone and Mineral Research* 7, no. 2 (1992): 170–185.

30. American College of Sports Medicine, Position Stand, Osteoporosis and Exercise, in *Medicine and Science in Sports and Exercise* 27, no. 4 (1995): i–vii.

31. M. Girodo et al., Deep Diaphragmatic Breathing: Rehabilitation Exercises for the Asthmatic Patient, *Archives of Physical Medicine and Rehabilitation* 73, no. 8 (1992): 717–720.

32. F.J. Cerny, Relative Effects of Bronchial Drainage and Exercise for In-Hospital Care of Patients with Cystic Fibrosis, *Physical Therapy* 69, no. 8 (1989): 633–639.

33. Goldberg and Elliot, *Exercise for Prevention and Treatment of Illness,* 99.

34. Goldberg and Elliot, *Exercise for Prevention and Treatment of Illness,* 89–90.

35. T.W. Pelham et al., The Effects of Exercise Therapy on Clients in a Psychiatric Rehabilitation Program, *Psychosocial Rehabilitation Journal* 16, no. 4 (1993): 75–84.

36. T.W. Pelham and P.D. Campagna, Benefits of Exercise in Psychiatric Rehabilitation of Persons with Schizophrenia, *Canadian Journal of Rehabilitation* 4, no. 3 (1991): 159–168.

37. R.S. Mazzeo et al., Exercise and Physical Activity for Older Adults, *Medicine and Science in Sports and Exercise* 30, no. 6 (1998): 992–1008.

38. L.R. Sauvage et al., A Clinical Trial of Strengthening and Aerobic Exercise To Improve Gait and Balance in Elderly Male Nursing Home Residents, *American Journal of Physical Medicine and Rehabilitation* 71, no. 6 (1992): 333–342.

39. J.O. Judge et al., Exercise To Improve Gait Velocity in Older Persons, *Archives of Physical Medicine and Rehabilitation* 74, no. 4 (1993): 400–406.

40. M.J. Lichtenstein et al., Exercise and Balance in Aged Women: A Pilot Controlled Clinical Trial, *Archives of Physical Medicine and Rehabilitation* 70, no. 2 (1989): 138–143.

41. Mazzeo et al., Exercise and Physical Activity for Older Adults.

42. Burton Goldberg Group, *Alternative Medicine,* 97–108.

43. D. Zuck, The Alexander Technique, in *Complementary Therapies in Rehabilitation,* ed. C. Davis (Thorofare, NJ: Slack, 1997): 161–187.

44. A.R. Stone, The Trager Approach, in *Complementary Therapies in Rehabilitation,* ed. C. Davis (Thorofare, NJ: Slack, 1997), 199–212.

45. S. Tse and D.M. Baily, T'ai Chi and Postural Controls in the Well Elderly, *American Journal of Occupational Therapy* 46, no. 4 (1992): 295–300.

46. A.E. Kirsteins et al., Evaluating the Safety and Potential Use of a Weight Bearing Exercise, Tai Chi Chuan, for Rheumatoid Arthritis Patients, *American Journal of Physical Medicine and Rehabilitation* 70, no. 3 (1991): 136–141.

47. Goldberg and Elliot, *Exercise for Prevention and Treatment of Illness*, 84.

48. S. Boots and C. Hogan, Creative Movement and Health, *Topics in Clinical Nursing* 3, no. 2 (1981):21–31.

49. P.A. Gillett et al., The Nurse as Exercise Leader, *Geriatric Nursing* 14, no. 3 (1993): 133–137.

50. N.K. Wenger, Modern Coronary Rehabilitation, *Postgraduate Medicine* 94, no. 2 (1993): 131–136, 141.

51. Boots and Hogan, Creative Movement and Health, 21–31.

VISION OF HEALING

Releasing the Energy of the Playful Child

The joy of playing and playfulness is a gift that we may lose as we grow out of childhood to take on the responsibilities of the adult. Illness may further deplete our ability to see the lighter side of life and take advantage of healthy hilarity. We must search out ways to reconnect with the joyful child within and use that energy to move to a higher level of wellness. When we laugh, our perception shifts. We release feelings of judgment, blame, and self-pity to embrace a more extended knowing of ourselves and others. Deliberately taking the time to amuse and be amused allows us to endure a great deal of change that would otherwise be overwhelming.[1]

Play is part of the richness of life; it enables us to live and grow. As infants and children, we play to learn. As adults, we play to relax, to enjoy interaction with others, to grow, and to gain a different perspective on our lives. Our play can be a variety of activities, from the simple experience of skipping or dancing for

the joy of movement, to the excitement of "playing to win" in a tournament or game.

Most animals play for at least some portion of their lives. The animals that play are those that can benefit from experience, those that can learn both step by step and on occasion by leaps of the imagination. The ones that play are those that must learn by discovery and practice, acquiring through trial and error (and trial and success) the skills they need to survive.[2]

> *There is more honest "belly laughter" in a Zen monastery than surely in any other religious institution on earth. To laugh is a sign of sanity; and the comic is deliberately used to break up concepts, to release tensions and to teach what cannot be taught in words. Nonsense is used to point to the beyond of rational sense.[3]*
>
> *Christmas Humphries*

NOTES

1. J. Segal, *Feeling Great* (Van Nuys, CA: Newcastle Publishing Co., 1981), 68.
2. M. Piers and G. Landau, *The Gift of Play* (New York: Walker and Co., 1980), 19.
3. T. Quereau and T. Zimmerman, *The New Game Plan for Recovery: Rediscovering the Positive Power of Play* (New York: Ballantine Books, 1992), 261.

Chapter 20

Humor, Laughter, and Play: Maintaining Balance in a Serious World

Patty Wooten

NURSE HEALER OBJECTIVES

Theoretical

- Define humor, laughter, and play and explain how they interrelate.
- Describe the psychosocial and physiologic benefits of laughter and play.
- Explain how humor, laughter, and play can aid in stress reduction.

Clinical

- Organize and integrate playful activities into your clinical practice.
- Document the psychophysiologic changes that occur in clients as they allow themselves to laugh and engage in playful activities.
- Develop a collection of humorous books, cartoons, games, and comedy videotapes and audiotapes that are appropriate for use in your area of nursing practice.

Personal

- Describe strategies for integrating a humorous perspective and playful activities into each day.
- Clarify and expand awareness of your personal humor preferences and favorite playful activities.
- Develop a heightened awareness of opportunities to insert humor and encourage playfulness.

DEFINITIONS

Humor: a quality of perception and attitude toward life that enables an individual to experience joy even when faced with adversity; a perception of the absurdity or incongruity of a situation.

Laughter: a physical behavior that occurs in response to something that is perceived as humorous, amusing, or surprising. This behavior engages most of the muscle groups and organ systems within the body. Laughter is often preceded by physical, emotional, or cognitive tension.

Play: a spontaneous or recreational activity that is performed for sheer enjoyment rather than to reach a goal or produce a product. Playfulness is a mood or attitude that infuses the individual with a sense of joy and positive emotions.

THEORY AND RESEARCH

Humor is a complex phenomenon that is an essential part of human nature. Anthropologists have never found a culture or society, at any time in history, that was completely devoid of humor. A sense of humor is both a perspective on life—a way of perceiving the world—and a behavior that expresses that perspective. As Moshe Waldoks declared: "A sense of humor can help you overlook the unattractive, tolerate the unpleasant, cope with the unexpected and smile through the unbearable."[1]

Humor is a word of many meanings. It is derived from the Latin word *umor*, meaning liquid or fluid. In the Middle Ages, humor referred to an energy that was thought to interact with a body fluid and an emotional state. This energy was believed to influence health and disposition (e.g., he's in a bad humor). A sanguine humor was cheerful and associated with blood. A choleric humor was angry and associated with bile. A phlegmatic humor was apathetic and allied with mucus. A melancholic humor was depressed and related to black bile.[2] This belief system was an early recognition of the energy links between the mind and the body.

One of the earliest and most extensive reviews of humor and its use by health professionals was compiled by nurse-educator Vera Robinson.[3] First published in 1977, then updated and released again in 1991, Robinson's work began as part of a doctoral thesis in the early 1970s. Today, almost 30 years later, it continues to be one of the most comprehensive studies of humor and its importance in nursing practice. Her review of the theories of humor is both comprehensive and concise. Her findings are summarized here.

Humor from Different Perspectives

The humanities and the literature of the world, from the time of the ancient Greeks to the present, have been concerned with the nature of comedy and laughter. Comedy reveals people's imperfections, gives them courage to face life, and leaves them more tolerant. Tragedy is idealistic and expresses "the pity of it," while comedy tends to be more skeptical and expresses "the absurdity of it."[4]

Early philosophers were concerned with the nature of humor in relation to the issues of good and evil and the nature of humans. Both Plato and Aristotle felt that laughter arose from enjoyment of the misfortunes of others and that comedy was an imitation of people at their worst. Other philosophers viewed laughter as a valuable asset in correcting the minor follies of society.

According to the psychoanalytic view of humor set forth by Sigmund Freud, civilization has led to repression of many basic impulses, and joking is a socially acceptable way of satisfying these repressed needs. Freud described four major types of joke: the sexual joke, the aggressive and hostile joke, the blasphemous joke, and the skeptical joke. This joking activity serves to preserve psychic energy. Freud differentiated between wit, the comic effect, and humor. The pleasure of wit comes from an economy of inhibition; the pleasure of the comic, from an economy of thought; and the pleasure of humor, from an economy of feelings.[5]

Psychologists go beyond Freud's interpretation to assert that humor is not simply determined by the present stimulus situation but depends on recollections of the past and anticipation of the future. A collective process is important in generating the pleasure of humor. Humor is cognitively based and involves information-processing and problem-solving ability. Psychologist Harvey Mindess proposed the liberation theory of humor. He viewed humor and laughter as the agents of psychologic liberation. They free us from the constraints and restrictive forces of daily living and, in doing so, make us joyful.[6]

Anthropologists have described the use of humor within various cultures or ethnic groups. They have identified a joking relationship that is a kind of "permitted disrespect" in which one person is required to tease or make fun of another, who is in turn required to take no offense. This kind of social relationship is widespread in different societies and provides a basis for comparative studies of social structures.[7] One of the first cross-cultural studies of humor found that humor is the result of cultural perceptions, both individual and collective; it is a cognitive experience that must have a cultural niche and cannot occur in a vacuum.[8] Humor is universal, but the culture, society, or ethnic group in which it occurs influences the style and content of humor and the situations in which humor is used and is considered appropriate.[9]

Many sociological studies have explored exactly how humor is used within society. Humor is a social relationship and occurs in a social environment. Research has shown that it promotes group cohesion, initiates relationships, relieves tension during social conflict, and can be a means of expressing approval or disapproval of social action. Joking relationships within organizations serve to minimize stress and release antagonism.[10,11]

The three major theories of humor are the superiority theory, the incongruity theory, and the release theory. The superiority theory asserts that people laugh at the inferiority, stupidity, or misfortunes of others so that they may feel superior to them. People watch the foolish actions of Lucille Ball or Charlie Chaplin and feel smart and dignified compared to them. This type of laughter may not be entirely cruel and scornful but may also reflect warmth and empathy. Essentially, people are laughing at themselves, at their own imperfections. For the moment, they feel superior. What they are laughing at did not happen to them, but it could have. This type of comedy demonstrates that "man is durable, even though he may be weak, stupid, and undignified."[12(p.24)] In the superiority theory, humor can be viewed as a continuum: from laughing at no one (nonsense jokes), to laughing at a specific person or group (jokes about morons or ethnic groups), to laughing with others in general at people's foibles (Charlie Chaplin's humor), to laughing at oneself, the most therapeutic of all.

The incongruity theory of humor holds that a sudden shock or unexpectedness, an incongruity, ambivalence, or conflict of ideas or emotions is necessary to produce the absurdity provoking a burst of laughter.

The relief or release theory of humor proposes that humor and laughter provide a release of tension. The relief can be cognitive—an escape from reality, from seriousness, from reason. The relief can be an emotional release of anxiety, fear, anger, or embarrassment from social conflict. It can also be a release of nervous energy and physical tension.

Many of these theories of and perspectives on humor obviously overlap. Some describe the nature of humor, while others describe the function of humor. However, this diversity of perspectives shows that humor, laughter, and play are very complex phenomena that serve people in many ways. The possibilities for the study of humor are endless. The importance and influence of humor have been examined from the perspectives of anthropology, psychology, literature, sociology, linguistics, religion, and so on. More information about the influence of humor in people's lives can be obtained from the International Society for Humor Studies (see the "Resources" section at the end of the chapter). The therapeutic value of humor and its beneficial influence on the body-mind-spirit are discussed below.

Therapeutic Humor

Modern dictionaries define humor as the quality of being laughable or comical, or as a state of mind, mood, and spirit. Our sense of humor gives us the ability to find delight and experience joy even when faced with adversity. Humor, then, is a flowing energy, involving and connecting the body, mind, and spirit.

Humor can take many forms: jokes, cartoons, amusing stories, outrageous sight gags, funny songs, whimsical signs, bloopers, "daffynitions," and physical slapstick antics. These humorous techniques stimulate the auditory, visual, or kinesthetic senses.

Therapeutic humor can be classified into three basic categories: hoping humor, coping humor, and gallows humor. Hoping humor gives the individual the courage to face challenges. Coping humor offers a release for physical and emotional tension. Gallows humor provides a protection from the emotional impact of witnessing tragedy, death, and disfigurement. Sharing humor and laughter with clients and colleagues can have profound healing potential. Finding a humorous perspective on one's problems or experiencing the relaxing effects of laughter can be an effective stress management technique that helps one stay healthy.

The term *to heal* comes from the Anglo-Saxon word *haelen*, which means to bring together and make whole. Bringing together the body, mind, and spirit can be healing. Humor, laughter, and the resulting emotion, mirth, unite the body, mind, and spirit. Humor is a cognitive activity engaging the mind. Laughter is a physical activity involving the body. Mirth is an emotional state that lifts the spirit.[13]

Hoping Humor: Courage to Face Challenges

The ability to hope for something better enables human beings to cope with difficult situations. Hoping humor laughs in spite of the overwhelming circumstances. It reflects an acceptance of life with all its dichotomies, contradictions, and incongruities. This type of humor is usually warm and gentle and accepts the reality of the situation. Consider the following example of hoping humor.

Janet Henry had breast cancer. After her mastectomy, she received chemotherapy. First she lost her breast, then she lost her hair, but Janet never lost her sense of humor. She wrote a little poem to describe her ritual as she prepared for bed each night.

The Nightly Ritual
I prop my wig up on the dresser
And tuck my prosthesis beneath
And I thank God

I still go to bed
With my man and my very own
teeth.

With whimsy and gratitude, Janet remembered the blessings in her life in spite of her losses.[14]

Hoping humor can also be used to sustain the spirit during the shock and trauma of natural disasters. People create humor to literally laugh in the face of their loss. Both disaster victims and those who offer professional assistance use humor to provide hope and courage as they deal with the overwhelming task of recovery. As Charlie Chaplin once noted, "To truly laugh, you must be able to take your pain and play with it."[15]

Sandy Ritz, a nurse from Hawaii, completed her doctoral thesis in public health on the topic of humor and disaster recovery.[16,17] Her research showed how humor changed as the stages of recovery progressed. After the devastating floods in the Midwest during 1997, a large billboard announced: "Concerned about the weather? Call 1-800-NOAH." After a tornado destroyed a house in Texas, the family moved across town to live with relatives. They placed a sign on their front lawn: "Gone with the wind." After an earthquake in Los Angeles, one house that had completely collapsed had this sign in front: "House for Rent. Some assembly required."

Nurses and other professional caregivers use hoping humor to acknowledge their own reality and to laugh in spite of the pressure and demands. For example:

How You Know It's Going To Be a Long Shift
1. You step off the elevator and emergency room gurneys are lined up in the hall.
2. The crash cart is not in its usual location.
3. There are too many people in the nursing station.

4. There is nobody in the nursing station.
5. Housekeeping is scrubbing a large area of the floor.
6. You get two admissions during report.[18]

Coping Humor: Release for Tension

Illness and trauma cause stress and suffering. They disrupt our ability to function smoothly and present many challenges. Coping describes what people do to minimize this disruption and attempt to regain some control. To cope effectively, people must change how they think and how they behave. Humor is often used as a coping tool to change perspective, release tension, and regain a sense of control. As Freud noted: "Humor has a liberating element, it is the triumph of narcissism. It is the ego's victorious assertion of its invulnerability. It refuses to suffer the slings and arrows of reality."[19] Clients use coping humor to laugh about uncomfortable and embarrassing moments. While they may not always be able to control their external reality, they can use humor to control how they perceive their situation and use their ability to laugh about it to provide some sense of empowerment,[20,21] as shown by the following example.

The nurse was caring for Barbara during her weeklong hospitalization for chemotherapy. The drugs were powerful with many uncomfortable side effects. Fortunately, the nurse had been successful in managing Barbara's nausea with antiemetic medications. However, when the nurse entered the patient's room on Thursday, she found her bending over the toilet bowl vomiting profusely. The nurse was surprised and, without thinking, blurted out, "What are you doing?" Barbara wiped her chin, looked up at the nurse, and said, "Well, I had a tuna sandwich for lunch and I began feeling sorry for the tuna, so I thought I'd return it to its natural habitat."

Barbara used humor to redefine her uncomfortable situation, took control of her perceptual process, and changed her attitude about the event.[22]

Coping humor often expresses anxiety or frustration about things that are out of one's control. Consider the following:

Handy Exercises You Can Do To Prepare for Hospitalization
1. Lie naked on the front lawn, covered with a napkin, and ask people to poke you as they go by.
2. Practice inserting your hand in a running garbage disposal and smile, saying "Mild discomfort."
3. Set your alarm to go off every 10 minutes between 11 PM and 7 AM, at which times you will awaken and stab yourself with a screwdriver.
4. Learn to urinate into an empty lipstick tube.[23]

Caregivers also create humor to help release feelings of hostility or frustration created by patients or other professionals.[24-30] Sometimes nurses enjoy making jokes about physicians. For example:

What do you call two orthopedic surgeons reading an electrocardiogram?
A double-blind study.

Why is a neurosurgeon just like a sperm?
One in 200,000 becomes a human.

What does it mean when a physician writes WNL on the History and Physical?
We Never Looked.

Sometimes, caring for patients who are noncompliant, combative, demanding, or ungrateful can be frustrating. These patients are sometimes referred to as gomers, an acronym created by a physician writing about his internship experience.[31] GOMER is an acronym for Get Out of My Emergency Room. Over the years, several versions and additions to the gomer criteria list have evolved.

> You know your patient is a gomer if
> 1. his old chart weighs more than 5 pounds
> 2. his previous address was the VA hospital
> 3. he keeps tying his pajama strings in with the Foley catheter
> 4. he can have a seizure and never drop his cigarette
> 5. he asks for a cigarette in the middle of his pulmonary function test
> 6. his blood urea nitrogen level is higher than his IQ

Coping humor is a socially acceptable form of expressing hostility, but it should be used with caution. It can be viewed as disrespectful and hurtful if overheard by someone who either identifies with the person being laughed at or feels that this type of humor is offensive and inappropriate for health professionals. Sharing any form of humor is always a risky adventure because people vary greatly in what they find funny and which topics they consider too serious to laugh about. What is funny to one person may be viewed as offensive by another.[32] Exhibit 20–1 shows guidelines for appropriate use of humor.

Gallows Humor: Protection from Pain

Gallows humor is often used by professionals who work in situations that are horrifying or tragic. Every day these people cope with the reality and horror of illness, suffering, and death. In this group are doctors, nurses, police, newspaper journalists, social workers, hospice workers, and many others. These professionals, because of their caring and compassion, are more likely to feel the impact of the suffering they witness. Caregivers often use humor as a means of maintaining some distance from the suffering to protect themselves from empathic pain.[33,34] Gallows humor acknowledges the disgusting or intolerable aspects of a situation and then attempts to transform it into something lighthearted and amusing. People's ability to laugh in this situation provides them with a momentary release from the intensity of what might otherwise be overwhelming. They are able to maintain their balance and professional composure so that they may continue to offer their therapeutic skills.

Consider the following example. One night, in the emergency room at a county hospital, an ambulance brought in a homeless person who had been found unconscious in an alley. The man was filthy, his breath reeked of alcohol, and he had lice crawling on his body. It took two nurses more than an hour just to clean the man up enough for admission. It was difficult work, and the nurses' senses were overwhelmed with unpleasant sights and smells. One of the nurses read the intern's admission note on the way up in the elevator. It said, "Patient carried into emergency room by army of body lice, who were chanting, 'Save our host. Save our host.'" The nurse laughed heartily at this amusing picture. Suddenly the struggles of the last hours were put into a humorous perspective, and she felt a lot less anger and a lot more compassion.

One study of the use of humor among hospital staff in emergency rooms and critical care units described how gallows humor was used as a coping tool.

> There is a goodness of fit between how the provision of care induces stress in the emergency care environment and how the use of humor intervenes in that process. Emergency personnel experience a wide spectrum of serious events—trauma, life-threatening illness, chaotic emotional situations—often all at the same time. There is no time to emotionally prepare for these events, and little time to ventilate afterwards or "decompress." The spontaneous way in which hu-

Exhibit 20–1 Concerns and Cautions about Using Humor in Health Care Settings

Concerns

- *Will clients or colleagues consider the use of humor unprofessional?*

  Offer a brief explanation of the health benefits of humor to counter this. You can maintain your professionalism and still adopt a lighter style of interaction with patients and staff.

- *Will I be seen as incompetent?*

  Establish your competence first (especially among other staff), then let your sense of humor emerge. Clients usually welcome a lighter style of interaction.

- *Will clients misinterpret humor as indifference about their condition?*

  Shared humor does not replace concern, care, and respect. It makes those qualities more personal and believable.

- *What should I do if I really don't think the client's humor is funny?*

  Don't laugh, but smile and acknowledge the joke.

- *What should I do if the client's humor is offensive?*

  Be honest and tell the client that you really don't enjoy that kind of humor. Be flexible, open, and supportive of the client's humor generally. There are limits to joking as with any other behavior.

Cautions

- Be sensitive to whether the client is responding positively or negatively to humor. Don't force your humor on the client if the client is not receptive. Think of humor as a medication. You must administer the right medicine, in the right dosage, at the right time for a therapeutic benefit to occur. Two clients with the same symptoms do not always get the same medication. Some clients have allergic reactions. Be sensitive to the client's humor allergies.

- Remember that clients may not respond to humor until they have come to accept the reality of their disease. Do not try to use humor to subdue their depression or anger. The time may come, however, when humor can help them turn the corner of acceptance.

- Remember that sometimes clients don't feel like laughing. They may be nauseated, in pain, or just not in the mood.

- Remember that many clients have no history of using humor under stress. It may be unrealistic to expect them to react favorably to humor when their health is threatened. People generally use the same coping mechanisms in the hospital that they have used in other stressful situations. This may include becoming angry, depressed, withdrawn, anxious, assertive, or demanding. Each of these coping styles is compatible with humor once you know the client well. Always be sensitive to how the client is responding to your playful style.

- Remember that some clients may have religious convictions that stress reverence for the seriously ill. This may be incompatible with any form of humor or light-hearted interaction.

- Humor is inappropriate when
  1. the patient needs time to cry
  2. the patient needs quiet time to rest, contemplate, or pray
  3. the patient is trying to come to grips with any emotional crisis
  4. the patient is trying to communicate something important to you
  5. the person in the adjacent bed is very sick or dying.

- Avoid humor that is
  1. ethnic, sarcastic, mocking
  2. at the expense of another person (laugh with, not at)
  3. joking about any client or that client's condition.

mor can be produced in almost any situation, and it's instantaneous stress-reducing effects are well suited to the emergency care experience.[35,36(p.40)]

It is important to note that gallows humor, so therapeutic for staff, may not be appreciated by clients or their families. One group of nurses hung the following sign in the visitor waiting room to reassure visitors that the staff's use of humor actually helped them provide better care for their loved ones:

> You may occasionally see us laughing,
> or even take note of some jest.

Know that we are giving your
    loved one
our care at it's very best.
There are times when the tension
    is highest.
There are times when our systems
    are stressed.
We've discovered humor a factor
in keeping our sanity blessed.
So, if you're a patient in waiting,
or a relative, or a friend of one
    seeing,
don't hold our smiling against us,
it's the way we keep from
    screaming.[37(p.26)]

Cathartic Laughter

Laughter is a smile that engages the entire body. At first, the corners of the mouth turn up slightly. Then the muscles around the eyes engage and a twinkling can be seen in the eyes. Next the person begins to make noises, ranging from controlled snickers, escaped chortles, and spontaneous giggles to ridiculous cackles, noisy hoots, and uproarious guffaws. The chest and abdominal muscles become activated. As the noises get louder, the person begins to bend the body back and forth, sometimes slapping the knees, stomping the feet on the floor, or elbowing another person nearby. As laughter reaches its peak, tears flow freely. All of this continues until the person feels so weak and exhausted that the person must sit down or fall down. Very strange behavior!

Of course, not everyone experiences such intense laughter every time they are amused. For example, if people are concerned about how others might judge this behavior; if they are concerned with maintaining a dignified image; if they feel others might be offended by their robust laughter; or if the culture places strong taboos on such behavior, then people may struggle to contain themselves.[38,39]

Sounds of Laughter

If we listen to the sound of someone laughing, we hear that the laughter has different tones and rhythms, almost as if the laughter were coming from different parts of the body. These sounds may give us a clue as to why the person is laughing. A "tee hee" laugh is often a high-pitched titter that seems to come from the top of the head. This laugh arises when a person is very nervous and tries to disguise his or her anxiety with laughter. Like the valve atop a pressure cooker, this laughter acts as a safety valve and allows the person to release a little steam before he or she explodes from built-up pressure. A "heh heh" laugh is a shallow, almost hollow sound that comes from the throat area. This laugh occurs when a person feels socially obligated to laugh at a joke that is not really considered funny. A "ha ha" laugh emanates from the heart space with a warm resonance and palpable sincerity. This laugh occurs when someone is truly amused or delighted by the humorous stimuli. It is also the kind of laugh that occurs during deep insight or peaceful, joy-filled moments, such as during meditation. A "ho ho" laugh is the deep belly laugh, the kind in which a person really begins to let go of control and surrender to the experience of deep joy and amusement. The whole body is engaged in movement, which usually continues until exhaustion. The person must put down whatever is being held, and must sit down to avoid falling down. Sometimes the laughter is so deep and so prolonged that the person is left gasping for air and exhausted from the activity. After the laughter, as the person becomes quiet, a warm glow fills the body. The person feels lighter, almost buoyant, and the mind is clear of worry, fear, and anger. The body feels energized yet relaxed. Usually, the person is no longer aware of any pain that was previously felt.

If this laughter was shared with others, the person feels a sense of connection and trust. During these moments one's problems do not feel oppressive; one feels safe and at peace with the world. The body is listening to this emotional weather report and making subtle or sometimes profound changes at a molecular level. These changes have a powerful impact on the immune system and can enhance the ability to heal. As Barry Sultanoff, a holistic physician, explained: "Laughing together can be a time of intimacy and communion, a time when we come forward, fully present and touch into each other's humanness and vulnerability. By joining in humor and acknowledging our oneness, we can have a profound experience of unity and cooperation. That in itself maybe one of the most profound expressions of healing energy of which we are capable."[40]

What is this healing energy? Where does it come from? What does it do? For thousands of years we have extolled that "laughter is the best medicine." In many cultures, religions, and societies, people speak of the healing power of humor. The Old Testament says, "A merry heart does good like a medicine, but a broken spirit dries the bones" (Proverbs 17:22). This universally accepted truth is just now being explained by scientific research. Norman Cousins enlightened the medical community about the healing potential of laughter in his book *Anatomy of an Illness*.[41] In 1968, Cousins was diagnosed with ankylosing spondylitis, a potentially life-threatening, degenerative disease involving the connective tissue of the body, which is essential in holding together the cells and larger structures of the body. Cousin's case was so extreme that he soon experienced great difficulty and pain in moving his joints. He was told that his prospect for recovery was very bleak. Because of discomfort and fatigue, he was unable to travel or play tennis, activities that brought him great joy and satisfaction.

Cousins refused to accept his grim prognosis and decided to take charge of his own treatment, working in partnership with his physician. He remembered reading about the adverse consequences of negative emotional states on the chemical balance of the body. He reasoned that, if negative emotions had played any part in predisposing him to illness, then perhaps positive emotions could aid in his recovery. He sought activities that increased his positive emotions, such as faith, hope, festivity, determination, confidence, joy, and a strong will to live. He knew that laughter helped create positive emotions. With this in mind, Cousins watched films of the Marx brothers and Candid Camera. He had nurses read to him from humorous books. He played practical jokes and told jokes. He began feeling better. Blood tests showed that his sedimentation rate (an index of the degree of infection or inflammation in the body) decreased after his laughter sessions, and they continued to fall as he gradually recovered.

After several months of this "humor therapy," his illness resolved and never returned. One could argue that Cousins would have recovered anyway, even without the laughter. Or one could comment that the results are not scientifically significant and represent the observations of a single case. However, Cousins continued his quest to understand just how his healing occurred.

Cousins spent the remaining 12 years of his life as an adjunct professor at the University of California at Los Angeles Medical School, where he established a "humor task force" to coordinate and support clinical research into laughter. Today, 25 years after Cousins' self-healing experience with laughter, there is scientific research providing evidence for the specific physiologic changes that his individual story suggested.[42-45] Cousins declared:

Each human being possesses a beautiful system for fighting disease. This system provides the body with cancer-fighting cells—cells that can crush cancer cells or poison them one by one with the body's own chemotherapy. This system works better when the patient is relatively free of depression, which is what a strong will to live and a blazing determination can help to do. When we add these inner resources to the resources of medical science, we're reaching out for the best.[46]

Physiologic Response to Laughter

The behavior called laughter creates predictable physiologic changes within the body. William Fry, Jr., Professor Emeritus of medicine at Stanford University, began his research into laughter in the 1950s.[47] As with other exercise, the body's response has two stages: the arousal phase, in which the physiologic parameters increase, and the resolution phase, in which they return to resting values or lower. With vigorous, sustained laughter, the heart rate is stimulated, sometimes reaching rates of above 120 beats per minute. The normal respiratory pattern becomes chaotic; respiratory rate and depth are increased, while residual volume is decreased. Coughing and hiccups are often triggered due to phrenic nerve irritation or the dislodging of mucus plugs. Oxygen saturation of peripheral blood does not significantly change during the increased ventilation that occurs with laughter. Conditions such as asthma or bronchitis may be irritated by vigorous laughter. Peripheral vascular flow is increased due to vasodilatation. A variety of muscle groups become active during laughter, including diaphragm, abdominal, intercostal, respiratory accessory, and facial muscles, and occasionally muscles of the arms, legs, and back.[48–51]

Some of the most exciting research exploring the potential healing value of laughter is in the area of psychoneuroimmunology.[52] Psychoneuroimmunology studies the connections and communication patterns linking the nervous, endocrine, and immune systems. Candace Pert, one of the most respected researchers in the area of mind-body medicine, notes that emotions, which are registered and stored in the body in the form of chemical messages, are the most influential connection between the mind and the body. The emotions one experiences in connection with one's thoughts and daily attitudes—and, more specifically, the neurochemical changes that accompany these emotions—have the power to influence health.[53–55]

The key, according to Pert, is found in complex molecules called neuropeptides, which are formed from amino acids. Peptides are found throughout the body, including in the brain and immune system. The brain contains more than 60 different neuropeptides. These neuropeptides carry messages between the brain and the body as well as within the brain and within the body. Individual cells, including brain cells, immune cells, and other body cells, have receptor sites that receive neuropeptides. As our emotions change throughout the day, the neuropeptides available to cells reflect these variations. Receptor sites are important as a communication link between the brain and the immune system. Emotions can trigger the release of neuropeptides from the brain. These chemicals then enter the bloodstream and plug into receptor sites on the surface of immune cells. When this occurs, the cells' metabolic activity can be altered in either a positive or a negative direction. The kind and number of emotion-linked neuropeptides available at receptor sites of cells influences the probability of staying well or getting sick.[56] As Pert explains: "Viruses use these same receptors to enter into a cell, and depending on how much of the natural peptide for that receptor is around, the virus will have an easier or harder time getting into the cell. So our emotional state will affect whether we'll get sick from the same loading dose of a virus."[57]

One of the first research teams to join Norman Cousins' humor task force was Lee Berk and Stanley Tan from Loma Linda University Medical Center. Berk, a psychoneuroimmunologist, and Tan, an endocrinologist, have measured changes in immune function stimulated by the experience of mirthful laughter. In an interview, Berk noted:

> Essentially, we found that mirthful laughter serves to modulate specific immune system components. By modulate, we mean that chemicals released during the emotional experience of mirth can connect to receptors on the surface of the immune cells. This connection stimulates a change in the molecular machinery inside the cell. Specific molecules known as immunoregulators are like plugs that fit into receptors and subsequently increase or decrease the immune cell activity. One metaphor for modulation of immune activity is the conductor of an orchestra. Although the conductor does not actually play an instrument, he influences the tempo, harmony and volume of the music produced by the orchestra. Mirthful laughter would be like the conductor who enhances sonic integration and brings out melodious harmony. Whereas distressful emotions would be like the conductor who brings out harsh, disharmonious sounds. Emotion, like a conductor, modulates the activity and effectiveness of the immune cells although it does not directly protect the body from insult or infection.[58(p.47)]

The findings of Berk and Tan during more than 10 years of research can be summarized as follows. Mirthful laughter has been shown to

1. increase the number and activity of natural killer cells, which attack viral-infected cells and some types of cancer cells
2. increase the number of "activated" T cells; these cells are "turned on and ready to go"
3. increase the level of the antibody IgA, which fights upper respiratory tract infections
4. increase the levels of gamma interferon, a lymphokine that activates many immune components
5. increase levels of complement 3, which helps antibodies to pierce infected cells

In addition to measuring specific immune system changes, the research of Berk and Tan also shows that levels of stress hormones, which constrict blood vessels and suppress immune activity, actually decrease in response to mirthful laughter. Levels of epinephrine, dopamine, and cortisol, which usually rise in response to stress, were all lowered with laughter.[59-65]

Stress has been shown to create unhealthy physiologic changes. The connection between stress and blood pressure elevation, muscle tension, immunosuppression, and many other changes has been known for years. There is now proof that laughter creates the opposite effects. It appears to be the perfect antidote for stress.

This research helps us to better understand the mind-body connection. The emotions and moods we experience directly effect our immune system. If, however, we have a well-developed sense of humor, we are more likely to appreciate the amusing incongruities of life and experience more moments of joy and delight. These positive emotions can create neurochemical changes that buffer the immunosuppressive effects of stress.

The Power of Playfulness

The key to improving our sense of humor is the rediscovery of the playfulness we had as children. The joyous laughter that accompanies children's play leaves no doubt that they are happy. When we become more playful, we automatically become more spontaneous and enjoy whatever we are doing more than we otherwise would. The dictionary defines *play* as activities that are amusing, fun, or otherwise enjoyable in their own right. When we truly play, we seek to impress no one, and we produce no product—we just enjoy being in the moment. Playing is as old as humankind, as evidenced by the remains of toys found in the ancient ruins of Egyptian, Babylonian, Chinese, and Aztec civilizations.[66] When children play, they use their imagination to invent a reality that meets their needs. If we allow ourselves to be children and distort or exaggerate a situation to its most absurd limits, we create an opportunity for laughter. As we grow older, our ability to open ourselves to moments of playfulness becomes constrained. A serious attention to the business at hand may replace a willingness to laugh and play, subsequently reducing our health-promoting behaviors. Sometimes it is difficult to incorporate play into our lives again because it does not always fit our image of what is necessary and proper for an adult. Erikson noted that some adults, through the ages, have been inclined to judge play to be neither serious nor useful, and thus unrelated to the center of human tasks and motives, from which the adult, in fact, seeks recreation when he plays.[67]

Yet recent research on animals shows that play makes a crucial contribution to brain development. Natalie Angier recently summarized this research as follows: "An animal plays most vigorously at precisely the time when its brain cells are frenetically forming synaptic connections, creating a dense array of neural connections that can pass an electrochemical message from one neighborhood of the brain to the next. . . . Scientists believe that the intense sensory and physical stimulation that comes from playing is critical to the growth of these cerebral synapses and thus to proper motor development."[68] Play, then, is essential for survival in the animal world. Early childhood play is one way that humans practice socialization skills and mimic cultural rituals. It is a way that people create connections with others and build trust. Creative people are playful, experimental, and willing to take risks. Therefore, in serious situations like illness, which may require a change in lifestyle or other adaptation, creative problem solving can be a great help. Creative solutions seldom emerge when people are concentrating on something in a solemn, practical mood; they are more likely to come when people are in a relaxed, even playful mood.

Humor and Stress Management

If play serves to build up skills that are essential to effective adaptation as an adult, how then does humor help one adapt? Why does humor exist? One of the main reasons humor exists may be that it helps people adapt to the stresses in their lives. It is because of a human being's superior intellectual capacities that they have such high stress in their lives. As Hans Selye noted that stress is not the event but rather our perception of the event.[69] It is people's interpretation of events that causes stress, not the events themselves. A sense of humor helps people to view difficult circumstances in a less stressful way.

Because different people respond differently to the same environmental stimuli, some people seem to cope with stress better than others.[70,71] Sociologist Suzanne Kobassa defined three "hardiness factors" that can increase a person's resilience to stress and prevent burnout: commitment, control, and challenge.[72,73] If one has a strong commitment to oneself and one's work, if one believes that one is in control of the choices in one's life (internal locus of control), and if one views change as challenging rather than as threatening, then one is more likely to cope successfully with stress.[74] A theme that is becoming more prominent in the literature is the idea that a sense of powerlessness is a causative factor in burnout.

In this context, humor can be an empowerment tool. Humor gives people a different perspective on their problems, and with an attitude of detachment, they feel a sense of self-protection and control in their environment. As comedian Bill Cosby is fond of saying, "If you can laugh at it, you can survive it." It is reasonable to assume that, if the locus of control is strongly internal, a person will feel a greater sense of power and thus be more likely to avoid burnout.[75,76]

Humor and Locus of Control

This author's research, presented in 1990 at the Eighth International Conference on Humor Studies in England, documented changes in locus of control and appreciation of humor related to a humor training course.[77] Using the Adult Nowicki-Strickland Scale,[78] which has proven reliability and validity, we assessed the locus of control in 231 nurses in Pennsylvania, Kentucky, and California. We then administered Svebak's Sense of Humor Questionnaire, using only the subscales that have proven to be reliable and valid.[79,80] The experimental group then completed a 6-hour humor training course in which they were given permission and techniques for appropriate use of humor with patients and coworkers. The control group had no such humor training. The same survey tools were readministered to each group 6 weeks later to determine changes in locus of control and appreciation of humor.

Using the Wilcoxon Matched Pairs Signed-Ranks Test, we found that there was a significant decrease in the score for external locus of control in the experimental group (P = .0063, two-tailed). Using the same analysis for the control group, we found no significant change. No significant differences were found in the initial locus of control scores for the experimental and the control groups when tested using the Mann-Whitney U and Kolmogorov-Smirnov tests. This study indicates that, if people are encouraged and guided in using humor, they can gain a sense of control in their lives. The use of humor represents what Kobassa calls cognitive control. We cannot control events in our external world, but we can control how we view these events and our emotional response to them.[81] Further research is needed to determine how long these effects persist.

Ho Ho Holistic Health

Humor, laughter, and play contribute to our health and well-being in many ways. Each, in its own way, touches our body-mind-spirit. Humor, as a cognitive process, is primarily a mental activity. The behavior of laughter affects the whole body, from cells to entire organ systems. Play and a playful spirit fill us with joy, connect us with others, and keep us focused on the present moment. The interaction of body-mind-spirit with humor, laughter, and play forms the "Aha, Ha Ha, Ahhhh" continuum. The mind says, "Aha! I get the joke." The body says, "Ha Ha!" And the spirit says, "Ahhhh, everything feels much better now."

HOLISTIC CARING PROCESS

Assessment

In preparing to use humor, laughter, and play interventions, the nurse assesses the following parameters:

- the client's ability and willingness to smile and laugh

- the client's attitude toward using laughter and play in the current situation
- the client's history of using humor, laughter, and play in other circumstances
- the client's visual, auditory, cognitive, and physical limitations
- the client's preferred style of humor (i.e., jokes, cartoons, stories, comedy movies, animated cartoons, stand-up comedy, funny songs)[82]
- the client's favorite comedy artists— performers, writers, cartoonists, and so on.
- the client's feelings about previous experiences with humor and play
- the client's preferred playful activities

Patterns/Problems/Needs

The following are the patterns/problems/needs compatible with the interventions for humor, laughter, and play that are related to the nine human response patterns of the Unitary Person framework (see Chapter 14):

- *Relating:* Altered parenting, actual or potential
  Social isolation
- *Choosing:* Ineffective individual and family coping
- *Moving:* Activity intolerance, actual or potential
  Deficit in diversional activity
  Impaired physical mobility
- *Perceiving:* Powerlessness
  Disturbance in self-concept: altered self-esteem, role performance, personal identity
- *Sensory-perceptual:* Altered sensation/perception: visual, auditory, kinesthetic, gustatory, tactile, olfactory
- *Knowing:* Altered thought processes
- *Feeling:* Anxiety
  Pain
  Fear
  Potential for violence: self-directed or directed at others

Outcomes

Exhibit 20–2 guides the nurse in outcomes, nursing prescriptions, and evaluation for the use of humor, laughter, and play as a nursing intervention.

Therapeutic Care Plan and Interventions

Before the Session

- Assess your own ease and comfort with using humor and play as a therapeutic intervention.
- Practice smiling in front of a mirror. First scowl, then smile. Feel the difference.
- Evaluate your ability to respond to humor or engage in playful activity for your own personal pleasure.
- Increase awareness of your own preferred humor style, artist, writer, performer.
- Allow yourself to laugh with abandon at things you find funny.
- Become familiar with the content and variety of humorous items and playful activities that are available for you to use.
- Ensure that all supplies and equipment are in working condition.
- Improve your ability to tell a good joke. Remember these tips: Keep it short—less than 2 minutes. Be sure you can remember the whole joke before you start. Let your body, face, and voice become animated as you tell the joke. Pause occasionally as you deliver the material; create a brief and concise setup for the punch line; pause before delivering the punch line;

Exhibit 20–2 Nursing Interventions: Play and Laughter

Client Outcomes	Nursing Prescriptions	Evaluation
The client will smile and/or laugh in response to humorous stimuli.	Introduce the client to the concept that humor, laughter, and play benefit health. Guide the client in identifying his or her own preferred humor style. Help the client to clarify any blocks to using humor, laughter, or play.	The client requested some humor resources from family or friends. The client laughed in response to a selected humorous intervention. The client laughed at a joke, story, or cartoon provided by the nurse. The client shared a joke or story with the nurse or family. The client sees some absurdity in a personal incident and shares with staff or family.
The client will engage in playful activities.	Guide client to select a playful activity that matches his or her preference and ability	The client was observed amusing self with toy. The client plays game with family during visiting hours. The client wears amusing item to greet staff or family.
The client will experience decrease in subjective severity of target symptom as a result of humor or playful intervention.	Guide client in grading the severity of a symptom on a scale of 1 to 10 before and after intervention.	Patient rated pain at 6 before humor intervention and graded pain at 3 after intervention.

speak the punch line clearly and with punch!

- Review the client's chart or consult with others to assess changes in the client's situation since you last met.
- Sense your own needs and stress level. Give yourself permission to be silly and playful.

At the Beginning of the Session

- Assess the client's status according to the assessment parameters.
- Record vital signs and ask the client to assess pain, anxiety, tension, or other target symptoms on a numerical scale (1 = comfortable, 10 = extremely uncomfortable).
- Describe to the client the benefits that humor, laughter, and play have on the body (physiologic), mind (psychologic), and spirit (emotional and energy level).

- Provide the client with appropriate materials to match his or her preference and some instructions for use.

During the Session

- Use all interventions with sensitivity to the client's needs, response, and difficulties.
- Provide support for the client through your physical presence, encouragement, or time alone if the client wants to read or watch a videotape.
- Remember that humor is contagious and social. Interventions may be most effective if used within a group (e.g., family and friends) rather than individually.
- Remember that humor and play are spontaneous and therefore are most successful when not precisely planned.

- Continue to evaluate the mood and response of the client and adapt the humor and play intervention to meet the client's perceived needs.

At the End of the Session

- Record vital signs and ask the client to reevaluate the pain, tension, or target symptom on a scale of 1 to 10.
- Discuss the intervention with the client and obtain feedback for future sessions.
- Answer any questions the client may have.
- Encourage the client to continue using the intervention at home and to explore other possible variations.
- Use client outcomes (Exhibit 20–2) and the client's subjective experiences (Exhibit 20–4) to evaluate the session.
- Schedule a follow-up session.

Specific Interventions: Humor, Laughter, and Play

Humor interventions can be packaged in many different ways—as humor rooms, comedy carts, humor baskets, laughter libraries, or caring clown programs. The individual caregiver can adapt these programs to meet the specific needs of clients.

- Create a scrapbook of cartoons. Place the cartoons in a photo album with peel-back pages to protect them and keep them clean. Consider the audience that will read this scrapbook. Try to find humor about situations or problems your clients will be facing. Be careful not to add any potentially offensive or shocking items to the scrapbook. Include a variety of cartoon artists.
- Develop a file of funny jokes, stories, cards, bumper stickers, poems, and songs. When you hear something funny, write it down immediately, before you forget! Many humorous resources are available on the internet.

Books of jokes are available in stores and libraries, but these are rather unreliable resources for usable material. Their jokes are often offensive, outdated, or just not funny. A better method of building a collection is to write down jokes you hear from friends, see on television, or read in magazines.

- Collect or borrow funny books, videotapes, and audiotapes of comedy routines. These can be found in libraries, humor sections of bookstores, mail-order catalogs, or at humor conferences. (See "Resources" section at end of chapter.) Create a lending library.
- Keep a file of local clowns, magicians, storytellers, and puppeteers. Invite them to entertain at your facility, at the patient's home, or at a group function.
- Collect toys, interactive games, noisemakers, and costume items. Keep them available for play. Small wind-up toys can be enjoyable. The author has a pair of little shoes that walk around when wound up and a large nose that does the same—it is called the "runny nose." If you will be sharing such toys with a client, keep in mind safety and infection precautions. (See Exhibit 20–3.)
- Create a humor journal or log to record funny encounters or humorous discoveries. On days when you really need a laugh but cannot seem to find anything funny, you will have a collection of amusing stories at your fingertips. A nurse in one of the author's workshops recounted that she had created a journal for the operating room where she worked. She called the book *The Days of Our Knives*.
- Establish a bulletin board in your facility or on your refrigerator at home. Post cartoons, bumper stickers, and funny signs. If the display is public, you must consider the sensitivities of the audience and be careful to exclude

potentially offensive (e.g., ageist, sexist, ethnic) material.

- Subscribe to a humorous newsletter or journal to collect new ideas and inspiration. See the "Resources" section at the end of the chapter for a list of resources.
- Educate yourself about therapeutic humor. Attend conferences, workshops, and conventions. More effective techniques are developed daily. New research is published, and better resources become available on a regular basis. Stay up to date in this rapidly growing field. (See the "Resources" section.)

Communication studies have shown that people take in 7 percent of other people's words, 38 percent of their vocal characteristics, and 55 percent of their nonverbal signals.[83] Applying these concepts in the creation and communication of humor can make the efforts even more effective. Because the client will notice less than 10 percent of your words, choose them carefully. Develop a collection of zingy one-liners, clever riddles, funny stories, and brilliant jokes for every occasion.[84,85] Vocal characteristics are five times more important than words alone. Try to change the pace and tone of your voice or speak with an accent, and your words will have more impact. The most powerful communication tool we have is the ability to communicate nonverbally. Facial expressions, physical gestures, costuming, props, and the way we walk or stand or reach for something are nonverbal communication techniques that provide the greatest impact on our audience. Clowns and other physical-comedy artists have perfected these skills and use their body language to deliver the humorous message.[86,87]

- Laughter libraries offer a selection of funny and informative books about humor and health. Audiotapes and videotapes are usually a part of this collection. These resources can be used either at home or within a facility. There are literally hundreds of books that can be included in a laughter library.
- A humor room is a place where clients, their families, and staff can gather to laugh, play, and relax together. These rooms are decorated with comfortable furniture, plants, and artwork. The furniture is arranged in clusters so that groups of three to five people can gather around a game table, television, or reading area.[88]
- A comedy cart is a mobile unit with many of the same supplies available in a humor room. It can be wheeled into a client's room to bring mirth aid alongside the frightening medical equipment and monitoring devices. These carts often have clever names such as Laughmobile, Jokes on Spokes, Humor on a Roll, or Humor à la Cart.[89]

Exhibit 20–3 Supplies for Humor Programs

Joke books	Kaleidoscopes	Wind-up toys
Large sunglasses	Goofy hats	Rubber noses
Giant pacifier	Clown nose	Magic wand
Puppets	Rubber chicken	Smile on a stick
Funny buttons	Funny pictures	Groucho glasses
Squirt guns	Hand-held games	Cartoon books
Bubbles	Funny Post-It notes	Stickers

- A humor basket is possibly the easiest therapeutic humor program to create and is an appropriate place to start if time and resources are limited. This basket is a smaller collection of some comedy toys, gadgets, and props. Hospital staff find that humor baskets provide quick and easy access to items with humor potential, stimulate their own creativity, and enhance their spontaneity. (See Exhibit 20–4.)
- Bedside clowning attempts to distract patients from their problems to help them forget their pain. Patients are given a chance to watch or participate in some fun and silliness. Clowns offer a momentary release from personal burdens, inspire joy, and stimulate the will to live.[90-92] The *Hospital Clown Newsletter* advises performers on routines and precautions that will enhance their bedside skills. (See "Resources" section.)
- Scan your local TV program schedule and create a list of humorous entertainment options. Post this list in a common area.
- When using closed-circuit video programs, be sure to obtain permission for use if the material is copyrighted. In some situations, a license must be purchased to show these films to large audiences.

Case Studies

Case Study No. 1

Setting:	Hospital room
Client:	R.T., a 52-year-old man awaiting open heart surgery
Nursing Diagnosis:	1. Anxiety
	2. Coping, ineffective individual
	3. Powerlessness
	4. Social isolation

R.T. lay quietly in his hospital bed. The doctors had visited and left, the nurses were finished with their morning care. It was quiet. He was alone and feeling lonely. His wife Sally and the kids would not be able to visit until later that evening. What could he do until then? It was hard not to worry about his surgery scheduled for the next day. The more he worried, the more he felt agitated, depressed, and simply scared to death. The next moment, he was given the perfect solution. Evelyn, a smiling hospital volunteer entered his room pushing a decorated cart. She wore a colorful smock and a funny hat labeled, "Humor Patrol—Department of Energy." R.T. smiled for the first time that day. "Looks like you could use some mirth aide, and we've got a wonderful selection today." R.T. was skeptical but curious. He asked for an explanation. "Well," she replied, "it's difficult for patients to lie around all day waiting for the next medical procedure. They worry and get depressed. These emotions have been proven to inhibit healing, so to prevent them, we provide a therapeutic humor program for our patients. It's part of the hospital's mission statement, to offer care and attention to the whole patient, body, mind, and spirit."

R.T. agreed that his spirits needed a lift and his mind could use some distraction. He asked to see more. First, Evelyn opened the "Yuk-a-Day Vitamin" jar and read a few jokes, riddles, and funny one-liners. Then she opened a drawer and pulled out a few wind-up toys and started them running on his over-bed table. She continued to pull out toys, games, props, puppets, cartoon books, puzzles, and costume items. Soon both of them were laughing, joking, and playing around like small children. After performing a few magic tricks, Evelyn gave R.T. a list of the humorous audiotapes, videotaped programs, and books that were available from the hospital's laughter library. R.T. chose an audiotape of Bob Newhart, his favorite comedian, and arranged for a comedy videotape to be delivered when his family arrived that evening. He selected a few toys to borrow as well as some rubber vomit to tease the nurses and a squirt gun to defend himself against unwanted interruptions.

R.T. felt like a kid again, filled with enthusiasm and ready to have fun. He looked forward to the fun and laughter he would experience and share with his family. As Evelyn left, she offered one more answer to a problem he had not yet solved. "If you like, we can schedule a clown to visit with you while you're in the hospital." "Great idea," he thought. His son's birthday was on Saturday, and instead of missing his party, now they could share a special celebration right there in the hospital. He scheduled the clown visit. Because of the therapeutic humor program, R.T. was now feeling energized, optimistic, and relaxed. Laughter *is* the best medicine!

Case Study No. 2

Setting:	Outpatient clinic
Client:	J.B., a 45-year-old woman
Nursing	1. Activity intolerance
Diagnoses:	2. Anxiety
	3. Breathing pattern, ineffective
	4. Fear
	5. Powerlessness
	(All related to adult-onset intrinsic asthma)

J.B. had visited the clinic for treatment of her asthma over a period of several months. Her bronchodilator medications had been adjusted, she was using a cool mist to thin secretions, her activity level had increased, and she had returned to full-time employment. In the process of teaching breathing techniques to J.B., the nurse noted that she had difficulty in maintaining prolonged exhalation. She was able to lengthen her expiratory time between attacks but would forget the intervention when under the stress of wheezing and shortness of breath.

J.B. arrived at the clinic in mild distress after using an inhaler to open her airways with only partial success. After sitting J.B. in a straight chair, the nurse began coaching her in her breathing pattern while applying gentle pressure on her shoulders with each exhalation. As her breathing became easier, the nurse opened a bottle of bubble solution and invited J.B. to blow bubbles. Although J.B. felt that this was a rather nontraditional approach to her condition, she agreed to participate.

In order to blow bubbles successfully, one must exhale slowly and for a long period of time. J.B. remembered this from her own childhood and from playing with her children. She was soon blowing long streams of fragile bubbles, and her wheezing disappeared as she did so. As the attack eased, the nurse coached J.B. to visualize the bubbles as carrying away her tension triggers. J.B. expressed her delight with her new application of an old skill. Her tension decreased, and she returned to work confident in her ability to apply her skill during stressful situations. Linking the skill with an unusual and playful activity made the breathing strategy stand out in her memory and made it easier to recall under stress.

Evaluation

With the client, the nurse determines whether the client outcomes for humor, laughter, and play (see Exhibit 20–2) were successfully achieved. To evaluate the session further, the nurse may again explore the subjective effects of the experience with the client using the evaluation questions in Exhibit 20–4.

DIRECTIONS FOR FUTURE RESEARCH

1. Determine the impact of humor and laughter programs on quality of life,

Exhibit 20-4 Evaluation of the Client's Subjective Experience with Humor, Laughter, and Play

1. Was this a new experience for you? Can you describe it?
2. Can you describe any physical or emotional shift that occurred during the exercise?
3. Were there any distractions or uncomfortable moments during the exercise?
4. How long has it been since you had this kind of experience?
5. How was this exercise different for you from the last time you took part in a similar one?
6. Would you like to try this again?
7. How could the experience be made more meaningful for you?
8. What are your plans to integrate this exercise into your daily life?

pain control, and symptom management.

2. Examine the cost effectiveness of humor programs in increasing patient satisfaction, decreasing length of stay, and achieving compliance with treatment plan.

3. Analyze the impact of laughter and play programs on the immune-compromised patient and the patient at risk for developing infection.

NURSE HEALER REFLECTIONS

After reading this chapter, the nurse healer will be able to answer or begin the process of answering the following questions:

- What is my inner sense of joy when I hear myself or another laugh?
- Do I nurture my ability and the ability of my patients to be playful?
- Can I laugh and play with a sense of freedom and without guilt, even when my work is not yet finished?
- Can I experience playful activities without competing or feeling that I must accomplish a particular goal?

NOTES

1. A. Klein, *Quotations to Cheer You Up When the World Is Getting You Down* (New York: Sterling Publishing Co., 1991).
2. R. Moody, *Laugh after Laugh* (Jacksonville, FL: Headwaters, 1978).
3. V. Robinson, *Humor and the Health Professions* (Thorofare, NJ: Slack, 1991).
4. L. Kronenberger, *The Thread of Laughter* (New York: Alfred A. Knopf, 1952).
5. S. Freud, Jokes and Their Relation to the Unconscious, in *The Complete Psychological Works of Sigmund Freud*, vol. 8 (London: Hogarth Press, 1905/1961).
6. H. Mindess, *Laughter and Liberation* (Los Angeles: Mansh Publishing, 1971).
7. A.R. Radcliffe-Brown, On Joking Relationships, in *Structure and Function in Primitive Society* (New York: Free Press, 1952).
8. M. L. Apte, *Humor and Laughter: An Anthropological Approach* (Ithaca, NY: Cornell University Press, 1985).
9. A. Ziv, *National Styles of Humor* (Westport, CT: Greenwood Publishing Group, 1988).
10. R.M. Stephenson, Conflict and Control Functions of Humor, *American Journal of Sociology* 56 (1959): 569–574.
11. J. Boskin, *Humor and Social Change in Twentieth Century America* (Boston: Trustees of the Public Library, 1979).
12. J.W. Meeker, *The Comedy of Survival: Studies in Literary Ecology* (New York: Charles Scribner's Sons, 1972).
13. A. Klein, *Healing Power of Humor* (Los Angeles: Jeremy P. Tarcher, 1989).
14. Personal communication.
15. A. Goodheart, *Laughter Therapy* (Santa Barbara, CA: Stress Less Press, 1994).
16. S. Ritz, Survivor Humor and Disaster Nursing, in *Nursing Perspectives on Humor*, ed. K. Buxman (Staten Island, NY: Power Publications, 1995), 197–216.

17. P. Wooten, *Compassionate Laughter* (Salt Lake City, ID: Commune A Key Pub., 1996), p. 15.

18. C. Edson, You Know It's a Long Shift When . . ., in *Whinorrhea and Other Nursing Diagnoses*, ed. F. London (Mesa, AZ: JNJ Pub., 1995), 56–57.

19. Freud, Jokes and Their Relation to the Unconscious.

20. C. Gullickson, Listening Beyond the Laughter, in *Nursing Perspectives on Humor*, ed. K. Buxman (Staten Island, NY: Power Publications, 1995), 19–25.

21. Robinson, *Humor and the Health Professions*, p. 49.

22. Wooten, *Compassionate Laughter*, p. 18.

23. K. Hammer, *And How Are We Feeling Today* (Chicago: Contemporary Books, 1993).

24. Stephenson, Confict and Control Functions of Humor.

25. F. London, ed., *Whinorrhea and Other Nursing Diagnoses* (Mesa, AZ: JNJ Pub., 1995).

26. C. Kenefick and A. Young, eds., *The Best of Nursing Humor*, vol. 2 (Philadelphia: Hanley and Belfus, 1999).

27. J. Cocker, ed., *Stitches* (Toronto: Stoddart Publishing Co., 1993).

28. C. Prasad, *Physician Humor Thyself* (Winston-Salem, NC: Harbinger Medical Press, 1998).

29. G. Bosker, *Medicine's the Best Laughter* (St. Louis, MO: Mosby, 1995).

30. J. Wise, *Tales from the Bedside* (St. Louis, MO: Mosby–Year Book, 1994).

31. S. Shem, *House of God* (New York: Dell Publishing, 1978).

32. C. Hageseth, *A Laughing Place* (Fort Collins, CO: Berwick Publishing Co., 1988).

33. A. Klein, *Courage to Laugh* (Los Angeles: Jeremy P. Tarcher, 1998).

34. Robinson, *Humor and the Health Professions*, p. 87.

35. L. Rosenberg, A Qualitative Investigation of the Use of Humor by Emergency Personal as a Strategy for Coping with Stress, *Journal of Emergency Nursing* 17, no. 4 (1991): 197–203.

36. L. Rosenberg, Sick, Black, and Gallows Humor among Emergency Caregivers, or—Are We Having Any Fun Yet? in *Nursing Perspectives on Humor*, ed. K. Buxman (Staten Island, NY: Power Publications, 1995), 39–50.

37. Wooten, *Compassionate Laughter*.

38. Goodheart, *Laughter Therapy*, p. 86.

39. Wooten, *Compassionate Laughter*, p. 25.

40. Personal communication.

41. N. Cousins, *Anatomy of an Illness* (New York: W.W. Norton & Co., 1979).

42. Cousins, *Anatomy of an Illness*.

43. N. Cousins, *Head First—the Biology of Hope* (New York: E.P. Dutton, 1989).

44. N. Cousins, Intangibles in Medicine: An Attempt at Balancing Perspective, *Journal of the American Medical Association*, 260, no. 2 (1988): 1610–1612.

45. N. Cousins, Anatomy of an Illness, *New England Journal of Medicine* 295 (1976): 1458–1463.

46. Cousins, *Head First*.

47. P. Wooten, Interview with William Fry, *Journal of Nursing Jocularity* 4, no. 4 (1994): 46–47.

48. Wooten, Interview with William Fry.

49. W. Fry, Humor, Physiology and the Aging Process, in *Humor and Aging*, ed. L. Nahamow (Orlando FL: Academic Press, 1986), 81–98.

50. W. Fry, Mirth and oxygen saturation of peripheral blood, *Psychotherapy and Psychosomatics* 19 (1971): 76–84.

51. W. Fry, Mirth and the Human Cardiovascular System, in *The Study of Humor*, ed. L. Mindess (Los Angeles: Antioch University Press, 1979).

52. R. Ader, *Psychoneuroimmunology*, 2d ed. (New York: Academic Press, 1991).

53. Institute of Noetic Sciences, *The Heart of Healing* (Atlanta, GA: Turner Publishing, 1993).

54. C. Pert, *Molecules of Emotion* (New York: Charles Scribner's Sons, 1997).

55. C. Pert et al., Neuropeptides and Their Receptors: A Psychosomatic Network, *Journal of Immunology* 135 (1985): 820s–826s.

56. P. McGhee, *Health, Healing and the Amuse System* (Dubuque, IA: Kendall-Hunt Publishing, 1997), p. 13.

57. C. Pert, The Chemical Communications, in *Healing and the Mind*, ed. B. Moyers (New York: Doubleday, 1993).

58. P. Wooten, Interview with Dr. Lee Berk, *Journal of Nursing Jocularity* 7, no. 3 (1997): 46–48.

59. L. Berk et al., Humor Associated Laughter Decreases Cortisol and Increases Spontaneous Lymphocyte Blastogenesis, *Clinical Research* 36 (1988): 435A.

60. L. Berk et al., Eustress of Mirthful Laughter Modifies Natural Killer Cell Activity, *Clinical Research* 37 (1989): 115A.

61. L. Berk and S. Tan, Neuroendocrine and Stress Hormone Changes during Mirthful Laughter, *American Journal of the Medical Sciences* 298 (1989): 390–396.

62. L. Berk and S. Tan, Immune System Changes during Humor Associated with Laughter, *Clinical Research* 39 (1991): 124A.

63. L. Berk and S. Tan, Eustress of Humor Associated Laughter Modulates Specific Immune System Components, *Annals of Behavioral Medicine* 15 (1993): S111.

64. L. Berk, The Laughter-Immune Connection: New Discoveries, *Humor and Health Journal* 5, no. 5 (1996): 1–7.

65. L. Berk, New Discoveries in Psychoneuroimmunology, *Humor and Health Journal* 13, no. 6 (1994): 1–8.

66. L. Frankel, Play, in *World Book Encyclopedia* (Chicago: Field Enterprises Educational Corp., 1975), 506.

67. E. Erikson, *Toys and Reasons* (New York: W.W. Norton & Co., 1977), 17.

68. N. Angier, The Purpose of Playful Frolics: Training for Adulthood,*The New York Times*, October 20, 1992.

69. H. Selye, *The Stress of Life* (New York: McGraw-Hill, 1956).

70. C. Maslach, *Burnout—The Cost of Caring* (Englewood Cliffs, NJ: Prentice-Hall, 1982).

71. E. McCranie, Work, Stress, Hardiness, and Burnout among Hospital Staff Nurses, *Nursing Research* 36 (1987): 374–378.

72. S.C. Kobassa, Personality and Social Resources in Stress Resistance, *Journal of Personality & Social Psychology* 45 (1983): 839.

73. S.C. Kobassa and S.R. Maddi, *The Hardy Executive: Health and Stress* (Homewood, IL: Dow-Jones-Irwin Pub., 1984).

74. H.M. Lefcourt, *Locus of Control: Current Trends in Theory and Research* (Hillsdale, NJ: Lawrence Erlbaum Associates, 1982).

75. Kobassa, Personality and Social Resources in Stress Resistance.

76. P. Wooten, Humor: An Antidote for Stress, *Holistic Nursing Practice* 10, no. 2 (1996): 49–55.

77. P. Wooten, Does a Humor Workshop Effect Nurse Burnout, *Journal of Nursing Jocularity* 2(2) (1992): 42–43.

78. S. Nowicki, A Locus of Control Scale for College as well as Non-College Adults, *Journal of Personality Assessment* 38 (1974): 136–137.

79. S. Svebak, Revised Questionnaire on the Sense of Humor, *Scandinavian Journal of Psychology* 15 (1974): 328–331.

80. H. Lefcourt and R. Martin, *Humor and Life Stress* (New York: Springer-Verlag, 1986).

81. M. Seligman, *Helplessness* (New York: W.H. Freeman, 1975).

82. S.M.I.L.E. (Subjective Multidimensional Interactive Laughter Evaluation) is a computer software program that obtains answers to questions about a person's humor preferences, attitudes, and history. It then accesses a database that will match a person's stated preference with the audio, video, or book source that is most likely to make the person laugh. The questionnaire can be viewed or the software ordered through the web site (www.touchstarpro.com) (see "Resources" section).

83. J. Sherman, *The Magic of Humor in Caregiving* (Golden Valley, MN: Pathway Books, 1995), 70.

84. M. Helitzer, *Comedy Writing Secrets* (Cincinnati, OH: Writer's Digest Books, 1987).

85. R. Bates, *How To Be Funnier, Happier, Healthier and More Successful Too!* (Minneapolis, MN: Trafton Publishing, 1995).

86. F. Fife, *Creative Clowning* (Colorado Springs, CO: Java Pub., 1988).

87. M. Stolzenberg, *Clown for Circus and Stage* (New York: Sterling Publishing, 1981).

88. K. Buxman, Make Room for Laughter, *American Journal of Nursing* 91, no. 12 (1991): 46–51.

89. L. Gibson, Carts, Baskets and Rooms, in *Nursing Perspectives on Humor*, ed. K. Buxman (Staten Island, NY: Power Publications, 1995), 113–124.

90. Mindess, *Laughter and Liberation*.

91. R. Snowberg, *The Caring Clown*, vol. 1 (LaCrosse, WI: Visual Arts, 1992).

92. R. Snowberg, *The Caring Clown*, vol. 2 (La Crosse, WI: Visual Magic, 1997).

RESOURCES

Associations
American Association for Therapeutic Humor
222 S. Meramec, Suite 303
St. Louis, MO 63105
Phone: (314) 863-6232
Fax: (314) 863-6457
Website: www.aath.org

International Society for Humor Studies
Don Nilsen, Arizona State University
Department of English
Tempe, AZ 85287-0302
Website: www.uni-duesseldorf.de/WWW/MathNat/
    Ruch/SecretaryPage.html
Email: don.nilsen@asu.edu

Publications
Humor and Health Journal
PO Box 16814
Jackson, MS 39236
Phone: (601) 957-0075
Website: www.intop.net/~jrdunn
Email: jrdunn@intop.net

Fellowship of Merry Christians, Inc.
PO Box 895
Portage, MI 49081-0895
Phone: (800) 877-2757
Website: www.JoyfulNoiseletter.com
Email: JoyfulNZ@aol.com

Funny Times
PO Box 18530, Department 2AAM
Cleveland Heights, OH 44118
Phone: (216) 371-8600, ext. 8002
Website: www.funnytimes.com

Hospital Clown Newsletter
PO Box 8957
Emeryville, CA 94662
Phone: (510) 420-1511
Email: ShobiDobi@aol.com

Supplies
Jest for You Catalogue
Patty Wooten
PO Box 8484
Santa Cruz, CA 95062
Phone: (408) 460-1600
Fax: (831) 460-1601
Website: www.jesthealth.com
Email: pwooten@jesthealth.com

Clown Supplies
The Castles, Tre. 101, Suite C-7C
Brentwood, NH 03833
Phone and fax: (603) 679-3311

Too Live Nurse
PO Box 58
Columbiaville, NY 12050-0058
Phone: (518) 828-3271
Website: http://www.vgernet.net/toolive/
toolive2.html
Email: efiebke@berk.com

Humor and Happiness Catalogue
PO Box 18819
Cleveland, OH 44118-0819
Phone: (800) 677-3256

Touchstar Productions
522 Jackson Park Drive
Meadville, Pennsylvania 16335
Phone: (800) 759-1294
Website: www.touchstarpro.com
Email: info@touchstarpro.com

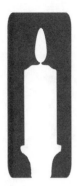

VISION OF HEALING
Creating Receptive Quiet

Be still and know that I am God.
                        Psalm 46

Moments of inner and outer quiet are the spaces and places in which we are most deeply in touch with ourselves and our true nature of being and with nature's true gift of restoring and renewing. As modern nurses entering the twenty-first century, we need to preserve and create sacred spaces of quiet, within ourselves and in our health care environments.

Quiet spaces help us to learn and deepen our practice of relaxation and meditation, to be present right here, right now, in this moment.

> *Breathing In, I Calm.*
> *Breathing Out, I Smile.*
> *Dwelling in this present moment*
> *I know this is a wonderful moment.*
>   *Thich Nhat Hanh*

Deceivingly simple, being in this moment offers a profound message that is increasingly important in our ever faster paced lives. Stopping, breathing, watching the sun set, a wave reach the shore, a baby sleeping, the wind in the leaves of a tree, can restore and renew our spirits as nurses and as healers.

> *In the beginning*
> *We attempt to cultivate Loving*
>   *Kindness*
> *Later Loving Kindness cultivates us.*
>   *Stephen Levine*

Cultivating a peaceful, compassionate heart, making time to relax and tend to our well-being, is a gift we give ourselves and impacts everything we do, every life we touch. Our spiritual path calls for nothing less.

Chapter 21

Relaxation: The First Step to Restore, Renew, and Self-Heal

Jeanne Anselmo and Leslie Gooding Kolkmeier

NURSE HEALER OBJECTIVES

Theoretical

- Learn the definitions of relaxation and self-regulation.
- Compare and contrast different relaxation exercises.
- List the body-mind-spirit changes that accompany profound relaxation.

Clinical

- Describe three different types of relaxation exercises and their appropriate clinical application.
- Identify a commonly used piece of equipment in your practice and describe how it can be used as a biofeedback device.
- Use breathing strategies with a client and record the subjective and clinical changes that occur with relaxed breathing.

Personal

- Pick one or a combination of relaxation and meditation practices and apply them to the stressful moment.

- Identify through focused awareness the places where you accumulate tension most often.
- Identify three personally meaningful therapeutic suggestions and use them as reminders to support your self-care relaxation practice and well-being.

DEFINITIONS

Autogenic Training: self-directed therapy that focuses on repetition of phrases about desired states of the body (e.g., heaviness and warmth).

Biofeedback: the use of instrumentation to mirror psychophysiologic processes which the individual is not normally aware and which may be brought under voluntary control; allows the person to be an active participant in health maintenance.[1]

Body Scanning: sequentially focusing awareness on various parts of the body for the purpose of consciously connecting body-mind and spirit. This fosters awareness of both subtle sensations and areas of accumulating tension.

Hypnosis: an approach for achieving a focused awareness and expanded consciousness with diminishing perception

---

Note: This chapter is an updated adaptation of Leslie Gooding Kolkmeier's original chapter that appeared in the previous edition of this book.

of peripheral sensations, thoughts, and feelings.

Mantra: a word or short phrase that is repeated either silently or aloud as a focus of concentration during the practice of meditation.

Meditation: originally based in spiritual traditions, the practice of focusing and concentrating one's attention and awareness while maintaining a passive attitude; a discipline that evolves with discipline and practice and is known for providing health benefits as well as for being a road to spiritual transformation.

Pain (Medical Definition): localized sensation of hurt or an unpleasant sensory and emotional experience associated with actual or potential tissue damage, or described in terms of such damage.

Pain (Nursing Definition): a subjective experience including both verbal and nonverbal behavior.[2]

Progressive Muscle Relaxation: the process of alternately tensing and relaxing muscle groups to become aware of subtle degrees of tension and relaxation; originally developed by Edmund Jacobson.

Relaxation: a psychophysiologic experience characterized by parasympathetic dominance involving multiple visceral and somatic systems; the absence of physical, mental, and emotional tension; the opposite of Canon's "fight or flight" response and Selye's general adaptation syndrome.[3]

Relaxation Response: an alert, hypometabolic state of decreased sympathetic nervous system arousal that may be achieved in a number of ways, including through breathing exercises, relaxation and imagery exercises, biofeedback, and prayer. A degree of discipline is required to evoke this response, which increases mental and physical well-being.

Self-Hypnosis: a learned approach for voluntarily achieving a state of consciousness for the purpose of changing one's thoughts, perceptions, or sensations.

Stress (Psychophysiologic Definition): the felt experience of overactivity of the sympathetic nervous system.

Transpersonal: transcending or going beyond personal, individual identity and meaning to include purpose, meaning, values, and identification with universal principles; spiritual.

THEORY AND RESEARCH

People are frequently told to "just relax," "take it easy," as part of their recovery from illness, as if everyone knew how to practice this skill. Yet the ancients knew that relaxation is a paradox: it is and is not that simple. Throughout the ages, in cultures around the world, practitioners of the sacred and healing arts and sciences developed and practiced stopping, quieting, and calming on a disciplined and regular basis, offering themselves deep rest to still the body-mind-spirit and emotions. They did this not only to access their natural ability to heal, restore, and renew their body-mind-spirit but also to open themselves to the divine, the oneness of being, the numinous. This oneness of being offered itself to these ancient spiritual voyagers as the waves of the mind stilled and the activity of the body quieted into a deep rest and relaxation found within their meditative refuge and relaxation practice.

Today we continue this voyage to touch shores beyond our unhealthy habit patterns and belief systems through the practice of the ancient arts of relaxation, meditation, yoga, Qi Gong, and breathing, and their modern counterparts autogenic training, progressive muscle relaxation, hypnosis, biofeedback, self-regulation, the relaxation response, and body scanning.

We now understand relaxation to be an ancient art with many modern interpretations, which has been anchored throughout nursing practice from childbirth education to pre- and postoperative teaching. Relaxation has been defined in medical and scientific terms as "a psychophysiologic state characterized by parasympathetic dominance involving multiple visceral and somatic systems; the absence of physical, mental, and emotional tension; the opposite of Canon's fight or flight response."[4]

Relaxation can also be described as an experience or process of deep rest, natural nurturing, inner connectedness, renewal, and openness that every living creature, from slumbering infants to creatures of the wild, knows instinctively and intuitively how to access. Unfortunately, this activity can be conditioned to become more an exceptional experience than the norm, thereby leading to the development of stress-related illnesses (which account for 75 to 80 percent of illness in modern life).

Therefore, the benefits of relaxation practice are great, especially for our hectic, modern, overscheduled lives. Relaxation interventions are useful for people in all stages of health and illness: the critically ill, expectant parents attending childbirth preparation classes, or bus drivers learning to regulate blood pressure while weaving through city traffic. Even in the acute phase of recovery from a myocardial infarction or during an examination in an emergency room after an accident, clients can derive the clinical benefits of relaxation by learning basic breathing and muscle relaxation exercises (Exhibit 21–1).

Modern nurses in all areas of practice have been offering relaxation, breathing, and some form of meditation to clients over the past four decades. Yet this is not new to nursing. Florence Nightingale counseled her nurses to support patient's rest and well-being by reducing unnecessary noise, not awakening patients out of their first sleep, protecting patients from unnecessary disturbances, such as conversations of doctors or friends within earshot and the disturbing rustling of crinolines. She advised that "all hurry or bustle is peculiarly painful to the sick."[5(p.28)] One wonders what Nightingale would say if she were visiting hospitals and health care settings today

and witnessing our efforts to follow her legacy in the chaos of our times.

These days, nurses offer relaxation practices in hospitals, community and adult education programs, outpatient clinics, and homeless shelters to promote a variety of personal benefits (Exhibit 21–2); they offer these practices to individuals, families, and groups, to children in classrooms, to clients and families in home care and hospice, and to workers and executives in workplaces and corporations.

Exhibit 21–1 Clinical Benefits of Relaxation

Relaxation training has the following clinical benefits:

- decreasing the anxiety accompanying painful situations, such as debridement or dressing changes
- easing the muscle tension pain of skeletal muscle contractions
- decreasing fatigue by interrupting the fight or flight response
- providing a period of rest as beneficial as a nap
- helping the client fall asleep quickly
- increasing the effect of pain medications
- helping the client dissociate from pain

Exhibit 21–2 Whole Self Benefits of Relaxation

Relaxation has the following benefits to self:

- decreasing pain
- decreasing anxiety
- improving immune system function
- quieting the fight or flight sympathetic response
- facilitating sleep
- providing rest
- increasing efficacy of pain medication
- reducing muscle tension, increasing blood flow
- improving sense of well-being
- offering insight and creativity

Cross-Cultural Context

Relaxation practices are found in all cultures around the world and throughout time. Whether these practices are mediated through the use of herbs, acupuncture, movement, or prayer, evidence of the power, impact, and importance of relaxation and the use of breath can be seen in shamanic healing, yoga, meditation, Chinese medicine, and other traditions across the globe. Modern research exploring the area of psychoneuroimmunology demonstrates the vital importance of relaxation in improving immune system function. Thus, psychoneuroimmunologic research suggests the importance of this ancient practice for our modern scientific world. (See Chapter 4 for further information.) Modern psychology has used relaxation as a dimension of systematic desensitization, in which clients learn to relax in the face of mild, then moderate, then intense stressors. Practitioners of biofeedback include relaxation practice with their therapy to help clients learn to self-regulate their peripheral temperature, muscle activity, and brain wave frequencies.

Jon Kabat-Zinn of the University of Massachusetts found relaxation breathing and body scanning to be a vital dimension of a mindfulness-based stress reduction practice used for dealing with pain and depression.[6] Dean Ornish includes relaxation, meditation, breathing, and yoga in his program to reverse heart disease.[7] Dolores Krieger and Dora Kunz guide nurses to perform centering, a practice of meditative inner connection and relaxed awareness, before entering into therapeutic touch practice with a client.[8]

These modern pioneers all continue to validate the importance of the ancient practice of relaxation through the use of its modern counterparts.

Caring for Ourselves, Caring for Others: A Spiritual Journey

These days the practice of relaxation in its many forms is even more important for nurses. In these challenging times of constant change, nurses need to walk a wellness path of self-care, self-healing, and spiritual awareness. Finding a relaxation practice can help nurses to restore and renew, to avoid burnout as well as model a personal wellness path for their clients. Living this path and sharing by example give nurses an inner understanding and appreciation for the challenges their clients face when clients start to integrate complementary practice into their everyday lives. Relaxation practice offers nurses an important refuge, a self-awareness foundation for deepening their spiritual journey as holistic caregivers. Whether individuals are being with themselves and with All That Is in meditation; exploring their own past issues, traumas, or painful life experiences in counseling and psychotherapy; or expanding their awareness in intuitive practices and energy healing, a foundation in deep relaxation of the body-mind-spirit is a fundamental step on the path. Long-time practitioners of healing arts continue to loop back, reconnect, and deepen their abilities to relax and renew with each step of their path (Exhibit 21–3).

The American psyche, poised to do everything with intensity and competitiveness, also enters with us into self-healing and spiritual practices. This intensity and competitiveness can be our undoing, especially if we forget the importance to our body-mind-spirit of "doing nothing." Holistic practice, whether offered within the allopathic health care system or explored in a retreat setting, offers health and healing benefits with clinical implications but remains in its essence an avenue of spiritual renewal.

> Do everything with a mind that lets go,
> Do not expect any praise or reward.
> If you let go a little, you will have a little peace.
> If you let go a lot, you will have a lot of peace.

If you let go completely, you will know complete peace and freedom.

Your struggles with the world will have come to an end.[9]

Achaan Chah*

Nurses must reclaim the legacy of caring by cultivating their compassion, wisdom, spirit of service, and heart-centered health care in their culture. Relaxation is a first step along this path. It is easy to learn and practice; its benefits are demonstrated quite readily; and it offers nurses an easy entree to a self-care plan for themselves, their colleagues, and their clients. Beverly Malone, president of the American Nurses Association, underscored the importance of self-care for nurses in her address to a nursing visioning conference:

> We've got to take care of ourselves in order to be there, to be poised for greatness, to be poised to help and to assist, to work with and just to be and to feel our greatness and to know our greatness. The world needs us right now, colleagues. The world needs us desperately, and it needs our compassion. It needs our energy. But we have to make sure that we are fueled up, that we are fired up, that we are ready. And we need to understand that it doesn't stay that way. The energy comes and it goes—and that's okay, that's life. And then we have to go back and get some more at our passion station, at our fueling station. Get up in the morning and move your body or meditate. We've got to start using

*Source: Achaan Chah, as quoted in The Fine Arts of Relaxation, Concentration, and Meditation, © Joel and Michelle Levey, 1987, 1991. Reprinted with permission of Wisdom Publications, 199 Elm St., Somerville, MA 02144 U.S.A.

Exhibit 21–3 Benefits of Relaxation for the Nurse and Holistic Nursing Practice

---

Relaxation
- is an essential element of self care
- cultivates a centered, calm presence
- as a self-care practice offers insights into challenges and benefits clients will experience
- offers a vehicle to modulate and self-regulate the nurses' own stress response within stress-filled work settings
- supports a therapeutic energetic bond and connectedness when practicing along with clients and/or colleagues
- creates opportunity for intuitive exploration, insight, and understanding of self and others, issues, and problems
- is an excellent vehicle for beginning professional gatherings and staff meetings; offers opportunity to be present, creative, open, and connected
- can be done anywhere, without any cost or equipment, is easily teachable and easily practiced
- can be a spiritual practice for opening ourselves to deeper ways of being

---

that opportunity to heal ourselves as nurses so we can be available for the moments of greatness, for the opportunities of greatness.[10]

The Stress Response

We are all familiar with the intense internal reaction that we experience when faced with an emergency: a truck cuts in front of us on the highway, a "code blue" comes over the loudspeaker, a child darts into the street. What some researchers refer to as an "adrenaline rush," the familiar fight or flight response, is actually a complex series of psychophysiologic processes that prepare us to deal with the real or perceived emergency. It is important to note that people respond to an imagined threat in the same way that they respond to an actual threat to their well-being.

The generalized stress response of the body, mind, and energy field is to

- constrict the blood flow to the hands and feet (cool extremities)
- tighten muscles
- constrict the energy field (closing down or blocking flow)
- increase heart rate
- increase oxygen consumption
- increase brain wave activity
- increase sweat gland activity
- increase blood pressure
- increase anxiety

This stress response readies the body-mind-spirit through this instinctive response pattern to prepare for a stress, shock, or trauma. In modern-day life, the body alerts or readies itself physically far beyond what is needed in order to deal with a fast-paced stressful life. Most people know how to turn on this stress response but have little familiarity with how to relax or turn off the stress response. Not only do people not know how to relax, but our society typically has a negative view of relaxed people.

The paradox is that masters of ancient practices have learned that, while instinctive responses such as the fight or flight response can put one on alert to help protect one in an emergency or a crisis, a more conscious relaxation discipline, practice, and philosophy offer deeper possibilities.[11]

An example for understanding this philosophy is the ancient Chinese hexagram for crisis. The two Chinese characters for crisis are *danger* and *opportunity*. Hidden within each crisis is an opportunity, not just a danger. People must learn to face the danger and seize the opportunity. Relaxation in practice offers people that possibility of turning a difficult situation around for the better.

Exercise. Imagine a relaxed person. Write as many words as you can to describe that image. After making your list, note how many of those words (1) you consider to represent a positive quality in a person, (2) society considers to represent a positive quality, (3) work environments consider to represent positive quality in a person. Log any awareness or insights you gain from this exercise in a journal. See if these insights help you when you are discussing relaxation practice with clients, your colleagues, your family, and others. This exercise may help you to become aware of conscious or unconscious positive and/or negative attitudes that can impact clients' interest and motivation to learn to relax.

MEDITATION

Relaxation Response Meditation

Though many people call the body-mind-spirit effects of relaxation the *relaxation response*, this phrase is attributed to Herbert Benson and his colleagues at Harvard University, who used a nonreligious form of meditation that is similar to transcendental meditation to produce the opposite of the fight or flight response. Their relaxation response meditation has been introduced into many health care settings and has been applied in a variety of studies that demonstrate its efficacy in treating hypertension and anxiety.[12,13] Both transcendental meditation and relaxation response meditation offer a practice consisting of 20 minutes of daily passive concentration focused on a neutral word, such as the sanskrit word *OM* in transcendental meditation or *ONE* in relaxation response meditation. In relaxation response meditation, slow repetition of the word with each exhalation has been shown to bring about the same psychophysiologic responses as other deep relaxation processes (see below). Further studies have documented a deep relaxation response when the client focuses on a short, personally meaningful religious statement or quotation, as was found in what Benson termed the "faith factor."[14]

The changes that occur when an individual reaches a deep level of relaxation are exactly the opposite of those that occur in the fight or flight response. Alterations take place in the automatic, endocrine, immune, and neuropeptide systems as follows:

- Deep relaxation increases
  - peripheral blood flow (warm extremities)
  - electrical resistance of skin (dry palms)
  - production of slow alpha waves
  - activity of natural killer cells (improved immune function)
- Deep relaxation decreases
  - oxygen consumption
  - carbon dioxide elimination
  - blood lactate levels
  - respiratory rate and volume
  - heart rate
  - skeletal muscle tension
  - epinephrine level
  - gastric acidity and motility
  - sweat gland activity
  - blood pressure, especially in hypertensive individuals[15]

Benson calls relaxation response meditation "a very simple technique."[16] For centuries, many elements of the relaxation response have been elicited within a religious context in cultures around the world.

Benson cites four basic elements that are common to all relaxation response practices: a quiet environment, a mental device, a passive attitude, and a comfortable position.[17] To incorporate these four factors, Benson recommends that the practitioner first create a quiet environment devoid of all noises and distractions. Next, the meditator is asked to choose a mental device, that is, the "constant stimulus of a single-syllable sound or word."[18] This word is repeated silently or in a low, gentle tone. To allow rest and relaxation, the person is invited to adopt a passive attitude, not forcing the relaxation response. The meditator also is counseled to simply disregard any distracting thoughts that enter the mind.[19] To reduce any stress or muscular effort, the meditator should adapt a comfortable position on the floor or use a chair. Incorporating

these elements and focusing on the mental device of the word one for 20 minutes each day facilitates the relaxation response.

The holistic nurse may wish to explore and experience each of the relaxation practices presented in this chapter and write his or her insights and experiences in a journal. See the "Notes" and "Suggested Readings" sections at the end of the chapter for further references on relaxation response meditation and other nonreligious meditation practices, such as Patricia Carringtons' Clinically Standardized Meditation.

Breathing In and Breathing Out

One of the simplest and deepest relaxation practices is right under our noses every moment of every day: breathing. We have special breathing practices to assist childbirth and we recognize special breathing patterns when we are dying. In between, we breathe each moment, and our breathing patterns reflect our lives' peaks and valleys, our stresses and our relaxing moments.

Beyond the unconscious breathing pattern that most people are involuntarily practicing is a conscious breathing practice described long ago in the ancient sacred texts of Yoga, the Buddha's Four Foundations of Mindfulness, Taoist Qi Gong practice, native shamanic practices, and spiritual teachings and practices from around the world.

Conscious awareness of breathing—whether the slow, deep, diaphragmatic breaths of hatha yoga or the mindful awareness of breathing in and out of mindfulness meditation—can be practiced in formal sessions of 20 to 45 minutes once or twice a day. Conscious awareness of breathing can also be practiced informally by breathing with mindfulness during everyday activities.

Jon Kabat-Zinn developed a mindfulness-based stress-reduction program that demonstrated how conscious awareness of breathing can help to relieve chronic pain, depression, and anxiety.[20] Participants in the 8-week program practice mindfulness meditation every day; they also practice body scanning (systematically bringing attention to each part of the body, letting the attention rest there, letting go of any judgment about how it is "supposed to feel" and just being with this part of the body, then moving on to the next place in the body), and yoga (performance of meditative asanas or postures combined with breathing to create a union of body, mind, and spirit). Several studies in clinics, communities, and prisons have demonstrated that Kabat-Zinn's program, as well as other modern forms of meditation, can improve quality of life and reduce symptoms. (See Table 21–1.)

Breathing and Energy Healing Practice

Breathing practice is also an integral dimension of yoga and Qi Gong. The breath or life force, called *prana* in yoga and *qi* (or chi or ki) in Chinese energy practice, is the vital force or energy that animates life. Nurses practicing therapeutic touch center themselves by conscious meditation on their intention to help or to heal, by letting go of outside distractions, and by opening themselves to allow the universal life force or prana to flow through them to their clients. They can use their breathing practice to help enhance their centeredness and their openness to this healing life force.[35]

The ancient Yogis knew that by learning consciously to control their breathing and their bodies through practicing a series of yoga postures (asanas), they could open and ready themselves for transcendent awareness. As mentioned previously, yoga practices have also been demonstrated to have great health benefits in the work of Kabat-Zinn[36] and Ornish.[37]

Qi Gong practices date back to about 5,000 BCE. Taoist and Buddhist Qi Gong masters channeled the flow of qi from nature and the universe through their bodies by practicing simple movements, combined with an awareness of breathing and meditation.

These ancient Chinese practices, which are one of the dimensions of traditional Chinese medicine, have long been renowned for producing health benefits and slowing the aging process. These effects are now being researched and documented in the scientific literature (see Table 21–1).

Yoga and Qi Gong practitioners consider these disciplines important self-care practices for the unitary body-mind-spirit. These practitioners offer a living legacy of self-care that not only offers healing to their patients but is the fundamental requirement for development of a healer and/or teacher. In contrast, the Western scientific course of study does not emphasize the cultivation of one's own personal wellness and spiritual development as a prerequisite for becoming a licensed health care professional.

Clinically Standardized Meditation

Patricia Carrington of Princeton University developed a form of meditation known as clinically standardized meditation. Her work is a forerunner of Kabat-Zinn's approach. Whereas Kabat-Zinn created a method based on Buddhist mindfulness practice, Carrington developed a meditation based on a classical Indian form of mantra meditation with a standardized set of instructions. This practice is more free flowing than Benson's relaxation response meditation, which asks the practitioner to link the repetition of a word with the breath. In clincally standardized meditation, the practitioner is instructed to allow "the mantra to proceed at its own pace, to get faster or slower, louder or softer, or even to disappear if it wants to."[38]

Other Forms of Meditation

As illustrated by transcendental meditation and the work of Benson and Kabat-Zinn,

Table 21-1 Research-Based Outcomes of Meditation

Practice	Modern Forms	Adapted by	Clinical Benefits	Researcher
Meditation	Mindfulness, insight meditation, vispassana		See list of deep relaxation changes in "Relaxation Response Meditation" section	
	Transcendental meditation (TM)	Maharashi Mahesh Yogi		
	Clinically standardized meditation	Patricia Carrington (1975)		
	Relaxation response meditation	Herbert Benson (1975)	Decreased hypertension	Benson et al. (1974)[21,22]
	Mindfulness-based stress reduction	Jon Kabat-Zinn (1977)	Decreased anxiety	Kabat-Zinn et al. (1992)[23] Miller et al. (1995)[24]
			Decreased chronic pain	Kabat-Zinn (1982)[25] Kabat-Zinn et al. (1987)[26]
			Improved psoriasis (as an adjunct to phototherapy and photochemotherapy)	Bernhard et al. (1988)[27]
Moving meditation	Yoga, meditation, stress reduction, nutrition, lifestyle	Dean Ornish	Reversal of heart disease	Ornish (1990)[28]
			Improved non–insulin-dependent diabetes mellitus	Ornish (1990)[29] Ornish (1990)[30]
	Qi Gong, Chi Kung		Improved atherosclerotic vascular disease	Ankun and Chong zing (1991)[31] Lim and Boone (1993)[32]
			Lowering of blood glucose levels	McGee et al. (1996)[33]
			Reduced stress	Ryu et al. (1996)[34]
	Therapeutic touch	Delores Krieger/ Dora Kunz		See Chapter 24

there are many forms of meditation. Some say that hundreds of practices can be listed under the heading of meditation. Each practice cultivates a qualitative state of mind that can induce a deep experience of relaxation and calm. In some meditative practices, such as transcendental meditation and relaxation response meditation, the individual focuses on an object of meditation in order to move away from and minimize thoughts. Other traditions, such as mindfulness meditation, insight meditation, and vispassana meditation, invite practitioners to cultivate greater awareness by returning to the breath as awareness of sensations, thoughts, and feelings are present.

Centering prayer, a Christian meditation practice developed by Father Thomas Keating, focuses on a word or sound in somewhat the same way that transcendental meditation uses mantras (sacred sanskrit syllables and words such as OM). Other meditation practices invite meditators to gaze at the flame of a candle, a sacred image, or a mandala; to chant aloud; or to concentrate on an unanswerable question (or Koan), as in Zen practice.

Janet Macrae calls therapeutic touch a moving meditation.[39] Sufi dancing is another form of moving meditation, as are Native American and shamanic ritual dance, which may continue for many hours or many days. The purpose of spiritually focused meditation is to awaken to a higher consciousness, to be at one with the sacredness of the All, to become one with the Divine. Individuals practice such meditation to open the body-mind-spirit to the qualities of compassion, wisdom, skillfulness, fearlessness, stillness, openness, and interconnectedness.

The healing arts are the underpinning of many culture's healing traditions. For example, Tibetan healers begin their education at an early age, studying sacred texts on healing and herbs as well as meditating and praying each day to cultivate a heart of compassion and loving kindness, to become one with the compassionate, healing energy and wisdom of the limitless realms. After years of study and apprenticeship (some apprentice from childhood), they practice their healing art and science of body-mind-spirit.

What would health care be like if nurses, physicians, and other health care practitioners began by cultivating a heart of compassion and service? What would the health care system be like? Would burnout exist? (See the section "Loving Kindness Meditation" below.)

Meditation Practices

This era will give birth to many distillations of ancient meditative practices, including intricate Tibetan meditative practices, because of their health benefits. Finding a meditation practice and learning to explore it deeply offers insight and a gift only committed practice can provide.

Mindful Breathing during Nursing Practice

Nurses who wish to be more present with their clients, to practice self-care, and to awaken to the simple sacredness of everyday nursing practice (e.g., hanging an intravenous bag, writing nursing notes, eating, walking down a hall, or feeding a patient) may want to practice mindful breathing each moment, as in the following exercises.

Breathing Exercise I
Script: *Breathing In, I am aware of Breathing In.*

Breathing Out, I am aware of Breathing Out.

Breathing In, I am aware of introducing this healing medication through this intravenous line.

Breathing Out, I send my healing intentions along with the medication to help support this patient's healing.

Breathing Exercise II
Script: *Breathing In, I am walking down this hall.*

Breathing Out, I smile, enjoying my steps.

Breathing In, I am fresh.

Breathing Out, I celebrate my aliveness.

Being with the breath, reminding one-self to offer self-care in each moment by consciously breathing with each activity, is a gift of self-renewal, freshness, and aliveness that deepens with practice. It is a gift nurses can give to themselves every moment.

Mindful Breathing Meditations

Exploring and practicing relaxation and meditation not only helps the nurse gain insight into specific methods and into the issues that clients may face as they work to integrate these techniques into their daily lives, but it also offers the nurse an opportunity for personal wellness, self-care, and spiritual development.

When choosing a meditation practice to explore, the nurse should commit to that practice for at least 4 to 6 weeks before trying another, while keeping a journal of his or her reflections along the way.

Mindfulness of the Breath Exercise I (Lying Down). Lie on the floor with your hands on your abdomen, close your eyes, and feel the movement of your body with every rise and fall of the breath. Follow the inhalation fully and the exhalation fully. With each inhale, repeat, in your mind, *"Breathing in, I am aware of breathing in,* and on each exhale, *Breathing out, I am aware of breathing out."* As you continue, you may shorten the phrase by repeating gently in your mind *"In"* on the in breath and *"Out"* on the out breath. As you are breathing and lying comfortably with your hands on your abdomen, allow a gentle smile to bloom on your lips and at the corners of your eyes. After all, this is supposed to be an enjoyable practice. Try this practice for 15 to 20 minutes. Observe and note any awareness, reflections, and insights in your personal journal.

To extend this practice during the next week, you may wish to continue lying down in a comfortable position, or you may choose a sitting meditation practice, as below.

Mindfulness of the Breath Exercise II (Sitting). In a quiet place, find a comfortable position sitting. Either sit on a chair with your feet on the floor and your back supported and straight, or sit on the floor using a meditation cushion (zafu) or a regular pillow folded in half to create a supportive lift under your buttocks. If you are sitting on the floor, find a comfortable way to place your legs, either (1) crossed in lotus or half-lotus position with or without pillows under your knees, (2) Indian style, or (3) straight out in front of you, with a pillow under your knees and your back supported against a back jack or against the wall.

Focus on a point on the floor in front of you and gently lower your lids until they are almost closed. Gently bring your attention to your breath.

> **Script:** *Breathing In, I am aware of*
> *Breathing In.*
> *Breathing Out, I am aware of*
> *Breathing Out.*
> *In.*
> *Out.*
> *Breathing In, I am calm.*
> *Breathing Out, I smile.*[40]
> Thich Nhat Hanh

Continue to bring your attention to your breath, allowing any thoughts, feelings, or awareness to pass through, then gently bringing your attention back to the breath and the repeated phrase.

Practice for approximately 15 to 20 minutes. After your practice, note your experience in your journal.

As you continue, you may want to note Kabat-Zinn's attitudinal foundations of mindfulness practice, which are relevant to all relaxation practice (Exhibit 21–4).

Walking Meditation

Walking as if one were planting peace with each step—this is the essence of walking meditation.[41] To practice, start with the left foot and begin walking slowly by syn-

Exhibit 21–4 The Attitudinal Foundation of Mindfulness Practices

- **Nonjudging:** Learning to become aware of judging and reacting to inner and outer experiences and develop an observing stance. Learning to witness or observe the judging mind and then return to the breath.
- **Patience:** Allowing each moment to unfold with its own fullness, at its own rate and pace. Discovering that each moment is a special moment to be with rather than rushing through it to get to a "better" one.
- **Beginner's mind:** Cultivating the freshness of seeing for the first time. Being receptive to new possibilities in every moment, experiencing well-worn practices as though they have never been experienced before. This is beginner's mind or don't know mind.
- **Trust:** Learning to cultivate trust in one's own basic wisdom, intuition, and goodness. Learning to listen first to one's own inner voice and trust its insights and awareness, even while being open and receptive to learning from other sources.

- **Nonstriving:** Nondoing, practicing without a goal other than for one to be oneself. The irony is that one already is. Nonstriving is trying less and being more by intentionally cultivating the attitude of nonstriving. Learning to be present with whatever emotion, experience, or sensation one is experiencing without trying to do anything either to enhance it or to reduce it. Nonstriving invites one to be with one's awareness and experience.
- **Acceptance:** Not denying or resisting what is, but cultivating being present with one's reality. Acceptance does not mean being satisfied with how things are or being resigned to this situation. Acceptance is a willingness to see things as they are.
- **Letting go:** Nonattachment to one's thoughts, experiences, feelings, and sensations. As we practice, we recognize our desire to hold onto certain types of feelings and experiences we deem pleasurable and to rid ourselves of those viewed as unpleasant and painful. Practicing letting go allows us to cultivate being with all our experience as it is and observing it moment to moment.

Source: From FULL CATASTROPHE LIVING by Jon Kabat-Zinn. Copyright © 1990 by Jon Kabat-Zinn. Used by permission of Dell Publishing, a division of Random House, Inc.

chronizing the breathing meditation practice of *In/Out* with each step. Sometimes you may take three steps to the *In* breath and three steps to the *Out* breath. Play with your practice, exploring how carefully you can become aware of the subtle sensations of slowly lifting, moving, and placing each step as you continue your awareness of breathing.

This practice can be interspersed between sitting practice sessions: 20 minutes of sitting, 10 minutes of walking, 20 minutes of sitting, 10 minutes of walking. This is also a wonderful meditation to practice at a more normal pace of walking at work, as well as going to and from work. *"Walking down the hall, I am aware of my footsteps and my breathing. Being in this present moment, I know this is the only moment."*

Cultivating the Heart of Compassion Meditations

Loving Kindness Meditation. This meditation* is adapted for helping professionals from Thich Nhat Hanh's Loving Kindness Meditation in *Teachings on Love.*[42]

Sitting peacefully, begin as in sitting meditation practice, then plant each phrase like a healing seed within your heart, following your breath and focusing on your intention to cultivate compassion. Say each line to yourself in your mind, or ask a friend to read this meditation aloud

---

Source: Adapted from a love meditation in *Teachings on Love* (1997) by Thich Nhat Hanh with permission of Parallax Press, Berkeley, California.

to you, pausing after each line so that you can slowly repeat it silently to yourself.

Part I: *May I be peaceful.*
May I be happy.
May I look to myself with the eyes of compassion and love.
May I be safe.
May I be free from accidents.
May I be compassionate with my anger and gentle with my fear.
May I be spacious and compassionate to the depths of my true heart.
May I be whole.
May I be well.
May I be free.
May I be peaceful.
May I be happy.

In Part II of this meditation, repeat the same meditation, while imagining that someone you care about and/or are having difficulty with is sitting in front of you, and centering your attention on cultivating and offering compassion while repeating silently in your mind:

Part II: *May you be peaceful.*
May you be happy.
May you look to yourself with the eyes of compassion and love.
May you be safe.
May you be free from accidents.
May you be compassionate with your anger and gentle with your fear.
May you be spacious and compassionate to the depth of your true heart.
May you be whole.
May you be well.
May you be free.
May you be peaceful.
May you be happy.

Then, in Part III, imagine offering compassion to all beings on earth, to the earth, to all the planets, and to all beings throughout the universe and beyond time and space:

Part III: *May all beings be peaceful.*
May all beings be happy.
May all beings look to themselves with the eyes of compassion and love.
May all beings be safe.
May all beings be free from accidents.
May all beings be compassionate with their anger and gentle with their fear.
May all beings be spacious and compassionate to the depths of their true heart.
May all beings be whole.
May all beings be well.
May all beings be free.
May all beings be peaceful.
May all beings be happy.

The St. Francis Prayer

A Simple Prayer
Lord, make me an instrument of your peace.
Where there is hatred . . . let me sow love.
Where there is injury . . . pardon.
Where there is doubt . . . faith.
Where there is despair . . . hope.
Where there is darkness . . . light.
Where there is sadness . . . joy.
O Divine Master, grant that I may not so much seek
To be consoled . . . as to console.
To be understood . . . as to understand.
To be loved . . . as to love.
For
It is in giving . . . that we receive.

It is in pardoning . . . that we are pardoned.
It is in dying . . . that we are born to eternal life.
St. Francis of Assisi

Quiet Heart Meditation

Meditation makes it possible to gain access to more of our human potential, to increase our ability to function in reality more effectively. In general, make 15 to 20 minutes available for this meditation.

Script: [Check first that the client is comfortable with this water image]: *Picture yourself sitting comfortably on the floor of a beautiful clear lake. Each time you experience a thought, feeling, or perception, picture it as a bubble rising slowly to the surface of the lake. Take 5 to 10 seconds to observe each thought, feeling, or perception rising until it passes from your sight. Do not explore or associate with any of the bubbles; simple notice them with a background of, "Oh, that's what I'm thinking (or feeling, or sensing) now. How interesting." As each bubble disappears, wait calmly for the next one.*

This is a single example of a meditation strategy. There are many variations, and no one is better than another. Each provides a different means to the same end: a voluntarily achieved, relaxed, hypometabolic experience, accompanied by a quiet body-mind-spirit. Most teachers recommend staying with a particular meditation path for a minimum of 1 month before contemplating a change. Individuals should follow what intuitively feels right, and spend time with the feelings experienced right after a period of meditation, and should know that, if they feel better and

less fragmented than they did before, they are on the right path.

Quiet Heart Prayer

Prayer is a way of eliciting the relaxation response in the context of one's deeply held personal, religious, or philosophic beliefs. Benson refers to this as incorporating the "faith factor" into relaxation. Many people are comfortable with prayer as a meditative strategy, and it requires only seconds to minutes. In the health care setting, the nurse should strive to accommodate the client's spiritual needs, either by calling on his or her personal background and resources or by enlisting the help of appropriate family, clergy, or chaplaincy staff.

MODERN RELAXATION METHODS

Progressive Muscle Relaxation

In 1935, Edmund Jacobson detailed a strategy leading to deep muscle relaxation.[43] The body is known to respond to anxious thoughts and stressful events with increased muscle tension. This physiologic tension further provokes subjective sensations of anxiety. In progressive muscle relaxation, the practitioner deliberately tenses muscle groups, focusing on the tightening sensations, and then slowly releases that tension; in this way, the individual learns to manage the levels of muscle tension. Progressive muscle relaxation allows the client to deepen the experience of comfort.

Several studies have demonstrated that progressive muscle relaxation reduces subjective feelings of anxiety and increases peak expiratory flow rates in asthmatic clients; it also helps clients with insomnia, headaches, ulcers, hypertension, and colitis (see Table 21–2).

In the original form of progressive muscle relaxation, clients learn to relax 16 of the body's muscle groups. They inhale while tensing their muscles and then ex-

Table 21–2 Research-Based Outcomes of Relaxation

Modern Form of Relaxation Practice	Developed by	Clinical Benefits	Researcher
Progressive muscle relaxation (PMR)	Jacobson	Chemotherapy symptoms: reduced pretreatment nausea and anxiety, lowered blood pressure, lowered post-treatment anxiety, depression, nausea (practiced once daily)	Lyles et al. (1982)[44]
		Immunocompetence in geriatric population: those practicing PMR demonstrated better immunocompetence (increased natural killer cell count and herpes antibodies) and decreased stress	Keicolt-Glaser et al. (1985)[45]
PMR and music		Myocardial infarction (acute): reduced apical pulses, increased peripheral temperatures, reduced incidence of cardiac complications (congestive heart failure, pericarditis, persistent chest pain)	Guzzetta (1989)[46]
PMR and meditation		Cardiac catheterization: reduced STAI scores and diazepam use	Wagner et al. (1992)[47]
Autogenic training	Schultz and Luthe	Reduced muscle tone, blood pressure, and skin resistance	Schultz and Luthe (1959)[48]
		Increased theta activity, decreased beta activity on electroencephalogram	Dierks et al. (1989)[49]
Autogenic biofeedback therapy		Reduced classical and common migraine	Blanchard et al. (1985)[50]
		Reduced idiopathic essential hypertension	Fahrion (1991)[51]
		Improved Raynaud's disease	Freedman (1987)[52]
Hypnosis		Preoperative hypnosis reduced postoperative vomiting after breast surgery	Enquist et al. (1997)[53]
		Self-hypnosis reduced anxiety following coronary artery bypass surgery	Ashton et al. (1997)[54]
Hypnosis/meditation		Improved quality of life in women with osteoporosis (phenomenologic study)	La Vorgna-Smith (1997)[55]
Biofeedback		Improved fecal incontinence and pelvic floor dyssynergia	Whitehead et al. (1996)[56]
Biofeedback-assisted relaxation		Lowered blood glucose levels, percentage of fasting blood glucose levels at target in type I diabetes	McGrady et al. (1991)[57]

hale and relax their muscles very slowly. Variations on progressive muscle relaxation, or modified progressive muscle relaxation, are integrated into many relaxation practices.

Progressive Muscle Relaxation Exercise: Tension Awareness

The purpose of a tension awareness exercise is to help the client identify subtle levels of mental tension and anxiety and the physical tension that accompanies these mental and emotional states. The client who is aware of the internal differences induced by this exercise can move to threshold levels of tension, holding just enough tightness in the muscle group to be aware of beginning tension and then relaxing the group. By moving from strong contractions to very subtle ones, the client becomes aware of the ability to fine-tune the relaxation process. This exercise requires 10 to 30 minutes.

Script: *First take a few moments to focus on your breathing. This will* *help you to focus better on internal cues of muscle tension and then relaxation. I will guide you as we begin to move through the muscles of your body. Become aware of how you can gain control over the tension found in those muscles. This process involves alternately tightening and relaxing muscle groups. Let yourself tighten each muscle group, hold the tension for 5 to 10 seconds or until mild fatigue is felt in the area, and then release the tension. . . . Begin with the muscles in your feet and calves; tighten that area as much as you can. Pull your toes up toward your head and become aware that, as the muscles tighten and as you continue to hold that tightness, your legs will perhaps tremble or shake a bit as they fatigue. . . . Now, let the tension slowly dissolve and feel the difference in your lower legs and feet. . . . Let your attention move up to your knees and thighs; tense those muscles by pressing your legs into the surface of the bed (couch, floor, chair). . . . When you are aware of how they feel, then allow the tension to drift away as you exhale.*

The exercise then proceeds to the following areas: hips and buttocks, abdomen and lower back, chest and upper back, shoulders and biceps, forearms and hands, neck and shoulders, jaw and tongue, and finally facial muscles. If the client is experiencing pain or difficulty with a particular part of the body, the exercise should begin as far away from the involved area as possible and conclude with the primary area of difficulty.

Clients should be coached to breathe throughout the session, thereby avoiding the temptation to hold their breath as they tighten their muscles. Clients may learn to exhale as they tighten muscle groups. Tension in muscles should be held short of true discomfort.

Progressive muscle relaxation is particularly effective for clients who are feeling physically tense, anxious, and perhaps agitated. Because it is an active intervention, it may be preferable to other passive exercises, especially early in client training. It should be used with caution for clients with ischemic myocardial disease, hypertension, and back pain, however.

Autogenic Training

In 1932, Johannes Schultz and his student, Wolfgang Luthe, developed a series of brief phrases designed to focus attention on various parts of the body and induce a mindbody shift in those parts.[58] The phrases that were developed are called *autogenic* because of their ability to assist a person in inducing self (auto) change from within. This approach to health care was a rather new one in the 1930s.

Although similar to self-hypnosis, autogenic strategies are a specific present-time-oriented means of gaining access to the natural restorative mechanisms of the mind. Autogenic training has been found to be effective in managing disorders in which cognitive involvement is prominent (see Table 21–2). These self-healing phrases can be combined with progressive muscle relaxation as an integrative approach to relaxation to help a broader spectrum of clients. Autogenic training is one of the most widely used approaches in teaching clients to warm their hands during biofeedback temperature training.

Autogenic Training Exercise

Clients may find autogenic training helpful to consciously rebalance the internal homeokinetic mechanisms of the cardiovascular and respiratory systems, which simultaneously affect the autonomic, endocrine, immune, and neuropeptide systems. The exercise generally lasts 10 to 20 minutes.

Script: *Slowly and silently repeat the following phrases to yourself as I say them out loud to you [repeat each phrase two to four times, pausing a few seconds between each repetition]: "I am beginning to feel quiet. . . . I am beginning to feel relaxed. . . . My feet, knees, and hips feel heavy. . . . Heaviness and warmth are flowing through my feet and legs. . . . My hands, arms, and shoulders feel heavy. . . . Warmth and heaviness are flowing through my hands and arms. . . . My neck, jaw, and forehead feel relaxed and smooth. . . . My whole body feels quiet, heavy, and comfortable. . . . I am comfortably relaxed. . . . Warmth and heaviness flow into my arms, hands, and fingertips. . . . My breathing is slow and regular. . . . I am aware of my calm, regular heartbeat. . . . My mind is becoming quieter as I focus inward. . . . I feel still. . . . Deep in my mind I experience myself as relaxed, comfortable and still. . . . I am alert in a quiet, inward way. As I finish my relaxation, I take in several deep, reenergizing breaths, bringing light and energy into every cell of my body."*

Autogenic training should begin in a warm (75° to 80°F) room to facilitate sensations of warmth. Clients can progress to cooler environments to generalize their training (to simulate being outside). Using the phrases while the mind is relaxed and receptive allows the peripheral circulation

to increase and cardiac and respiratory rates and rhythms to slow and stabilize. Several weeks may be required for the client to feel sensations of heaviness and warmth, although the client usually achieves restful heart rate and respiratory patterning much sooner.

Quieting Response Exercise: The Golden Moment

It is helpful for clients to become aware of external stressors and their internal responses to these stressors on a frequent basis. With the quieting response, clients can learn to manage and change their internal responses while continuing with daily activities.

The following is an abbreviated version of a quieting response that can be performed frequently during the day and takes only 5 to 10 seconds.

Script: *Check your breathing. Notice what is bothering you at this moment. Smile at yourself and say to yourself, "What a silly thing to do to my body!" Take a slow, deep breath to a count of 1-2-3-4, and breathe out slowly to a count of 1-2-3-4. Again, slowly breathe in. As you breathe out, let your body, particularly your lips and jaw, go as limp as possible. Imagine warmth and heaviness flowing down your body to your toes. Allow your eyes to dance and inwardly smile. Go on with your activities, alert and relaxed.*

Developed by Charles Stroebel, a biofeedback clinician and researcher, this intervention is an eclectic combination of stressor identification, breathing techniques, progressive relaxation, changing self-talk, and autogenics. The strategy has been modified into a program called "QR for Kids" to help children identify their body responses to stressors and replace them with relaxation.[59] In this program, children learn to identify what is bothering them, let their eyes sparkle, breathe in through imaginary holes in their feet, and allow their bodies to become warm and relaxed as they exhale. This intervention is reinforced with a variety of imagery exercises.[60]

Effects of Relaxation Therapies

Over the past three decades, practitioners involved in stress reduction, relaxation training, and biofeedback have questioned whether all the various techniques elicit a single relaxation response, as hypothesized by Herbert Benson in 1975, or whether specific practices render specific effects.[61] The latter view proposes that specific cognitive effects are produced by the use of cognitively oriented methods (see the section "Autogenic Training"), autonomic effects are produced by autonomically oriented methods, and muscular effects are produced by muscularly oriented methods (see the section "Progressive Muscle Relaxation"). (See Table 21–3.)

Holistic Nurse Learning Experiment I

One of the most effective tools for understanding relaxation is self-exploration and self-experimentation. Within him- or herself, the nurse is a minilaboratory able to explore these various methods and do his or her own inner research. All that is needed is a journal and the commitment to inner exploration and personal and professional self-development.

A commitment must be made to practice the method for at least 4 to 8 weeks to explore beyond initial positive or negative reactions. Practice each day following your script or tape and keep a journal of your awareness observations: how you felt in your body before and after the session, any areas of comfort or discomfort you noted before or after the session, and so on. (See Exhibit 21–5.)

After practicing, exploring, and writing a journal about your selected practice, you may want to explore another practice in a similar fashion and compare and contrast their effects.

Table 21–3 Hypothesized Effects of Relaxation Techniques

Relaxation Technique	Hypothesized Effect	Researcher
Progressive muscle relaxation (PMR)	Modified PMR might be expected to develop muscular skill.	Davidson and Schwartz (1976)[62]
Autogenic training (AT)	AT might generate both cognitive and somatic effects because it emphasizes body awareness through repeated self-suggestion.	Linden (1993)[63]
AT vs. PMR	AT is particularly effective in cultivating specific sensations suggested in the self-suggestion statements and has much greater effects in that realm than does PMR.	Lehrer et al. (1980)[64] Shapiro and Lehrer (1980)[65]
Relaxation response meditation	Relaxation response elicited is hypothesized to be universal (i.e., all relaxation techniques are considered equivalent).	Benson (1975)[66]

Exhibit 21–5 Inner Laboratory Journal

Name _____

Date _____   Practice method _____

Session no. _____   _____

Place of practice _____

Method of practice: Tapes ☐ _____

Script ☐ _____

Read aloud ☐ _____

Memorized ☐ _____

Other ☐ _____

Pre-Session Awareness

High comfort,   **Low comfort,**
high well-being   **low well-being**

10   0

Describe areas of comfort:

_____

_____

_____

No pain   **High pain**

0   10

Where? (Describe) _____

Post-Session Awareness

Note areas of: ____ Tingling   ____ Heaviness
                      ____ Pulsing   ____ Lightness
                      ____ Throbbing   ____ Calm
                      ____ Warmth   ____ Inner Peace
                      ____ Numbness   ____ Energy Flow

____ Arms   ____ Head   ____ Abdomen
____ Hands   ____ Neck   ____ Back
____ Legs   ____ Face   ____ Chest
____ Feet   ____ Jaw   ____ Shoulders
____ Hips   ____ Eyes   ____ Pelvis

continues

Exhibit 21–5 Continued

Describe any images, thoughts, feelings:

_____

_____

_____

_____

_____

_____

_____

_____

_____

High comfort,	**Low comfort,**
high well-being	**low well-being**
10	**0**

Describe areas of comfort:

_____

_____

_____

No pain	**High pain**
0	**10**

Where? (Describe) _____

Another method of exploration is to invite others to join you in experimenting with the same practice or different ones. Holding periodic group meetings to review your observations and your inner laboratory journals can help you to explore variations in experiences with the same practice and compare and contrast differences in and preferences for various practices.

Selecting Relaxation Interventions for Clients

No formula exists for determining which relaxation intervention is best for which client. The approach must be tailored to the individual based on his or her condition, personal preferences, and available time. A few clients may initially resist the idea of relaxation practice in spite of the nurse's best efforts to present it in a positive manner. In this situation, the issue need not be forced, for the client may accept the intervention at a later time. Taking some time to explore the client's experience and the source of the resistance may reveal misconceptions or myths that further dialogue can dispel. Recall your list of descriptors of a relaxed person and its implications for motivation and client participation from the beginning of this chapter.

The use of tapes that present relaxation instructions in a nonthreatening, gentle manner, often accompanied by soothing music, may hasten acceptance of the intervention. Relaxation videotapes of calming scenes may be left playing on a television set or tranquil music can be played on the home or business audio system as gentle background for daily activities. The following are guidelines for the client in the use of relaxation tapes:

1. Listen to an exercise at least once a day, preferably twice a day.
2. Never listen to a tape when you are driving or operating a vehicle.
3. Arrange to have uninterrupted privacy while you listen to the tape.
4. Listen with headphones to help block out distracting noises from the environment.
5. Listen to the tape in a relaxing position in which your body is supported.

Hypnosis and Self-Hypnosis

Most people misunderstand the use of trance and hypnosis, and associate it with stage professionals and entertainment. However, hypnosis and trance have been used for healing and therapeutic purposes from the times of ancient Egypt and Greece. In these ancient societies, priest healers in healing temples helped their patients evoke a healing trance. Native shamans evoke a trance to seek healing guidance and wisdom for themselves and members of their tribes. In the late eighteenth century, Viennese physician Franz Mesmer offered "magnetic" treatments to his patients that included hypnosis. The word *mesmerized* is now part of our language—an indication of the impact of Mesmer's work.

Hypnosis has been defined in many ways, but most authorities agree that hypnosis brings about some sort of altered awareness and behavior compared with the presumably normal state. In hypnosis, attention can be more focused or more mobile, and there is a tendency for greater responsiveness to suggestion. Once the visual, behavioral, and thinking processes and cues associated with hypnosis are understood, they may be seen to occur spontaneously under a variety of circumstances. According to David Cheeks, an expert in the study of trance and altered states, "hypnotic states may occur when people are frightened, disoriented in space, unconscious, very ill, or stammering."[67] All of these states are states that patients and clients of nurses experience every day, and thus most nurses first encounter their clients and patients in an already altered state of hypersuggestibility. This naturally occurring trance state opens up the client to the influence of nurses' therapeutic presence and therapeutic suggestions.

Remember Cheeks's description of the hypnotic trance of frightened and ill patients and consider how clients and patients are given the news of their diagnosis and prognosis by their physicians in that state of fear and hypersuggestibility. Many patients today still are told that they have only a few months to live or that nothing can be done for them. This nontherapeutic suggestion is being instilled in a patient in a suggestible moment by one of his or her most trusted authorities, the physician. What outcome could be expected? How might the process differ if the client were offered more positive therapeutic suggestions? Nursing experts have been interested in exploring and integrating hypnosis, trance, and therapeutic suggestions because of the history of hypnosis in healing throughout the cultures of the world, because of its natural availability due to client hypersuggestibility during health care crisis, and because of its ease of use and practicality.[68] Dorothy Larkin and many other nurse experts in hypnosis have explored ways in which therapeutic suggestion can enhance patient cooperation and comfort.[69]

Nurses can recognize a hypnotic experience in clients who have a faraway stare, glazed eyes, or fixed attention. Larkin notes that nurses "can utilize this receptive state by offering therapeutic suggestion, reassurance, and health-promoting education. Continual assessment will need to be observed so if the subject's attention suddenly shifts, the nurse can concurrently change the offered therapeutic strategy to meet the patient's needs and altered perceptions."[70(p.88)]

Learning how to use therapeutic suggestion is not foreign to nurses who have used health education to focus clients on healing and health-promoting phrases in order to help them reframe their experiences. Norman Cousins described a reframing experience in which he supported a man on the street who was having a myocardial infarction. Holding the man's hand, Cousins whispered in his ear that the paramedics were on the way and that the man's body was already beginning to heal itself. He helped the patient begin relaxation breathing and continued to reframe the situation through the use of therapeutic suggestion by introducing simple information about the body's ability to restore, rebalance, and heal during a crisis.[71] Imagine how Cousins' approach contrasts with what usually happens with clients who have heart attacks and do not get any information about their condition, have people speak in terms they can't understand, or have others speak in the room as if they were not present.

Therapeutic suggestion is also a vital accompaniment in disbursing medication. For example, the nurse might say, "This medication will help to quiet your nervous system so you can relax more comfortably into sleep." Rather than having the nurse say, "This pill is for your insomnia." Suggestion and hypnosis have been used in a wide variety of clinical settings. Hypnosis has been used by nurses in hospice care, palliative care, home care, and critical care, as well as in burn units and oncology, obstetrics, medicine, and surgery units, to name only a few areas. (See Table 21–2.)

All nurses can learn to use reframing and positive therapeutic suggestion, and to recognize an everyday hypnotic trance state in clients in crisis (also see the section "Cryptotrauma" later in this chapter). Some nurses may want to pursue hypnosis as an area of expertise by receiving reputable training and exploring the "Resources" and "Suggested Readings" sections at the end of the chapter, which offer sources for further information. Nurses can also practice self-hypnosis and therapeutic suggestion as part of their personal self-care, in addition to teaching clients this practice so that they can continue self-care at home.

Biofeedback

Another modern form of the ancient healing art of relaxation uses modern technological equipment that most nurses employ daily to monitor psychophysiologic change. This combination of ancient awareness practice and technology is called biofeedback. Biofeedback was termed the "yoga of the West" by Elmer and Alyce Green, researchers and early biofeedback pioneers at the Menniger Institute in Topeka, Kansas.[72] When the devices monitoring the unitary body-mind-spirit are turned so that clients can see their displays, clients learn how to read their bodies' signals more accurately and are empowered to make therapeutic changes. Educating clients about how their bodies respond to stress and teaching them how to react more healthfully is the work of biofeedback.

Recall what has just been explored with regard to therapeutic hypnotic suggestion and reframing and imagine how this new knowledge and awareness might be used to empower clients as they encounter the monitors and other technical equipment in the health care setting. If you can imagine turning your monitors around and teaching clients the positive meaning of the monitor's signals so that they can understand how their bodies respond to thoughts and feelings, then you have already begun to understand the impact and usefulness of biofeedback. Biofeedback machines can measure many functions of the unitary body-mind-spirit. Whether the biofeedback comes from a temperature monitor measuring hand temperature or from Kirlian photography showing the energy field as displayed on a computer, clients are learning something that, prior to the use of this technology, may have been hidden from their perception. With practice, clients can tune their inner awareness to become like the Yogis and learn to influence and control these previously imperceptible and seemingly uncontrollable signals.

The most widely used biofeedback monitors include temperature-sensing units for measuring vasodilatation of extremities, electromyographs for monitoring motor neuron activity of the muscles, electroencephalographs for measuring brain-wave frequencies and patterns, and electrodermal response units for measuring electrical activation of the sweat glands. Heart rate and blood pressure monitors are also widely used in biofeedback (Exhibit 21–6).

Biofeedback has been practiced since the 1960s. Its focus is to teach clients to create "psychosomatic health," as Elmer Green would put it, instead of psychosomatic illness.[73] This goal is accomplished with the assistance of the biofeedback equipment and the nurse therapist. Specialized training and certification in biofeedback is available through the Association for Applied Psychophysiology and Biofeedback and the Biofeedback Certification Institute of America (see "Resources" section). Both organizations are established multidisciplinary groups that integrate the sciences and arts of engineering, psychology, neuroscience, research, education, healing, meditation, and yoga.

Exhibit 21–6 Clinical Indicators for Biofeedback

Neuromuscular disorders
  Chronic muscle contraction
  Movement disorders
  Spasticity
Central nervous system disorders
  Stroke
  Some epilepsies
Vascular disorders
  Raynaud's disease
  Migraine
Pain
  Headache
  Back pain
Gastrointestinal and genitourinary disorders
  Urinary and fecal incontinence
  Urinary and fecal retention
Stress reduction
  Insomnia
  Anxiety
  Phobias
  Alcoholism/addiction
  Attention-deficit hyperactivity disorder
  Procedure-related anxiety

Holistic Nurse Learning Experiment II

Biofeedback can offer nurses the opportunity for independent professional practice, whether in private practice or in institutional settings. Many nurses integrate biofeedback into relaxation therapy, stress management, health counseling, and teaching. Other nurses specialize in neurofeedback applications for the care of insomnia, depression, addictions, and attention-deficit hyperactivity disorder. Another area of particular interest to nurses is the use of electromyography to help clients manage urinary and fecal incontinence (see Table 21–2). All these areas of specialization require extensive study, practice, and mentoring. However, every nurse can benefit from using simple biofeedback principles and techniques in everyday nursing practice. Learning to understand these biofeedback principles from the inside out is the purpose of the following series of experiments. One or two psycho-physiologic monitors, paper, and a pen are required. Any monitors available—pulse oximetry, blood pressure, heart rate, incentive spirometer—can be used, or an inexpensive temperature-sensing unit can be purchased (see "Resources" section).

Allow 30 minutes for the exercise. Make yourself comfortable. Make sure the environment is relaxing and is as quiet as possible, and that there will be no interruptions. Set up the biofeedback equipment and attach the leads to yourself so you can easily monitor your responses. Pick only one or two types of equipment, such as an extremity temperature monitor and an automatic blood pressure and/or oxygen saturation rate monitor. If you are setting up a temperature unit, begin by attaching the ceramic end of the wire (called the thermister) to the fleshy, palmar surface of your fingertip (see Figure 21–1). Run the

wire down along the length of the finger and attach the thermister with paper tape so the tape covers the end of the ceramic tip. You should begin to see changes in the temperature as the heat of your finger warms the thermister. Do not use plastic tape when attaching a thermister because it creates a greenhouse effect and can alter the accuracy of the readings.

The warmer the hands, the greater the blood flow and circulation to the extremities, indicating quieting of the sympathetic nervous system and quieting of the fight or flight response. Cooling extremities demonstrate the opposite: decrease in blood flow and circulation in the extremities, and an increase in the fight or flight response. Normal hand temperature readings can range from 65°F to 99°F.

Sit quietly for 3 to 5 minutes, then notice your readings on the temperature unit and any other unit you have chosen to monitor.

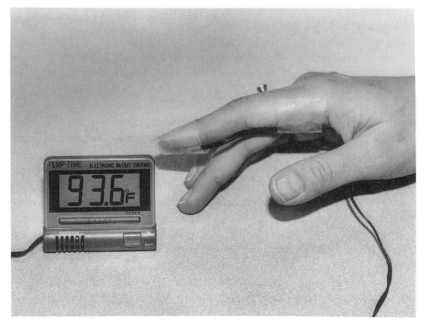

Figure 21–1 Biofeedback Temperature Unit. Finger with Thermister Attached. Ceramic tip of biofeedback thermal probe (thermister) is attached to palmar tip of finger. Tip of thermister is covered with paper tape and wire is attached to finger as demonstrated in photograph (clear tape is used in the photograph so that placement of thermister is visible).

Try to check your readings with as little disturbance to the quiet of the experience as possible. These primary or initial readings are called your baseline readings. Write down these baseline readings. If you are comfortable, remain attached to the biofeedback monitors. Make sure that your body is supported and that you can easily see the monitors with as little movement as possible. Next, perform one of your favorite relaxation or meditation practices for 10 to 20 minutes.

Take readings immediately at the end of the session in a quiet, unhurried way so as not to disturb your relaxation. Notice any difference in your readings before and after the practice. What did the readings demonstrate about your practice experience? What change did you experience inside? Were these changes reflected in your biofeedback readings?

If you notice a drop in the temperature of your hands during or after a relaxation practice, check the following:

1. Did you feel hurried?
2. Were you trying too hard to relax?
3. Were you thinking about something other than the relaxation practice or wondering what the monitors would show?
4. Was the room warm enough?
5. Were there any interruptions, expected or unexpected, such as people entering the room, phones ringing, etc.?

Whatever the results are, they can only help to deepen your understanding of the internal awareness and responses involved in these special practices. Remember to adopt the attitude of nonjudgmental observer and explore your inner awareness. Examine Exhibit 21–7 to determine whether any of these factors can help to explain your response. With practice, you may notice an increase in your prerelaxation or postrelaxation temperature reading.

Exhibit 21–7 Important Factors in Relaxation Practice

- **Passive volition:** Letting go, being without doing or striving, allowing, being with the process as it unfolds rather than making it happen; planting a seed in the mind of wanting to relax and then letting go and watching the process.
- **Attention to the here and now:** Being oriented toward the present, not caught up in what happened or what might happen.
- **Altered perception of time:** Experiencing time as expanded or contracted. Relaxation practice can change the perception of time so that a very short practice session feels like a long time or a long practice session is experienced as a few moments.
- **Enjoyment of practice:** Committing to practice and, even more importantly, enjoying practice. Most traditional healers and teachers of the restorative arts ask their students if they are enjoying their practice. Finding a practice that helps one weather the storms of life and enhances one's inner connection is a joy.

Holistic Nursing Experiment II (Variations)

Variation A: Client Practice

Try the biofeedback experiment described above on a client. Use an abbreviated form of the experiment (5 to 10 minutes) with clients, taking readings before and after relaxation practice. Explore and explain the meanings of the readings and invite the client to describe what he or she felt inside and what he or she feels the readings mean.

This technique provides an opportunity for health care teaching and counseling to move from client compliance into client empowerment. Teaching clients how anxiety, worry, and stress can produce higher blood pressure, cooler hands, and tenser muscles, and how relaxation can produce the opposite responses, is an easy way to begin a dialogue providing clients with insight into the stressors of their lives and how they respond to them.

Variation B: Group Self-Care Experiment

Try relaxation/biofeedback in a group (Figure 21–2). Start with a group of colleagues rather than a group of clients. Later you can begin to introduce this technique to a group of clients as you gain experience and knowledge with the practice. Schedule a relaxation break for your unit. Take 15 minutes at the beginning of a staff meeting or schedule the relaxation practice during a lunch break every week or month. A relatively quiet room with chairs arranged in a circle, flowers for the center of the circle, and some music will be required. Invite each person to bring a small journal and pen and obtain a biofeedback temperature monitor for each person. Small alcohol thermometers are the least expensive temperature monitors; liquid crystal cards, dots, or bands also work. If electronic temperature units or finger alcohol thermometers are used, attach the unit to the palmar surface of the finger with paper tape (see Figure 21–1). Agree as a group to meet on a regular basis, keep a journal of individual progress, and begin and end on time so that people can easily return to work or finish lunch.

Set up the room in advance so that the flowers are in the center of the circle of chairs. Have members of the group attach their temperature monitors. Allow 1 to 2 minutes before taking the first baseline reading. Next, introduce a relaxation exercise. You can continue to play music or turn the music down or off, while one of the group members offers a relaxation practice. The role of relaxation leader can be rotated. Depending on the interests of the group, the same practice can be carried out at each meeting or different practices can be offered each week.

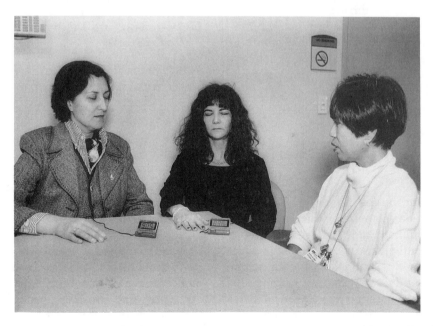

Figure 21–2 Nursing Group Practicing Biofeedback. Nurses practice biofeedback hand-warming as part of self-care/patient care as they are led in a guided meditation by their nurse colleague.

After the relaxation practice, group members take another monitor reading and write journal entries on their experiences and responses. A few minutes should be left for group members to explore and share their experiences with one another. Observe what happens over time. Invite group members to track their medication use and observe overall changes in blood pressure, headaches, pain, anxiety, and so on.

Special Issues. "I don't have time. I'm too busy. I could be/should be catching up on my work, not relaxing." Sandy O'Brien and Jeanne Anselmo developed a staff wellness project using the practices described above.[74] The answer they found to the challenge of "I don't have time to practice" is that we cannot afford *not* to take time to center ourselves and care for ourselves in order to do the best for our own health while offering the best of care to our clients and families.

While relaxation practice does take time and commitment, most groups learn to avoid giving in to the work-and-hurry sickness and begin to enjoy the benefits of stopping, calming, and letting go.

Cautions and Contraindications for Relaxation, Meditation, and Biofeedback

Medications. Clients who take insulin, thyroid replacement medication, antihypertensives, cardiac medications, antianxiety agents, and sleep medications must be monitored for a change in their symptoms and medication needs as they learn to deepen their relaxation response. As clients learn to regulate their stress response, their medication requirements may change. Work closely with clients' prescribing providers to ensure that their medications are titrated properly.[75]

Education and Information. Discussing issues and experiences associated with relaxation before and after each session helps to involve the client, positively empower them, and reframe any of the anticipatory anxiety or questions they may have.

Mental Health History. Clients with a history of dissociative experiences, acute psychosis, borderline personality, and posttraumatic stress disorder are best cared for by nurses and professionals skilled in treating such clients. Check your client's mental health history before beginning relaxation practice.[76]

Cryptotrauma. Many patients have experienced undiagnosed physical and/or psychologic trauma. Many times patients are reluctant to disclose these problems, and many times health professionals are unskilled in or uncomfortable with exploring these issues. Domino and Haber reported that 66 percent of women at a multidisciplinary pain center with chronic headaches had a prior history of physical and/or sexual abuse (61 percent had experienced physical abuse; 11 percent, sexual abuse; and 28 percent, both physical and sexual abuse). The average duration of abuse was 8 years.[77]

The term *cryptotrauma* indicates that the trauma which is the cause of the patient's pain is hidden or has not been revealed. Signals to watch for in clients with posttraumatic stress disorder and/or cryptotrauma include

- hypervigilance
- difficulty falling or staying asleep
- irritability or outbursts of rage
- difficulty concentrating
- exaggerated startle response
- dissociation
- addiction
- flashbacks
- numbing
- panic attacks
- disturbed self-perception, denigration
- isolation
- inability to be comfortable with touch
- nightmares[78]

Even with the most sensitive and careful history taking and preparations, clients with such disorders can have flashbacks related to the underlying trauma. If this occurs, first, do not panic. Remember your intention to help and support, and trust your therapeutic bond with the client. Second, center and ground yourself. Clients in a panic state related to anxiety or flashback are supersensitive to people around them; centering, calming, and grounding yourself will deeply help them. Third, reassure the client, speak to the client in a calm, soothing voice. Have the client open his or her eyes, feel their feet on the floor, or touch the furniture; if possible, have the client tighten and release their hands and feet and be aware of their body and of being with you in the present. If appropriate, hold the client's hand; use your judgment. Fourth, remember that the information with which the client is getting in touch is important for the client's wholeness and healing. A simple, short statement explaining this to the client helps to reframe the situation and plant therapeutic suggestions during these most open and suggestible moments. Seek appropriate referrals for the client as needed.

Restorative Practices

As explored above, relaxation practice can help the individual to center and open to loving-kindness, inner awareness, and connectedness in meditation, to cultivate the relaxation response, and to develop self-regulation abilities through biofeedback. Relaxation practice also brings the gifts of restoring, opening, and renewing.

Yoga

In restorative yoga, practitioners open themselves more deeply to the healing energies that flow through them in each posture (asana). They accomplish this by supporting their bodies in yoga poses using bolsters, pillows, and blankets.[79]

Yoga is a philosophy of living that unites physical, mental, and spiritual health. When practiced for the purpose of relaxation, it involves breathing and stretching exercises and postures. The exercises vary greatly in difficulty. Because yoga starts with very gentle stretches and breathing techniques, it is ideally suited for clients with stiff muscles and decreased activity levels who are attempting to begin an active relaxation and exercise program. Clients need not embrace the philosophy to benefit from the activity.

Daily practice of restorative yoga (even 10 to 15 minutes a day) creates more energy, restorative rest, and calm. Restorative yoga is a wonderful practice to perform during a break at work. (See the "Resources" section for more information.)

Qi Gong

Seasonal Qi Gong practices restore and renew, and center and open meridians as the energy field and body changes with the seasons. Some techniques of Chinese Qi Gong have been practiced for at least 5,000 years. Simple movements are combined with breath and meditation in a flow with nature's healing qi. Restoration and healing come from daily practice. Qi Gong practices are a part of Chinese medicine, which includes acupuncture, external Qi Gong (receiving healing energy from a healer or master), herbal medicine, diet, massage, and self-care. (See "Resources" section.)

Restorative Gardens

"Nature alone heals"[80] is one of Nightingale's most famous quotes. What Nightingale knew, gardeners and nature lovers also know, that nature can heal and cure. Many hospitals and health care centers are creating healing gardens, restorative gardens, greenhouses, meditative gardens, and labyrinths in their plazas, lobbies, rooftops, and other inner and outer spaces to help cultivate relaxation, renewal, and peace. Bringing nature inside the healing environment is not at all new and dates back to medieval monastic healing sanctuaries. The medieval architectural designs included low windows so that patients could look out at nature's beauty.

Simply helping clients to be with nature amid the high-tech health care system can improve well-being, reduce anxiety, and calm fears. Nurses themselves can benefit from resting in a garden or creating natural spaces within the health care setting.[81]

HOLISTIC CARING PROCESS

Assessment

In preparing to use relaxation interventions, the nurse assesses the following parameters and lived experiences:

- the client's perception of personal tension levels and need to relax
- the client's readiness and motivation to learn relaxation strategies, because relaxation is a very subjective and personal endeavor
- the client's past experience with the process of relaxation, hypnosis, or meditation
- the client's personal definition and lived experience of what it means to be relaxed
- the client's ability to remain comfortably in one position for 15 to 30 minutes
- the client's hearing acuity, so that the nurse can speak at an appropriate level while guiding the client in relaxation exercises
- the client's religious beliefs, so that the nurse can present the relaxation process in a way that will meld comfortably with the client's belief system
- the client's level of pain or discomfort, anxiety, fear, or boredom

- the client's perception of reality, history of depersonalization states, and locus of control, because deep relaxation may exacerbate the symptoms of psychotic and prepsychotic individuals
- the client's medication intake, particularly of medications that may alter response to relaxation or may need to be titrated as relaxation progresses

A questionnaire may be used to complete the assessment. The information gathered in the questionnaire provides starting points for discussion and further exploration.

Patterns/Problems/Needs

The following are the patterns/problems/needs compatible with relaxation interventions that are related to the nine human response patterns (see Chapter 14):

- **Relating:** Social isolation
- **Choosing:** Altered coping; ineffective individual and family
- **Moving:** Activity intolerance, actual or potential
  Deficit in diversional activity
- **Perceiving:** Powerlessness
  Altered self-concept; disturbance in self-esteem, role performance, personal identity
  Altered sensation/perception: visual, auditory, kinesthetic, gustatory, tactile, olfactory
- **Knowing:** Altered thought processes
- **Feeling:** Anxiety
  Altered comfort: pain
  Fear
  Potential for violence: self-directed or directed at others

Outcomes

Exhibit 21–8 guides the nurse in client outcomes, nursing prescriptions, and evaluations for the use of relaxation as a nursing intervention.

Therapeutic Care Plan and Interventions

Before the Session

- Become personally familiar with the experience of the relaxation intervention before approaching the client.
- If the client has previous positive experience with a particular relaxation intervention, encourage further practice and use of that intervention.
- Review with the client his or her lived experience and gather information from the chart, diaries, and/or verbal

self-report concerning pain, anxiety, and activity levels since last session.

Preparation of the Environment (Ideal)

- Arrange medical and nursing care to allow for 15 to 45 minutes of uninterrupted time.
- Keep the room warm and ventilated, not cold.
- Shut the door or otherwise decrease extraneous noise and distraction. Place a note on the door indicating a need for privacy until a designated time.
- Unplug the telephone or ask a family member or roommate to answer the telephone should it ring during the relaxation training session.
- Reduce the lighting to a low level.
- Use natural or incandescent lighting if possible; fluorescent lighting can cause headaches in some patients.

Exhibit 21–8 Nursing Interventions: Relaxation

Client Outcomes	Nursing Prescriptions	Evaluation
The client will demonstrate decreased anxiety, tension, and other manifestations of the stress response as a result of the relaxation intervention.	Guide the client in the relaxation exercise. Evaluate for decrease in anxiety, tension, and other manifestations of the stress response as evidenced by heart rate within normal limits, decreased respiratory rates, return of blood pressure toward normal, resolution of anxious facial expressions and mannerisms, decrease in repetitious talking or behavior and inability to sleep or restlessness.	The client exhibited decreased anxiety, tension, and other manifestations of the stress response as evidenced by normal vital signs; a slow, deep breathing pattern; and decreased anxious behaviors.
The client will demonstrate a stabilization or decrease in pain as a result of the relaxation intervention.	Evaluate for decrease in pain as evidenced by reduction or elimination of pain control medication and increased activities or mobility.	The client's intake of pain medication stabilized and then decreased with relaxation skills practice. The client began to participate in activities previously limited by pain.
The client will link breathing awareness to a commonly occurring cue and use this combination to reduce tension.	Teach awareness of breathing patterns and habitual linking of relaxing breathing to a cue in the environment.	The client used turning in bed as a cue to take a slow, deep breath and relax jaw muscles.

Client Comfort Measures

- Have the client empty his or her bladder before starting the intervention.
- Help the client find a comfortable sitting or reclining position with hands resting by the sides or on the thighs.
- Ensure the client's comfort by providing a blanket or by adjusting the thermostat to a comfortably warm setting; have small, soft pillows available for positioning.

Timing of the Session (Ideal)

- Hold the training session before meals or more than 2 hours after the last meal. A full stomach coupled with relaxation may lead to sleep.

Support Tools

- Have available music tapes and a tape recorder/player.
- If the session is to be followed by drawing, have paper, crayons, or markers available.
- Tell the client that you may be asking simple yes or no questions during the session to check the comfort level of the music or to confirm the client's understanding of verbal instructions. The client may answer these questions by raising a preestablished yes finger or no finger or nodding the head.

At the Beginning of the Session

- Review briefly the potential benefits of relaxation intervention and enlist the client's cooperation. Explore client's lived experience of relaxation and stress.
- Explain to the client that relaxation may be easier if practiced with the eyes closed. The client may drift off to sleep, but this position allows the client to focus attention inward while remaining awake. This may take practice to accomplish, and many times clients fall asleep due to exhaustion or lack of sleep. In such a case, the restorative dimension of relaxation is at work.

- Explain that one purpose of breathing and relaxation exercises is to experience inward relaxation and become aware of the body-mind-spirit connections associated with relaxation.
- Emphasize that you are merely a guide and that any therapeutic results obtained from the session are due to the client's involvement, interest, and practice.
- Let go of outcomes. There is an ebb and flow to the learning experience. Encourage the client to practice for comfort and awareness, noting shifts in breathing, anxiety, and sensations.
- Arrive at mutually agreeable goals for the session, such as reduction of pain, decreased time to sleep onset, or reduction of anxiety.
- Have the client quantify the level of the parameter to be changed; for example, "My pain or anxiety level right now is 7 on a scale of 0 (none) to 10 (extreme pain)." Record the level before and after the session.
- Record baseline vital signs; if biofeedback equipment is used, record baseline readings.
- Assure the client that sensations of heaviness, warmth, floating, or lightness are naturally occurring indications of deep relaxation; explain that the client can end the experience at any moment he or she desires by opening the eyes, tightening the fists, and/or stretching; this will orient the client and enable the exercise to continue.
- Begin soft background music. (See Chapter 23 for suggestions regarding music selection.)
- Guide the client through a basic breathing relaxation exercise. Breathing exercises may be repeated slowly for several minutes as an introduction to deeper relaxation.

- Start the session with short breathing or relaxation exercises (5 minutes); lengthen the exercises (to 10 to 20 minutes) as the client becomes better able to relax and attend to inner thoughts and feelings.

During the Session

- Phrase all therapeutic suggestions and self-statements in a positive form. For example, say "I am aware of comfort moving down my arm and into my hand," rather than, "I am not in pain." These suggestions enhance the process and reframe the experience.
- Speak in a relaxed manner. Ask the client for feedback concerning the appropriateness of the practice and his or her ability to hear the background music and instructions. Have the client respond with a finger movement (using signals established before the session) or nod of the head, and make adjustments as necessary.
- Pace your instructions according to the following visual cues from the client. Each indicates a deepening of relaxation.
  - change in breathing pattern: slower, deeper breaths progressing to slow, somewhat shallower breathing as relaxation deepens
  - more audible breathing
  - fluttering of eyelids
  - blanching of the skin around the nose and mouth
  - easing of jaw tightness, sometimes to the extent that the lips part and the jaw drops slightly
  - if client is supine, pointing of toes outward rather than straight up
  - complete lack of muscle holding (ask client's permission to lift arm gently by the wrist; no resistance should be felt and the arm should move as easily as any other object of similar weight
- Modify your instructions and strategies to fit the situation. Encourage an intubated and ventilated patient who cannot control respiratory rate or volume to drop the jaw and allow the rhythm of the ventilator to soothe tight muscles, for example. Gently placing your hand over the clavicle or holding the person's hand as you speak can increase the human bond for relaxation.
- Intersperse your instructions with therapeutic suggestions of encouragement that the client can use after the session as cues to recapture aspects of the relaxation experience. Examples of such phrases are:
  - Perhaps you are noticing a softening of your muscles.
  - As you take your next breath, become aware of how the warmth is flowing down your arm.
  - Deep breathing helps to replenish the oxygen and energy of the body and helps the body heal, relax, restore, and renew.
- As the client relaxes, he or she may experience a release of emotional life issues, which can surface in the conscious mind. Be alert for signs of emotional discomfort or letting go, such as tears or a change in breathing to deeper, faster breaths. If such a sign occurs, ask gentle questions (e.g., "Can you put those feelings into words and express them safely?") and allow time for the client to express and deal with the material before continuing with or concluding the session. See the section on cryptotrauma for more information on helping clients stay grounded if they tap into emotion-laden material. Often, clients in a deeply relaxed state gain insight into how to resolve problems or which directions to take in their lives.

At the End of the Session

- Bring the client gradually into a wakeful state by suggesting that he or she take deep, energizing breaths, begin to move hands and feet, and stretch;

orient the client to the room, talking with the client about the comfort he or she created.

- Have the client reevaluate, on the scale of 0 to 10 used earlier, the level of comfort or severity of the parameter previously selected to be changed. Record the level.
- Allow time for discussion of the experience, including discussion of the techniques that seemed especially effective and the client's physical, emotional, and energy awareness. Invite the client to express his or her experience by writing, making a journal entry, or drawing. Different clients will prefer different methods, such as creating an abstract drawing, offering a story, or writing poetry, to express their experience.
- Ensure that medication changes, if indicated, are appropriately monitored.
- Engage the client in continuing practice on an individually assigned basis until the next session.
- Help the client choose supportive measures for practicing his or her relaxation skill.
- Review a log or journal in which the client records relaxation practice, symptoms, medications, time, and results.

Case Studies

Case Study No. 1

Setting:	Outpatient; multidisciplinary holistic health care center
Client:	S.D., a 47-year-old African-American man with family history of stroke
Medical Diagnosis:	Progressive essential hypertension, unresponsive to any antihypertensive therapy
Current Medications:	Catapres, Lasix, Valium, Minipress, potassium chloride
Nursing Diagnoses:	1. Altered physical regulation (essential hypertension)
	2. Anxiety

3. Fear
4. Powerlessness
5. Ineffective coping related to anxiety, stress of job, and parenting of five children
6. Self-esteem disturbance, situational

S.D. had been diagnosed with severe uncontrollable essential hypertension. He scrupulously took his antihypertensive medications and had had an extensive clinical workup to rule out any secondary causes. S.D. was very frustrated, because his father had died of a stroke and S.D. did not want to have a stroke or "die young." He and his wife cared for their five children. He worked at a job that required him to perform physical labor and walk up and down three flights of stairs.

His physician sent him to learn biofeedback-assisted relaxation as an adjunctive therapy. His blood pressure at rest while on medication ranged from 160/100 to 200/120 millimeters of mercury (mm Hg). To reduce S.D.'s fear and feeling of powerlessness, the nurse explored his lived experience of his condition and used health care teaching and stress management counseling to reframe his understanding of what was happening in his body.

The nurse explained to S.D. that his body knew very well how to respond to stress, but that he needed the opportunity and the time to recover from stress and learn less physically distressing ways to respond. S.D. was shown how to use the temperature trainer and a small galvanic skin response unit that indicated sympathetic outflow by measuring sweat gland response. He was taught simple breathing exercises and autogenic phrases while he learned to monitor his body-mind-spirit response on the biofeedback displays.

Because of the urgency and critical nature of his situation, he was invited to participate in three practice sessions a week for 1 month instead of the usual one session per week. He was asked to practice the relaxation two times a day. Within the first two weeks, he had brought his blood pressure down to 140/100 mm Hg. He continued sessions each week during the second month and then continued practice on his own. After 3 months, his blood pressure was 140/80 mm Hg while he continued on the same level of medication.

After 1 year, his medication level was reduced, and blood pressure was maintained at 140/80 mm Hg. The nurse scheduled a meeting with S.D., his wife, and all their children to explore their needs, fears, and concerns about S.D.'s health. The family agreed to help support S.D. in his health care practice by making sure he was not disturbed during his practice time. The opportunity to share their love and support and to understand how their loved one was working to help himself offered them a new understanding of their father/husband, his health care issues, and how they could be active in his wellness plan.

Case Study No. 2

Setting:	Home care and hospital preoperative and postoperative care
Client:	M.D., a 76-year-old European American woman undergoing surgery for renal tumor
Nursing Diagnoses:	1. Altered physical regulation (renal tumor)
	2. Anxiety
	3. Fear
	4. Ineffective coping related to renal tumor, possible cancer
	5. Powerlessness

M.D. complained of back pain. A sonogram revealed a large renal tumor. The surgeon told M.D. and her husband the results of the sonogram and recommended surgery within the next 5 days. M.D. and her husband were very upset after their visit to the surgeon and consulted with a nurse in private practice about methods of readying for surgery.

Because of M.D.'s shock and anxiety, and her fear about the possible outcome of the surgery, the nurse discussed with the cli-

ent, her family, and the surgeon whether or not the surgery had to be performed immediately. The surgeon had determined that the tumor was a slow-growing mass that had been present for at least 2 years. The surgeon agreed that the surgery could be scheduled 2 weeks later to give M.D. time to prepare her body-mind-spirit for the experience.

M.D. was taught breathing and meditation exercises, began receiving Reiki energy sessions, and, with preoperative teaching, began to create visualizations of surgery as a healing experience. The 2-week delay gave her a chance to reduce the shock and include her family and her parish in her preparation. Members of her women's group at the church prayed for her and were "breathing toward her," sending spiritual energy, love, and support. Her family from out of town had an opportunity to come and escort her to the hospital. Most importantly, she was able to prepare and practice her relaxation healing surgery experience so that, in the preoperative room, she was so relaxed that she told the nurse she was resting on the "breath of God."

Her relaxation practice included quiet meditation, prayer, deep breathing, and visualization of each of the steps that would occur, from the night before the surgery through the ride to the hospital, the preoperative preparation, surgery, and recovery.

Interspersed throughout her educational preparation were the therapeutic suggestions that there would be very little pain or bleeding and no infection from the surgery, and that everyone who was in contact with her could be a vehicle for sending healing light and energy. Every intravenous line, medication, procedure, and caretaker became a part of her visualization.

M.D.'s holistic nurse went with her into the preoperative area and helped her practice her relaxation strategies; the nurse also informed the rest of the surgical team of M.D.'s plan to practice during the surgery. The staff wanted to know if their other patients could learn these practices, since M.D.'s response was so positive.

Exhibit 21–9 Evaluation of the Client's Subjective Experience of Relaxation

1. Was this a new experience for you? Can you describe it?
2. Did you have any physical or emotional responses to the relaxation exercises? If so, can you describe them?
3. Do you feel different after this experience? How?
4. How does your bodymind communicate with you when your stress level is at an uncomfortable point?
5. Would you like to do this again?
6. Were there any distractions to your relaxation?
7. What would make this a more pleasant experience for you?
8. How do you see yourself integrating relaxation skills into your daily life?

M.D.'s surgery went well. She did have cancer, but she continued to use the practices she had learned and extended them into an ongoing wellness plan. These practices improved her well-being, energy, and spirit; enhanced her immune function; and slowed the progression of the disease. She died 4 years later, practicing relaxation through to the moment of her death. These practices wove together her spiritual life, her desire to be an active participant in her care, and her understanding of her health, wellness, and well-being.

Evaluation

With the client, the nurse determines whether the client outcomes for relaxation interventions (see Exhibit 21–8) were successfully achieved. To evaluate the session further, the nurse may again explore the subjective effects of the experience with the client (Exhibit 21–9). Because the accomplishment of these interventions may take place over a period of days or weeks, they must be reviewed and reevaluated periodically. Continuing support and encouragement are necessary.

Relaxation exercises can be taught to clients under almost any circumstances. They not only reduce the fear and anxiety associated with many medical and nursing interventions but, once learned, may be used in all aspects of a client's life. They increase the overall movement toward wholeness and balance for both client and nurse, and they facilitate other interventions by allowing the client to move toward learning and participating more fully in his or her own health promotion.

DIRECTIONS FOR FUTURE RESEARCH

1. Correlate the changes in psychophysiology with the specific relaxation interventions used to determine the most effective interventions and their presentation.
2. Conduct tightly structured studies to evaluate relaxation techniques, using control groups to validate changes brought about by relaxation exercises.
3. Monitor and validate the effect of the "compassionate guide" in the relaxation process.
4. Conduct qualitative studies to explore the meaning of the client's lived experience of phenomena relevant to nursing.

NURSE HEALER REFLECTIONS

After reading this chapter, the nurse healer will be able to answer or begin the process of answering the following questions:

- How does my inner experience of tension or anxiety shift when I release my muscle tightness?
- How do I model relaxation to my family, friends, colleagues, and clients?
- What is my kinesthetic experience of letting go of tension, concerns, and physical and emotional stresses?
- What cues about my inner experience of tension or relaxation do I receive from my breathing pattern?
- How do I cultivate peace of mind as I move through my potentially stressful job activities?
- Am I aware that my attitudes toward my tasks are contagious to my clients?

NOTES

1. G. Fuller, *Biofeedback: Methods and Procedures in Clinical Practice* (San Francisco: The Biofeedback Institute of San Francisco, 1977), 1.

2. N. Meinhart and M. McCaffery, *Pain: A Nursing Approach to Assessment and Analysis* (East Norwalk, CT: Appleton-Century-Crofts, 1983), 377.

3. K. Phillips, Biofeedback as an Aid to Autogenic Training, in *Mind and Cancer Prognosis*, ed. B. Stoll (New York: John Wiley & Sons, 1979), 153.

4. M. McCaffery, Relieving Pain with Noninvasive Techniques, *Nursing 80*, no. 12 (1980): 57.

5. F. Nightingale, *Notes on Nursing, Commemorative Edition* (Philadelphia: J.B. Lippincott Co., 1992), 28.

6. J. Kabat-Zinn, *Full Catastrophe Living: Using the Wisdom of Your Body and Mind To Face Stress, Pain, and Illness* (New York, NY: Bantam Doubleday Dell Publishing Group, 1990).

7. D. Ornish, *Dr. Dean Ornish's Program for Reversing Heart Disease* (New York: Random House, 1990).

8. D. Kreiger, *Accepting Your Power To Heal: The Personal Practice of Therapeutic Touch* (Santa Fe, NM: Bear and Co. Publishing, 1993), 17–20.

9. A. Chah, The Fine Arts of Relaxation, Concentration, and Meditation, © Joel and Michelle Levey, 1987, 199. Reprinted with permission of Wisdom Publications, Somerville, MA.

10. B. Malone, presentation at the Nursing Visioning Summit II: Celebrating Our Diversity, Our Wisdom, and Our Community, Omega Institute, Rhinebeck, NY, October 1998.

11. Kabat-Zinn, *Full Catastrophe Living*, 248–273.

12. H. Benson et al., Decreased Premature Ventricular Contraction through the Use of the Relaxation Response in Patients with Stable Ischemic Heart Disease, *Lancet* 2, no. 7931 (1975): 380.

13. M. Frenn et al., Reducing the Stress of Cardiac Catheterization by Teaching Relaxation, *Dimensions of Critical Care Nursing* 5, no. 2 (1986): 108–116.

14. H. Benson, *Beyond the Relaxation Response* (New York: Times Books, 1984).

15. Benson, *Beyond the Relaxation Response*.

16. H. Benson, Your Innate Asset for Combating Stress, in *Relax: How You Can Feel Better, Reduce Stress, and Overcome Tension*, ed. J. White and J. Fodeman (New York: Confucian Press, 1976), 53–54.

17. Benson, Your Innate Asset for Combating Stress.

18. Benson, Your Innate Asset for Combating Stress.

19. Benson, Your Innate Asset for Combating Stress.

20. J. Kabat-Zinn, *Full Catastrophe Living*.

21. H. Benson et al., Decreased Blood Pressure in Borderline Hypertensive Subjects Who Practiced Meditation, *Journal of Chronic Diseases* 27 (1974): 163–169.

22. H. Benson et al., Decreased Blood Pressure in Pharmacologically Treated Hypertensive Patients Who Regularly Elicited the Relaxation Response, *Lancet* 1 (1974), 289–291.

23. J. Kabat-Zinn et al., Effectiveness of a Meditation-Based Stress Reduction Program in the Treatment of Anxiety Disorders, *American Journal of Psychiatry* 149, no. 7 (1992): 936–943.

24. J. Miller et al., Three Year Follow Up and Clinical Implication of Mindfulness Meditation-Based Stress Reduction Intervention in the Treatment of Anxiety Disorders, *General Hospital Psychiatry* 17 (1995): 192–200.

25. J. Kabat-Zinn, An Outpatient Program in Behavioral Medicine for Chronic Pain Patients on the Practice of Mindfulness Meditation: Theoretical Considerations and Preliminary Results, *General Hospital Psychiatry* 4 (1982): 33–47.

26. J. Kabat-Zinn et al., Four-Year Follow Up of a Meditation-Based Program for the Self Regulation of Chronic Pain: Treatment Outcomes and Compliance, *Clinical Journal of Pain* 2 (1987): 154–173.

27. J. Bernhard et al., Effects of Relaxation and Visualization Technique as an Adjunct to Phototherapy and Photochemotherapy of Psoriasis [correspondence], *Journal of the American Academy of Dermatology* 19, no. 3 (1988): 572–573.

28. D. Ornish et al., Can Lifestyle Changes Reverse Coronary Artery Disease? *Lancet* 336 (1990): 129.

29. Ornish et al., Can Lifestyle Changes Reverse Coronary Artery Disease?

30. Ornish, *Dr. Dean Ornish's Program for Reversing Heart Disease*.

31. K. Ankun et al., Research on "Anti-Aging" Effect of Qi Gong, *Journal of Traditional Chinese Medicine* 2, no. 2 (1991): 153.

32. Y. Lim et al., Effects of Qi Gong on Cardiorespiratory Changes: A Preliminary Study, *American Journal of Chinese Medicine* 21, no. 1 (1993): 106.

33. C.T. McGee et al., Qi Gong in Traditional Chinese Medicine, in *Fundamentals of Comple-*

mentary and Alternative Medicine, ed. MS. Micozzi (New York: Churchill Livingstone, 1996).

34. H. Ryu et al., Acute Effect of Qi Gong Training on Stress Hormonal Levels in Man, *American Journal of Chinese Medicine* 24, no. 2 (1996): 193.

35. Krieger, *Accepting Your Power to Heal*, 17.

36. Kabat-Zinn, *Full Catastrophe Living*.

37. Ornish, *Dr. Dean Ornish's Program for Reversing Heart Disease*.

38. P. Carrington, *Freedom in Meditation* (Kendall Park, NJ: Pace Educational System, 1984).

39. J. Macrae, *Therapeutic Touch: A Practical Guide* (New York: Alfred A. Knopf, 1987).

40. T. Nhat Hanh, *The Blooming of a Lotus: Guided Meditation Exercises for Healing and Transformation* (Boston: Beacon Press, 1993), 17.

41. T. Nhat Hanh, *The Long Road Turns to Joy: A Guide to Walking Meditation* (Berkeley: Parallax Press, 1996), 8.

42. T. Nhat Hanh, *Teachings on Love* (Berkeley, CA: Parallax Press, 1997), 21.

43. E. Jacobson, *Progressive Relaxation* (Chicago: University of Chicago Press, 1938).

44. J. Lyles et al., Efficacy of Relaxation Training and Guided Imagery in Reducing the Adverseness of Cancer Chemotherapy, *Journal of Consulting and Clinical Psychology* 50 (1982): 509–529.

45. J. Keicolt-Glaser et al., Psychosocial Enhancement of Immunocompetence in a Geriatric Population, *Health Psychology* 4 (1985): 25–41.

46. C.E. Guzzetta, Effects of Relaxation and Music Therapy on Patients in a Coronary Care Unit with Presumptive Acute Myocardial Infarction, *Heart and Lung* 18 (1989): 609–616.

47. C.D. Wagner et al., The Effectiveness of Teaching a Relaxation Technique to Patients Undergoing Elective Cardiac Catheterization, *Journal of Cardiovascular Nursing* 6, no. 2 (1992): 65–75.

48. J. Schultz and W. Luthe, *Autogenic Training: A Psychophysiologic Approach in Psychotherapy* (New York: Grune & Stratton, 1959).

49. T. Dierks et al., Brain Mapping of EEG in Autogenic Training (AT), *Psychiatry Research* 29 (1989): 433–434.

50. E. Blanchard et al., Behavioral Treatment of 250 Chronic Headache Patients: A Clinical Replication Series, *Behavior Therapy* 16 (1985): 308–327.

51. S. Fahrion, Hypertension and Biofeedback, *Primary Care* 18 (1991): 663–682.

52. R. Freedman, Long Term Effectiveness of Behavioral Treatments for Raynaud's Disease, *Behavior Therapy* 18 (1987): 387–399.

53. B. Enquist et al., Preoperative Hypnosis Reduces Postoperative Vomiting after Surgery of Breasts: A Prospective Randomized and Blended Study, *Acta Anaesthesiologica Scandinavia* 41, no. 8 (1997): 1028–1032.

54. C. Ashton et al., Self-Hypnosis Reduces Anxiety following Coronary Artery Bypass Surgery: A Prospective, Randomized Trial, *Journal of Cardiovascular Surgery* 38, no. 1 (1997): 69–75.

55. M. La Vorgna-Smith, Hypnotherapy/Meditation and Mind/Body Healing: A Phenomenological Study of Women with Osteoporosis [Abstract presented at the Second Annual Alternative Therapies Symposium, Orlando, FL, 1997].

56. W. Whitehead et al., Biofeedback for Disorders of Elimination: Fecal Incontinence and Pelvic Floor Dyssynergia, *Professional Psychology: Research and Practice* 27, no. 3 (1996): 234–240.

57. A. McGrady et al., Biofeedback-Assisted Relaxation in Insulin Dependent Diabetes: A Replication and Extension Study, *Annals of Behavioral Medicine* 28, no. 3 (1996): 185.

58. Schultz and Luthe, *Autogenic Training*.

59. E. Stroebel, *Kiddie QR*, audiotape and workbooks (Wethesfield, CT: QR Publications, 1987).

60. Stroebel, *Kiddie QR*.

61. R. Davidson et al., The Psychobiology of Relaxation and Related States: Multiprocess Theory, in *Behavioral Control and the Modification of Physiological Processes*, ed. D.J. Mostofsky (Englewood Cliffs, NJ: Prentice-Hall, 1976).

62. Davidson et al., The Psychobiology of Relaxation and Related States.

63. W. Linden, The Autogenic Training Method of J.H. Schultz, in *Principles and Practice of Stress Management*, 2d ed., ed. P.M. Lehrer et al. (New York: Guilford Press, 1993).

64. P. Lehrer et al., Effects of Progressive Relaxation and Autogenic Training on Anxiety and Physiological Measures with Some Data on Hypnotizability, in *Stress and Tension Control*, ed. F.J. McGuigan et al. (New York: Plenum Publishing, 1980).

65. S. Shapiro et al., Psychophysiological Effects of Autogenic Training and Progressive Relaxation, *Biofeedback and Self-Regulation* 5 (1980): 249–255.

66. H. Benson, *The Relaxation Response* (New York: William Morrow and Co., 1975).

67. D. Cheeks, Hypnosis, in *The Complete Guide to Holistic Medicine Health for the Whole Person*, ed. A. Hastings et al. (New York: Bantam Books, 1981), 141–156.

68. B. Rogers, Therapeutic Conversation and Posthypnotic Suggestion, *American Journal of Nursing* 72 (1972): 714–717.

69. D. Larkin, Therapeutic Suggestion, in *Relaxation and Imagery: Tools for Therapeutic Communication and Intervention*, ed. R. Zahorek (Philadelphia: W.B. Saunders Co., 1988).

70. Larkin, Therapeutic Suggestion.

71. N. Cousins, invited address, Institute of Noetic Sciences, New York Chapter, NYU Medical Center Dental School, New York, Fall 1988.

72. E. Green and A. Green, *Biofeedback the Yoga of the West* (Cos Cob, CT: Hartley Film Foundation, 1970).

73. Green and Green, *Biofeedback the Yoga of the West*.

74. S. O'Brien, Staff Wellness Program Promotes Quality Care, *American Journal of Nursing* 98, no. 6 (1998): 16B.

75. M. Schwartz, Selected Problems Associated with Relaxation Therapies and Guidelines for Coping with the Problems, in *Biofeedback*, ed. M. Schwartz et al. (New York: Guilford Press, 1987), 171.

76. Schwartz, Selected Problems Associated with Relaxation Therapies, 170.

77. J. Domino et al., Prior Physical and Sexual Abuse in Women with Chronic Headaches: Clinical Correlates, *Headache* 27 (1987): 310–314.

78. D. Harness, Cryptotrauma and Post Trauma Stress Disorders, *Biofeedback*, 5–6.

79. J. Laster, *Relax, Renew: Restful Yoga for Stressful Living* (Berkeley, CA: Rodwell Press, 1995).

80. Nightingale, *Notes on Nursing*, 74.

81. N. Gerlach-Spriggs et al., *Restorative Gardens: The Healing Landscape* (New Haven, CT: Yale University Press, 1998).

SUGGESTED READINGS AND VIDEOTAPES

J. Anselmo, Awareness, Self Healing and Self Care, in *Conference Proceedings: Healing the Mind: Western and Buddhist Approach*, ed. A. Bini (New York: Tibet Center, in publication 1999).

J. Anselmo, Dancing with the Chaos: A Grassroots Approach to Transformation and Healing in Nursing, in *Policy and Politics in Nursing and Health Care*, 3d ed., ed. D. Mason and J. Leavitt (Philadelphia: W.B. Saunders Co., 1998).

J. Anselmo, Holistic Nursing Practice and Complementary Modalities, in *Psychiatric Nursing: An Integrative Approach of Theory and Practice*, ed. P. O'Brien and K. Ballard (New York: McGraw-Hill Book Co., 1999).

J. Anselmo, Self Healing, Awareness and Self Regulation, in *Introduction to Holistic Nursing Process Workbook* (New York: Holistic Nursing Associates, 1992).

At the Heart of Healing: Experiencing Holistic Nursing, 2-vol. interactive videocassette with workbook, 18.5 AACN, CEU's (Holistic Nursing Associates and Kineholistic Foundation, Relaxation, Self Care, Biofeedback, Imagery, and Therapeutic Touch, 1994). (800) 225-1914 ext. 275.

T. Nhat Hanh, *The Blooming of the Lotus, The Miracle of Mindfulness: A Manual on Meditation* (Boston: Beacon Press, 1976).

T. Nhat Hanh, *Peace Is Every Step: The Path of Mindfulness in Everyday Life* (New York: Bantam Books, 1991).

T. Nhat Hanh, *Teachings On Love* (Berkeley, CA: Parallax Press, 1997).

J. Kabat-Zinn, *Full Catastrophe Living: Using the Wisdom of Your Body and Mind To Face Stress, Pain, and Illness* (New York: Bantam Doubleday Dell Publishing Group, 1990).

D. Larkin, Nursing, in *Medical Hypnosis: An Introduction and Clinical Guide*, ed. R. Tames (New York: Churchill Livingstone, 1999).

P. Lehrer and R. Woolfork, *Principles and Practice of Stress Management*, 2d ed. (New York: Guilford Press, 1993).

J. Levey and M. Levy, *The Fine Arts of Relaxation, Concentration, and Meditation* (Boston: Wisdom Publications, 1987).

M. Schwartz and Associates, *Biofeedback: A Practitioners Guide* (New York: Guilford Press, 1987).

J. Spencer and J. Jacobs, *Complementary/Alternative Medicine: An Evidence Based Approach* (St. Louis, MO: Mosby, 1999).

M. Snyder and R. Lindquist, *Complementary/Alternative Therapies in Nursing*, 3d ed. (New York: Springer Publishing, 1998).

Restorative Practices

Restorative Yoga

J. Lasater, *Relax, Renew: Restful Yoga for Stressful Living* (Berkeley: Rodwell Press, 1995).

Restorative Gardens

N. Gerlach-Spriggs et al., *Restorative Gardens: The Healing Landscape* (New Haven: Yale University Press, 1998).

Qi Gong

M. Chia, *Chi Self Massage: The Taoist Way of Rejuvenation* (Huntington, NY: Healing Tao Books, 1986).

S. Wang and J. Liv, *Qi Gong for Health and Longevity: The Ancient Chinese Art of Relaxation, Meditation and Physical Fitness* East Health (Tustin, CA: Development Group, 1995).

RESOURCES

The Relaxation Response
The Mind Body Medicine Institute
Division of Behavioral Medicine
New England Deaconess Hospital
185 Pilgrim Road
Boston, MA 02215
(617) 732-9530

Biofeedback Workshops
Association for Applied Psychophysiology and
   Biofeedback
10200 West 44th Avenue #310
Wheat Ridge, CO 80033
(303) 422-8436

Biofeedback Certification
Biofeedback Certification Institute of America
10200 West 44th Avenue #304
Wheat Ridge, CO 80033
(303) 420-2902

Mindfulness Meditation
Stress Reduction Clinic
University of Massachusetts Medical Center
Worcester, MA 01655
(508) 856-1616

Subtle Energy and Energy Medicine
Institute for the Study of Subtle Energy and Energy
   Medicine
356 Goldco Circle
Golden, CO 80403
(303) 278-2228

Yoga, Relaxation, Qi Gong
Check local holistic education institutes, universities, continuing education programs, Chinese energy medicine centers, yoga ashrams, and health food stores for resources in your area.

Hypnosis
American Society of Clinical Hypnosis
2200 East Devon Avenue, Suite 291
Des Plaines, IL 60018

New York Milton H. Erickson Society for
   Psychotherapy and Hypnosis
Pain and Stress Management Program
(914) 576-5213

Biofeedback Temperature Units, Stress Dots, Alcohol Thermometers, Stress Cards
Call Association for Applied Psychophysiology and Biofeedback for full listing of distributors, also.
American Biotech Corporation
24 Browning Drive
Ossining, NY 10562
(914) 762-4646

VISION OF HEALING

Modeling a Wellness Lifestyle

Nurses must first identify their own state of wellness and then model a wellness lifestyle if they are to be effective teachers. Wellness is an evolving process that does not just happen. It requires ongoing self-assessments in all areas of human potential, as well as investigation of one's values and beliefs. Nurses should reflect on these questions about their state of wellness:

- Do I see wellness as a fluctuating state that I can continuously participate in creating?
- Do I see my health as affected and determined by family, friends, job, and environment?
- Do I think that I can learn new wellness behaviors?
- Is the responsibility for my staying well mine or someone else's?

Self-responsibility for wellness resides within each of us. The key elements of a wellness program should include all areas of the circle of human potential (see Chapter 15). Through these areas, we focus on maximizing wellness. In planning a wellness program, we must develop and incorporate four basic and critical factors: (1) a positive self-image, (2) a positive attitude, (3) self-discipline, and (4) integration of body-mind-spirit. Each person will develop and incorporate these factors in his or her own unique way.

A positive self-image is a view of oneself as a worthy human being. We must continue to develop keenly all of our senses and see ourselves as well in all respects—physical, mental, emotional, social, and spiritual. A positive attitude means that we like and respect ourselves in all that we do. To thrive in this life, we must learn to respect our body-mind-spirit. We also must learn self-discipline, which embodies the idea of being calm and consistently following positive wellness patterns, such as relaxation, exercise, play, and good nutrition. Body-mind-spirit integration means that we see ourselves as a whole. We learn to "walk our talk" of integration in both the personal and the professional aspects of our lives. We must learn to be more humane to ourselves. We are part of a whole universe, and we must see this relationship in terms of interacting wholes that are different from the sum of the parts. We must feel a keen sense of balance and relatedness between who we are, where we are, and how we interact with everyone.

Application of the wellness model to our own lives can assist us in feeling whole and inspired about life. To apply the model, we need to

- search for patterns and antecedents or precipitants of stress and anxiety
- identify positive feelings and emotions
- emphasize our human values

- *assess any pain and disease as valuable signals of internal conflict, not as totally negative events*
- *emphasize the achievement of maximal body-mind-spirit wellness*

- *view the elements of the body-mind-spirit as equal factors, with one element never more important than the others*

Chapter 22

Imagery: Awakening the Inner Healer

Bonney Gulino Schaub and Barbara Montgomery Dossey

NURSE HEALER OBJECTIVES

Theoretical

- Define and contrast the different types of imagery.
- Discuss the different theories of imagery.
- Explain different imagery interventions.

Clinical

- Incorporate imagery interventions into your clinical practice.
- Learn techniques to empower your spoken words.
- Train your voice so that your tone of voice and the pacing of selected words and phrases convey the qualities of calmness, reassurance, openness, and trust.

Personal

- Bring awareness of your own imagery process into your daily life.
- Choose a special healing image to focus on throughout the day.
- Learn to trust and interpret the meaning of your images.

DEFINITIONS

Body-Mind Imagery: the conscious formation of an image that is directed to a body area or activity that requires attention or increased energy.

Clinical Imagery: the conscious use of the power of the imagination with the intention of activating biologic, psychologic, or spiritual healing.

Correct Biologic Imagery: biologically accurate images that are visualized to send messages to physiologic processes.

End-State Imagery: images that contain specified imagined hopes and goals (e.g., a healed wound).

Guided Imagery: a highly structured imagery technique.

Imagery Process: internal experiences of memories, dreams, fantasies, inner perceptions, and visions, sometimes involving one, several, or all the senses, serving as the bridge for connecting body, mind, and spirit.

Imagery Rehearsal: an imagery technique designed to rehearse behaviors or prepare for activities or procedures.

Impromptu Imagery: the nurse's introduction of his or her spontaneous, intuitive images or perceptions into the therapeutic intervention.

Packaged Imagery: commercial tapes that have general images.

Relationship Imagery: imagery technique designed to explore relationships.

Spontaneous Imagery: the unexpected reception of an image, as if it "bubbled up," entering the stream of consciousness.

Symbolic Imagery: inner images that represent a person's deeper knowledge. Occurring in the form of metaphors or symbols, they may be immediately translatable to rational verbal thought, or their meaning may slowly emerge over time.

Transpersonal Imagery: images that connect one to expanded (i.e., beyond personality) levels of consciousness, such as imagining one's body as a mountain and beginning to feel an inner quality of immovable strength and solidity.

Visualization: the use of external images (e.g., religious painting, written word, nature photograph) to evoke internal imagery experiences that energize desired emotions, qualities, outcomes, or goals.

THEORY AND RESEARCH

Imagery is an essential aspect of holistic nursing practice, as it brings the natural powers of the mind into the process of health and healing. Distinct from thinking, imagery as a technique interacts with the image-making function of the brain, which in turn acts on the entire physiology. Imagery can be used on its own or in conjunction with therapeutic touch, meditation, biofeedback, reiki, reflexology, and other holistic practices. Imagery is an independent nursing intervention, a nurse-initiated action performed by nurses to bring about patient outcomes falling within the scope of nursing practice.[1]

The research definition of imagery is a perception of a stimulus in the absence of that stimulus. For example, if a person imagines a lemon and begins to taste lemon juice, they are having a perception (tasting the juice) of a stimulus (lemon) that is not present. This "absence of stimuli" definition is relevant to the crucial issue of the placebo effect, a phenomenon in which the patient thinks (imagines) he or she is receiving a potent medicine and experiences the anticipated effects, both positive (placebo) and negative (nocebo), of that medication, when in fact a neutral substance was administered. This effect was demonstrated in a study that followed the progress of 303 patients medicated with a placebo for benign prostatic hyperplasia over a 25-month period. The study demonstrated rapidly significant improvements in urinary output and relief of symptoms of benign prostatic hyperplasia, but some patients also experienced negative side effects of the inert placebo "medication."[2]

In a study on the effect of a placebo in the relief of postsurgical pain, researchers found that the experience of an analgesic effect with the administration of a placebo was most effective with those patients who had prior successful outcomes with opioid exposure. For example, some patients experienced respiratory depression from the placebo, if they had previously experienced this effect from the opioid.[3]

A practitioner's suggestions regarding an expected outcome influence the effect of a placebo. In a study where subjects were instructed to place their hands in ice water, one group was informed of the beneficial effect of this practice, one group was told of the possible hazards, and the control group was given a neutral suggestion. The pain threshold, tolerance, and endurance of the three groups were compared. The tolerance of participants given the positive suggestion was significantly greater than that of the other two groups. In contrast, the group given the negative suggestion had significantly decreased tolerance and endurance of the test condition.[4]

This information challenges the holistic nurse to understand and work with the power of a patient's imagination when providing care. The expectation of sickness, and the feelings of fear associated with this expectation, may actually contribute to illness.[5] Therefore, the interpersonal skills of the nurse, his or her self-awareness and focus, and positive outlook are all factors that help the patient imagine well-being and healthy outcomes.[6]

If a patient can physically benefit from imagining good results, then the imagination is a powerful healing tool in health care. Clinical imagery is the application of the conscious use of the power of the imagination with the intention of activating biologic, psychologic, or spiritual healing. The key word in this definition is *conscious*. The power of the imagination, for good or bad, is always affecting people. People imagine negative futures and employ their intelligence to worry about that negative future. Their life becomes focused around a negative future that they imagine to be true. Imagery's clinical focus is to use the imagination to promote life-affirming behaviors and goals.

The effectiveness of imagery in healing has been recognized and used cross-culturally for thousands of years.[7,8] As more nurses gain an understanding of the benefits of imagery and use it to complement traditional nursing interventions, it will revolutionize the practice of nursing. It will change nursing because it engages the nurse and the client/patient at a higher level of consciousness than traditional nursing does. With imagery, the nurse introduces proven ancient methods of healing into modern health care. This cross-fertilization of ancient and modern methods is creating a new form of practical spirituality in U.S. health care.[9] In assisting this development, nurses play a key role in contributing to the scientific basis for imagery.

Imagery and States of Consciousness

Several important psychology research findings about the ongoing imagery process, or "stream of consciousness," have implications for the nursing care of patients and clients. Sensory deprivation research in the early 1960s spurred the study of the ongoing imagery process. Initially, the purpose of this research was to examine the functioning of the brain in the absence of sensory input. Much of this research resulted from the space program's need to understand the impact on astronauts of the sensory deprivation, isolation, and confinement of space travel.[10] These studies indicated that an ongoing imagery process is a vital element in human mental experience, particularly when perceptual stimulation is reduced as it is in those who have a sensory impairment; those who are dealing with the monotony of hospitalization, particularly those in intensive care units; and those who work in monotonous environments.

Research conducted on the process of daydreaming has also provided nurses with insights helpful in their work with imagery. Foulkes and Fleisher applied a simple technique, previously used in sleep research, to study waking mental activity.[11] Subjects reclined in moderately lit rooms in bed but stayed awake. They were isolated from the researchers, and electroencephalogram (EEG) monitors were used to make sure they did not fall asleep. At randomly selected times, subjects were asked to describe their mental activity. In 84 of 120 "arousals," subjects reported awareness of imagery; in more than a quarter of these instances, the images were extremely vivid. The researchers concluded that relaxed, waking thought is fairly susceptible to momentary intrusions of extremely vivid and at times unusual content. The research of Foulkes and Fleisher, along with that of Singer and Antrobus,[12,13] point to the richness and variety of imagery content in mentally healthy subjects. This information can allow the nurse to be comfortable with the wide variety of material evoked during an imagery session. It is the value and nature of working with imagery to encounter creative and novel perspectives on the issues being explored.

Another significant aspect of imagery work is its potential to tap into memory at very deep levels. Wilder Penfield, a Canadian neurosurgeon working in the middle of the twentieth century, did extensive experimentation with direct electrical stimulation and mapping of the brain during surgery. In his research on locally anesthetized, conscious subjects, he identified an area of the brain he labeled the "interpretive cortex." Upon electrostimulation of this region, he discovered that there is a brain mechanism "capable of bringing back a strip of past experience in complete detail without any of the fanciful elaborations that occur in a man's dreaming . . . a record that has not faded but seems to remain as vivid as when the record was made."[14(p.34)] Penfield went on to indicate that, although the memories recalled in this manner were predominantly visual or auditory, the memory record included all the sensory information that had entered consciousness (e.g., smells, tastes, sounds, tactile sensations). In addition, there was a sense of familiarity about the event. Simultaneous with the experience of these memory records, Penfield's subjects retained an awareness of their present situation, namely that they were on an operating table having their brain probed by a surgeon.

Penfield's studies illustrate the capacity of consciousness to be absorbed in multiple activities at the same time. Penfield's patients were conscious of complete sensory recall of memories, were conscious of being on an operating room table, and were able to verbalize their experiences to Penfield and his staff. Appreciating the potentials of human consciousness is a key element in imagery work.

Clinical Effectiveness of Imagery

In a comprehensive review of the research on the physiologic effects of imagery,[15] Graham cited studies demonstrating the impact of mental imagery on a wide range of systems:

- Vasomotor activity resulting in alterations in skin temperature
- Increasing internal blood flow, demonstrated by increased temperature in specific skin areas
- Decreased external bleeding in hemophiliacs during oral surgery
- Increases in heart rate resulting from imaging sexually or emotionally arousing situations
- Heart rate reduction in response to images of relaxation
- Increases in systolic blood pressure in response to images of fear and anger

Other physiologic responses to imagery include salivary gland activation, changes in blood sugar, gastrointestinal activity, and blister formation.[16]

Jacobson demonstrated imagery's effect on motor responses in 1929 when he showed that subtle tensions of small muscles or sense organs result from imagining movement (see Chapter 21).[17] In addition, imagined activity stimulates the appropriate motor neurons. A recent study demonstrated the effectiveness of imagery rehearsal as practice in the learning of motor skills.[18] This is the "ideo-motor" aspect of imagery that has been applied in the use of imagery rehearsal for improving athletic performance.[19] In fact, the research on motor responses has been extensively applied in athletic training,[20-22] but it also holds rich possibilities for application in rehabilitation nursing and in any setting where people are experiencing limitations in movement and activity. This aspect of imagery was applied in working with patients affected with Parkinsonism. Mental images of movement were used to help in freeing movement in "frozen" body parts.[23]

Simonton and associates explored the effect of imagery on immune function and the application of this information in the treatment of cancer,[24] as did Achterberg and Lawlis.[25,26] Hall studied the effect of hypnosis and imagery on immune modulation, noting increases in the number of lymphocytes and general increased immune system responsiveness.[27,28] Schneider and associates demonstrated enhanced immune responsiveness in subjects working with imagery of "white blood cells attacking germs."[29] Schneider and associates also successfully used imagery to increase adherence, or "stickiness," of neutrophils.[30] Two factors affected the successful use of imagery in these studies. First, the biologic accuracy of the imagery appeared to be significant. Second, the ability to work with the imagery without straining at it played a part in significant outcomes. In yet another study, healthy subjects were able to reduce the release of the "stress hormones" (corticosteroids) that reduce immune function when using images of relaxation.[31]

Clinical imagery has been applied for pain reduction during cancer treatment,[32] and imagery interventions alone were found to be as effective as the combination of imagery and teaching of cognitive behavioral skills to reduce anxiety during magnetic resonance imaging (MRI) diagnostic procedures.[33] A clinical study on the use of imagery as a coping strategy for perioperative patients had participants listen to imagery tapes for 3 days preoperatively; during anesthesia induction; during surgery; in postanesthesia care; and for 6 days postsurgery. Patients treated with guided imagery required 50 percent less narcotic medication and experienced significantly lower levels of anxiety and perception of pain.[34]

In a review of the application of imagery in cardiovascular disease, Luskin and associates cited imagery as a helpful tool in several issues: altering behaviors associated with cardiac risk, such as bringing about smoking cessation; reducing heart rate reactivity over a 28-week follow-up period; decreasing anxiety responses in male automatic defibrillation recipients.[35]

Many studies have demonstrated imagery's therapeutic effect in reducing anxiety and improving quality of life.[36-39] People can learn to produce positive healing results through imagery process. The effectiveness of imagery in reducing anxiety was found to be positive even if the imagery recipients were not vivid imagers.[40] Nursing students who were taught imagery-based stress management interventions were able to apply the imagery techniques successfully for their self-care, as well as to use them in their medical/surgical, maternity/gynecology, community, home care, and psychiatric clinical rotations.[41]

In conclusion, research findings on imagery and physiology include the following:

- Images relate to physiologic states.
- Images may either precede or follow physiologic changes, indicating that they have both a causative and a reactive role.
- Images can originate in conscious, deliberate behaviors, as well as in subconscious acts (e.g., electrical stimulation of the brain, reverie, dreaming, brain wave biofeedback).
- Images can be the hypothetical bridge between conscious processing of information and physiologic change.
- Images can influence the voluntary (peripheral) nervous system, as well as the involuntary (autonomic) nervous system.
- Imagery is not about mental pictures, but is a resource for gaining access to the imagination and more subtle aspects of inner experience. It may involve all sensory modalities: visual, olfactory, tactile, gustatory, auditory, and kinesthetic.[42]

Clinical Imagery Theories

Eidetic Psychotherapy

Ahsen developed a theory of imagery called eidetics.[43] He posited that there are three unitary, interactive modes of awareness available:

1. Image (I)
2. Somatic response (S)
3. Meaning (M)

This triad of image–somatic response–meaning (ISM) defines the eidetic image that is stored in the mind as an experiential unit. The somatic response and meaning components are repressed in the image, constituting what Ahsen labeled "the consciousness–imagery gap." Ahsen theorized that alterations in the image alter the corresponding somatic responses and meanings of past events. This theory can be related to the previous cognitive and biologic explanations of imagery. Ahsen developed an elaborate and broadly applicable theory for working with eidetic images in the clinical setting. The implication of this theory is that any work at the somatic level (e.g., therapeutic massage) or work at the meaning level (e.g., counseling) must include awareness of the images evoked by these practices.

Psychosynthesis

Roberto Assagioli was an Italian psychiatrist who introduced meditation and imagery into clinical practice beginning in 1909.[44,45] His theory of the wholeness of human consciousness, called psychosynthesis, has been extensively applied in the helping professions since 1965. He was personally most interested in developing a science of the higher self, a term that he used to describe the aspect of each person that holds inner wisdom and connection with life purpose. He saw the higher self as a developmental step latent inside each person.

Assagioli used imagery in three forms:

1. Inner images to explore the various levels of human experience, including biologic, social, and transpersonal experience
2. Inner images to represent the intentions and goals of the patient
3. External images—the actual paintings and statues of his city, Florence, Italy—

to help encourage transpersonal feelings in his patients. He often suggested that his patients go to a particular museum or church to meditate on a particular work of art because of the spiritual insights and feelings that the artist expressed in the work.

Assagioli viewed imagery within a body-mind-spirit context. He developed a set of principles that he referred to as "psychological laws" to describe the interactive effects among images, ideas, emotions, physical responses, behaviors, attitudes, and impulses. According to one such law, "Images or mental pictures tend to produce the physical conditions and the external acts that correspond to them." According to a second law, "Attitudes, movements, and actions tend to evoke corresponding images and ideas; these, in turn, evoke or intensify corresponding emotions."[46] In these and other laws, Assagioli was seeking to outline the ability of the mind through imagery and intention to interact with, and positively affect, the mind/body for healing and growth.

In a recent study that follows the spirit of Assagioli's work, researchers began with the observation that directing attention to the body is part of the effectiveness of techniques such as imagery and meditation in producing psychophysiologic harmonious states.[47] They wondered what the measurable effect would be of directing attention to particular body organs. Their studies focused specifically on the heart. When simultaneously measuring heart rhythm by electrocardiogram (ECG) and brain wave rhythm by EEG, they instructed subjects to focus attention on their heart beat. In doing this, they discovered a state of heart–brain electrical wave synchronization. They then postulated that a process emerges as a result of the synchronization occurring from this focused direction of consciousness: self-attention—connection—self-regulation—order—ease. They proposed that this existed in contrast to a process of disatten-tion—disconnection—disregulation—dis-order—disease. It was also observed that the synchronization was more effective when participants practiced with eyes closed.

CLINICAL TECHNIQUES IN IMAGERY

It is clear that imagery affects our gen-eral physical state and our sense of emo-tional well-being. Patients with negative imagery will go into physical states of fear and nervous vigilance. If instead they choose to focus their minds on specific positive imagery, all of their physical sys-tems will move toward states of ease and harmony. Imagery interacts with physi-ologic processes, sending messages and information from the right brain to the cen-tral nervous system.

Nurses may use specific, highly struc-tured, guided body-mind, correct biologic, and end-state imagery techniques. The use of symbolic drawing can be introduced in the exploration process. Perhaps the most available use of imagery is the nurse's own impromptu imagery. Im-promptu imagery is the nurse's unplanned use of an image that arises in her own im-agery process during a clinical interac-tion. For example, an emergency room nurse, caring for a woman who had badly injured arms as a result of a car accident, was unable to establish an intravenous (IV) line because the woman's veins were collapsing. The situation was urgent, and there was discussion about the possible need to amputate an arm. The nurse, who had recently started studying clinical im-agery, suddenly had an image of this woman holding a baby. She immediately suggested that the woman take a few mo-ments and embrace her injured arm as if it were a tiny baby. She said, "Hold your arm, and send it loving energy." Within mo-ments, the woman was calm, and the nurse was able to start the IV infusion.

Another nurse became aware of a patient's anxiety as she was preparing to administer a transfusion of packed cells. The woman had recently experienced a number of transfusion reactions and was very fearful about the procedure. The nurse, who was meeting the patient for the first time, noticed that the cells had come from a source in Florida. She had an image of the blood donor basking on a warm Florida beach. The nurse told the woman where the blood supply had originated and suggested that she imagine these cells bringing the healing energy of the Florida sun and the gentle breeze of the beach to soothe and calm her. The patient immedi-ately responded favorably to this sugges-tion, happy to have a calming image with which to engage her mind. The transfusion was a success.

Imagery in Holistic Health Counseling

Imagery clearly taps a deeper level of self-knowledge in the patient. One ex-ample of this occurs in relationship imag-ery. In one instance, when a patient was asked to describe his relationship with his father, he offered a few familiar comments. But when he was asked to get an *image* of his father, the patient suddenly got in touch with the feelings of sadness and hopeless-ness that his father stimulates in him. This deeper level of self-knowledge allowed the patient to appreciate why he struggles with hopelessness in himself.

The remarkable ability of imagery to of-fer intimate information to the patient, im-mediately and directly, is its special contri-bution to holistic health counseling. Such information may be helpful in making health decisions, in rehearsing new behav-iors, in understanding relationships, and in making life choices.

Values and Spirituality

Nurses are often caring for patients at a stage in their lives when values and spirituality have become a central concern. Illness, divorce, ethical dilemmas, deaths, or other life crises often cause people to slow down and ask basic questions about how they are going to conduct their lives. Changes in physical capacities, the need to find different employment, decisions about education and lifestyle, and retirement all call upon people to reassess their deepest values and their sense of spiritual purpose in life. Such a stage of life is a time of "crossroads decisions," in which there is a need to have a larger vision of life's path. Immediate reasons for one decision or another are only relatively helpful. People know that their "crossroads decision" will be affecting them for a long time, and they need to be aware of their values and spiritual perspective to help with decisions.

At these times, rational thought processes are not enough, because they do not reveal the big picture. Imagery allows someone to imagine the actual results of a decision. For example, a nurse counseling a 59-year-old elementary schoolteacher struggling with a decision about retirement suggested that she close her eyes, focus on her breath, and imagine herself retired. After a few moments, the woman experienced an image of herself at home, looking bored and unhappy. She was frustrated with this image. She then tried to imagine her retirement as a time of new growth. She went back into the imagery, trying to imagine herself retiring and going back to school to study something new—but she was. Her imagination literally refused to see it. She then imagined herself doing service work in the community. Suddenly, during this imagery, she felt a peace and an ease settle into her experience.

Imagining pictures of the future makes specific behavioral and emotional information available. This information is in-valuable for decision making because it provides a holistic level of information that is not available at the purely verbal level.

Transpersonal Use of Imagery

The transpersonal (beyond personality) level of human nature is a fact. Cultures throughout the world have used prayer, meditation, imagery, diet, physical training, study, ritual, art, and many other methods to experience transpersonal states of consciousness. People seek these states because they tend to provide a subtler understanding of the universal patterns of reality and a more peaceful perspective on the "little self" living in the immensity of creation. Holistic nurses frequently cite transpersonal experiences as one of the reasons that they became interested in introducing holistic methods into their work. Motivated by their own development through such experiences, they desire to pass the potentials of transpersonal experiences on to others.

The role of imagery in transpersonal experience is a crucial one. Holistic nurses can use transpersonal imagery to introduce patients safely to the transpersonal level of consciousness.[48] This imagery is referred to as transpersonal because it links and identifies the individual experience to universal processes. Transpersonal imagery taps into an expanded experience of the self, an experience that draws on human beings' capacity to connect deeply with the flow of life energy and creation. This connection, and the imagery that emerges from it, can be interpreted as a connection with God, with all of humanity, with a higher power, with the wonder of the universe and nature, or connection with the mysterious, nonverbal communication that occurs between people at the level of intuitive knowing and caring (see Chapters 2 through 6).

Visualization practice can be helpful for energizing and eliciting transpersonal experiences. Art images, photographs, and picture postcards are all sources for images that can be used in work with transpersonal symbols. The nurse can begin to collect art cards and other images that can be used to help patients. For example, one elderly woman hospitalized with advanced heart disease was feeling very lonely, depressed, and fearful. She expressed fear that she was going to die. In sharing this with the nurse, she said she was confused by spirituality and did not know what she believed. The nurse asked if she would like to explore these feelings with imagery, and the woman agreed. The nurse led her in a brief relaxation and then suggested that she experience herself in a place that she felt was sacred. The woman was silent for a long time. The nurse sat silently with her. After a while, the woman opened her eyes. She was very surprised by her imagery. She felt herself in Florence, Italy, a place she had never visited. She imagined walking the streets, looking at the beauty of the churches and feeling deeply connected to the sacredness of the art. She said she always imagined Florence as a sacred place. She deeply loved Renaissance art and imagined the magic of a place where so much beauty had been created. She realized that her love of art was the closest thing she could identify as a spiritual feeling. Recognizing the importance of this imagery for the patient, the nurse said she would bring her a postcard of Florence. This pleased the woman, and the nurse told her that it would be important to honor this inner experience by keeping a reminder of it where she could connect with it over the course of the day.

Working with metaphors and symbols of transcendent experiences is an effective way to help a patient who is experiencing spiritual distress, hopelessness, and helplessness. Bringing a client into deep relaxation and then introducing one of these metaphors in an open-ended, exploratory way can be deeply meaningful. The patient can choose the symbol that he or she wants to explore, or the nurse can create the journey based on information from the patient. In times of illness and crisis, people may have spontaneous spiritual experiences and images. It is advisable to learn about these images so that patients can be supported and derive benefit from their experience (Table 22–1).

Imagery with Disease/Illness

Much emphasis is placed on treating disease, the pathologic changes in organic form either observed or validated by laboratory tests. There is also a great need to address the individual's personal experience of his or her illness, general state of being, anxiety level, state of hopefulness or despair, and the meaning attributed to the situation. The nurse, using imagery, can promote a sense of well-being in clients and help them change their perceptions about their disease, treatment, and their inner resources and innate healing ability.

Fear and negative imagery are not unusual in an individual with an undiagnosed or even a known illness. For example, a woman who discovers a palpable breast lump may conjure up frightening images before any tests or diagnoses. These images may include cancer, mastectomy, chemotherapy, radiation, hair loss, nausea/vomiting, severe pain, metastatic disease, the deathing process, funeral, and the actual moment of dying. This process may be conscious or preverbal. It may be noticed in dreams, daydreams, spontaneous images, and kinesthetic sensings.

Concrete Objective Information

Nursing research has been conducted over the last 20 years in the use of imagery in preparing patients for difficult procedures. This technique, referred to as concrete objective information, is broadly applicable in nursing practice.[49] It is a form of

Table 22-1 Symbols and Metaphors of Transformation

Symbol or Metaphor	Transformative Experience
Introversion	Exploration of the true self; self-knowledge; inner journey to the soul, to beingness
Deepening/descent	Journey to the underworld of the psyche; confronting the difficult aspects of the self, the shadow; entering a cave; the heroic journey of facing fears
Ascent/elevation	Climbing a mountain to reach a higher plane of awareness
Expansion/broadening	Enlarging perspective; taking in the wholeness and seeing beyond one's small, individual perspective
Awakening	Awakening from the dream or from illusions; opening to the truth or reality of what really matters
Illumination	Bringing in the light of the human soul; spiritual light to transform or "enlighten" a situation; moving from darkness to light; bringing in life energy
Fire	Purification; spiritual alchemy; candles, lanterns, bonfires, ceremonies of transformation
Development	Growth, blossoming; potentials waiting to become real
Love	Opening the heart; compassion and generosity, forgiveness
Path/pilgrimage	"Mystic way;" the journey of outward exploration; seeking to be changed by new experience or knowledge
Rebirth/regeneration	Birth of the new being; resurrection
Freedom/liberation	Liberation of psychic, physical, and spiritual energy to align with creation and creativity

Source: Adapted by permission of Sterling Lord Literistic, Inc. Copyright © 1965 by Robert Assagioli.

---

imagery rehearsal, and its effectiveness lies in the importance of the "prepared mind." People are fearful of the unknown and of feeling out of control. This technique addresses both these fears.

Concrete objective information explores the client's subjective and objective experiences of the upcoming event. Clients who receive information about both subjective and objective components of tests, procedures, and surgery recover more quickly. They are able to plan and use more effective coping strategies than clients who receive only one of the components. A surgical patient's subjective experience includes what will be felt, heard, seen, smelled, or tasted before, during, or after the procedure. In addition, it includes the sensory experiences of a postsurgical healing incision (e.g., pressure, smarting, tingling), as well as sensations over time (e.g., fleeting sharp sensations from the incisional area

when turning in bed or when coughing). Table 22-2 lists sensations evoked by selected procedures.

Objective experiences are observable and verifiable by someone other than the person going through the procedure. Thus, for the surgical patient, an objective experience may include the time and place of the presurgery nurse's visit, the matters to be discussed in the visit, the preoperative preparation of the skin, placement on the stretcher to go to surgery, awakening in the recovery room, and expected sensations. This process reduces the likelihood that the patient will interpret normal sensations or events as signs that "something's wrong." It also allows the nurse and patient to plan specific ways for the patient to handle difficult parts of the event.

The following procedural points related to the use of concrete objective information originate in science-based nursing practice:

Table 22–2 Documented Subjective Experience Descriptors by Stressful Health Care Event

Stressful Event	Descriptors
Gastroendoscopic examination	Intravenous medication; feel needle stick, drowsiness As air is pumped into stomach, feeling of fullness like after eating a large meal Feel physician's finger in mouth to guide tube insertion
Nasogastric tube insertion	Feeling passage of tube Tearing Gagging Discomfort in nose, throat, mouth Limited mobility
Cast removal	Hear buzz of saw Feel vibrations or tingling See chalky dust Feel warmth on arm or leg as saw cuts cast; will not hurt or burn Skin under padding looks and feels scaly and dirty Arm or leg may feel a little stiff when first trying to move it Arm or leg may feel light because cast was heavy
Barium enema	Lying on hard table Table feels hard Feel fullness Feel pressure Feel bloating Feel uncomfortable Feel as if might have a bowel movement
Abdominal surgery	Preoperative medications: feel sleepy, light-headed, relaxed, free from worry, not bothered by most things, dryness of mouth Feel incision: tenderness, sensitivity, pressure, smarting, burning, aching, sore Sensations might become sharp and feel like they are traveling along incision when moving Arm with intravenous tube feels awkward and restricted but not painful Feel tired after physical effort Feel bloating in abdomen Cramping due to gas pains Pulling and pinching when stitches are removed
Tracheostomy	When moving about, swallowing, or during suctioning: feel hurting, pressure, choking
Mastectomy— mean of 5.5 years postoperative	Arm or chest wall pain, "pins and needles," numbness, weakness, increased skin sensitivity, heaviness Phantom breast sensations, such as twinges, itching
4-vessel arteriography	Before contrast medium: table is hard, head taping is uncomfortable, cleansing solution is cold After contrast medium: hot, burning sensation in face, neck, chest, or shoulders

Source: Adapted from *Nursing Interventions: Essential Nursing Treatments*, 2d ed., by G. Bulechek and J. McCloskey, p. 145, with permission of W.B. Saunders Company, © 1992.

- Identify the sensory features of the procedure to be used.
- Determine the individual's perception of the procedure/treatment/test to be experienced.
- Choose words that have meaning for the person.
- Use synonyms that have less emotional impact, such as "discomfort" instead of "pain."

- Select specific experiences when giving examples rather than abstract experiences (see Table 22-2).
- Help individuals reframe any negative imagery. For example, patients often fear chemotherapy and think of it as a poison because of all the precautions and side effects associated with it. It is very important to have a way of framing the experience that is positive and focuses on healing. For example, the nurse may say, "Chemotherapy is powerful and effective in fighting the most vulnerable cells, the confused and incomplete cancer cells. The healthy cells, most of the cells in your body, are strong and protected."
- Plan specific strategies to be used at different stages of the procedure, such as using a breathing technique while waiting for the procedure to begin and using imagery of a safe place during the procedure as a distraction from uncomfortable sensations.

Fears in Imagery Work

There are three predictable and understandable fears encountered in imagery work: (1) nothing will happen; (2) too much will happen; or (3) it will be done wrong.

Nothing will happen. Patients fear that they will not be able to imagine anything in response to the nurse's imagery suggestion. Coincidentally, the nurse may share the same fear. The nurse may be afraid that the imagery method will produce nothing of worth for the patient.

The answer to this fear is to be curious about any experience that occurs during the course of the imagery. If, for example, the patient reports that her breathing became faster as soon as she heard the nurse's suggestion to relax, the nurse should be curious about why the patient believes her breathing became faster. The patient may respond that she was afraid of relaxing. On the surface, this may seem a strange statement. How can anyone be afraid of relaxing? In fact, relaxation can be frightening, for example, for someone who has experienced trauma in childhood and feels the importance of maintaining vigilance. Such information can be invaluable in actually helping the patient to enter states of relaxation safely and to engage in imagery work.

Too much will happen. Patients fear that the imagery will evoke difficult or even overwhelming thoughts and feelings. Coincidentally, the nurse may share the same fear. The nurse may fear the imagery method will be too evocative and will have negative consequences for the patient.

The answer to this fear is that imagery does not take away a person's defenses. If the imagery suggestion is too evocative, the patient will simply fail to hear it, will ignore it, will change it into a suggestion that is easier to work with, or will simply open his or her eyes and stop the process. If a patient does have difficult thoughts and feelings in response to the imagery suggestion, these thoughts and feelings will develop because the patient is ready to receive them.

These statements presuppose that the nurse is skilled in imagery and is not imposing a manipulative imagery practice. Each patient has the potential for important new knowledge and new feeling. The nurse is not using imagery to make something happen. Rather, the nurse is using imagery to evoke what is already present in the patient. Carried out in this spirit, the nurse will not evoke any experiences for which the patient is not ready. The imagery suggestion will instead open the patient to the interior world of latent intuition, knowledge, and creative problem solving already present in the patient's imagination.

It will be done wrong. Anxious to please the nurse, patients fear they cannot do imagery the "right way." Coincidentally, the nurse may also harbor the fear that there is a "right way" to do imagery and that his or her personal skills are inadequate for the "right way."

The answer to this fear is to realize that there is no right way. The processes of the imagination are unique to each person; thus, each imagery experience is unique. Furthermore, a nurse may use the same imagery suggestion twice, and the same patient may experience two totally different responses to the imagery. It is very important to realize that the patient's experience is the center of all imagery work. The nurse may suggest imaging a walk in an open field, and the patient may respond by imaging the atmosphere in a dark room. The dark room becomes of importance. The original suggestion of an open field is no longer significant. The meaning of the dark room for the patient becomes the source of interest and new learning. The nurse's imagery suggestion is simply that—a suggestion—to evoke the latent powers and intelligence of the imagination into the service of the patient. Imagery techniques can be studied for many years, imagery skills can be honed, and yet it remains the unique response of the patient that is central to the work.

HOLISTIC CARING PROCESS

Assessment

In preparing to use imagery as a nursing intervention, the nurse assesses the following parameters:

- the client's potential for organic brain syndrome or psychosis in order to determine if general relaxation techniques should be used instead of imagery techniques.
- the client's anxiety/tension levels in order to determine which types of relaxation inductions will be most effective.
- the client's hopes in regard to the session and reason for seeking help.
- the client's wants, needs, desires, or recurrent/dominant themes.

- the client's understanding that it is not necessary to literally hear, see, feel, touch, or taste when working with imagery, that it is best to trust the inner experience in whatever form the information comes.
- the client's primary sensory modalities.
- the client's understanding that imagery is basically a way in which we communicate with ourselves at a deep level.
- the client's understanding that imagery can bring us into contact with our body and find out what it needs.
- the client's previous experiences with the imagery process.
- the client's emotional comfort level with closing eyes, bringing attention inside and opening to states of internal awareness. If the client is not comfortable with closing the eyes, the nurse can suggest just lowering the eyes and gazing at a point on the floor approximately 1 or 2 feet in front of him or her. This will cause the client's peripheral vision to blur, eyelids will usually get heavy, and then the eyes will close effortlessly. Some clients need to learn to trust that it is safe to relax, that they are experiencing a natural phenomenon.
- the client's knowledge of relaxation skills. If not skilled in relaxation, the client may need an explanation of what the normal sensations will be and time to shift to the "letting go" state. Once the client becomes skilled at entering a relaxed state, a selected word, phrase, or hand posture can become a signal to relax.
- the client's ability to maintain attention and not drowse off in the session.

Patterns/Problems/Needs

The following patterns/problems/needs compatible with imagery interventions relate to the human response patterns of unitary person (see Chapter 14) as follows:

- **Exchanging:** All diagnoses
- **Relating:** Social isolation
  Role performance
  Caregiver role strain
  Parental role strain
- **Valuing:** Spiritual well-being
  Spiritual distress
- **Choosing:** Altered effective coping
  Impaired adjustment
  Ineffective denial
  Potential for growth
  Decisional conflict
  Health-seeking
    behaviors
- **Moving:** Sleep pattern
    disturbance
  Relocation stress
    syndrome
- **Perceiving:** Altered self-concept
  Disturbance in body
    image
  Disturbance in self-
    image
  Potential hopelessness
  Potential
    powerlessness
- **Feeling:** Pain
  Anxiety
  Fear
  Post-trauma response
  Grief

Outcomes

Table 22–3 guides the nurse in client outcomes, nursing prescriptions, and evaluations for the use of imagery as a nursing intervention.

Therapeutic Care Plan and Implementation

Before the Session

- Become calm and centered. Let your bodymind release any tension and tightness. Prepare to guide the client with relaxation and imagery.
- Focus on the client's baseline feelings/emotions as revealed during the assessment process.
- Prepare the room to ensure quietness and the client's comfort.
- Have the client empty the bladder before the session begins.
- Place a sign on the door stating that the session is in progress in order to avoid interruptions.
- Have the client sit, recline, or lie down, depending on client preference and clinical situation.
- Have a selection of music tapes available from which the client can choose (see Chapter 23).
- Have a light blanket available in case the client should feel cool.
- Have blank paper, crayons, and colored markers available should the client wish to draw before or after the session.

At the Beginning of the Session

- Give the client a general definition of imagery: "Imagery is a natural way to connect body-mind-spirit by quieting the busy mind and body. This helps you tap into the power of the imagination."
- Have the client develop a positive expectation of what is to occur using bodymind and/or end-state imagery directed toward a successful outcome. Help the client clarify his or her intention and focus on the healing efforts.
- Assist the client in experiencing the imagery process and making friends with the experience of inner wisdom. This process is a key aspect of self-empowerment and creativity.
- Have the client center awareness on the present moment, focusing on breath or other sensory experience, in order to facilitate the imagery process.
- Instruct the client to let spontaneous images emerge from the inner self with-

Table 22–3 Nursing Interventions: Imagery

Client Outcomes	Nursing Prescriptions	Evaluation
The client will demonstrate skills in imagery.	Following an assessment, guide the client in an imagery exercise.	The client participated in imagery exercise by choice.
	Assess the client's levels of anxiety with this new process.	The client demonstrated no signs of anxiety with imagery process.
	After the imagery process experience, assess effectiveness through client dialogue.	The client stated that the imagery experience was helpful.
	Encourage the client to recognize daily self-talk and the images that lead to balance and inner peace.	The client reported using self-dialogue with imagery.
	Help the client to create images of desired health habits, feelings, desires for daily living.	The client reported creating images of desired health habits, feelings, and desires for daily living.
	Teach the client coping, power over daily events, ability to move toward healthy lifestyle.	The client reported increased coping with daily stressors.
	Teach the client to recognize images leading to self-defeating lifestyle habits.	The client reported recognition of negative images leading to self-defeating behavior; the client creates positive images.
The client will participate in drawing, if appropriate.	Encourage the client to draw images and symbols as a communication process with self.	The client used drawing as a communication process with self.

out judging or analyzing them, allowing the stream of consciousness to flow. Release expectations of logically working the images through to resolving conflicts at this time. Help the client to trust inner experience and to approach it with curiosity and compassion.

- Tell the client that, in following guided relaxation and imagery scripts, different images will appear. If any images appear that the client is unwilling or unready to deal with, it is perfectly all right to open his or her eyes and discuss it. This is valuable information to understand and clarify. When the client is ready, the session can proceed.
- After giving an induction, and a state of deep relaxation is demonstrated, the nurse can suggest to the client that

he or she "allow images to emerge from this relaxed state."

During the Session

- With your guidance, let the client create his or her own images.
- Assess the state of relaxation throughout the session. Notice decreased tension in the face, chest, torso, and legs. The changes can range from subtle to dramatic. Respirations become deeper, with more space between the breaths. The eyelids may flicker (especially with very vivid imagers), and the lips and face may change to a paler color.
- Determine if the client is following the imagery process. The nurse may instruct the client, "If you are following the imagery, raise a finger to indicate

yes." Similarly, the nurse may ask if the client needs a slower pace or would like to get more comfortable. Clients who are used to working with inner imagery can usually focus more easily than novices. If the client cannot clear the mind, suggest returning to breath awareness.

- Determine the length of the session based on the client's needs, body responses, and session outcomes. The sessions can last from 10 or 15 minutes to an hour or longer.
- Allow your personal intuition to emerge while guiding. It helps you to recognize subtle cues from the client that something special is present in the imagery process.
- Continually assess the client's body language and facial expressions for resistance to the imagery process. If there is resistance, the imagery should be kept simple and more directed: "Focus on your right hand . . . and notice sensations in your right hand. . . ." At other times, a less direct, guided imagery approach is needed, such as "At your own pace, . . ." "In your own way. . . ." Resistance to, or blocking the experience is not failure. It becomes useful information to help the client to recognize that the body-mind-spirit needs some healing.

At the End of the Session

- Bring the client to an alert state gradually, allowing time for silence before discussion. Observe and take cues from the client as to the appropriate time to begin the discussion. The moments following a session are a time for personal insight. This opportunity may be lost if talking begins too soon. Both the client and the guide need to be immersed in the healing of silence, even if only for 20 to 30 seconds.

- If appropriate, have the client finish the session by drawing or writing down some impressions.
- Discuss the experience with the client, and encourage the client to interpret the imagery. The nurse can facilitate the interpretation by weaving imagery questions into conversational interaction and asking open-ended questions that guide the client in further contemplation.
- Provide the client with appropriate educational materials. Give written guidelines for integrating imagery skills and bodymind communication into daily life.
- Encourage the client to integrate relaxation and imagery daily. Instruct the client to notice patterns of tension at different times during the day. Then show the client how to replace tension patterns with relaxation and different types of imagery.
- Encourage the client to notice constant inner self-talk, focusing on introducing positive images and statements into this inner dialogue.
- Introduce the idea of "constant instant practice," using some frequent activity of daily life (e.g., telephone calls) as a reminder to practice imagery.
- Have the client use the images that come forth from inner awareness as guides for practice. Suggest the use of a journal or diary for recording images and their interpretation.
- Emphasize that practice is the key to successful imagery interventions. Have the client establish a scheduled time to practice, just as he or she takes medication on a schedule.
- Experiment with different exercises.
- Use the client outcomes (see Table 22–3) that were established before the imagery session and the questions shown in Exhibit 22–1 on the client's

Exhibit 22-1 Evaluating the Client's Subjective Experience with Imagery

1. Was this a new kind of imagery experience for you? Can you describe it?
2. Did you have a visual experience? Of people, places, or objects? Can you describe them?
3. Did you see colors while being guided? Did the colors change as the guided imagery continued?
4. Were you aware of your surroundings? Were you able to let the imagery flow?
5. Did you like the imagery?
6. Did the imagery produce any feelings or emotions?
7. Did you notice any textures, smells, movements, or taste while experiencing the imagery?
8. Was the experience pleasant?
9. Did you feel relaxed and refreshed after the experience?
10. Would you like to try this again?
11. What would make this a better experience for you?
12. What is your next step (or your plan) to integrate this on a daily basis?

subjective experience with imagery to evaluate the session.
• Schedule a follow-up session.

Specific Interventions

Facilitation and Interpretation of the Imagery Process

It is essential for nurses to become aware of their own imagery process and familiarize themselves with the rich variety and individuality of imagery experiences. When nurses come together in a group to listen and share personal and professional stories, they hear many perspectives. They can train themselves to listen to the use of metaphors and images and learn from the different types of imagers.

In order to facilitate the imagery process, the nurse serves as a guide. There is absolutely no way to predict what will surface in a client's imagination. Every experience is different, even when the same script is used.

Nurses who are unfamiliar with imagery and guiding should learn a few basic relaxation and imagery scripts and practice on themselves by making tapes of their own voice and following their own guiding. This will help build confidence with the intervention. It is helpful to learn a variety of scripts pertaining to common problems in clinical practice, such as preoperative anxiety, recovery from surgery, postoperative coughing, effective wound healing, fear, anxiety, pain, and relationship problems. For scripts not frequently used, some nurses keep a notebook or reference book handy. In studying clinical imagery, the nurse needs to be willing to open up and learn it from the inside out, using imagery for personal change and development.

Each individual is the best interpreter of his or her own imagery process.[50] Symbolic information that surfaces in the imagination is rich with personal meaning. Many people have been closed off from or afraid of their imagination. Nurses should encourage clients to record their images in a diary or journal for further exploration. It is easy to lose symbolic imagery in the conscious thoughts that dominate someone's attention during a busy day.

When teaching imagery, the nurse listens to the way that a client tells his or her story to get a sense of the client's outlook and orientation to the world. Does the client have a materialistic, concrete outlook on problem solving and life in general, or a more intuitive, spontaneous perspective? For the logical, concrete thinker, written information is useful. For example, if using imagery for hand warming, the nurse may prepare an imagery teaching sheet that includes specific physiologic information and instructions such as

- an explanation of normal blood flow physiology
- a drawing of blood flow to the hands via radial and ulnar arteries that branch into intricate blood vessel networks of the hands and the fingers
- examples of images that warm the hands.

Less structure is necessary for the more intuitive patient. The nurse can go directly to working with imagery and use the teaching sheets to support what the vivid imager has learned.

There is no need to follow teaching sheets explicitly. Suggested images are adapted to fit what feels right to the client. Teaching sheets refresh and reinforce the teaching–learning session and provide additional information to be mastered. Clients can add their own notes about specific images and personalize their practice. The nurse can help clients rework weak or erroneous imagery so that it more accurately reflects healthy outcomes (e.g., images focusing on weak, confused, cancer cells and a strong immune system instead of vice versa).

Guided Imagery Scripts

The guidelines that follow will help the nurse in the effective implementation of imagery scripts as nursing interventions:

- Start the session with an induction, a general relaxation—focusing on breath, shortened passive progressive relaxation, or body awareness, for example.
- Reaffirm that there is no right or wrong way for the client to do imagery, that whatever occurs is useful information, and that the client has complete control over the process (e.g., deciding whether to go further or to stop).
- Follow the induction instructions for yourself so that you communicate a calming presence.
- Personalize the imagery by using the client's name or other specific references several times during the process.

- Speak slowly and smoothly, allowing for pauses and silence after each suggestion.
- Observe the client's body language and breathing rhythm to assess responses to suggestions.
- If there are signs of tension such as shallow breathing, tightness of muscles, or tense facial muscles in response to an imagery suggestion, ask, "What are you experiencing now?"
- If the client appears to be struggling to get into the imagery, pause in the script and suggest that the client reconnect with breath and go more deeply into relaxation.
- Avoid saying "yes" or "right" or other words that communicate evaluative reactions to the client's experience. A more supportive comment such as "stay with your experience" can be made.
- Provide encouragement and guidance for those with less vivid imagery. Vivid imagers, on the other hand, prefer more silence: words may be distracting or intrusive to them. Extremely vivid imagers may prefer to keep their eyes partially open to prevent feeling overwhelmed.
- End the session by bringing the person's awareness back to the room (e.g., "At the count of 5, you will be fully awake and alert . . . 1 . . . 2 . . . 3 . . . 4 . . . 5").

Induction for Imagery. A simple breathing technique or other relaxation technique may be useful to focus the client's mind inward and induce imagery. This allows awareness of subtler aspects of experience to become available to the person. This inward focus can be thought of as reducing external stimuli so that the inner awareness is enhanced.

The following induction script can be used as a preparation for most imagery interventions. It is especially appropriate for a person who needs assistance quieting the body.

Resting the hands on the lower abdomen and breathing into the belly (diaphragmatic breathing) is an effective calming posture. In this position, the palms of the hands are resting on the body's energy center. By noting the slowing of breathing, relaxation of facial muscles, and changes in skin color, the nurse can assess the effectiveness of the relaxation technique. The induction for imagery can take 5 to 10 minutes.

> **Script:** *Make yourself comfortable and close your eyes. . . . Put your hands gently on your lower abdomen, just below your navel. . . . Bring all your attention to the sensations in your hands. . . . Notice the slight rise and fall of your hands as they move with your breathing. . . . Notice the tactile sensations of the surfaces of your hands and fingers. . . . Bring all your awareness into these sensations. . . . [Pause.] Now notice the temperature of your hands. . . . [Pause.] Notice their weight. . . . [Pause.] Now notice any sensations inside the skin, perhaps tingling or pulsing. . . . [Pause.] Now bring your attention to the center of your chest and be aware of the sensations . . . noticing the movement of your chest with each breath . . . the passage of breath into your lungs . . . the tactile sensations of your skin . . . perhaps an awareness of your heartbeat. . . . [Pause.] Now bring your awareness to your nose and be aware of breath passing through your nostrils. . . . Notice the slight cool sensations of the air touching the inside of your nose. . . .*

Connecting with Life Energy. This imagery, which draws upon a person's sense of his or her inner energy, focuses on the fact that the body is not just sick. The life force is operating without any conscious effort. This awareness can reframe a person's attitude, bringing a connection with inner healing mechanisms and with what is functioning healthfully, as opposed to focusing on the disease process.

> **Script:** *Bring your awareness to your imagination and take a moment to reflect on all the systems that are functioning in your bodymind at this moment . . . your heart and your circulatory system . . . [pause] your immune system . . . [pause] your respiratory system . . . [pause] your senses. . . . [Pause.] Be aware of all of these. . . . [Pause.] Realize that you don't need to do anything to make these systems function. . . . They are part of your body's wisdom. . . . [Pause.] And now be aware that deep within you is a source of life energy . . . a vital spark that has been a part of you since the moment of your conception. . . . It has always been a part of you . . . guiding and energizing your body and mind. . . . Use your imagination to get in touch with this source of life energy. . . . Trust whatever information your imagination gives you. . . . Locate this source in your body. . . . Feel its strength and energy. . . . [Pause.] Allow your intuition to give you an image or symbol for this source and when you have the image, spend some time with it. . . . [Pause.] If it feels right, communicate with it . . . What does it need from you? . . . [Pause.] If there is anything*

else that needs to happen in relation to this image, let it happen.... Take your time.... When you feel ready, bring your awareness back to the room....

Special/Safe Place. Clients need to identify a special place that is a safe retreat. This is an easy place for novices to start. It takes 10 to 20 minutes. Several different approaches can be useful.

Scripts:

- *Let your imagination choose a place that is safe and comfortable ... a place where you can retreat at any time. This is a healthy technique for you to learn.... This place will help you survive your daily stressors. [If the client is in the hospital, ...] This safe and special place is very important, particularly while you are in the hospital.... Any time that there are interruptions, just let yourself go to this place in your mind.*
- *Form a clear image of a pleasant outdoor scene, using all of your senses.... Breathe ... smell the fragrance of flowers or the breeze. Feel ... feel the texture of the surface under your feet. Hear ... hear all the sounds in nature, birds singing, wind blowing. See ... see all the different sights around as you let yourself turn in a slow circle to get a full view of this special space. [Include taste, if appropriate.]*
- *Let a beam of light, such as the rays of the sun, shine on you for comfort and healing. Allow yourself to experience the warmth and relaxation. Form an image of a meadow. Imagine that you are in the meadow.... The meadow is full of beautiful grass and flowers. In the meadow, see yourself sitting by a stream ...*

watching the water ... flowing by ... slowly and gently.

- *Imagine a mountain scene. See yourself walking on a path toward the mountain. You hear the sound of your shoes on the path ... smell the pine trees and feel the cool breeze as you approach your campsite. You have now reached the foothills of the mountain. You are now higher up the mountain ... resting in your campsite. Look around at the beauty of this place.*
- *Imagine yourself in a bamboo forest.... You are walking in a large bamboo forest. The bamboo is very tall.... You lean against a strong cluster of bamboo ... hear the swaying ... and hear the rustling of the bamboo leaves, gently moving in the wind.... Look into the sky of your mind.... See the fluffy clouds. A cloud gently comes your way, ... and the cloud surrounds your body. You climb up on the cloud and lie down. Feel yourself begin to float off gently in a gentle breeze.*

Worry and Fear. Some images can help clients change the internal experience of worry and fear. Clients should set aside 10 to 20 minutes a day to worry, preferably in the morning before they start their daily routines. This approach reassures the subconscious that it *has* worried, and the person has greater success at stopping the habitual worry during the rest of the day.

Script: *Let worries come one by one ... just watching as one replaces the other. As you do this for a short period of time, feel the experience that occurs with each of those worries and fears. Notice how just having a worry or fear changes your state right now.*

Stop the images. Focus on your breathing ... in ... and out. ... Allow yourself to have three complete cycles of breathing before continuing. ... In your relaxed state, become aware of these feelings of relaxed bodymind. This time, take your relaxed state with you into your imagination. Let one worry come to your mind right now. See and feel it. ... See yourself in that situation relaxed and at ease.

Right now, just say to yourself, "I can stop this worry." Imagine yourself functioning without that worry or fear. See yourself waving good-bye to that worry and fear. See yourself completely free of that worry and fear. Look at the decisions that you can make for your life that will lead you in new directions. Feel your energy as you breathe in. As you exhale, let go of all of the worry, fear, tension, and tightness.

Experience your comfortable bodymind. Know that you can work with many of your worries and fears that surface daily. Whenever they come, let the dominant worry surface. ... Then feel what it is like as you gradually give up portions of the worry ... until it is completely gone. If that seems impossible right now, decide which part of that worry and fear you need to keep and which part you can let go. And now, see yourself waving good-bye to the part that you can let go.

Now, feel what it is like in your mind with part of that worry or fear gone. Experience that and feel the changes within the body. Assess the part of the worry or fear that remains. Again, allow a portion of that worry or fear to move away. See yourself waving good-bye. Feel the change inside as more is released.

Let yourself now be in a place where the worry and fear are diminished. Assess what part remains and see if you can now begin to give up that part. Pay attention to the experiences inside your body as you do this.

This script has many variations: writing worries/fears on a seashell and watching a seagull pick up the shell and drop it into the sea; running along a road, dropping the worries/fears by the road, and watching the wind blow them away; letting a picture of worries and fears flow forward in a moving stream. This basic script can also be individualized by putting into words what the client revealed before the session.

Inner Guide. The nurse can assist the client in creating purposeful self-dialogue that gains access to inner wisdom and personal truth that always resides within one's being. It is advisable to allow 10 to 20 minutes for this exercise.

Script: *As you begin to feel even more relaxed now ... going to a deeper place within ... feeling deeply relaxed ... peaceful and safe ... let yourself become aware of a sense of not being alone. With you right now is a guide ... who is wise and concerned with your well-being. Let yourself begin to see this wise being with whom you can share your fears or your joys. You have a trust in this wise being.*

If you do not see anyone, let yourself be aware of hearing or feeling this wise being, noticing the presence of care and concern. In whatever way seems best for you, . . . proceed to make contact with this wise inner guide. Let yourself establish contact with your guide now . . . in any way that comes. Your guide may appear to you in any form, such as a person, an animal, an inner presence/ peace . . . or as an image of the very wisest part of you.

Notice the love and wisdom with which you are surrounded. This wisdom and love are present for you now. . . . Let yourself ask for advice . . . about anything that is important for you just now. Be receptive to what emerges. . . . Let yourself receive some new information. This inner guide may have a special message to share with you. . . . Listen with openness and pure intention to receive.

Allow yourself to look at any issue in your life. It may be a symptom, a choice, or decision. . . . Tell your wise guide anything that you wish. . . . Listen to the answers that emerge. Imagine yourself acting on the answers and directions that you received. . . . Imagine yourself calling upon the wisdom and love of this wise guide to help you in the days to come. Now in whatever way is best for you . . . bring closure to the visit with this inner guide. You can come back here any time that you wish.

All you have to do is take the time.

This script helps clients gain an awareness of their own inner wisdom. It is best to introduce this exercise after a client has done several imagery sessions. Word choices should take into account the client's dominant sense. If a client prefers the visual, for example, the nurse uses the word *see*; if the client prefers the auditory, the word *hears*; if the client prefers the kinesthetic, the word *feels*.

Seeking an inner guide can be done over many sessions. The client should be aware that many different guides or advisors will surface over time. The guide may also appear as a traditional religious figure such as a shaman, the Virgin Mary, a saint, Moses, or Buddha. It can be interesting and surprising when someone meets a spiritual figure not from their own religious tradition. The guide may also emerge as an admired historical or living person such as a favorite author or artist, a philosopher, or a heroic leader such as Martin Luther King.

There are many versions of this script, so the nurse can add, invent, and explore. Much detail can be added to this imagery script to lengthen the session. When time is extended, a wealth of insight can emerge for the client. The nurse should pause frequently and let a few moments pass in silence during the guiding, as indicated by his or her intuition.

Red Ball of Pain. To decrease psychophysiologic pain, clients can learn to use distraction. This kind of imagery is good for both acute and chronic pain, as well as for the discomfort or pain of procedures. It takes 10 to 20 minutes.

> **Script:** *Scan your body. . . . Gather any pains, aches, or other symptoms up into a ball. Begin to change its size. . . . Allow it to get bigger. . . . Just imagine how big you can make it. Now make it*

smaller.... See how small you can make it.... Is it possible to make it the size of a grain of sand? Now allow it to move slowly out of your body, moving further away each time you exhale.... Notice the experience with each exhale ... as the pain moves away.

Give suggestions to the client to change the size of the ball several times in both directions. This serves as a distraction and an exercise in manipulating the pain experience rather than being trapped or overwhelmed by it. This imagery provides a tremendous sense of control as well as pain relief for the client. The person's body cues indicate how many times to go in each of the opposite directions.

Pain Assessment. Imagery helps access and control both acute and chronic psychophysiologic pain. The following exercise can be done in 10 to 20 minutes.

Script: *Close your eyes and let yourself relax.... Begin to describe the pain in silence to yourself. Be present with the pain.... Know that the pain may be either physical sensations ... or worries and fears. Let your pain take on a shape ... any shape that comes to your mind. Become aware of the dimensions of the pain.... What is the height of your pain? ... The width of the pain? ... And the depth of the pain? Where in the body is it located? ... Give it color ... a shape.... Feel the texture. Does it make any sound?*

And now with your eyes still closed, ... let your hands come together with palms turned upward as if forming a cup. Put your pain object in your hands. [Once again, the nurse asks these questions about the pain, preceding each question with this phrase, "How would you change the size, etc.?"]

Let yourself decide what you would like to do with the pain. There is no right way to finish the experience.... Just accept what feels right to you. You can throw the pain away ... or place it back where you found it ... or move it somewhere else. Let yourself become aware ... of how pain can be changed.... By your focusing with intention, the pain changes.

It is not unusual for the pain to go completely away or at least lessen after this exercise. The client also learns to manipulate the pain so that it is not the controlling factor of his or her life. The exercise is also effective with severe pain. After giving pain medication, the nurse can have the client relax during the imagery process.

Correct Biologic Imagery Teaching Sheets and Scripts

Clients who are given specific information about the role of bodymind connections, correct biologic healing images, and stress management strategies have fewer complications and shorter recovery times.[51-53] The nurse elicits from a client/patient images and symbols that have special healing meaning and value, then makes an audiocassette for the client/patient that includes correct biologic images, specific concrete objective information, specific symbols, and specific types of imagery. (See Chapter 23 for guidelines on making an audiocassette tape and establishing an audio/video library.)

It may seem that the following scripts are suitable only for well educated, sophisticated individuals, but this is not the case. It is necessary, however, for the nurse to assess the individual's education level and adapt these scripts to fit the person's needs and cultural beliefs. Imagery is an important tool, particularly for those clients who do not read.

Bone Healing.[54] An imagery exercise for bone healing may be done in 20 to 30 minutes. Prior to imagery, to teach basic biologic imagery of bone healing, the nurse explains

- reaction (cellular proliferation). Within the hematoma surrounding the fracture, cells and tissues proliferate and develop into a random structure (Figure 22–1A).
- regeneration (callus formation). At 10 to 14 days after the fracture, the cells within the hematoma become organized in a fibrous lattice. With sufficient organization, the callus becomes clinically stable. The callus obliterates the medullary canal and surrounds the two ends of bone by irregularly surrounding the fracture defect (Figure 22–1B).
- remodeling (new bone formation). Approximately 25 to 40 days after the fracture, calcium is laid down within bone that has spicules perpendicular to the cortical surface (Figure 22–1C). Osteonal bone gradually replaces and remodels fiber bone. The fracture has been bridged over by new bone (Figure 22–1D). Conversion and remodeling continue up to 3 years following an acute fracture.

Script: *In your relaxed state, [name], allow yourself to imagine a natural process that is occurring within your body.... New cells are gathering very fast at the site of your fracture [cellular proliferation]. This is an important process as it lays the foundation for your bone healing. With your next breath in ... become aware of the fact ... that right now your body is allowing those new cells to multiply rapidly [positive suggestion]. Your blood cells ... at the site of your fracture are arranging themselves in a special healing pattern You can relax ... even more ... if you want to ... as you continue with this very natural healing process.*

In a few days, ... your wise body will begin to create a strong lattice network of new bone [regeneration]. This will allow your bone to become stable, bridging the new bone that is forming. As you focus in a relaxed way, ... you help in your healing, ... for relaxation increases this natural process. Imagine your relaxation to be like a gentle breeze of wind that flows over and throughout your body.

In a few more weeks, your new bone will be formed.... Natural deposits of calcium from your body will be taken into the place of healing [remodeling]. Allow an image to come to your mind now of beautiful, healed bone. In about 6 weeks, you will have a beautiful bridge where the calcium has formed new bone.... Can you imagine a healing light within you right now? Allow this healing light to radiate throughout your body, bringing its loving energy to every cell in your body.... Stay with this experience for as long as you want, and then whenever you feel ready,

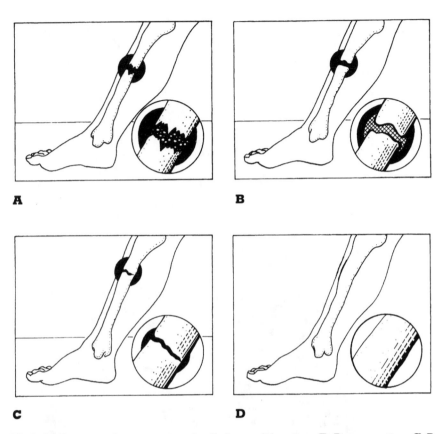

Figure 22–1 A, Reaction: hematoma and cellular proliferation. **B**, Regeneration. **C**, Remodeling: calcium ossification. **D**, Healed bone. *Source:* Reprinted with permission from J. Achterberg, B. Dossey, and L. Kolkmeier, *Rituals of Healing,* © 1994, Bantam Books.

slowly bring your awareness back to the room. . . .[55]

Burn Graft Healing. In 20 to 30 minutes, the nurse can teach patients about the normal burn graft healing process with correct biologic images (Figure 22–2A).

- Day 1: The adhesion of surfaces and the bridging of the space between the graft bed and the graft begin (Figure 22–2B).
- Day 2: The vessels from the patient grow into the graft (Figure 22–2C).
- Day 3: The vessels establish vascular continuity (Figure 22–2D).

    Script: *In your relaxed state now, . . . let's begin a journey into your body. . . . Begin to identify the capacity that you have to work with the healing process with your new graft. In your mind, go to the area where you have been burned. I am going to describe the healing process . . . that is taking place with your new graft. In your mind, go to the area of your body where you have received your new graft. If you begin to feel any tension, . . . just take a deep breath, and know that you can let yourself relax and release any tension at this time. . . . Notice how you can deepen your state of relaxation . . . releasing the ten-*

A

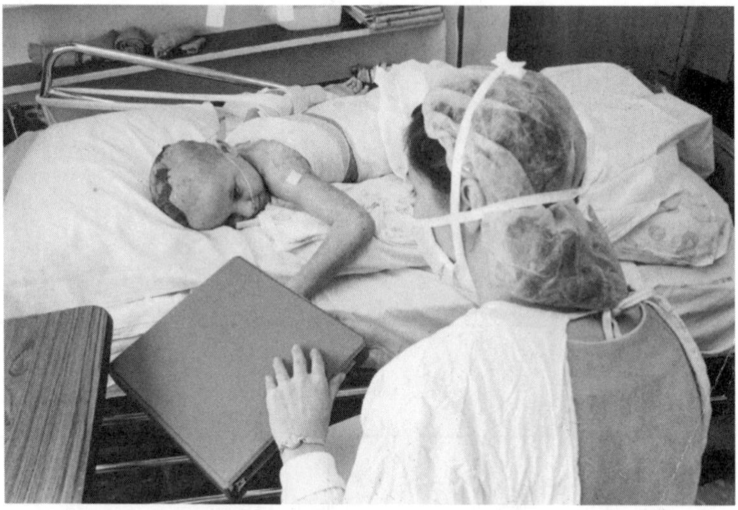

B

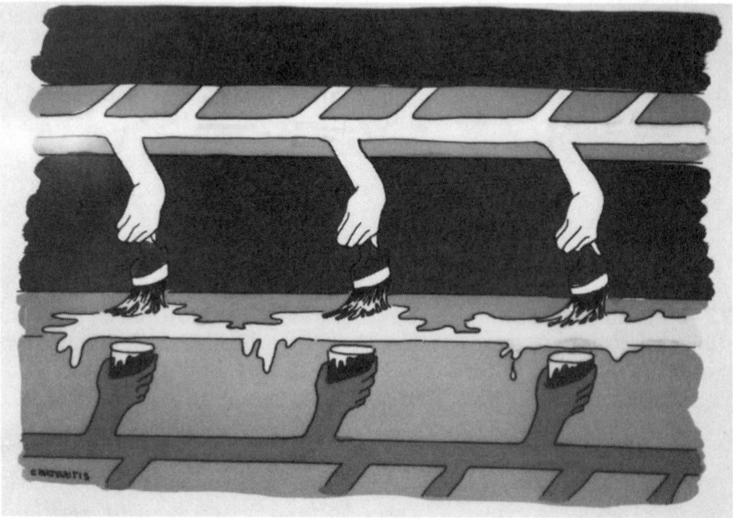

Figure 22-2 A, A child who has been severely burned is provided process images just prior to his surgery. **B**, Skin grafts, using the boy's own healthy skin, will be placed over the burned areas. He is shown these pictures and told that, on the first day, something like glue will come out of his body to stick on the graft. *Source:* Reprinted with permission from J. Achterberg, B. Dossey, and L. Kolkmeier, *Rituals of Healing,* © 1994, Bantam Books.

sion as you breathe out [positive suggestion]. . . . *Imagine relaxation is like a still mountain lake. Experience the gentle wind forming ripples on the surface of the lake. . . . As the ripples widen, . . . realize they are ripples of relaxation flowing* through your body and mind [metaphor]. *Before your graft, the area where you were burned was gently cleansed. . . . In this clean area, the graft was gently placed and covered with a thick layer of dressings.*

C

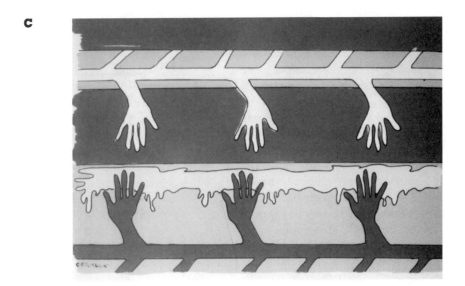

D

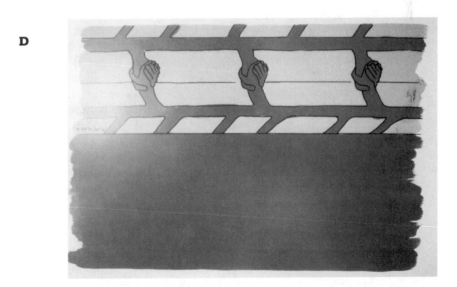

Figure 22–2 continued. **C**, On the second day, blood vessels (like hands) will reach out toward each other. **D**, Finally, if all goes well, on the third day, his skin graft will be complete. *Source:* Reprinted with permission from J. Achterberg, B. Dossey, and L. Kolkmeier, *Rituals of Healing,* © 1994, Bantam Books.

In your mind, begin to imagine the healing process. On Day 1, imagine that your own skin secretes a kind of glue. This glue is very important, because it will allow your new graft to stick and hold in a healthy way. Just take several relaxing breaths now ... in ... and out, ... feeling the pause between each of those breaths. As you go deeply into relax-

ation, feel yourself . . . partici-pating in natural healing processes, . . . your skin secreting a glue, and your new graft sticking to it and becoming part of your body . . . part of your healing. During this first day, you will also remember to move gently and work with the nurses as they help you with your comfort . . . your heal-ing . . . your recovery. . . .

Now begin to move to Day 2. On this day, after receiving your graft, your body continues the healing process. Your body is sending nutrients to the graft, small blood vessels are sprouting out . . . like little hands moving out, sending nu-trients to every cell in this area, nourishing and caring for you. Remember to stay as still as possible and let the nurses help you move. [Adapt this phrase as needed if working with a small child.] *This is important, . . . for it also helps those tiny blood vessels grow in a very healthy manner. Dur-ing this time, you will continue to increase your relaxation to that particular area where your grafts will take hold. And as you exhale, let go of any ten-sion and tightness.*

Now move to Day 3 of your recovery process. By Day 3, the blood vessels from your own body . . . and the blood vessels from your graft actually grow together. Imagine . . . blood vessels joining hands, uniting . . . [metaphor]. *As you feel this experience of your blood vessels joining hands, just imagine now this graft is part of your body . . . just like*

all the other cells of your body Imagine this is happening now, . . . the graft is now a part of you. . . .

Again, let us go over these three important areas that will occur after your graft. On Day 1, your skin secretes a glue, and the glue sticks to your own skin. On Day 2, blood vessels from your own skin and the blood vessels from the graft be-gin to grow together. By Day 3, those blood vessels have joined together, and this graft is now a part of your body. [If the graft is from the patient, the nurse may continue.] *Spend some time now focusing on that area where the graft came from your body. The natural healing abil-ity is also occurring there, with the new skin now being formed.* [Repeat information in the script on wound healing, but substitute the words "new skin" for "graft."][56]

Wound Healing.[57] To teach the normal wound healing process with correct bio-logic images, the nurse explains

- reaction. Fluid leaks into tissue at the time of the injury, causing swelling and inflammation; white blood cells migrate to the wound. Inflammation continues from injury to 72 hours (Fig-ure 22–3A).
- regeneration. Granulation and de-posit of fibrous collagen protein tissue continue for as long as 3 weeks follow-ing the injury (Figure 22–3B).
- remodeling. Healing of a wound takes 3 weeks to 2 years for severe wounds (Figure 22–3C).

A wound healing intervention may last 20 to 30 minutes.

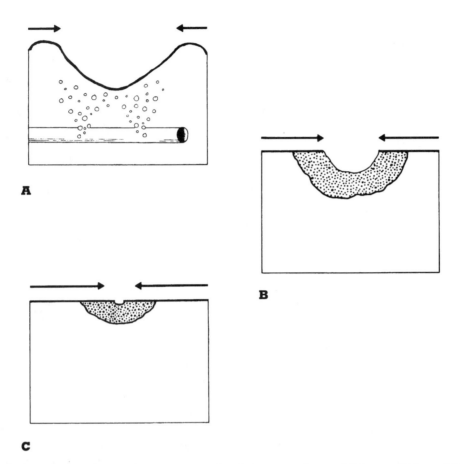

Figure 22–3 A, Reaction: inflammation and stabilization of wound (injury to 72 hours). **B**, Regeneration: granulation and deposit of fibrous collagen protein tissue (up to 3 weeks). **C**, Remodeling: healed wound (3 weeks to 2 years). *Source:* Reprinted with permission from J. Achterberg, B. Dossey, and L. Kolkmeier, *Rituals of Healing,* © 1994, Bantam Books.

Script: *Focus on calmness and rhythmic breathing . . . and become aware of your ritual . . . for cleansing your wound. Let it be done slowly . . . without hurry. To avoid holding your breath, . . . take several rhythmic breaths prior to cleansing your wound. When you are ready to begin the cleansing of your wound, . . . take a breath in . . . and, on the exhale, place the hydrogen peroxide or other solutions on the wound and surrounding area or along suture lines. Next, on the area that has been cleansed and patted dry, place the ointment in the same area to help speed the healing process. Now is the time to place a clean dressing on the wound.*

Allow yourself to imagine a natural process that is occurring within your body. . . . New cells are being made in the open skin area . . . to allow a stable place for repair and new growth. Now your blood flow is surging to this area. . . . Special white blood cells, your macrophages, are recognizing any foreign material and carrying it away. Remember . . . be with the special healing process of your wound. . . . If your wound is superficial, it heals from the edges toward the center. . . . A deep wound will heal from the inside to the outside.

A beautiful area is now forming. . . . you might imagine it like looking down into a lovely shallow bowl. Within this area . . . your body now places soft, healthy, delicate fibrous protein tissue . . . like a network of beautiful lights . . . the beginning of a strong scar that starts below the surface of the skin.

Become more aware . . . of the fact . . . that your own special cells, the fibroblasts, are producing this collagen protein. Many small buds of new tissue continue to be laid down and grow stronger and fuller, creating healthy new skin and scar tissue. The opening shrinks and becomes smaller as healing occurs.

Let an image or feeling of the new healed skin surface emerge. . . . Your skin has healed from the inside to the outside. See, hear, and feel your healed, smooth, new skin that is strong and healthy.

Immune System Odyssey.[58] Patients can be taught correct biologic images of the normal process of the immune system. (For more details, see Chapter 4 on mind modulation of the immune system.) The nurse may explain the following:

- **Neutrophils.** The most numerous cells, billions of neutrophils swim in the bloodstream; when they sense unhealthy tissue, they pass through the blood vessel, move to the unhealthy tissue or cells, surround it, shoot caustic chemicals, and destroy the unhealthy tissue or cells (Figure 22–4).
- **Macrophages.** Moving throughout the body, ever ready to eat, macrophages travel in hoards, each one swells up, consuming the enemy (e.g., bacteria, viruses, yeast, cancer cells).
- **T-cells.** Born in the bone marrow, millions of T-cells go from infancy to adolescence each minute. They go to the thymus gland, where they get a special imprint; some are designated killer cells, while others become helpers or suppressors. All these specialized cells keep a watchful vigil in the lymph nodes and tissue until needed.
- **B-cells.** For years, B-cells wait and mature in the bone marrow until needed. They can change like caterpillars to butterflies, becoming plasma cells that manufacture magic bullets, the protein called antibodies. Operating like a guided missile, they can shoot the target, paralyze the enemy, shoot caustic chemicals, and explode the bad cells and tissue. B-cells can clone themselves and create whatever number it takes to do the battle.

In 20 to 30 minutes, the nurse can guide the client through an intervention, modifying the script as needed.

Script: *You are about to embark on the most incredible journey imaginable, a journey through your own immune system, touching your body's healing forces with your mind; you will sense, feel, envision a miracle. A miracle of defense and protection, a miracle of the billions of honor-*

able, persistent warriors within that have but one mission: to guard you from disease and injury and invasion.

To fully appreciate this odyssey, which is as complex as it is magnificent, it is important to clear and focus your mind, to relax your body. The bridge between your mind and body is easily crossed when distractions are released, when a sense of peace and calm spreads warmly from the top of your head to your toes. As you let go of stress, your immune system is activated. Relax, now, as you participate and observe your own healing process.

As your mind becomes clearer and clearer, feel it becoming more and more alert. Somewhere deep inside of you, a brilliant light begins to glow. Sense this happening. . . . The light grows brighter and brighter and more intense. . . . This is your bodymind communication center. Breathe into it. . . . Energize it with your breath. The light is powerful and penetrating, and the beam begins to grow from it. The beam shines into your body into any area you wish. It is your searchlight, your bridge into the glorious mysteries about to unfold. Practice shining it into your body. Sometimes this is easier to do than other times. Just allow it to happen.

The immune journey begins inside your bones. So take this most intelligent beam of light and shine it into a long bone . . . a leg bone perhaps. Penetrate deeply into the marrow. This is the birthing center

for all your blood cells. Just imagine if you can, . . . feel if you can, . . . billions . . . of young cells being born . . . many kinds, each with a task to nurture and protect you. As we go through this exercise, we will focus on a few types of cells that are vital to defending you. They have names: neutrophils, macrophages, T-cells, B-cells, natural killer cells. One by one, we'll shine the light on them, watching them work to guard and protect and remove cells that no longer serve you.

The most numerous cells are called neutrophils. They eat and engulf the invaders in a most ingenious way. Imagine them maturing, moving into your bloodstream, floating, ever alert for a call to work in your defense. As a call warns them of an invader, they become exceedingly alert. No longer swimming freely, millions, billions of them sense the danger and move methodically, directly, preparing for attack. The blood vessels become sticky, attracting the neutrophils to their surface. The small opening in the blood vessel walls dilates in the vicinity of the attack. Imagine the neutrophils being attracted to the walls. They move quickly along the vessel walls until they know with absolute certainty that the invader is near. Now, they extend a small foot, a pseudopod, into the walls, and changing shape, they slither through, entering your tissues. Moving forward now, as they approach the invader, they send another small foot out, surrounding the

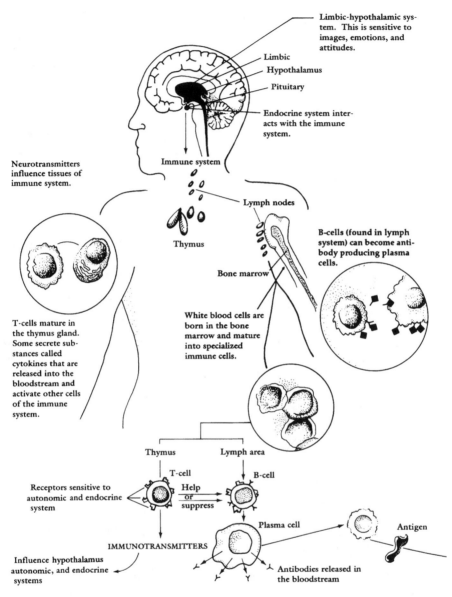

Figure 22-4 Immune system components. *Source:* Reprinted with permission from J. Achterberg, B. Dossey, and L. Kolkmeier, *Rituals of Healing,* © 1994, Bantam Books.

enemy, shooting caustic chemicals into it, wearing it thin. The enemy is halted, destroyed, may even explode into harmless bits. Imagine this happening, constantly, protecting you from the dangers of living in a hostile world. Billions and billions of neutrophils are born every day.

Now, shining the beam of light back into the bone marrow, imagine the macrophages, or the giant eaters . . .

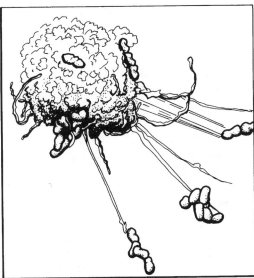

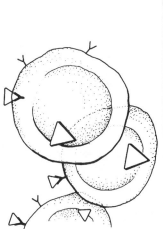

Neuropeptides produced
in the brain lock onto
specific receptors of
immune cells.

Phagocytes, such as neutrophils and the macrophage
pictured here literally eat bacteria, viruses, cancer cells,
and other foreign particles or destroyed tissue and
contain chemicals that break down and destroy the
invaders.

The immune system pro-
duces memory cells when
exposed to an antigen, and
the immune system then
remembers that encounter
and becomes more efficient
against it the next time it
gets invaded by micro-
organisms that produce
antigens.

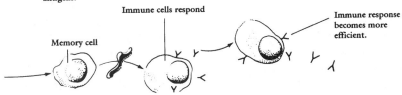

Immune cells respond

Immune response
becomes more
efficient.

Memory cell

Figure 22–4 continued

fewer of them, but long-lived
with many talents. As they mature, watch them move into tissues and organs and blood.
They line the walls of the lungs
and liver . . . waiting, survey-
ing, watching, ever ready to

move. Bacteria, viruses, yeast
cells, even cancer cells trigger
the alarm. As the warning of an
invader sounds, the macrophages swell up, becoming large
and powerful. They may even
mesh together with the other

macrophages, moving rapidly in a powerful, connecting flank. They reach out for the enemy; lasso it with their armlike extensions, and bring the invader into their bodies, injecting it with potent enzymes. With lightning speed, they consume an enemy. What they can't destroy, they encircle and preserve, protecting you from its dangerous acts. The macrophages are also your scavengers. They can and will digest anything and everything in your body that you no longer have use for. Imagine this happening for a moment.

The macrophages and neutrophils are nonspecific, nondiscriminating in their attack and clean-up activities. Other cells, the lymphocytes, or the T-cells and the B-cells, have an assigned function, a target that they spend their entire lives stalking. It might be a special virus, or bacteria, or cancer cell, or other foreign tissue. Let's look at these cells in action.

Shining the beam, again, into the bone marrow, observe the T-cells being born. Millions . . . more than you could possibly count . . . move from infancy to adolescence each minute. The T-cells will each be given a special task as they are processed in the thymus gland. Shine your imagery light into the middle of your chest, here is the thymus gland. Feel it pulsating with energy. Watch, now, as the adolescent T-cells flow in rapidly, each touched with a spark of wisdom, each challenged with a mission. Some will be killers,

assassins with a single target. Others will be helpers for your B-cells. Still others will be suppressors, signaling that the battle is over, protecting your body from excessive immune activity. Imagine these, the killers, the helpers, the suppressors, maturing quickly and with glorious specificity in your thymus. When each has been imprinted, they leave the thymus to go about their tasks. The T-cells keep a wakeful vigil in your lymph nodes, your spleen, other lymph tissue. Think of this for a time. . . .

Back in the bone marrow once again, the B-cells are highlighted by the beam. They mature and move into the lymph tissues and blood, waiting for the encounter. Each has a specific enemy to protect you from, and they can wait patiently for years, patrolling, waiting, and watching. When the encounter finally takes place, the B-cells change, like cocoons into butterflies, becoming a plasma cell. The plasma cells manufacture magic bullets, which are proteins called antibodies. Each antibody is like a guided missile. . . . It moves directly for its target and hooks on to it, like a key in a lock. The enemy is paralyzed and its surface damaged. Other chemicals are liberated in the blood by this action, and they burn holes in the wall of the enemy, causing an explosion. The B-cells also clone themselves, creating whatever number is needed to do pure and perfect battle in your defense.

One last time, peering into the birthing center of the immune system, the light shines onto natural killer cells. The natural killers are wondrous defenses against cancer. Like viruses and bacteria, cancer cells are not especially unusual in the human body. The body simply recognizes them as invaders and sends out the forces of defense. Only in the most unusual circumstances (e.g., when cancer cells wear a disguise) does the immune system fail to find them. Watch now, as the natural killer cells are born and move into the bloodstream. Take the light and shine it on one cell, and watch its action. Ever alert, it senses a cancer cell in the vicinity. Moving at lightning speed, it collides with the cancer cell. Its mere touch paralyzes the cell. Fingers of the natural killer cell reach into the cancer cell, oozing in its power and might. Then a small cannonlike structure within the natural killer cell tilts, aims, and fires deadly chemicals into the cancer cell. Already paralyzed, the cancer cell develops blisters, peels like an orange. Its cellular matter dissolves, leaving only harmless skeletal remains. The natural killer cell, alive and well, continues its alert patrol of your body.

Before you end this exercise, go over the immune process once more, sensing all the immune cells working in a superbly coordinated team of defense. In the bone marrow, billions of cells are being born each minute, in exactly the number and combinations that you need to stay healthy. As the white blood cells mature, each develops a remarkable intelligence. Each has a dedicated task. Witness these cells moving out of the bone marrow, into blood tissue, watching and waiting for the opportunity to protect and cleanse you. Feel the presence of these magnificent guardians, and sense their power. These dedicated warriors, this system of defense has a universe of its own. That universe is you. By relaxing, as you have just done, and concentrating on this process, you have actively participated in keeping yourself healthy.[59]

Drawing

In the imagery process, drawing is an effective way to open up communication with the self and others. It externalizes previously internal mental images and emotions. The emphasis in this intervention is not on how well the client can draw, but on the client's ability to get in touch with feelings and healing potential through drawing. When clients are overwhelmed with emotions, drawing images of the feelings can be therapeutic. Drawing is also helpful with children who are not verbally sophisticated. Tremendous insight can be gained in this process with both adults and children who are going through painful procedures or are experiencing certain concerns, fears, or problems in daily life.

Drawing after being guided through an imagery exercise can bring further insights. The creativity that is evoked is different from the logical mode of explaining the experiences in words. Drawing works very well when a client is crying and is unable to talk easily, but wants to express what he or she is experiencing. When using drawing as an intervention, the nurse can suggest the following general ideas:

- Express yourself with a few images. There is no one best way to draw. Drawings can be either realistic or symbolic. The most important thing is that you express yourself in a nonlogical way. This can bring new awareness and understanding into your life.
- If you find that you are too focused on the result of the drawing exercise, use your nondominant hand. With your eyes closed, allow yourself to get into the expressive quality of drawing.
- Do not judge your drawing. Allow your body, mind, and spirit to connect as you begin simply to be with the paper and crayons in the present moment.
- Notice the energy flow from you. Let your body energy resonate with your imagery/spirit energy. Let the energies slowly begin to resonate together. Do not try to control the process, because this inner quality comes from being immersed in the imagery and drawing experience.
- On the blank piece of paper, allow an image to begin to form that represents your feelings and thoughts in this moment. Choose colors that speak to you. If you wish to change the color that you started working with, feel free to do so.
- After you have drawn, you might want to write some details of your images. Often, what you felt or heard during the imagery drawing may surface into conscious awareness and provide new insights about your important images.

When working with drawing for a client's specific disease/symptoms, it is helpful for the nurse to educate the client about the body processes that are being affected. It is therapeutic for the client to have an understanding of, and an image for, the healthful state, the disease/symptoms and its medication, treatments, and associated procedures, and his or her personal belief systems. Asking the client to draw the disease/symptoms in the way that has self-meaning often reveals a client's constricted view of healing possibilities or misunderstanding of the disease/symptoms, either of which may impair recovery. The drawing process helps the client recognize that the disease need not control his or her life. Insight from drawing helps the client reframe experiences of illness, let go of the inner judgments and struggles, and mobilize his or her creativity for achieving desired outcomes.

The challenge for nurses is to develop innovative teaching worksheets, booklets, and verbal descriptions of bodymind healing; to integrate imagery as part of each nursing interaction and intervention; and to develop assessment tools.[60] The nurse and client should identify the following elements for the best outcome:

- Disease or disability: the vividness of the client's view of the disease, illness, or disability and, if the process is ongoing, the strength of the disease/illness to decrease health or the client's focus on the reverse—the vividness and the strength of the client's ability to stabilize the disease/illness or stop the process
- Internal healing resources: the vividness of the client's perception of his or her healing ability and the effectiveness of this ability/action to combat the disease
- External healing resources: the vividness of the treatment description and the effectiveness of the positive mechanism of action

Case Study

Setting:	Coronary care unit (CCU), followed by outpatient cardiac rehabilitation program
Patient:	J.D., a 48-year-old male, with acute myocardial infarction

Patterns/ Problems/ Needs

complicated by congestive heart failure and pericarditis secondary to the infarction

1. Decreased cardiac output related to mechanical factors (congestive heart failure)
2. Altered comfort related to inflammation (pericarditis)
3. Anxiety related to acute illness and fear of death

The nurse asked J.D. several questions in order to explore with him his psychospiritual state. Following the interaction, the nurse felt that further exploration of the meaning and negative images that he conveyed was essential to his recovery. She asked him if he wanted to pursue some new ideas that might help him access his inner healing resources and strengths. He said that he would.

Nurse: In your recovery now with your heart healing, how do you experience your healing?

J.D.: There is this sac around my heart, and every time I take a deep breath, my breath is cut off by the pain [*pericarditis*]. My heart is like a broken vase. I don't think it is healing.

Nurse: I can understand why you are discouraged. However, some important things that are present right now show that you are better than when you first came to the CCU. Your chest pain is gone, and your heartbeats are now regular. If you focus on what is going right, you can help your heart and lift your spirits. Let me help you learn how to think of some positive things.

J.D.: I don't know if I can.

Nurse: I would like to show you how to breathe more comfortably. Place your right hand on your upper chest, and your left hand on your belly. I want to show you how to do relaxed abdominal breathing. With your next breath in, through your nose, let the breath fill your belly with air. And as you exhale, through your mouth, let your stomach fall back to your spine. As you focus on this way of breathing, notice how still your chest is.

J.D.: (*After three complete breaths*) This is the easiest breathing I've done today.

Nurse: As you focused on breathing with your belly, you let go of fearing the discomfort with your breathing. Can you tell me more about the image you have of your heart as a broken vase?

J.D.: I saw this crack down the front of my heart right after the doctor told me about my big artery that is blocked, that runs down the front of my heart, that caused my heart attack.

Nurse: (*Taking a small plastic bag full of crayons out of her pocket and picking up a piece of paper*) Is it possible for you to choose a few crayons and draw your broken heart using those images you just talked about?

J.D.: I can't draw.

Nurse: This exercise has nothing to do with drawing, but something usually happens when you draw an image of your words.

J.D.: Do you mean the image of a broken vase? (*When halfway through with the drawing*) I know this sounds crazy, but my father had a heart attack when he was 55. I was visiting my parents. Dad hadn't been feeling well, even complained of his stomach hurting that morning. He was in the living room, and as he fell, he knocked over a large Chinese porcelain vase that broke in two pieces. I can remember so clearly running to his side. I can see that vase now, cracked in a jagged edge down the front. He made it to the hospital, but died 2 days later. You know, I think that might be where that image of a broken heart came from [*Figure 22–5A*].

Nurse: Your story contains a lot of meaning. Remembering this event can be very helpful to you in your healing. What are some of the things that you are most worried about just now?

J.D.: (*Tears in his eyes*) Dying young. I have this funny feeling in my stomach just now. I don't want to die. I'm too young. I have so much to contribute to life. I've been driving myself to excess as far as work. I need to learn to relax and manage my stress, even drop some weight, start exercising, and change my life.

Nurse: J., each day you are getting stronger. You might even consider that this time of rest after your heart attack can be a time for you to reflect on what are the most important things in life for you. Whenever you feel discouraged, let images come to you of a beautiful vase that has a healed crack in it. This is exactly what your heart is doing right now. Even as we are talking, the area that has been damaged is healing. As it heals, there will be a solid scar that will be very strong, just in the same way that a vase can be mended and become strong again. New blood supplies also come into the surrounding area of your heart to help it heal. Positive images can help you heal, because you send a different message from your mind to your body when you are relaxed and thinking about becoming strong and well. You help your body, mind, and spirit function at their highest level. Let yourself once again draw an image of your heart as a healed vase, and notice any difference in your feelings when you do this.

With a smile, he picked up several crayons and began to draw a healing image to encourage hope and healing (Figure 22–5B).

When J.D. entered the outpatient cardiac rehabilitation program following his acute myocardial infarction, he was motivated to lower his cholesterol, lose weight, learn stress management skills, and express his emotions. Two weeks into the program, J.D. did not appear to be his usual extroverted self. The cardiac rehabilitation nurse engaged him in conversation, and before long, he had tears in his eyes. He stated that he was very discouraged about having heart disease. He said, "It just has a grip on me." The nurse took him into her office, and they continued the dialogue. After listening to his story, she asked J.D. if he would like to explore his feelings further. He very shyly nodded yes.

In order to facilitate the healing process, she thought it might be helpful to have J.D. get in touch with his images and their locations in his body. She began by saying, "If it seems right to you, close your eyes and begin to focus on your breathing just now." She guided him in a general exercise of head-to-toe relaxation, accompanied by an audiocassette music selection of sounds in nature. As his breathing patterns became more relaxed and deeper, indicating relaxation, she began to guide him in exploring "the grip" in his imagination.

Nurse: Focus on where you experience the grip. Give it a size, . . . a shape, . . . a sound, . . . a texture, . . . a width, . . . and a depth.

J.D.: It's in my chest, but not like chest pain. It's dull, deep, and blocks my knowing what I need to think or feel about living. I can't believe that I'm using these words. Well, it's bigger than I thought. It's very rough, like heavy jute rope tied in a

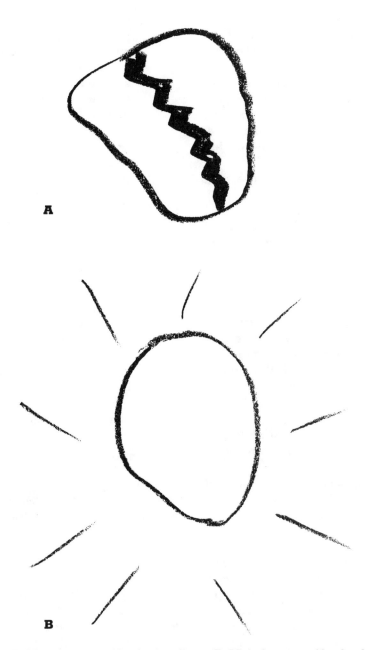

Figure 22-5 A, J.D.'s drawing of his broken heart. **B**, J.D.'s drawing of his healed heart.

knot across my chest. It has a sound like a rope that keeps a sailboat tied to a boat dock. I'm now rocking back and forth. I don't know why this is happening.

Nurse: Stay with the feeling, and let it fill you as much as it can. If you need to change the experience, all you have to do is take several deep breaths.

J.D.: It's filling me up. Where are these sounds, feelings, and sensations coming from?

Nurse: From your wise, inner self, your inner healing resources. Just let yourself stay with the experience. Continue to use as many of your senses as you can to describe and feel these experiences.

J.D.: Nothing is happening. I've gone blank.

Nurse: Focus again on your breath in . . . and feel the breath as you let it go. . . . Can you allow an image of your heart to come to you under that tight grip?

J.D.: It is so small I can hardly see it. It's all wrapped up.

Nurse: In your imagination, can you introduce yourself to your heart as if you were introducing yourself to a person for the first time? Ask your heart if it has a name?

J.D.: It said hello, but it was with a gesture of hello, no words.

Nurse: That is fine. Just say, "Nice to meet you," and see what the response might be.

J.D.: My heart seems like an old soul, very wise. This feels very comfortable.

Nurse: Ask your heart a question for which you would like an answer? Stay with this and listen for what comes.

J.D.: (*After long pause*) It said practice patience, that I was on the right track, that my heart disease has a message, don't know what it is.

Nurse: Just stay with your calmness and inner quiet. Notice how the grip changed for you. There are many more answers to come for you. This is your wise self that has much to offer you. Whenever you want, you can get back to this special kind of knowing. All you have to do is take the time. When you set aside time to be quiet with your rich images, you will get more information. You might also find special music to assist you in this process. . . . Your skills with this way of knowing will increase each time you use this process . . . now that whatever is right for you in this moment is unfolding, just as it should. In a few moments, I will invite you back into a wakeful state. On five, be ready to come back into the room, wide awake and relaxed. One . . . two . . . three . . . four . . . eyelids lighter, taking a deep breath . . . and five, back into the room, awake and alert, ready to go about your day.

J.D.: Where did all that come from? I've never done that before.

Nurse: These are your inner healing resources that you possess to help you recognize quality and purpose in living each day. In our future sessions, we will teach and share more of these skills.

Evaluation

With the client, the nurse determines whether the client outcomes for imagery were successful (Table 22–3). To evaluate the session further, the nurse may again explore the subjective effects of the experience with the client (see Exhibit 22–1).

Imagery is a tool for connecting with the unlimited capabilities of the bodymind. It is a nonverbal modality and a rich resource for information about all life processes. Using imagery, a nurse can help a client make changes in perceptions, behaviors, and attitudes that can promote healing.[61] The client experiences more self-awareness, self-acceptance, self-love, and self-worth. Nurses and clients come to know themselves in a new way as they create and communicate in the symbolic language of the imagination.

DIRECTIONS FOR FUTURE RESEARCH

1. Determine whether a client's specific images increase the client's psychophysiologic healing.
2. Develop valid and reliable tools that measure imagery.
3. Compare the stress level, attitudes, and work spirit of nurses who routinely use imagery as a nursing intervention to those of nurses who do not use imagery.
4. Evaluate the relationship of imagery scripts, physiologic responses, and healing in different clinical settings.
5. Determine if subjects can learn through manipulation of both imagery scripts and their verbal reports to eliminate or modify negative psychophysiologic responses.
6. Examine cultural diversity through specific types of imagery and symbols.

NURSE HEALER REFLECTIONS

After reading this chapter, the nurse healer will be able to answer or begin a process of answering the following questions:

- How do I feel about my imagination?
- When I work with imagery, what inner resources can assist me in my life processes?
- How am I able to remove the barriers to my imagery process?
- In what way do I recognize the nonrational part of myself?
- Can I allow my clients to interpret their own imagery to facilitate their own healing?

NOTES

1. J. Giedt, Guided Imagery: A Psychoneuroimmunological Intervention in Holistic Nursing Practice, *Journal of Holistic Nursing* 15, no. 2 (1997): 112–127.

2. J. Nickel, Placebo Therapy of Benign Prostatic Hyperplasia: A 25 Month Study, Canadian PROSPECT Study Group, *British Journal of Urology* 81, no. 3 (1998): 383–387.

3. F. Benedetti et al., The Specific Effects of Prior Opioid Exposure on Placebo Analgesia and Placebo Respiratory Depression, *Pain* 75, no. 2–3 (1998): 313–319.

4. P. Staats et al., Suggestion/Placebo Effects on Pain: Negative As Well As Positive, *Journal of Pain Symptom Management* 15, no. 4 (1998): 235–243.

5. R. Hahn, The Nocebo Phenomenon: Concept, Evidence, and Implications for Public Health, *Preventive Medicine* 26, no. 5 (1997):607–611.

6. M. Wall and S. Wheeler, Benefits of the Placebo Effect in the Therapeutic Relationship, *Complementary Therapies in Nursing and Midwifery* 2, no. 6 (1996): 160–163.

7. J. Achterberg, *Imagery in Healing* (Boston: Shambhala, 1985).

8. A. Sheikh et al., Healing Images: From Ancient Wisdom to Modern Science, in *Eastern and Western Approaches to Healing*, ed. A. Sheikh and K. Sheikh (New York: John Wiley and Sons, 1989), 470–515.

9. R. Schaub, Alternative Health and Spiritual Practices, *Alternative Health Practitioner* 1, no. 1(1995):35–38.

10. J. Singer, *Imagery and Daydream Methods in Psychotherapy and Behavior Modification* (New York: Academic Press, 1974).

11. D. Foulkes and S. Fleisher, Mental Activity in Relaxed Wakefulness, *Journal of Abnormal Psychology* 84, no. 1 (1975):66–75.

12. J. Singer and J. Antrobus, Daydreaming, Imaginal Processes and Personality: A Normative Study, in *The Function and Nature of Imagery*, ed. P. Sheehan (New York: Academic Press, 1972).

13. J. Singer, *The Inner World of Daydreaming* (New York: Harper Colophon, 1975).

14. W. Penfield, *The Mystery of the Mind* (Princeton, NJ: Princeton University Press, 1975).

15. H. Graham, *Mental Imagery in Health Care* (London: Chapman & Hall, 1995), 2–4.

16. Graham, *Mental Imagery in Health Care.*

17. E. Jacobson, Electrical Measurements of Neuro-muscular States during Mental Activities: Imagination of Movement Involving Skeletal Muscle, *American Journal of Physiology* 91 (1929):597–608.

18. L. Yaguez et al., A Mental Route to Motor Learning: Improving Trajectorial Kinematics through Imagery Training, *Behavior and Brain Research* 90, no. 1 (1998):95–106.

19. W. James, *Principles of Psychology*, Vol. 2 (New York: Henry Holt, 1890).

20. R. Suinn, Imagery and Sports, in *Imagery: Current Theory, Research, and Application*, ed. A. Sheikh (New York: John Wiley and Sons, 1983), 507–534.

21. D. Smith, Imagery in Sport: A Historical and Current Overview, in *Mental Imagery*, ed. R. Kunzendorf (New York: Plenum Press, 1991), 215–224.

22. R. Weinberg et al., Effects of Visuo-Motor Behavior Rehearsal, Relaxation, and Imagery on Karate Performance, *Journal of Sports Psychology* 3 (1981): 228–238.

23. M. Quintyn and E. Cross, Factors Affecting the Ability To Initiate Movement in Parkinson's Disease, *Physical and Occupational Therapy in Geriatrics* 4 (1986): 51–60.

24. O. Simonton et al., Psychological Intervention in the Treatment of Cancer, *Psychosomatics* 21, (1980): 226–227.

25. J. Achterberg and G.F. Lawlis, *Imagery and Disease* (Champaign, IL: Institute for Personality and Ability Testing, 1978).

26. Achterberg, *Imagery in Healing*.

27. H. Hall, Imagery, PNI and the Psychology of Healing, in *The Psychobiology of Mental Imagery*, ed. R. Kunzendorf and A. Sheikh (Amityville, NY: Baywood, 1990).

28. H. Hall, Voluntary Immunomodulation, *The Challenge* 12, no. 4 (1990): 18–20.

29. J. Schneider et al., Guided Imagery and Immune System Function in Normal Subjects: A Summary of Research Findings, in *Mental Imagery*, ed. R. Kunzendorf (New York: Plenum Press, 1991), 179–191.

30. J. Schneider et al., Psychological Factors Influencing Immune System Function in Normal Subjects: A Summary of Research Findings and Implications for the Use of Guided Imagery (Paper presented at the Tenth Annual Conference of the American Association for the Study of Mental Imagery, 1988). New Haven, CT.

31. M. Rider et al., The Effect of Music, Imagery and Relaxation on Adrenal Corticosteroids and the Re-Entrainment of Circadian Rhythms, *Journal of Music Therapy* 22 (1985): 46–58.

32. K. Syrjala et al., Relaxation and Imagery and Cognitive-Behavioral Training Reduce Pain during Cancer Treatment: A Controlled Clinical Trail, *Pain* 63, no. 2 (1995): 189–198.

33. M. Quirk et al., Evaluation of Three Psychological Interventions To Reduce Anxiety during MRI Imaging, *Radiology* 173 (1989): 759–762.

34. D. Tusek et al., Guided Imagery As a Coping Strategy for Perioperative Patients, *American Operating Room Nurse Journal* 66, no. 4 (1997):644–649.

35. F. Luskin et al., A Review of Mind-Body Therapies in the Treatment of Cardiovascular Disease, Part 1: Implications for the Elderly, *Alternative Therapies in Health and Medicine* 4, no. 3 (1998):46–61.

36. M. Richardson et al., Coping, Life Attitudes, and Immune Responses to Imagery and Group Support after Breast Cancer Treatment, *Alternative Therapies in Health and Medicine* 3, no. 5 (1997):62–70.

37. Giedt, Guided Imagery.

38. C. Holden-Lund, Effects of Relaxation with Guided Imagery on Surgical Stress and Wound Healing, *Research in Nursing and Health* 11 (1988): 235–244.

39. B. Rees, Effect of Relaxation with Guided Imagery on Anxiety, Depression, and Self-Esteem in Primiparas, *Journal of Holistic Nursing* 13, no. 3 (1995):255–267.

40. K. Kwekkeboom et al., Imaging Ability and Effective Use of Guided Imagery, *Research in Nursing and Health* 21, no. 3 (1998):189–198.

41. B. Stetson, Holistic Health Stress Management Program: Nursing Student and Client Health Outcomes, *Journal of Holistic Nursing* 15, no. 2 (1997): 143–157.

42. Achterberg, *Imagery in Healing*, 115–116.

43. A. Ahsen, *Psycheye* (New York: Brandon House, 1977).

44. R. Assagioli, *Psychosynthesis: A Manual of Principles and Techniques* (New York: Hobbs, Dorman, 1965).

45. R. Assagioli, *Act of Will* (New York: Viking, 1973).

46. Assagioli, *Act of Will*, 51–52.

47. L. Song et al., Heart-Focused Attention and Heart–Brain Synchronization: Energetic and Physiological Mechanisms, *Alternative Therapies in Health and Medicine* 4, no. 5 (1998): 44–62.

48. B. Schaub and R. Schaub, *Healing Addictions* (Albany, NY: Delmar, 1997).

49. N. Christman et al., Concrete Objective Information, in *Nursing Interventions: Essential Nursing Treatments,* 2d ed., ed. G. Bulechek and J. McCloskey (Philadelphia: W.B. Saunders, 1992), 140–149.

50. B. Schaub et al., Clinical Imagery: Holistic Nursing Perspectives, in *Mental Imagery,* ed. R.G. Kunzendorf (New York: Plenum Press, 1991), 207–213.

51. J. Achterberg et al., *Rituals of Healing* (New York: Bantam Books, 1994).

52. Achterberg, *Imagery in Healing.*

53. Achterberg and Lawlis, *Imagery and Disease.*

54. Achterberg et al., *Rituals of Healing.*

55. Achterberg et al., *Rituals of Healing,* 131–132.

56. B. Dossey et al., Psychophysiologic Self-Regulation, in *Critical Care Nursing: Body-Mind-Spirit,* 3d ed., ed. B. Dossey et al. (Philadelphia: J.B. Lippincott, 1992), 37–38.

57. Achterberg et al., *Rituals of Healing,* 124–128.

58. Achterberg et al., *Rituals of Healing,* 317–328.

59. Achterberg and Lawlis, *Imagery and Disease.*

60. Achterberg et al., *Rituals of Healing.*

61. K. Brown-Saltzman, Replenishing the Spirit by Meditative Prayer and Guided Imagery, *Seminars in Oncology Nursing* 13, no. 4 (1997): 255–259.

RESOURCES

At the Heart of Healing: Experiencing Holistic Nursing
3½-hour, two-volume video set, including workbook. Sections on imagery, hypnosis, polarity therapy, biofeedback, therapeutic touch, and other aspects of holistic nursing practice.
Kineholistic Foundation
P.O. Box 719
Woodstock, NY 12498

Mind-Body Program for Patients, Professional Training, Audiotapes, and other resources
Getting Well
P.O. Box 2628
Orlando, FL 32802
Telephone: 1-800-426-8662
E-mail: gtngwell@magicnet.net

Life-Sciences Institute of Mind-Body Health
2955 SW Wanamaker Drive, Suite B
Topeka, KS 66614
Telephone: 785-271-8686
Fax: 785-271-8698
E-mail: lifesci@cjnetworks.com

Certification Program in Clinical Imagery and Clinical Meditation
New York Psychosynthesis Institute
2 Murray Court
Huntington, NY 11743
Telephone: 516-673-0293
Fax: 516-423-2684
E-mail: rschaub@ix.netcom.com

VISION OF HEALING

Composing the Harmony

Grown-ups love figures. When you tell them that you have made a new friend, they never ask you any questions about essential matters. They never say to you, "What does his voice sound like? What game does he love best? Does he collect butterflies?"

Instead they demand: "How old is he? How many brothers has he? How much does he weigh? How much money does his father make?" Only from figures do they think they have learned anything about him.[1]

And we must learn that to know a man is not to know his name but to know his melody.[2]

Moisture from the drops of music nurtures and supplies vital nutrients to our physical and emotional well-being. We become healthy. We flourish as a species. We prosper. We grow. We laugh. We cry. We dance. We sing. We love. We live. We become one.[3]

Music therapy is personal power made manifest. It's a map to the place where strength and well-being and love lie buried deep inside us all. It is a force to create change from within, to find the healer in all of us.[4]

The ancients knew it; our bodies know it. The emerging physician, the new doctor of balance, fullness, and resonance, rests on a new understanding of the physics of harmonics and the powers in sound. The overture is sounding for the twenty-first century. The ancient healers are calling forth our deeper senses. Orpheus, Apollo, Tubal-cain, Aesculapius, David, St. Gregory, St. Francis, Saraswati, and St. Cecilia are sounding their calls. How soon will we be able to use the beauty of musical sound to compose ourselves into perfect octaves of harmony in mind, body, and spirit?[5]

NOTES

1. A. De Saint Exupery, *The Little Prince* (New York: Harcourt, Brace, & World, 1971), 16.

2. Unknown Oriental Philosopher.

3. B.J. Crowe, Music—The Ultimate Physician, in *Music: Physician for Times To Come*, ed. D. Campbell (Wheaton, IL: Quest Books, 1991), 118.

4. Crowe, Music.

5. D. Campbell, Introduction: The Curative Potential of Sound, in *Music: Physician for Times to Come*, ed. D. Campbell (Wheaton, IL: Quest Books, 1991), 8.

Chapter 23

Music Therapy: Hearing the Melody of the Soul

Cathie E. Guzzetta

NURSE HEALER OBJECTIVES

Theoretical

- Evaluate the principles of sound.
- Analyze the psychophysiologic theories that explain why music therapy works as a bodymind modality.

Clinical

- List the factors to be considered in choosing music selections that are relaxing for clients.
- Develop a music library for use with clients.
- Develop several different music therapy techniques, and use them in clinical practice.
- Explore with clients their internal responses when listening to music in a relaxed state.

Personal

- Participate in "experimental listening."
- Record your responses to various types of music in a music notebook.
- Participate in a "music bath."
- Participate in a toning and groaning exercise before listening to music.
- Practice focused and conscious hearing each day to recognize subtle differences in sound.

DEFINITIONS

Cymatics: the study of patterns of shape evoked by sound.

Frequency: the number of vibrations or cycles per unit of time.

Music Therapy: the behavioral science concerned with the systematic application of music to produce relaxation and desired changes in emotions, behavior, and physiology.

Oscillation: the fluctuation or variation between minimum and maximum values.

Resonance: the vibration of a structure at a frequency that is natural to it and most easily sustained by it.

Sonic: of or having to do with sound.

Sound: that which is produced when some object is vibrating in a random or periodic repeated motion.

Sympathetic Resonance: the reinforced vibration of an object exposed to the vibration at about the same frequency as another object.

THEORY AND RESEARCH

Music, which is a vital part of all societies and cultures, has been linked to medicine throughout history. According to Greek mythology, Orpheus was given a lyre by the god Apollo and was instructed in its use by the muses; hence, the word *music*. Apollo was the god of music and his son, Aesculapius, was the god of healing and medicine. The Greeks believed music had the power to help heal the body and soul. Music has been used in spiritual ceremonies and in celebrations. Armies march to battle with music, and mothers lull their infants to sleep with song. Music is played during rites of initiation, during funeral ceremonies, and on harvest and feast days. There is something about the power of music that has been used throughout time. It is of no surprise then that music is currently being applied as a complementary therapy in health care.

Sound, Frequency, and Intensity

It is necessary to appreciate the principles and theories of sound to understand fully its tremendous capacity to achieve therapeutic psychophysiologic outcomes. Sound is produced when some object is vibrating in a random or periodic repeated motion. It can be heard by the human ear when it ranges in frequency or pitch from 16 to 20,000 cycles per second. Within this vibratory range, we can hear 1,378 different tones.[1] We also hear and perceive sound by skin and bone conduction. Our other senses, such as sight, smell, and touch, allow us to perceive an even wider range of vibrations than those sensed by hearing. Thus, we are sensitive to sounds in ways that most people do not even consider.

The interrelationship between wave forms and matter can be understood by rendering vibrations into physical forms. When scattered liquids, powders, metal filings, or sand are placed on a disk with a vibrating crystal, repeatable patterns form on the disk. As the pitch is changed, the harmonic pattern formed on the disk also changes. Thus, matter assumes certain shapes or patterns based on the vibrations or frequency of the sound to which it is exposed. The study of patterns of shapes evoked by sound is called cymatics.[2] The forms of snowflakes and faces of flowers may take on their shape because they are responding to some sounds in nature.[3] Likewise, it could be possible that crystals, plants, and even human beings are, in some way, music that has taken on visible form.

The human body also vibrates. The ejection of blood from the left ventricle during systole distends the aorta with blood. The pressure produced by aortic distension causes a pressure wave to travel down the aorta to the arterial branches. The pressure wave travels faster than the flow of blood and creates a palpable pulse called the pressure pulse wave.[4] Waves are a series of advancing impulses set up by a vibration or impulse. The pressure pulse wave is composed of a series of waves that have differing frequencies (i.e., number of vibrations per unit of time) and amplitude. In the arterial branches, there is one fundamental frequency and a number of harmonics that usually have a smaller amplitude than the fundamental frequency. The arterial vessels resonate at certain frequencies (fundamental frequency), thereby intensifying some waves while other waves are damped and disappear. This phenomenon is called resonance.[5]

The human body vibrates, from its large structures, such as the aorta and arterial system, down to the genetically preprogrammed vibrations coded into our molecules. Our atoms and molecules, cells, glands, and organs all have a characteristic vibrational frequency that absorbs and emits sound. Thus, the human body is a system of vibrating atomic particles acting as a vibratory transformer that gives off and takes in sound.

Because the human body absorbs sound, the concept of resonance has implications for everyone. Sympathetic vibration, or sympathetic resonance, refers to the reinforced vibration of an object exposed to the vibration at about the same frequency as another object.[6] For example, if two tuning forks are designed to vibrate at approximately the same pitch, striking one of the tuning forks produces a sound that spontaneously causes the second tuning fork to vibrate and produce the same sound—even though the second fork was not physically struck. Actually, the sound wave from the first fork does physically strike the second fork, causing the second to resonate responsively to the tune of the first. This sympathetic resonance occurs because the vibratory characteristics of the two forks allow energy transfer from one to the other. When two objects have similar vibratory characteristics that allow them to resonate at the same frequency, they form a resonant system.

The atomic structure of our molecular system is also a resonant system. Nuclei vibrate, and the electrons in their orbit vibrate in resonance with their nucleus. Moreover, as long as the atom, cell, or organ contains an appropriate vibrational pattern, it can be "played" by outside stimuli in harmony with its vibrational makeup.[7] The phenomenon of entrainment happens when 2 or more vibrating objects come into step or in phase with each other to create a sympathetic resonant system. Thus, environmental sounds, such as those emitted from a dishwasher, television, or computer or those hospital sounds associated with structural (e.g., open, closely located patient rooms), mechanical (e.g., beepers, monitors, alarms, and equipment), and personnel noise may be capable of stimulating or producing sympathetic vibrations in the molecules and cells of the body.[8] Music can act as a natural pacemaker, speeding up or slowing down the heart rates, brain waves, and respirations to achieve a gradual entrainment with the music and a change in the individual's psychophysiologic state.[9]

The human body vibrates at an inaudible fundamental frequency of approximately 8 cycles per second when it is in a relaxed state. During relaxed meditation, the frequency of brain waves produced is also about 8 cycles per second. Furthermore, the earth vibrates at this same fundamental frequency of 8 cycles per second. This phenomenon, called Schumann's resonance, is a function of electromagnetic radiation and the earth's circumference. Thus, there is a sympathetic resonance between the electrically charged layers of the earth's atmosphere and the human body, and, therefore, "being in harmony with oneself and the universe" may be more than a poetic concept.[10]

The intensity or loudness of a sound is measured in decibels (dB). The gentle rustling of leaves can be measured at 10 dB, a whisper at 30 dB, and a quiet home or work environment at 40 to 50 dB. Loud sounds such as jackhammers and motorcycles can register at 100 dB, car horns and loud music at 115 dB, while a rocket launch can register at 180 dB. Pain begins at 125 dB.[11] The Environmental Protection Agency has recommended that the noise level of hospitals be less than 45 dB during the day and less than 35 dB at night.[12] The average noise levels of most hospitals, however, has been found to be in the range of 50 to 75 dB during the day, with little reduction at night.[13]

Purposes of Music Therapy

Defined as a behavioral science that is concerned with the use of specific kinds of music to effect changes in behavior, emotions, and physiology,[14] music therapy can reduce psychophysiologic stress, pain, anxiety, and isolation. It also is useful in helping clients achieve a state of deep relaxation, develop self-awareness and creativity, improve learning, clarify personal values, and cope with a variety of psychophysiologic dysfunctions.[15,16] Music therapy complements traditional therapy, providing clients with integrated body-mind experiences and encouraging them to become active participants in their own health care.

Appropriate music is an important vehicle in achieving the relaxation response;

it removes a person's inner restlessness and quiets endless thinking. It can be used as a healing ritual to stop the mind from running away and to achieve inner quietness. The healing capabilities of music are intimately bound to the personal experience of inner relaxation.[17]

Psychophysiologic Responses to Music Therapy

Music alters a person's psychophysiology. The goal of music therapy and the type of music played (i.e., soothing or stimulating) determine the direction of the psychophysiologic changes. Soothing music can produce a hypometabolic response characteristic of relaxation in which autonomic, immune, endocrine, and neuropeptide systems are altered. Similarly, music therapy can produce desired psychologic responses, such as reductions in anxiety and fear.

Shifting States of Consciousness

When appropriately used, music can serve as a vehicle for reaching nonordinary levels of human consciousness.[18] Music makes it possible to alter ordinary states of consciousness to achieve the mind's fullest potential. With music therapy, individuals are able to shift their perception of time from virtual time, which is perceived in a left brain mode and is characterized by hours, minutes, and seconds, to experiential time, which is perceived through the memory.[19]

Experiential time exists because people experience both a state of tension and a state of resolution.[20] The memory perceives tensions and resolutions in a linear sequence that is called a disturbance or an event. An emotion or a sound, for example, is a disturbance that can produce tension (i.e., psychophysiologic effects), which is followed by a return to equilibrium or resolution. The rate of these linear sequences or events influences the perception of time. Slow-moving music lengthens the perception of time because one's memory has

more time to experience the events (tensions and resolutions) and the spaces between the events. Thus, clock time becomes distorted, and clients can actually lose track of time for extended periods, enabling them to reduce anxiety, fear, and pain.

Music can assist the individual in moving through the six states of consciousness: (1) normal waking state, (2) expanded sensory threshold, (3) daydreaming, (4) trance, (5) meditative states, and (6) rapture.[21] During relaxation, music is first perceived in a normal wakeful state. Continued relaxation reduces sensory thresholds and expanded awareness states predominate. The individual can then continue to move through the daydreaming, trance, and meditative states and progress to rapture, depending on the level of involvement with the music and the depth of the relaxation.

Hemispheric Functioning

Right brain functioning is concerned with the intuitive, creative, and imaging way of processing information. The right hemisphere is employed differently in the musical process than is the left. The right "metaphoric" hemisphere is responsible for the major aspects of musical perception and music behavior (i.e., the recognition of pitch, a Gestalt sense of melody, rhythm, style, and musical memory).

The commonalities between the components of speech and music are a basis for the perceptual processes of the brain's right hemisphere that influence language functions and behavior. The left hemisphere is predominantly involved with analytic thinking, especially in verbal and mathematical functions.[22] Music may activate the flow of stored memory material across the corpus callosum so that the right and left hemispheres work in harmony rather than conflict.

As one's musical knowledge grows, the brain's response to music shifts from a holistic to a more sequential and linear experience.[23] Music students and musicians tend to analyze the music to which they listen, classify the instruments, and critique the compositional techniques. Instead of integrating right and left brain functioning while listening to music in a relaxed state, such individuals tend to remain in or change to the left brain mode. With practice, however, they can let go of these conditioned responses to integrate the functioning of both hemispheres.[24]

Because music is nonverbal in nature, it appeals to the right hemisphere, whereas the traditional verbalization that the nurse uses in therapy with a client has its primary effect on the logical left brain. Music therapy, therefore, establishes a means of communication between the right and left brain.[25] The more connections that can be made in the brain, the more integrated the experience is within memory[26] (Figure 23–1).

Music, even more than the spoken word, "lends itself as a therapy because it meets with little or no intellectual resistance and does not need to appeal to logic to initiate its action . . . is more subtle and primitive, and therefore its appeal is wider and greater."[27] In a relaxed state, individuals can let go of preconceived ideas about listening to music and its patterns, instruments, and rhythm and shift their thinking to the right side of the brain to alter their states of consciousness.[28]

It has been suggested that listening to complex music (e.g., Mozart's Sonata for Two Pianos in D Major) can produce the Mozart effect, which "warms up the brain" much like physical exercise, to organize and facilitate the firing patterns of neurons in the cerebral cortex. As a result, right brain functioning related to temporal–spatial reasoning may improve.[29] It is believed that the Mozart effect is responsible for enhancing concentration, intuition, intelligence, and healing.

Emotions, Imagery, and the Senses

Music elicits a variety of different experiences in individuals. Clients reaching an

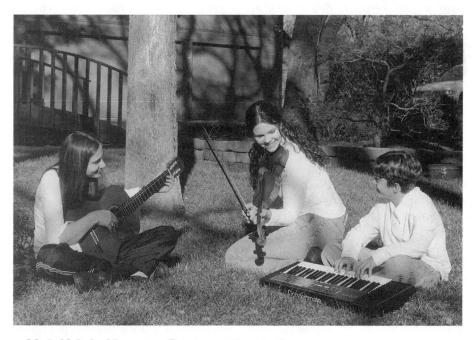

Figure 23–1 Melodic Memories. Courtesy of Angela Guzzetta.

altered state of consciousness during relaxation and music therapy may visualize settings, peaceful scenes, or images, or they may experience various sensations or moods.[30] Music passages can evoke scenes from fantasy to real life. Not only can melodic patterns evoke such positive emotions as love, joy, and deep peace, but also they can reduce negative emotions such as hostility and sadness.[31]

During relaxation and music therapy, individuals can be guided in experiencing synesthesia, or a mingling of senses.[32] Musical tones can evoke color and movement, or tastes can evoke shapes. Many children spontaneously "see" sounds and "taste" textures.[33]

Music and color can be expressed in terms of vibrations. When color is translated into musical vibrations, the harmonies of color are 40 octaves higher than the ear can hear. A piano spans approximately 7 octaves. If the piano keyboard could be extended another 50 octaves higher, the keys played at these higher octaves would produce color rather than audible sound.[34]

The musical selection entitled "Spectrum Suite" (see Steve Halpern Sound Rx in Resources at the end of chapter) is designed to evoke colors. While listening to this selection, clients are guided in focusing on seven main energy centers known to exist in the body. In Eastern culture, these centers are called chakras. Each energy level is then associated with a specific musical tone and a specific color. For example, while focusing on the spine (the first energy center), the client is guided to hear and feel the keynote of C resonating in the spinal area and to visualize the vibrations of the color red bathing this area of the body.[35]

Limbic System

Music therapy evokes psychophysiologic responses through the influence of musical pitch and rhythm on the limbic system (the seat of emotions, feelings, and sensations) and by stimulating the release of endorphins (meaning endogenous morphine), which act on specific receptors in the brain to alter emotions, mood, and physiology.[36-38] The quieting and calming effect of music can also produce other desired autonomic, immunologic, endocrine, and neuropeptide changes (see Chapter 4). Thus, the immediate influence of music therapy is on the mind state, which, in turn, influences the body state, producing a psychophysiologic response and a balance of body-mind-spirit.

The Human Body

Our entire body responds to sound, whether we consciously hear the sound or not. Even though our minds can tune out the sounds of airplane or automobile traffic, our bodies cannot. Many sounds assault our body because they are not in harmony with our fundamental vibratory pattern. On the other hand, musical vibrations that are in tune with our fundamental vibratory pattern may have a profound healing effect on the entire human body and mind, affecting changes in emotions and in organs, enzymes, hormones, cells, and atoms. Theoretically, musical vibrations may help restore regulatory function to a body out of tune (i.e., during times of stress and illness) and help maintain and enhance regulatory function to a body in tune. The therapeutic appeal of music may lie in its vibrational language and ability to align the body-mind-spirit with its own fundamental frequency.[39]

Research has demonstrated that music can affect physiologic outcome measures such as heart rate,[40,41] heart rate variability,[42] blood pressure,[43] respiratory rate,[44] galvanic skin response,[45,46] vasoconstriction,[47,48] muscle tension,[49,50] immune function,[51-53] and levels of stress hormones such as cortisol, epinephrine, and norepinephrine.[54]

Music Therapy Applications

Music has been used to foster a variety of desired outcomes.[55] For example, music enhances creativity by the development of new ways of association. Creativity is determined by how one approaches and considers things.[56] It incorporates the unexpected, the unknown, and the peculiar. It can be enhanced by relaxation wherein the busy mind settles into a more quiet and receptive state. Through visualization, the mind can envision new ideas and ways of thinking. Listening to appropriate music can also stimulate the brain to produce alpha and theta waves, which are known to stimulate creativity.[57]

Music and movement and/or tonal exercises help clients become aware of their bodies and the energies released in them. Such techniques are employed to achieve bodymind balance and release blocked energies. Therapists have used musical instruments in another form of music therapy, particularly with disabled individuals. Clients play various instruments during the therapy to develop the qualities of perseverance, perceptiveness, concentration, and initiative, as well as to promote perceptual–motor coordination and group interaction.[58]

Music has been used to improve learning. High psychophysiologic stress levels inhibit or block learning. When music and relaxation are combined, students learn better. Their learning can become more fun, and they become more fully involved in the experience. Music also has been used as a catalyst during the process of accelerated learning.

Audiotapes are now available in the marketplace to correct and reprogram unhealthy, unconscious thought patterns. Music enhances such tapes, as their aim is to put the listener in a relaxed and balanced state. During relaxation, the reprogramming message reaches the deeper unconscious mind where the new thought pattern will ultimately reside. Such self-help tapes frequently include desired affirmations or suggestions, combined with meditative music or white noise.[59]

Similarly, music has been used to facilitate reframing of past memories and experiences.[60] In achieving an altered state of consciousness, the unconscious mind can remember details of an individual's past experiences that the conscious mind may have forgotten. When the conscious mind remembers such experiences, the client can be helped to reframe or reorganize the memories to produce a more healthy and positive experience.[61]

To enhance learning and facilitate self-help, music has been combined with subliminal suggestions. The subliminal technique involves the delivery of verbal messages to the individual at a volume so low or, through a change in speed or frequency, so fast that the conscious mind cannot perceive them. The conscious mind responds to the music while the unconscious mind absorbs and responds to the verbal suggestion.[62]

Music has been used to evoke imagery for a number of therapeutic ends (see Chapter 22). Clients who have difficulty with the imagery process may find relaxing background music helpful. Appropriately selected music can activate right hemisphere functioning and release a flow of images.[63]

Bonny has developed an innovative approach called guided imagery and music (GIM).[64] By means of the conscious use of imagery that is evoked by relaxation and music,[65,66] GIM is a method of self-exploration, self-understanding, growth, healing, and transformation. In this approach, the client listens to classical music in a relaxed state, allowing the imagination to come to conscious awareness and sharing these experiences with a guide. The guide helps integrate the experience into the client's life.

Music thanatology is a new field in which music therapy addresses the complex needs of the dying. The primary focus of the music is to help the person complete the transition between life and death. It helps patients let go of the physical body during the last hours before death by enhancing peace, acceptance, and a calm anticipation of death. Specially trained therapists, using the media of harp and voice, implement music thanatology.[67]

Music Therapy in Clinical Settings

Music can act as a catalyst to facilitate mental suggestion and enhance a client's own self-healing capacities. Thus, music has potential usefulness in the treatment of many health problems.[68] For example, it can reduce stress and anxiety in

- healthy adults[69]
- hospital employees[70]
- mechanically ventilated patients[71]
- patients with cardiovascular disease[72-79]
- patients with cancer[80]
- surgical patients in the perioperative care setting[81]
- newborn infants in the nursery[82]
- low-birthweight infants in the neonatal intensive care unit[83]
- pediatric patients undergoing needle sticks[84]
- patients undergoing gastrointestinal endoscopic procedures[85]

Likewise, music has been used to reduce pain in pediatric burn patients undergoing debridement;[86] patients undergoing coronary artery bypass graft,[87] and abdominal surgery,[88,89] bone marrow transplant patients;[90] patients with rheumatoid arthritis;[91] and adult and pediatric patients with cancer.[92-94] Music can also help to reduce the nausea and vomiting associated with chemotherapy.[95,96]

The effects of music also have been used to induce relaxation in patients prior to and after chiropractic procedures,[97] in surgical patients in the postanesthesia care unit,[98] and in mechanically ventilated patients.[99,100] In addition, music has been used to reduce symptoms or improve recovery for

- patients with brain damage following head trauma[101]
- elderly and demented patients[102-106]
- patients with Alzheimer's disease[107-109]
- patients undergoing general anesthesia[110,111]
- pediatric patients in intensive care units[112]
- patients with asthma,[113] eating disorders,[114] acquired immunodeficiency syndrome (AIDS),[115] hypertension, migraine headaches, gastrointestinal ulcers, Raynaud's disease[116]

Selection of Appropriate Music

It is an important and challenging task to select appropriate music for use in music therapy, as the selections can influence the outcomes.[117] Most music, however, is not composed for the purposes of relaxation and healing. Individuals often associate events in their lives, both pleasing and displeasing, with certain kinds of music.[118] This conditioned learning response influences their music preferences and perceptions. Likewise, the acceptability and perceptions of calming music differ among cultures and age groups.[119,120] Thus, the particular individual must choose the music which is appropriate for them.[121]

A variety of soothing selections should be available for working with clients (Table 23–1) because it is difficult to predict a client's music preference and response to a particular selection. Musical selections that are relaxing and meditative to one client can be disruptive and annoying to another. Moreover, the music that some individuals identify as relaxing may not be physiologically relaxing at all.[122] Researchers and music experts tend to agree that rock and grunge music, characterized by fast tempos, heavy drums, and repeating bass lines, do not evoke psychophysiologic relaxation[123,124]—even if the individual thinks it does. Classical, spiritual, or popular music may not be relaxing or soothing either.[125]

Musical selections without words are preferable, as clients may concentrate on the words, their messages, and their meaning rather than allowing themselves to concentrate and flow with the music.[126] Some music has been designed to shift brain waves to more relaxed patterns (see designer music in Table 23–1). During ordinary consciousness and daily activities, beta brain waves predominate at a range of 14 to 20 cycles per second. Alpha waves, which occur at 8 to 13 cycles per second, characterize states of heightened awareness and calm. During periods of sleep, creativity, and meditation, theta waves occur at 4 to 7 cycles per second. Delta waves ranging from .5 to 3 cycles per second occur during unconsciousness, deep sleep, and deep meditation.[127] It is believed that any music such as baroque, or slow-moving selections that have a pulse of 60 beats per minute can be used to shift consciousness from the beta to the alpha range to improve alertness and reduce tension.[128]

Different types of music can have different effects on individuals. The categories of music outlined in Table 23–1 present a wide variety of selections that can be made available for clients. Each category of music incorporates an extensive array of styles and effects, ranging from fast-moving and active to slow-moving and relaxing selec-

Table 23–1 Categories of Music

Category	Composer Sources	Characteristics
Classical music	e.g., Mozart, Haydn, Bach	Embodies clarity, elegance, and transparency. It can improve concentration, memory, and spatial perception.
Slower baroque music	e.g., Bach, Handel, Vivaldi, Corelli	Imparts a sense of stability, order, predictability, and safety and creates a mentally stimulating environment for study or work.
Romantic music	e.g., Schubert, Schumann, Tchaikovsky, Chopin, Liszt	Emphasizes expression and feeling, often invoking themes of individualism, nationalism, or mysticism; can enhance sympathy, compassion, and love.
Impressionist music	e.g., Debussy, Fauré, and Ravel	Is based on free-flowing musical moods and impressions and evokes dreamlike images. It is suggested that a quarter hour of musical daydreaming followed by a few minutes of stretching can unlock creative impulses and put the individual in touch with his or her unconscious.[a]
Gregorian chant		Uses the rhythms of natural breathing to create a sense of relaxed spaciousness; can be used for quiet study, meditation, and stress reduction.
Religious and sacred music	e.g., shamanic drumming, church hymns, gospel music, and spirituals	Is useful for grounding the individual in the moment, facilitating feelings of deep peace and spiritual awareness, transcending and releasing pain.
Nontraditional, meditative, ambient, attitudinal, or new age music	e.g., Steven Halpern or Brian Eno	Elongates the sense of space and time and can induce a state of relaxed alertness. Has a wide appeal because it transcends personal taste and involves no intellectual analysis nor emotional recollections. There is no recognizable melody or harmonic progressions; frequently, there is no central rhythm or natural beat. It helps the bodymind attune itself with its own pattern or resonance. The music tends to flow endlessly and serves as a vehicle for relaxation, self-absorption, and contemplation.[b]

continues

Table 23–1 Continued

Category	Composer Sources	Characteristics
Designer music	e.g., medical Resonance Therapy Music® (MicroMusic-Laboratories)	Is a new category of music designed to produce significant changes in the individual's psychophysiology.[c,d] It is composed to alter the brain by stimulating the person's inherent regeneration processes.[e] Other compositions have been developed to improve mental and emotional states, promote autonomic nervous system balance, increase hormonal immunity, and enhance creativity, decision making, and physical energy.[f–h] Some designer music has built into the musical soundtracks simulated brain wave sound frequencies related to distinctive mind states (e.g., sleep, relaxation) to affect the listener's psychophysiology.[i–k]
Jazz, the blues, Dixieland, soul, calypso, reggae	i.e., music and dance forms that came out of the expressive African heritage	Can uplift and inspire, release deep joy and sadness, convey wit and irony, and affirm our common humanity.
Salsa, rhumba, maranga, macarena	i.e., music and dance forms of South America	With a lively rhythm and beat, can increase heart rate, respirations, and body movement. Samba, however, has the rare ability to soothe and awaken at the same time.
Big Band, pop and Top 40, and Country Western		Can inspire light to moderate movement, arouse the emotions, and create a sense of well-being.
Rock music	e.g., Elvis Presley, the Rolling Stones, Michael Jackson	Can stir the passions, stimulate active movement, release tension, mask pain, and reduce the effect of other loud, unpleasant sounds in the environment and provide a source of distraction. It can also create tension, dissonance, stress, and pain in the body if the listener is not emotionally receptive to be energetically entrained.
Heavy metal, punk, rap, hip hop, and grunge		Can excite the nervous system, leading to dynamic behavior and self-expression. It can also signal to others the depth and intensity of the listener's inner turmoil and need for release.

Source: From THE MOZART EFFECT by Don Campbell. Copyright © 1997 by Don Campbell. By permission of Avon Books, Inc.

[a]D. Campbell, The Mozart Effect (New York: Avon Books, 1997), 79.

[b]P.M. Hamel, Through Music to the Self (Boulder, CO: Shambhala Press, 1979), 142.

[c]R. McCraty et al., The Effects of Different Types of Music on Mood, Tension, and Mental Clarity, Alternative Therapies in Health and Medicine 4, no. 1 (1998): 75–84.

[d]Medical Resonance Therapy Music®—Scientific Research/Clinical Observations (Edermunde, Germany: AAR Edition, Scientific Information Service, 1996).

[e]P. Hubner, The Harmony Laws of Nature in the Microcosm of Music (Edermunde, Germany: AAR Edition, Scientific Information Service, 1995).

[f]R. McCraty et al., Music Enhances the Effect of Positive Emotional States on Salivary IgA, Stress Medicine 12 (1996): 167–175.

[g]D.L. Childre, Speed of Balance—A Musical Adventure for Emotional and Mental Regeneration (Boulder Creek, CA: Planetary Publications, 1995).

[h]W. Tiller et al., Cardiac Coherence: A New Noninvasive Measure of Autonomic System Order, Alternative Therapies in Health and Medicine 2, no. 1 (1996): 52–65.

[i]McCraty et al., The Effects of Different Types of Music.

[j]J. Thompson, Brainwave Suite (Pine Bush, NY: Natural Wellness).

[k]S. Halpern, In the Key of Healing (Pine Bush, NY: Natural Wellness).

tions.[129] The various categories and specific selections should be evaluated for their relaxing or active qualities before using them in music therapy sessions.

Hospital Music

Several companies and individuals have developed relaxing musical selections for use in the clinical setting (see Resources at the end of the chapter). These tapes are designed for patient use in hospitals before, during, and after surgery; during childbirth; and for all healing and recovery stages to reduce stress and enhance healing and well-being.[130]

For example, Halpern has created nontraditional long-playing musical selections that provide up to 8 hours of continuous relaxing music.[131] Likewise, Bonny has developed a set of music tapes, called Music Rx, for use in various hospital settings. The tapes consist of classical selections designed to reduce stress, provide a pleasant diversion, and promote quiet mood states. Testing of Music Rx with intensive care and surgical patients at two hospitals showed that patients who participated in the Music Rx program had reduced heart rates, greater relief from pain, and positive psychologic ratings.[132] Music Rx is recommended for patients in the critical care units and operating and recovery rooms, as well as other inpatient and outpatient settings. As we learn more about how vibratory frequencies and patterns affect our bodymind, healing music will be composed to realign our altered vibratory patterns and bring them back to balance.

Mazer and Smith have developed the Sondrex System®, which delivers soothing music through a high-quality compact disk (CD) player and provides a microphone for caregivers to communicate directly with the patient while the music is playing.[133] This system has been recommended for use in the perioperative and obstetrics/gynecology settings, endoscopy and cardiac catheterization laboratories, emergency medicine departments, and physician offices (see Resources at the end of the chapter).

Individual Musical Preference

Individuals need to evaluate their responses to various types of music. Although different musical selections can produce various effects, the fullest effect occurs when the listener is appropriately prepared to experience the sounds. The therapeutic effect of music is lessened when the listener is angry, distracted, critical, analytic, or resistant. With a relaxed and receptive bodymind, however, music has the potential to enter the body and play through it rather than around it. Thus, some form of relaxation exercise is recommended before the music experience.

Depending on the individual's physiology, mind state, and mood, music can produce different feelings at different times. An important rule to follow when listening to music is the iso-principle,[134] which states that matching the individual's mood to the appropriate music helps achieve an altered state of consciousness. When the mind and feelings are vibrating at a certain frequency, the music should be in resonance with that frequency.

Individuals can create their own tapes to match their moods and musical preference. If their mood is tense or angry and a relaxed outcome is desired, they may start out with a short selection (3 minutes or less) of music that resonates with the mood and then add selections that progress to a relaxed state.

Before creating a personal tape, an individual should spend some time experimenting with music—trying a variety of musical selections and learning what happens when listening to specific selections under a variety of circumstances. The kind of music that one uses to relax after a stressful day a work, for example, may be very different from the selection that one chooses while undergoing a painful dental procedure. "Experimental listening" involves listening to various types of music at different times of the day and week.[135] For example, an individual may spend 20 minutes listening to each type of music and then systematically evaluate his or her response to the selection, according to the following procedure:

1. Set aside 20 minutes of relaxation time.
2. Find a comfortable position.
3. Find a quiet place where there will be no interruptions.
4. Check your pulse rate.
5. Observe your breathing pattern (e.g., fast, slow, normal).
6. Assess your muscular tension (e.g., pain, muscle tightness, shoulder stiffness, jaw and neck tension or loose, limp, sleepy?).
7. Evaluate your mood state (e.g., angry, happy, sad).
8. Listen to the music for 20 minutes. Let your body respond to the music as it wishes: loosen muscles, lie down, dance, clap, hum.
9. Following the session, assess your heart rate and breathing pattern again.
10. Assess your muscular tension (e.g., more relaxed? more stimulated? tighter? tenser? calmer?).
11. Evaluate your mood state.
12. Record the name of the music selection and your before-and-after responses in a music notebook for use when developing your own therapeutic tapes.
13. On a separate page in your notebook, recall and write down the many ways that music has empowered your life psychologically, physically, and spiritually. Include your most dramatic, intimate, and emotional memories associated with music. You will begin to realize the importance of sound in your life and recognize its healing potential.
14. Based on your response, create your own relaxation music tape of 20 to 30 minutes in length. The more regularly you use the tape, the more effective it will become.

Listening to music can be a holistic experience. As more individuals come to realize that music can be a principal source of healing and stress reduction, they will take great care to select their music. Music therapy may be incorporated into daily living activities, such as taking a "music bath" after a morning shower as a means of balancing the bodymind for the events of the day.[136]

HOLISTIC CARING PROCESS

Assessment

In preparing to use music therapy interventions, the nurse assesses the following parameters:

- the client's music history and the types of music that the client prefers (e.g., classical, popular, country, folk, hymns, jazz, rock, blues, other)
- the client's ability to identify types of music that make him or her happy, excited, sad, or relaxed
- the client's ability to identify types of music that are distasteful and make him or her tense
- the client's awareness of the importance of music in life: Is music played at home? In the car? At work? For relaxation? For excitement? For enjoyment? During times of stress? As a means of coping with stress?
- the client's frequency of music listening (per day or per week)
- the client's preference for music listening, such as radio, phonograph, cassette or CD player
- the client's previous participation in relaxation/imagery techniques combined with music: How long? How regularly?
- the client's use of some type of music for relaxation purposes; if so, ask the

client to describe the bodymind responses evoked by music
- the client's insight into the use of music to produce psychophysiologic alterations
- the client's mood (iso-principle) that will determine the type of music to choose and the goals of the session.

(Assessment parameters outlined in Chapter 21, Relaxation, and Chapter 22, Imagery, should also be included, because relaxation, imagery, and music cannot be separated.)

Patterns/Problems/Needs

The following patterns/problems/needs compatible with music therapy interventions relate to the nine human response patterns (see Chapter 14) are as follows:

- **Exchanging:** All diagnoses
- **Relating:** Social isolation
  Loneliness
- **Valuing:** Spiritual distress
- **Choosing:** Ineffective individual coping
  Impaired adjustment
  Noncompliance
- **Moving:** Sleep pattern disturbance
  Sleep deprivation
  Fatigue
  Adult failure to thrive
  Disorganized infant behavior
- **Perceiving:** Body image disturbance
  Self-esteem disturbance
  Hopelessness
  Powerlessness
- **Knowing:** Confusion
  Altered thought processes
  Impaired memory
- **Feeling:** Pain
  Nausea

Chronic sorrow
Risk for violence
Post-trauma syndrome
Anxiety
Death anxiety
Fear

Outcomes

Table 23–2 guides the nurse in client outcomes, nursing prescriptions, and evaluation for the use of music therapy as a nursing intervention.

Therapeutic Care Plan and Implementation

Before the Session

- If in the clinical area, inform others of need for minimal noise (may also post sign on patient door requesting no interruptions for 30 minutes).
- Establish the goals for the session with the client.
- Discuss how music therapy quiets the bodymind and facilitates relaxation and self-healing.
- Discuss the length of the session, usually 20 to 30 minutes.
- Ask the client to empty his or her bladder, if necessary.
- Ask the client to remove eyeglasses.
- Prepare the environment for optimal relaxation:
  —Close the drapes.
  —Dim the lights.
  —Turn off any potential environmental noises (e.g., monitor, alarms, beepers, phones).
- Ask the client to sit or lie in a comfortable position. It is sometimes helpful to place a small pillow under the knees to relieve lower back strain. Have a light blanket available for warmth, if needed.
- Spend a few moments centering yourself to be fully present with the client.

Table 23-2 Nursing Interventions: Music Therapy

Client Outcomes	Nursing Prescriptions	Evaluation
The client will select music of choice and will participate in music therapy sessions to achieve a relaxed response and facilitate healing.	Provide the client with various musical taped selections to facilitate selecting music of choice. Guide the client in music therapy sessions and help the client to establish the routine of listening to music once or twice a day.	The client chose music of choice for listening and reported enjoying the music. The client participated in music therapy sessions twice a day to facilitate healing.
The client will demonstrate positive physiologic outcomes in response to the music therapy session, such as: • decreased respiratory rate • decreased heart rate • decreased blood pressure • decreased muscle tension • decreased fatigue	Assess the client's physiologic outcomes in response to music therapy before and immediately after the session. Evaluate the client's: • respiratory rate • heart rate • blood pressure • muscle tension • level of fatigue	The client demonstrated: • decreased respiratory rate • decreased heart rate • decreased blood pressure • decreased muscle tension • decreased fatigue
The client will demonstrate positive psychologic outcomes in response to the music therapy session such as: • positive emotions and relaxed feeling • decreased restlessness and agitation • decreased anxiety/depression • increased motivation • increased positive imagery • decreased isolation	Assess the client's psychologic outcomes in response to music therapy before and immediately after the session. Evaluate the client's: • emotions and level of relaxation • level of restlessness and agitation • level of anxiety/depression • level of motivation • type of imagery experienced • level of social isolation	The client demonstrated or verbalized: • positive emotions and more relaxed feeling • reduced restless and agitated behaviors • decreased levels of anxiety (or depression) • increased motivation to accomplish life's daily tasks • increased positive imagery • decreased feelings of social isolation

At the Beginning of the Session

Script: *The purpose of the session is to relax in a wakeful state and have a quiet experience listening to music. First, I will guide you in a few exercises to relax. Then I will guide you in how to listen to music (of your choice). Then try to let the music relax your body-mind-spirit even more as you listen to the music for 20 minutes. Now close your eyes if you wish. Find a comfortable position with your hands at the side of your chest or on your body—whatever is most comfortable. At any time, you may change positions, scratch, or swallow. There may be noises around, but these will not be important if you concentrate on my voice.*

Guide the client in a general relaxation or imagery script (see Chapters 21 and 22).

During the Session

Script: *Now, as you continue to relax, I will turn on the music. Listen to the music. Tell yourself that you would like to go wherever the music takes you. Allow yourself to follow the music. Let the music suggest to you what to think and what to feel. Do not try to analyze the music or the melody. If you find distracting thoughts occurring, simply let go of them and come back to concentrating on the music. Allow the music to relax you even more than you are now. The music will play for 20 minutes, and I will leave the room. I will quietly come back into the room before the music is over. Now continue to relax your body-mind-spirit; let the music help you.*

At the End of the Session

Script: *Now that the music is over, I will guide you in counting back from 5 to 1. You will come back into the room easily and quietly. You will feel very relaxed, calm, and peaceful. You will remember the pathway that led you to this new experience, and you will be able to find it quickly whenever you wish to return.*

Close the session as follows:

- While the client is in a self-reflective state, lead him or her in further guided imagery exercises, or journal entries, if desired.
- Use the client outcomes (see Table 23–2) that were established before the session and the client's subjective experience (Exhibit 23–1) to evaluate the session.
- Schedule a follow-up session.

Exhibit 23-1 Evaluating the Client's Subjective Experience with Music Therapy

1. Was this a new kind of music listening experience for you? Can you describe it?
2. Did you have any visual experiences? Of people, places, or objects? Can you describe them?
3. Did you see any colors while listening? Did the colors change as the music changed?
4. Did you notice any textures, smells, movements, or taste while experiencing the music?
5. Were you less aware of your surroundings? Were you able to flow with the music?
6. Did you like the music?
7. Did the music produce any feelings or emotions?
8. Was the experience pleasant?
9. Did you feel relaxed and refreshed after the experience?
10. Would you like to try this again?
11. What would be helpful to make this a better experience for you?

Specific Interventions

Development of Audiocassette/ Videocassette Library

Nurses can develop an audiocassette/ videocassette library on each clinical unit or in each practice area. Relaxation, imagery, and music therapy audiotapes and videotapes are recommended for use in all clinical settings from the birthing to the dying process. Audiotapes and videotapes can be developed and collected that are of specific benefit to the particular client/patient population with which the nurse is working. Following are suggestions for building a successful audiotape/videotape library:

1. **Equipment**
   - Have several tape/CD players with comfortable headsets per unit.
   - Place all equipment in a safe and convenient location.

- Establish a method of headset disinfection to be done after each patient finishes with the equipment.
- Have a variety of music tapes available. Commercial tapes are relatively inexpensive and readily available. A complete tape library will include music, relaxation, imagery, and stress management tapes, as well as specific tapes for smoking cessation; pre-, intra-, and postoperative surgery; weight reduction; pain management; insomnia; self-esteem; subliminal learning; and so on. Consider different types of music, such as easy listening, light and heavy classical, popular, jazz, operatic, folk, country, hymns, choral, nontraditional, and designer selections (see Table 23–1).
- Ask staff members to donate one favorite relaxation tape to the library.
- Write different companies (see Resources at the end of the chapter) and request a catalogue of their selections.
- Encourage nurses to develop tapes for specific client/patient problems that can help with procedures, tests, and treatments. The tapes may or may not have soothing background music.
- Have brochures and catalogues of recording companies available upon request from the patient.
- Encourage use of different tapes for further relaxation, imagery, and stress management training.

2. **Procedures**
   - If tapes/CDs are checked out on an outpatient basis, have the client make a deposit to cover the cost of the tape/CD in case it is not returned.
   - Label all equipment and materials with owner's name, telephone number, and return address.
   - Establish who will have authority to check out the tapes and equipment. If

in the hospital, a volunteer could assist in checking out the equipment for the patient after the nurse has assessed the patient's needs and selected the appropriate tape/CD.
- Prepare a sign-out log that records the patient's name, room, date, and check-out time for inpatients or address and telephone number for outpatients.
- Instruct the patient in the use of the equipment and tapes, if necessary.
- Allow 20 to 30 minutes of listening without interruption twice a day. Place a sign on the patient's door stating, "Relaxation Session in Progress—Please Do Not Disturb."
- Following the listening session, evaluate the patient's response to the music and answer any questions.
- Chart the type of music selected and the patient's specific response to the therapy. For example, were the desired outcomes achieved (e.g., lowered respiratory rate, decreased heart rate and blood pressure, decreased muscle tension and anxiety)? Identify the client's subjective evaluation of the experience (e.g., found the experience relaxing, helped with sleep, assisted in coping with pain, assisted with painful procedure).
- Return the equipment and tapes/CD to the library and record the check-in information in the log.

Music Therapy Scripts

Training for Skillful Listening. Music therapy sessions of 15 minutes may help clients improve the art of listening and train them consciously to hear sounds clearly.

> **Script:** *Concentrate on the sounds around you. Let your ears hear every possible sound. Explore the subtle sounds, breathing,*

distant cars, wind blowing, hum of the lights. . . . *Limit your sensations. Keep your eyes closed. Avoid touching. Heighten and isolate your perception of sound. Listen to the parts of sound. Listen to a sound. Imagine that the sound makes a line. Bend the line that the sound makes. Does it go up? Does it go down? Does it curve or have humps? The word—bend—itself has a bend. Notice the height of the bend. Imagine the top and bottom of the bend. . . .*

Imagine the grain of the sound. Is it rough or smooth? Rough like sandpaper or smooth like silk or something in between? What is the volume? High or low? What is the intensity? Loud or soft? What color do you associate with the sound? What emotions do you notice as you listen to this sound?

Now use your voice to imitate sound. Imitate the sound of a jet flying high through the air. . . . Now imitate the sound of a helicopter flying through the air. . . . Imitate the sound of a soft wind. . . . Imitate the sound of an autumn leaf falling. The point of this exercise is not to become an expert jet imitator, but to realize there is more to the art of listening and hearing than we think. When you practice focused and conscious hearing, you will recognize subtle differences in sound. You will expand your skills in the art of listening.

Expanding the Senses. Listening to music for 10 to 20 minutes can help clients to ex-

pand awareness, open up the senses, and participate in a mingling of the senses. The nurse (1) explains the purpose of the session to the client, (2) conducts a general relaxation session with the client, (3) turns on the music, and (4) begins slowly, pacing the words with the client's increased relaxation.

Script: *Let the music take you to a soothing peaceful place that is filled with various textures, sights, colors, and sounds. . . . Take a moment to find this place. . . . You feel comfortable and relaxed in this peaceful place. Slowly begin to explore the surface and texture of your surroundings. Permit the music to help you experience softness, smoothness, and gentleness. . . .*

As you continue to explore, discover the colors associated with the shape, texture, and feelings of things. Let the music suggest the sound of the colors and textures.

Touch the things in your environment. Let your fingers, tongue, and cheeks experience the textures. Take time to enjoy each feeling. Do not feel rushed as you explore. . . .

As you touch each thing in your surroundings, take time to investigate its source. Where did it come from? Why does it feel as it does? And why is it here?

With each surface, explore its color, its sound. The deeper you travel into the essence of your surroundings, the richer the experience will be. . . .

Continue this experience for another 10 to 20 minutes. Gradually come back into the room awake, alert, and ready to continue the day.

Toning and Groaning. By participating in this exercise for 10 to 20 minutes, clients can prepare for meditation, release intensive emotions, or induce an altered state of consciousness.

> **Script:** *Lie comfortably on your back. Begin with an audible groan such as "oh-h-h" or "ah-h-h." Let the groan be as deep as possible without forcing it. Let it give you a feeling of release, of emptying out any tension. Feel your skin and bones vibrate with the sound.*
>
> *Many people spontaneously groan when they have taken off a tight belt or tight shoes. Your groaning should be a comparable release of and freedom from constraint. Let it be loud and natural without forcing the sound. . . . You might even feel a bit silly about groaning. You might giggle or laugh. That's okay. Just let it out. . . .*
>
> *Stretch your arms and legs now. Then let your body relax and groan again. Notice the sound becoming effortless, relaxing, and deeper. . . . Be sure to let the groan come from deep down in your feet. Notice the vibrations starting up your body. As you continue to groan, feel a weight being lifted from you. Heaviness is being lifted while a sense of lightness sets in. . . . Groaning is a healing process. Allow it to happen. Enjoy the feeling of release. . . .*
>
> *You will notice a tendency for your voice to rise as your tensions are allowed to leave. Let your voice do what it wants as you continue to groan. It will*

find its natural place. When your body reaches its tone, it will be satisfied, and you will sigh a deep satisfying sigh.

> *At this point you are toning. You have found your tone. You are sounding your tone. You are resonating with your body. This is your own music.*

The nurse ends the session or prepares for imagery scripts, meditation, or music listening.

Taking a Music Bath. Listening to music for 20 minutes can help clients to prepare for a balanced day, prevent stress, and reduce stress. The nurse first explains the purpose of the session to the client. It is also important to conduct a general relaxation session with the client before proceeding with the script. After turning on the music, the nurse begins slowly, pacing the words with the client's increased relaxation.

> **Script:** *As the music begins, you will begin a music bath. Allow the sound to wash over you, letting the music touch every surface of your body. Permit the sound to rinse off any tension, unpleasant emotions, and any sound pollution to prepare for the day. . . .*
>
> *Allow yourself to be immersed in the musical sounds as if you were in a warm, relaxing tub of water or standing under the warm water in a shower. Imagine the water filled with soothing, relaxing sounds. The sounds are cleansing your body and calming your emotions. . . .*
>
> *As you allow your entire body to become immersed in the sounds, notice how the music*

resonates in different parts of your body. As you become more relaxed, notice how much more you are enjoying the music. . . .

As the music rinses away your tension, permit yourself to feel refreshed. The music bath has reached every part of your body. You have renewed and refreshed energy. . . .

Allow any remaining tension to be washed away, permitting you to feel balanced, calm, and refreshed.

Continue listening to the music now for 20 minutes. As the music ends, gradually come back into a wakeful, relaxed, and refreshed state.

Merging the Bodymind with Music. A quiet listening experience that mingles the senses and induces relaxation may last 20 minutes. Nontraditional music, with nonmetered beat and periods of silence between sounds is suggested. (See Steve Halpern Sound Rx for nontraditional selections in Resources at the end of this chapter.) After conducting a general relaxation session with the client, the nurse turns on the music and begins, pacing the words with the client's increased relaxation.

Script: *Visualize your ears. Explore your ears. Feel your ears expanding and becoming larger. Permit your ears to become channels in the sides of your head that open and lengthen throughout your body and into your feet. Allow these channels to hear all parts of your body.*

Think of the sounds you are hearing as something more than a pleasant hearing sensation. The sounds are nourishment and energy for your body—your mind—your

spirit. . . . Let the sound of the music move in you, around you, above you, below you. The sound is everywhere, and you can hear it throughout your body. . . .

See sound, taste it, feel it, smell it, hear it. Turn the sound into light and color and see it. Concentrate your attention on the sounds and the silence between the sounds. . . .

Open your ears. You have beautiful, big ears—channels throughout your body. Let the sounds pass through these channels to experience the event totally. Merge with the music. There will no longer be music and a listener, rather a state of total experiencing of the sound. Total concentration of the sound . . . moment-by-moment and on the silence between. . . . You can go beyond. . . . You will experience the soundless sound, the state where sound becomes silence, silence becomes sound, and they merge together.

Continue the experience for another 10 to 20 minutes. Gradually come back into the room awake, alert, and ready to continue the day.

Case Study

Setting:	Coronary care unit (CCU)
Patient:	W.R., a 62-year-old man who was admitted at 3:00 A.M. with the presumptive diagnosis of acute myocardial infarction
Patterns/ Problems/ Needs	1. Chest pain related to acute myocardial infarction
	2. Anxiety related to cardiovascular stressors and hospitalization

Prior to admission, W.R. had experienced severe, substernal chest pain that radiated to the left shoulder, arm, and hand. It was associated with nausea, vomiting, and shortness of breath. The chief of military police at a local military base, he stated that he worked 10 to 12 hours every day and was a hard-driving individual. He had been in excellent health before this episode and denied any previous hospitalization.

Following admission to the CCU, W.R. had no current chest pain, and his vital signs and cardiac rhythm were stable. However, he was assessed to be highly anxious, with clenched fists and jaw, obvious muscle tension, startle reactions to minor noise, and flight of ideas with constant talking. When asked by the nurse if he wanted to participate in a relaxation exercise that would help him cope better with his admission to the CCU and his illness, W.R. was reluctant, but agreed because he said he did not have much else to do.

After providing a music history, the patient selected a soothing classical music tape from the CCU's audiocassette library. The patient was supplied with a tape recorder and comfortable headsets. The music was checked for the appropriate volume and turned off, and the headset was placed beside the patient's pillow. A small finger thermistor was taped to the patient's left index finger, and his apical heart rate and peripheral temperature were recorded. The nurse guided the patient with a head-to-toe relaxation script and continued with the Merging the Bodymind with Music script. The headsets were then placed on the patient, and he continued the relaxation exercise while listening to music for 20 minutes.

Following the first session, W.R. said that he was sure he was not doing it "right" and that he did not wish to try it again. The nurse said that she understood. She also explained that there is no "right" way to experience relaxation and that everyone

experiences it a little differently. She added that relaxation is a skill to be learned, like riding a bike, and that the more people practice the technique, the better and richer is their response. She encouraged W.R. to try one more session, and he agreed. The nurse observed that there had been no change in W.R.'s finger temperature or heart rate following this first session.

Following the second session, W.R. was noticeably quiet. When the nurse inquired how he perceived the session, W.R. said, "It was OK—see you tomorrow." Following the third session, the nurse identified an 8-degree increase in finger temperature and a 10-beat/minute decline in heart rate from pre-session readings. W.R. had a small grin on his face and stated, "I can't believe what just happened to me. This stuff really works. I felt really relaxed. You know, I have a tough job. I work 10 hours a day. For me, relaxing means having a beer after work or going on a vacation 1 week a year. I have been walking around for 62 years with a stiff neck, and I never knew it. No one ever told me how to really relax. After this [session], I know now that, when I thought I was relaxing, I really wasn't. I have never felt like this in 62 years."

W.R. was transferred from the CCU to the telemetry unit that afternoon. He stated that he planned to continue his music therapy sessions twice a day during the remainder of his hospitalization and after his return home. He was given catalogues on relaxation music tapes and informed that such tapes could also be purchased from the hospital's gift shop.

Evaluation

With the client, the nurse determines whether the client outcomes of music therapy (see Table 23–2) were successfully achieved. To evaluate the session further, the nurse may again explore the subjective effects of the experience with the client (Exhibit 23–1).

It is important to ask clients to share their experiences, as the sharing helps evaluate the experience and clarify any misconceptions. Some people may report that their experiences were totally different from any previous experience and they discovered previously unknown mind spaces. Others may not perceive any beneficial effects of the therapy after the first or second session. They may worry if they cannot image, see colors, or feel relaxed.[137] These clients need reassurance that there is no right response and that not everyone experiences the same type of sensations, feelings, sights, or sounds in the same way. They also need encouragement to continue to practice the technique a few more times before drawing any conclusions regarding its effectiveness. The desired outcomes of music therapy in reducing stress are relaxation and a psychophysiologic quieting of the body-mind-spirit. Clients should understand that relaxation is an acquired skill and the effectiveness of such therapy is usually a function of practice. The more they practice relaxation skills, the better they become in producing changes in their psychophysiology.

Some people may feel that they need "two or three more" sessions with the nurse before they have acquired the skills to practice the technique themselves. In reality, no guide can teach the client relaxation skills. Any changes happen because of the individual's motivation, involvement, and skill—not because a guide is present. As soon as clients realize that they can make similar suggestions to themselves to induce relaxation, they are ready to continue the technique alone. Some people may wish to make an audiocassette of the guide's voice during the session or record their own script. The audiocassette then serves as the guide.

DIRECTIONS FOR FUTURE RESEARCH

1. Pre-test and post-test various types of "relaxing" music to validate that clients perceive such music as relaxing.
2. Create a sound-and-color healing room within a hospital setting, and evaluate its effects on patient recovery.
3. Evaluate several music scripts to determine whether one script is more effective than another in achieving specified outcomes.
4. Compare the effectiveness of music therapy with that of other relaxation techniques in various client groups to determine which technique is the most effective for which type of clients.
5. Develop valid and reliable evaluation tools that assess a client's subjective response to music therapy.
6. Evaluate the effects of a music audiocassette library on hospitalized patients' length of stay, recovery, and complications.
7. Compare the attitudes, stress levels, feelings of empowerment, and retention rates of nurses who routinely use music as a nursing intervention with those of nurses who do not use music.

NURSE HEALER REFLECTIONS

After reading this chapter, the nurse healer will be able to answer or will begin a process of answering the following questions:

- How do I feel about music as a healing ritual?
- When I listen to music, how do I allow myself to let go into the music?
- Am I able to use music with my clients to facilitate the healing process?

NOTES

1. R. Leviton, Healing Vibrations, *Yoga Journal* (1994, January–February): 59–60.

2. H. Jenny, *The Structure and Dynamics of Waves and Vibrations* (Basel, Switzerland: Basilius Press, 1967).

3. S. Halpern and L. Savary, *Sound Health: Music and Sounds That Make Us Whole* (New York: Harper & Row, 1985), 33.

4. C.E. Guzzetta, Physiology of the Heart and Circulation, in *Cardiovascular Nursing: Bodymind Tapestry*, ed. C.E. Guzzetta and B.M. Dossey (St. Louis: C.V. Mosby, 1984), 104–153.

5. Guzzetta, Physiology of the Heart and Circulation, 115–116.

6. Halpern and Savary, *Sound Health*, 33–37.

7. Halpern and Savary, *Sound Health*, 37.

8. D. Campbell, *The Mozart Effect* (New York: Avon Books, 1997).

9. Campbell, *The Mozart Effect*, 125.

10. Halpern and Savary, *Sound Health*, 39.

11. Campbell, *The Mozart Effect*, 32.

12. US Environmental Protection Agency. Information on Levels of Environmental Noise Requisite to Protect Public Health and Welfare with an Adequate Margin of Safety (Washington, DC: US Government Printing Office, 1974, #550/9-74-004).

13. D.O. McCarthy et al., Shades of Florence Nightingale: Potential Impact of Noise Stress on Wound Healing, *Holistic Nursing Practice* 5 (1991):39–48.

14. C. Schulbert, *The Music Therapy Sourcebook* (New York: Human Sciences Press, 1981), 13.

15. P.M. Hamel, *Through Music to the Self* (Boulder, CO: Shambhala Press, 1979), 166.

16. H. Bonny and L. Savary, *Music and Your Mind* (New York: Harper & Row, 1973), 15.

17. Hamel, *Through Music to the Self*, 174.

18. Bonny and Savary, *Music and Your Mind*, 14.

19. R. McClellan, Music and Altered States of Consciousness, *Dromenon* 2(1979):3–5.

20. McClellan, Music and Altered States of Consciousness.

21. S. Krippner, *The Highest State of Consciousness* (New York: Doubleday, 1972), 1–5.

22. D.G. Campbell, *Introduction to the Musical Brain* (St. Louis: MMB Music, 1984), 14–65.

23. Campbell, *Introduction to the Musical Brain*, 45.

24. Bonny and Savary, *Music and Your Mind*, 90.

25. R. Beebe, Synesthesia with Music, *Dromenon* 2 (1979):7.

26. Campbell, *Introduction to the Musical Brain*, 14.

27. I. Altshuler, A Psychiatrist's Experience with Music As a Therapeutic Agent, in *Music as Medicine*, ed. D. Schullian and M. Schoen (New York: Henry Schuman, 1948), 267.

28. McClellan, Music and Altered States of Consciousness, 4.

29. Campbell, *Introduction to the Musical Brain*, 15–16.

30. Bonny and Savary, *Music and Your Mind*, 30.

31. R. McCraty et al., The Effects of Different Types of Music on Mood, Tension, and Mental Clarity, *Alternative Therapies in Health and Medicine* 4, no. 1 (1998):75–84.

32. J. Page, Roses Are Red, E-flat Is, Too, *Hippocrates* (1987, September–October):63–66.

33. J. Houston, *The Possible Human* (Los Angeles: Jeremy P. Tarcher, 1982), 47–48.

34. Halpern and Savary, *Sound Health*, 183.

35. Halpern and Savary, *Sound Health*, 185.

36. Campbell, *Introduction to the Musical Brain*, 20–22.

37. C.B. Pert, *Molecules of Emotion* (New York: Charles Scribner's Sons, 1997).

38. McCraty et al., The Effects of Different Types of Music, 75.

39. Halpern and Savary, *Sound Health*, 39–43.

40. C.E. Guzzetta, Effects of Relaxation and Music Therapy on Patients in a Coronary Care Unit with Presumptive Acute Myocardial Infarction, *Heart and Lung* 18(1989):609–616.

41. C. Webster, Relaxation, Music and Cardiology: The Physiological and Psychological Consequences of Their Interrelation, *Australian Occupational Therapy Journal* 20(1973):9–20.

42. R. McCraty et al., Music Enhances the Effect of Positive Emotional States on Salivary IgA, *Stress Medicine* 12 (1996): 167–175.

43. Webster, Relaxation, Music and Cardiology.

44. Webster, Relaxation, Music and Cardiology.

45. P.O. Peretti and K. Swenson, Effects of Music on Anxiety As Determined by Physiological Skin Responses, *Journal of Research Music Education* 22 (1974): 278–283.

46. G.H. Zimny and E.W. Weidenfeller, Effects of Music upon GSR of Children, *Child Development* 33 (1962): 891–896.

47. Guzzetta, Effects of Relaxation and Music Therapy.

48. V.E. Kibler and M. Rider, Effects of Progressive Muscle Relaxation and Music on Stress as Measured by Finger Temperature Response, *Journal of Clinical Psychology* 39, no. 2(1983):213–215.

49. J.P. Scartelli, The Effect of EMG Biofeedback and Sedative Music, EMG Biofeedback Only and Sedative Music Only on Frontalis Muscle Relaxation Ability, *Journal of Music Therapy* 21, no. 2(1984):67–78.

50. S.B Reynolds, Biofeedback, Relaxation Training and Music: Homeostasis for Coping with Stress, *Biofeedback Self Regulation* 9, no. 2 (1984):169–177.

51. McCraty et al., Music Enhances the Effect of Positive Emotional States on Salivary IgA.

52. M. Rider, Imagery, Improvisation, and Immunity, *Psychotherapy* 17(1990):211–216.

53. M.S. Rider et al., Effect of Immune System Imagery on Secretory IgA, *Biofeedback Self Regulation* 15(1990):317–333.

54. M. Mockel et al., Stress Reduction through Listening to Music: Effects on Stress Hormones, Hemodynamics and Mental State in Patients with Arterial Hypertension and in Healthy Persons, *Deutsche Medizinische Wochenschrift* 120, no. 21 (1995): 745–752.

55. B.J. Crowe, Music—The Ultimate Physician, in *Music: Physician for Times To Come*, ed. D. Campbell (Wheaton, IL: Quest Books, 1991), 111.

56. Halpern and Savary, *Sound Health*, 115.

57. Campbell, *Introduction to the Musical Brain*, 62–63.

58. Schulbert, *The Music Therapy Sourcebook*, 104.

59. Halpern and Savary, *Sound Health*, 136.

60. Halpern and Savary, *Sound Health*, 129.

61. Bonny and Savary, *Music and Your Mind*, 31.

62. Halpern and Savary, *Sound Health*, 137.

63. Halpern and Savary, *Sound Health*, 96–97.

64. H. Bonny, Guided Imagery and Music Brochure (Port Townsend, WA: Institute for Music and Imagery, 1986).

65. S.J. Stokes, Letting the Sound Depths Arise, in *Music and Miracles*, ed. D. Campbell (Wheaton, IL: Quest Books, 1992), 187–188.

66. K. Bruscia, Visits from the Other Side: Healing Persons with AIDS through Guided Imagery and Music, in *Music and Miracles*, ed. D. Campbell (Wheaton, IL: Quest Books, 1992), 195–207.

67. T. Schroeder-Sheker, Music for the Dying: A Personal Account of the New Field of Music Thanatology—History, Theories, and Clinical Narratives, *Journal of Holistic Nursing* 12, no. 1 (1994): 83–99.

68. D. Aldridge, The Music of the Body: Music Therapy in Medical Settings, *Advances* 9, no. 1 (1993): 17–35.

69. C.H. McKinney et al., Effects of Guided Imagery and Music (GIM) Therapy on Mood and Cortisol in Healthy Adults, *Health Psychology* 16, no. 4 (1997): 390–400.

70. O. Quintino et al., Job Stress Reduction Therapies, *Alternative Therapies in Health and Medicine* 3, no. 4 (1997): 54–56.

71. L.L. Chlan, Psychophysiologic Responses of Mechanically Ventilated Patients to Music: A Pilot Study, *American Journal of Critical Care* 4, no. 3 (1995): 233–238.

72. Guzzetta, Effects of Relaxation and Music Therapy.

73. C.A. Bolwerk, Effects of Relaxing Music on State Anxiety in Myocardial Infarction Patients, *Critical Care Nurse Quarterly* 13, no. 2 (1990):63–72.

74. P. Updike, Music Therapy Results for ICU Patients, *Dimensions of Critical Care Nursing* 9, no. 1 (1990):39–45.

75. J.M. White, Music Therapy: An Intervention To Reduce Anxiety in the Myocardial Infarction Patient, *Clinical Nurse Specialist* 6(1992):58–63.

76. D. Elliott, The Effects of Music and Muscle Relaxation on Patient Anxiety in a Coronary Care Unit, *Heart and Lung* 23, no. 1 (1994):27–35.

77. L.M. Zimmermann et al., Effects of Music on Patient Anxiety in Coronary Care Units, *Heart and Lung* 17(1988):560–566.

78. J.F. Byers and K.A. Smyth, Effect of Music Intervention on Noise Annoyance, Heart Rate, and Blood Pressure in Cardiac Surgery Patients, *American Journal of Critical Care* 6, no. 3 (1997):183–191.

79. S. Barnason et al., The Effects of Music Interventions on Anxiety in the Patient after Coronary Artery Bypass Grafting, *Heart and Lung* 24, no. 2 (1995):124–132.

80. Aldridge, The Music of the Body.

81. M.F. Cunningham et al., Introducing a Music Program in the Perioperative Area, *AORN Journal* 66, no. 4 (1997):674–682.

82. J. Kaminski and W. Hall, The Effect of Soothing Music on Neonatal Behavioral States in the Hospital Newborn Nursery, *Neonatal Network* 15, no. 1 (1996):45–54.

83. J.M. Standley and R.S. Moore, Therapeutic Effects of Music and Mother's Voice on Premature Infants, *Pediatric Nursing* 21, no. 6 (1995):509–512.

84. A.B. Malone, The Effects of Live Music on the Distress of Pediatric Patients Receiving Intravenous Start, Venipunctures, Injections, and Heel Sticks, *Journal of Music Therapy* 33, no. 3 (1996):231.

85. P. Bampton and B. Draper, The Effects of Relaxation Music on Patient Tolerance of Gastrointestinal Endoscopic Procedures, *Journal of Clinical Gastroenterology* 25, no. 1 (1997):243–245.

86. J. Edwards, You Are Singing Beautifully: Music Therapy and the Debridement Bath, *Arts in Psychotherapy* 22, no. 1 (1995):53–55.

87. L. Zimmerman et al., The Effects of Music Interventions on Postoperative Pain and Sleep in Coronary Artery Bypass Graft (CABG) Patients, *Scholarly Inquiry for Nursing Practice* 10, no. 2 (1996):153–170.

88. M. Good, A Comparison of the Effects of Jaw Relaxation and Music on Postoperative Pain, *Nursing Research* 44, no. 1 (1995):52–57.

89. L.K. Taylor et al., The Effect of Music in the Postanesthesia Care Unit on Pain Levels in Women Who Have Had Abdominal Hysterectomies, *Journal of Perianesthesia Nursing* 13, no. 2 (1998):88–94.

90. S. Boldt, The Effects of Music Therapy on Motivation, Psychological Well-Being, Physical Comfort, and Exercise Endurance of Bone Marrow Transplant Patients, *Journal of Music Therapy* 33, no. 3 (1996):164–188.

91. J.A. Schoor, Music and Pattern Change in Chronic Pain, *Advances in Nursing Science* 15, no. 4 (1993):27–36.

92. M.M. Stevens et al., Pain and Symptom Control in Paediatric Palliative Care, *Cancer Surveys* 21 (1994):211–231.

93. G. Kerkvliet, Music Therapy May Help Control Cancer Pain, *Journal of the National Cancer Institute* 82 (1990):350–352.

94. L.B. Zimmerman et al., Effects of Music in Patients Who Had Chronic Cancer Pain, *Western Journal of Nursing Research* 11 (1989):298–309.

95. L. Kammrath, Music Therapy during Chemotherapy: Report on the Beginning of a Study, *Krakenpflege-Frankfurt* 43(1989):282–283.

96. J. Frank, The Effects of Music Therapy and Guided Visual Imagery on Chemotherapy Induced Nausea and Vomiting, *Oncology Nursing Forum* 12 (1985):47–52.

97. J.M. Strauser, The Effects of Music versus Silence on Measures of State Anxiety, Perceived Relaxation, and Physiological Responses of Patients Receiving Chiropractic Interventions, *Journal of Music Therapy* 34, no. 2 (1997):85–105.

98. R.M. Heiser et al., The Use of Music during the Immediate Postoperative Recovery Period, *AORN Journal* 65, no. 4 (1997):777–785.

99. D.K. Fontaine, Nonpharmacologic Management of Patient Distress during Mechanical Ventilation, *Critical Care Clinics* 10, no. 4 (1994):695–708.

100. L. Chlan, Effectiveness of a Music Therapy Intervention on Relaxation and Anxiety for Patients Receiving Ventilatory Assistance, *Heart and Lung* 27, no. 3 (1998):169–176.

101. C.M. Lucia, Toward Developing a Model of Music Therapy Intervention in the Rehabilitation of Head Trauma Patients, *Music Therapy Perspectives* 4 (1987):34–39.

102. G.C. Mornhinweg and R.R. Voignier, Music for Sleep Disturbance in the Elderly, *Journal of Holistic Nursing* 13, no. 13 (1995):248–254.

103. D. Prinsley, Music Therapy in Geriatric Care, *Australian Nurses Journal* 15 (1986):48–49.

104. M.A. Steckler, The Effects of Music on Healing, *Journal of Long Term Home Health Care* 17, no. 1 (1998):42–48.

105. M. Snyder and J. Olson, Music and Hand Massage Intervention To Produce Relaxation and Reduce Aggressive Behaviors in Cognitively Impaired Elders: A Pilot Study, *Clinical Gerontologist* 17, no. 1 (1996):64–69.

106. M. Brotons et al., Music and Dementias: A Review of Literature, *Journal of Music Therapy* 34, no. 4 (1997):204–245.

107. Brotons et al., Music and Dementias.

108. J. Tyson, Meeting the Needs of Dementia, *Nursing of the Elderly* 1 (1989):18–19.

109. M. Brotons and P. Pickett-Cooper, The Effects of Music Therapy on Agitation Behaviors of Alzheimer's Disease Patients, *Journal of Music Therapy* 33, no. 1 (1996):2–18.

110. L. Keegan, Holistic Nursing, *Journal of Post Anesthesia Nursing* 4 (1989):17–21.

111. W. Lehmann and D. Kirchner, Initial Experiences in the Combined Treatment of Aphasia Patients Following Cerebrovascular Insult by Speech Therapist and Music Therapists, *Zeitschrift Altenforschung* 41 (1986):123–128.

112. B. Dun, A Different Beat: Music Therapy in Children's Cardiac Care, *Music Therapy Perspectives* 13, no. 1 (1995):35–39.

113. P.M. Lehrer et al., Relaxation and Music Therapies for Asthma among Patients Prestabilized on Asthma Medication, *Journal of Behavioral Medicine* 17, no. 1 (1994):1–24.

114. R.W. Justice, Music Therapy Interventions for People with Eating Disorders in an Inpatient Setting, *Music Therapy Perspectives* 12, no. 2 (1994):104–110.

115. Bruscia, Visits from the Other Side.

116. Campbell, *The Mozart Effect*.

117. G.C. Mornhinweg, Effects of Music Preference and Selection on Stress Reduction, *Journal of Holistic Nursing* 10, no. 2 (1992):101–109.

118. Hamel, *Through Music to the Self*, 169.

119. M. Good and C.C. Chin, The Effects of Western Music on Postoperative Pain in Taiwan, *Kao-Hsiung i Hsueh Ko Hsueh Tsa Chih* 14, no. 2 (1998):94–103.

120. McCraty et al., The Effects of Different Types of Music.

121. K. Allen and J. Blascovich, Effects of Music on Cardiovascular Reactivity among Surgeons, *Journal of the American Medical Association* 272 (1994):882–884.

122. Halpern and Savary, Sound Health, 46.

123. McCraty et al., The Effects of Different Types of Music.

124. M.A. Wooten, The Effects of Heavy Metal Music on Affects Shifts of Adolescents in an Inpatient Psychiatric Setting, *Music Therapy Perspectives* 10, no. 2 (1992):93–98.

125. Hamel, *Through Music to the Self*, 169.

126. Tyson, Meeting the Needs of Dementia.

127. Campbell, *The Mozart Effect*, 65.

128. Campbell, *The Mozart Effect*, 66.

129. Campbell, *The Mozart Effect*, 78–80.

130. D. Aldridge, An Overview of Music Therapy Research, *Complementary Therapies in Medicine* 2(1994):204–216.

131. Halpern and Savary, Sound Health, 203.

132. H. Bonny, Sound Spaces: Music Rx Is Proven in the ICU, *ICM West Newsletter* 2, no. 4 (1982), 1–2.

133. S. Mazer and D. Smith, Sound Choices: Using Music To Design Your Environments (Carlsbad, CA: Hay House, 1999).

134. Bonny and Savary, Music and Your Mind, 43.

135. B. Wein, Body and Soul Music, *American Health* (1987, April):67–74.

136. Halpern and Savary, Sound Health, 150.

137. Campbell, *The Mozart Effect*, 258–259.

RESOURCES

Relaxation, Music, and Imagery Tapes

Institute for Music, Health, and Education
Don G. Campbell, Director
P.O. Box 4179
Boulder, CO 80306
Telephone: 314-531-4756

Mind/Body Health Sciences
393 Dixon Road, Goldhill
Salina Star Route
Boulder, CO 80302
Telephone: 303-440-8460

Music Design
4650 N. Port Washington Road
Milwaukee, WI 53212
Telephone: 1-800-862-7232

Natural Wellness
P.O. Box 1139
Pine Bush, NY 12566-1139
Telephone: 1-800-364-5722

New Era Media
425 Alabama Street
San Francisco, CA 94110
Telephone: 415-863-3555

Nightingale Conent
7300 N. Nehigh Avenue
Niles, IL 60617
Telephone: 1-800-525-9000

Sounds True
413 S. Arthur Avenue
Louisville, CO 80027
Telephone: 1-888-303-9185

Spring Hill Music
P.O. Box 800
Boulder, CO 80306
Telephone: 1-800-427-7680

Steve Halpern Sound Rx
P.O. Box 2644
San Enselmo, CA 94979
Telephone: 1-800-909-0707

Music Therapy Tapes Designed for Hospital Use

Healing HealthCare Systems
(Susan Mazer and Dallas Smith)
P.O. Box 8010
Reno, NV 89503
Telephone: 1-800-348-0799

Music RX
P.O. Box 173
Port Townsend, WA 98368
Telephone: 206-385-6160

Spring Hill Music (Music for the Mozart Effect, Vol. II, Heal the Body, Music for Rest and Relaxation by Don Campbell)
P.O. Box 800
Boulder, CO 80306
Telephone: 1-800-427-7680

Steven Halpern (Hospital Suite)
P.O. Box 2644
San Enselmo, CA 94979
Telephone: 1-800-909-0707

Surgical Audiotape Series
(for pre-, intra-, and postoperative experiences)
70 Maple Avenue
Katonah, NY 10536

Additional Resources

American Association of Music Therapy
P.O. Box 80012
Valley Forge, PA 19484
Telephone: 215-265-4006

Association for Music and Imagery
331 Soquel Avenue, Suite 201
Santa Cruz, CA 95062

The Bonny Foundation
2020 Simmons Street
Salinas, KS 67401

CAIRSS for Music (Computer-Assisted Information Retrieval Service System)
A bibliographic data base of over 11,000 music
    research literature in music education, music
    psychology, music therapy, and music medicine.
http://imr.utsa.edu

Institute for Consciousness and Music
7027 Bellona Ave.
Baltimore, MD 21212

Institute for Music and Neurologic Function
Beth Abraham Hospital
612 Allerton Avenue
Bronx, NY 10467
Telephone: 718-920-4567

International Society for Music in Medicine
Dr. Ralph Springe, Executive Director
Sportkrankenhaus Hellersen
Paulmannshoher, Strasse 17
D-5880 Ludenscheid, Germany

Mid-Atlantic Institute for Guided Imagery and Music
P.O. Box 4655
Virginia Beach, VA 23454
Telephone: 757-498-0452

MuSICA (Music and Science Information Computer Archive)
c/o Dr. Norman M. Weinberger
Center for the Neurobiology of Learning and
    Memory
University of California, Irvine
Irvine, CA 92717
E-mail: mbic@mila.ps.uci.edu

National Association of Music Therapy
8455 Colesville Road, Suite 930
Silver Spring, MD 20910
Telephone: 301-589-3300

VISION OF HEALING

Using Our Healing Hands

Imagine being transported into a dimension that bathes your entire being in a delicious sensation, one that stimulates and/or relaxes your physical sensory receptors and taps into mental and spiritual domains. Many people report this kind of opening, something that feels akin to floating on a cloud, when they experience hands-on healing for the first time. Subsequent sessions build upon and augment the initial effect.

Stroking and enfolding, kneading manipulation, light touch, pressure point, and working within an energy field are just some of the phrases that come to mind when thinking about the modality of touch. Within a single generation, the phenomenon of touch as a nursing intervention has evolved from the basic bedside back rub into an expansive variety of full-body hands-on techniques.

Many practitioners and recipients of the various touch modalities believe that the end result is more beneficial than simply the obvious physical effect. Numerous hands-on therapies are designed to awaken the recipient's psyche and heighten spiritual awareness while producing both overt and covert physical changes. The environment, the centeredness of the practitioner, the specific modality selected, and the receptivity of the client all contribute to an experience that has

the power to embrace both psyche and soma and result in a positive alteration of body, mind, and spirit.

Nurses refer to the hands-on aspects of nursing as touch therapy, therapeutic touch, healing touch, therapeutic massage, or bodywork, as well as a variety of other labels. Despite the different names, the intent is always the same: to care for another through some mode of physical touch or energy field manipulation. Although the techniques vary among practitioners, the objectives of the various therapies are similar: to relax; soothe; stimulate; relieve physical, mental, emotional, and/or spiritual discomfort; or aid in the transition of the client to a heightened plateau of being. Those who use touch as a therapeutic modality do so from a calm, centered place and believe that focused intention facilitates the transference of healing energy. However, just as not all nurses relate well to the technical nature of an intensive care unit or operating room, not all nurses have the ability or desire to use the medium of touch. Generally, both practitioners and recipients know after a few encounters if this approach works for them. When it does, the nurse who develops hands-on therapeutic skills can become a practitioner of a whole new array of powerful healing modalities.

Chapter 24

Touch: Connecting with the Healing Power

Karilee Halo Shames and Lynn Keegan

NURSE HEALER OBJECTIVES

Theoretical

- Learn the definitions of the various types of touch techniques.
- Compare and contrast the various touch therapies.
- Observe subjective and objective changes in the client after the touch therapy session.
- Compare and contrast your responses to touch therapy with the published descriptions of other nurses.

Clinical

- Develop your abilities to center and become calm before you use touch therapies in your practice.
- Learn to calm, soften, and steady your voice as you use it as an adjunct to touch therapy.
- Experiment with soothing music or guided imagery (spoken or from audiotapes) as an adjunct to the touch session.
- Create opportunities to practice touch therapies in your clinical area.
- Notice whether there are any changes in your emotions during or after you use touch therapy.
- Notice whether there is any change in your sense of time when you use touch. Does time slow down or speed up?

Personal

- Become aware of how you use touch in your everyday life.
- Examine the significance of touch in your personal and professional relationships.

DEFINITIONS

Acupressure: the application of finger and/or thumb pressure to specific sites along the body's energy meridians for the purpose of relieving tension, reestablishing the flow of energy along the meridian lines, and restoring balance to the human energy system.

Body Therapy and/or Touch Therapy: the broad range of techniques that a practitioner uses in which the hands are on or near the body to assist the recipient toward optimal function.

Caring Touch: touch performed with a genuine interest in the other person, as well as empathy and concern.

Centering: a sense of self-relatedness that can be thought of as a place of inner being, a place of quietude within oneself where one can feel truly integrated, unified, and focused.[1]

Energy Center: specific center of consciousness in the human energy system that allows for the inflow of energy from the Universal Energy Field as well as for outflow from the individual's energy field. There are seven major energy centers in relation to the spine and many minor centers at bone articulations in the palms of the hands and the soles of the feet. Also called *chakra*.

Energy Meridian: an energy circuit or line of force. Eastern theories describe meridian lines flowing vertically through the body culminating at points on the feet, hands, and ears.

Foot Reflexology: the application of pressure to points on the feet held to correspond to other parts of the body.

Grounding: the process of connecting to the earth and the earth's energy field to calm the mind and focus one's inner flow of energy to enhance healing endeavors.

Human Energy System: the entire interactive, dynamic system of human subtle energies, consisting of the energy centers, the multidimensional field, the meridians, and acupuncture points.

Intention: the motivation or reason for touching; the direction of one's inner awareness and focus for healing; the state of being fully present in the moment.

Procedural Touch: touch performed to diagnose, monitor, or treat an illness; touch that focuses on the end result of curing the illness or preventing further complications.

Shiatzu: the systematic use of the thumb and/or heel of the hand for deep pressure work along the energy meridian lines.

Therapeutic Massage: the use of the hands to apply pressure and motion to the recipient's skin and underlying muscle to promote physical and psychologic relaxation, improve circulation, relieve sore muscles, and accomplish other therapeutic effects.

Therapeutic Touch: a specific technique of centering intention used while the practitioner moves the hands through a recipient's energy field for the purpose of assessing and treating energy field imbalance.

THEORY AND RESEARCH

Touch in Ancient Times

Healing through touch is as old as civilization itself. Practiced extensively in all ancient cultures, this oldest form of treatment was to "rub it if it hurts."[2] The Egyptians used bandages, poultices, touch, and manipulation. Pyramids from the earliest times in Egypt show representations of a person holding hands near another, with waves of energy depicted moving from the hands to the body nearby. The oldest written documentation of the use of body touch to enhance healing comes from Asia. The *Huang Ti Nei Ching* is a classic work of internal medicine that was written 5,000 years ago. The *Nei Ching*, a 3,000- to 4,000-year-old Chinese book of health and medicine, records a system of touch based on acupuncture points and energy circuits. The ancient Indian Vedas also described healing massage, as did the Polynesian Lomi practice and the traditions of Native Americans.

During the height of Greek civilization, Hippocrates wrote of the therapeutic effects of massage and manipulation; he also gave instructions for carrying out these practices. He wrote during the time of the great Aesculapian healing centers, at which many whole-body therapies included touch. Touch therapies were also employed at the healing centers to assist individuals who wished to make the transition to a higher level of function. Massage was used as a mode of preparation for dream work, which was a significant part of therapy in the healing rites. The Roman historian Plutarch wrote that Julius Caesar was treated for epilepsy by being pinched over his entire body every day.

Both shamans and traditional practitioners used touch widely until the rise of the Puritan culture during the 1600s and the shift from primitive healing practices to modern scientific medicine.[3,4] Puritan culture equated touch with sex, which was associated with original sin. During the late nineteenth and early twentieth centuries, health care moved away from anything associated with superstition and primitive healing, and was directed toward scientific medicine. All unnecessary touch was discouraged because of the association of touch with primitive healing and because of the prevailing strong Puritan ethic. Consequently, touch as a therapeutic intervention remained undeveloped in U.S. health care until research into its benefits began in the 1950s.

Cultural Variations

The fact that many cultures, both ancient and modern, have developed some form of touch therapy indicates that rubbing, pressing, massaging, and holding are natural manifestations of the desire to heal and care for one another. However, attitudes toward touch vary from culture to culture.[5] One society may view touch as necessary, whereas another may view it as forbidden. The nurse must be aware of personal and cultural views and reactions to touch.

Philosophic and cultural differences have influenced the development of touch in various areas of the world. The Eastern world view is founded on energy, whereas the Western world view is based on reductionism of matter. This basic cultural difference has led to the evolution of widely differing approaches to touch. The Eastern world view holds that qi (or chi), also described as energy or vital force, is the center of body function. A meridian is an energy circuit or line of force that runs vertically through the body.[6] Magnetic or bioelectrical patterns flow through the microcosm of the body in the same way that magnetic patterns flow through the planet and the universe. Meridian lines and zones are influenced by pressure placed on points along those lines. Expert practitioners in acupuncture or Shiatzu purport to direct healing energy to the recipient via an en-

ergy flow that moves through the body and out through their hands.[7] In contrast, the Western world view holds that it is the physical effect of cellular changes occurring during touch that influences healing. For example, massage stimulates the cells to aid in waste discharge, promotes the dilation of the vascular system, and encourages lymphatic drainage. Swedish and therapeutic massage were developed to produce these physical changes.

A blending of Eastern and Western techniques has resulted in an explosion of new and widely practiced modalities. The modern-day renaissance in body therapies is probably a healthy response to the fast-paced technologic revolution that has swept our culture, bringing back a sense of balance and caring.

Modern Concepts of Touch

Research is finally beginning to document what healers have always intuitively known. Some of the first studies documenting the significance of touch involved infant monkeys and surrogate mothers.[8] In the 1950s, Harlow caged one group of infant monkeys with a monkey-shaped wire form serving as a surrogate mother and a second group with a soft cloth mother surrogate. When frightened, the monkeys housed with the wire form reacted by running and cowering in a corner. The other group reacted to the same stimuli by running and clinging to the soft cloth surrogate for protection. These infant monkeys even preferred clinging to an unheated cloth surrogate mother to sitting on a warm heating pad. Although the cloth surrogate was unresponsive, the offspring raised with it developed basically normal behavior. This and other classic studies conclusively documented the significance of touch in normal animal growth and development.

Studies of human development soon followed. One study of abandoned infants and infants whose mothers were in prison found that infants whom the nurses held and cuddled thrived, but those who were left alone became ill and died.[9] These studies led to the development of the concept of touch deprivation. Other studies have shown that touch has a positive effect on the immune system.[10]

These early studies in the 1950s and 1960s awakened scientific interest in the phenomenon of healing touch. Bernard Grad, a biochemist at McGill University, was one of the first to investigate healing by the laying on of hands. He conducted a series of double-blind experiments with the renowned healer Oskar Estebany.[11] In these studies, wounded mice and damaged barley seeds were separated into control and experimental groups. After Estebany used therapeutic touch to manipulate the energy fields of the mice and seeds in the experimental groups, these groups demonstrated a significantly accelerated healing rate in comparison to the control groups. In a subsequent study, an enzymologist worked with Grad using the enzyme trypsin in double-blind studies.[12] After the trypsin was exposed to Estebany's treatments, its activity was significantly increased.

Nursing Studies

Although touch therapy is as old as civilization, documentation of how, why, and where it works is relatively new in the nursing literature. Hand holding has been described as a positive means of communication that seems to break down barriers.[13] Through the mechanism of touch, a nurse can convey feelings of caring and understanding to the client.[14] One study of 52 hospitalized patients addressed three universal issues regarding nonprocedural touch; 70 percent of patients felt that touch was emotionally comforting, 87 percent agreed that the nurse's touch was soothing and comforting, and 75 percent agreed that the use of touch made them feel valued and personalized their care.[15] In a review of the subject, Bottorff concluded that, because of the dearth of studies, little is known with certainty about nurse-patient touch.[16]

Critical Care

The anxiety level of myocardial infarction patients in coronary care units is known to be high. The coronary care nurse is in a position to manipulate the client's environment to reduce or eliminate anxiety. Glick carried out a quasi-experimental study to determine the relationship between the type of touch and the anxiety experienced by myocardial infarction patients in an intermediate cardiac care unit.[17] Those receiving the greatest benefits from the caring touch of nurses were patients with preexisting coronary artery disease and men under the age of 60 years. Those experiencing the least benefit were women who were touched both by significant others and by the investigator.

McCorkle investigated the effects of touch as nonverbal communication on a group of seriously ill middle-aged adults and found that the nurse's touch increased the duration of verbal responses.[18] These findings confirmed the results of another study in which the use of touch was found to increase verbal interactions between nurses and patients.[19] Still another study demonstrated that touch slowed the heart rate, decreased diastolic blood pressure, and reduced anxiety.[20] The beneficial effects of touch for surgical patients in the perioperative area have also been documented.[21] Despite the growing evidence that touch is beneficial, a natural field study by Schoenhofer of 30 nurse-patient dyads in hospital critical care units found that touch is seldom used as a nursing comfort measure.[22]

Care of the Elderly

Our culture has been described as suffering from "skin hunger," a form of malnutrition that has reached epidemic proportions in the United States.[23] Rozema notes that the elderly need touch as much as or more than any other age group; however, skin hunger or poverty of touch is often acute among elderly adults.[24] It is an unfortunate coincidence that elderly people often have fewer family members or friends to touch them at a time when touch could be an enhanced form of communication because other senses might be reduced.

A study of the use of touch by health care personnel found that clients between the ages of 66 and 100 years received the least amount of touch.[25] Clients in geriatric institutions show not only their hunger for affection but also the great value that they place on the smallest gesture, the simplest touch.[26] An experimental study that examined anger and hostility among nursing home residents found that the less mobile patients responded more positively to touch and were less angry than their more mobile counterparts when touched.[27,28] Clearly, touch helped patients them feel more connected to those around them and to their environment.

Professionals must examine their own feelings about the meaning of touch before using it as a therapeutic tool. Our cultural emphasis on youth may play an important role in perpetuating the touch deprivation of elderly people. In a study of their perceptions of touch and their feelings about infants and nursing home residents, student nurses were asked to describe the tactile and affective sensations of touching in five words.[29] The students described the infants as cuddly, small, warm, soft, and smooth, but they described the elderly patients as wrinkled, loose, flabby, bony, and cold. The students were more comfortable touching newborns than they were touching geriatric patients. A nurse who reacts adversely to the skin changes of older people may find it difficult to touch an elderly client.[30] The nurse's reluctance may then communicate a negative message to the elderly person. Relatively little expressive touch actually takes place between nurses and elderly patients.[31]

Not all clients want to be touched. A study of 24 nursing home residents with high agitation and severe cognitive impairment found that touch was related to an increase in aggressive behaviors. The researchers believed that the cognitively impaired elderly patients may have viewed touch as a violation of their personal space.[32] Other research reported that 2 percent of nursing home patients were uncomfortable with touching.[33] Two factors were associated with the discomfort: the gender of the nurse and the part of the body that was touched. Female patients were not comfortable being touched by older male nurses. Hand or arm holding did not evoke a negative reaction, but many patients reported feeling discomfort or pain when the nurse placed an arm around their shoulders. An older female nurse's touch to the face was well accepted by almost all patients, however.

The art of touch, as well as when to touch and when not to touch, can be learned. Nursing students can and should be taught the importance of touch as therapy. They need exposure and experience to overcome their cultural conditioning against touching adults, especially unfamiliar ones, to increase their ease in initiating this intervention. They also need guidance in developing a sensitivity to those who desire or may decline touch.

Care of Children

A study comparing the effectiveness of therapeutic touch and casual touch for stress reduction in hospitalized children aged 2 weeks to 2 years demonstrated that therapeutic touch reduced the time needed to calm children after stressful experiences.[34] Most hospitalized children are suffering from separation anxiety. Nurses find that connecting with them through touch invites their cooperation and relaxation.

Obstetrics

Thirty women who experienced a normal spontaneous vaginal birth attended by a nurse-midwife were interviewed during the immediate postpartal period. They perceived touch as therapeutic most frequently during the transition phase of labor. Hand holding was the type of touch most consistently valued throughout labor. The findings showed that touch helped women in labor cope with the experience.[35]

Touching Styles

Data collected by in-depth interviews with eight experienced intensive care nurses revealed two substantive processes, the touching process itself and the acquisition of a touching style, neither of which had been previously reported in the literature. Estabrooks and Morse note that the touching process is more than skin-to-skin contact; it involves entering the patient's space, connecting, talking, following nonverbal cues, and eventually touching. Nurses learn about touch from their culture, family, street learning, personal experience, and nursing school.[36]

Effects of Therapeutic Touch

Therapeutic touch, a movement of the practitioner's hands through the recipient's energy field without body contact, has gained increasing attention during the past decade. A controlled study of 90 patients in the cardiovascular unit of a large medical center showed a significant decrease in anxiety in those patients who received therapeutic touch, compared with those who received only casual touch or no touch at all.[37] Another study demonstrated an average reduction of 70 percent in tension headache pain over 4 hours after therapeutic touch, more than twice the average pain reduction following placebo touch.[38] Krieger and others continue to document the importance of therapeutic touch and encourage its investigation using controlled studies.[39,40]

Bodymind Communication

Touch is perhaps one of the most frequently used, yet least applauded, of the five recognized senses. It is the first sense to develop in the human embryo, and the one most vital to survival. Touch can vary from subtle fleeting brush strokes to violent physical attacks. Touch evokes the full range of emotions from hatred to the most intimate love relationship. Figuratively, touch is used in literature and even daily conversation to describe emotions. For example, "That speech really touched me," or "This workshop will allow you to touch one another heart to heart." These figurative expressions signify the deep importance and value of touch.

As the largest and most ancient sense organ of the body, the skin enables us to experience and learn about the environment.[41] Through the skin, we perceive the external world. The skin, particularly the skin of the face, not only communicates to the brain knowledge about the external world but also conveys to others information about the state of an individual's bodymind-spirit.

A piece of skin the size of a quarter contains more than 3 million cells, 12 feet of nerves, 100 sweat glands, 50 nerve endings, and 3 feet of blood vessels. There are estimated to be approximately 50 receptors per 100 square centimeters—a total of 900,000 sensory receptors.[42] Viewed from this perspective, the skin is a giant communication system that, through the sense of touch, brings messages from the external environment to the attention of the internal environment—the bodymind.

Because health care is increasingly being delivered in very complicated technologic settings, nurses are concerned with ensuring that the human spiritual and social needs of patients not be overlooked.[43] Yet nurses must take into account social contexts and cultural differences before engaging in energetic efforts to provide touch therapy. A nurse should never assume that a client will find touch comforting but should always ask before touching. If the suggestion evokes no response or a pained expression, the nurse may try a tentative touch and observe the client's response carefully. To be truly effective, touch must be given authentically by a warm, genuine, caring individual to another who is willing to receive it. It cannot and should not be packaged and dispensed. Phony touching may be more upsetting than none at all.

Like any other nursing intervention, hugging and touching demand careful assessment. Nurses need to recognize their own feelings, as well as to consider the client's age, sex, and ethnic background.[44] A few key questions (e.g., "Would a back massage help you relax?" "Would it help if I held your hand?") can help the client clarify his or her own beliefs and values regarding different types, locations, and intensities of touch.

There are many variations in and names for the touch therapies available for use as nursing interventions. Some are basic human contacts, such as hand holding and hugging. Others are more complex. Some clients will react strongly to touch, especially if they have been exposed to inappropriate or uncomfortable touch at other times. The touch therapies described below are used by holistic practitioners who often advocate and teach healthy lifestyle behavior patterns to their clients to augment well-being during the course of the touch therapy treatments. The addition of guided imagery and/or music before and during treatment may heighten the relaxation response elicited during touch therapies. The setting—be it acute care, long-term care, home care, rehabilitation center, or wellness center—will also affect the focus and length of the treatment.

TOUCH INTERVENTIONS AND TECHNIQUES

A variety of techniques are included under the heading of body therapies. Except for therapeutic touch, all body therapies involve actual physical contact. The contact usually consists of the practitioner's touching, pushing, kneading, or rubbing the recipient's skin and underlying fascia tissue. Each of the therapies has its own body of knowledge, history, and technique.

Touch can be used therapeutically in nursing in a great variety of ways. Some methods require special licensure or certification, while others can be incorporated after minimal introduction via videotape or classroom presentation. All begin with the nurse's receiving permission to touch, followed by the nurse's efforts to center and set intentionality for the client's healing. Touch therapies can be classified into several categories: somatic and musculoskeletal therapies; Eastern, meridian-based, point therapies; energy-based therapies; emotional bodywork; manipulative therapies; and other holistic touch therapies. Many programs have been developed to teach these therapies.

Somatic and Musculoskeletal Therapies

The category of somatic and musculoskeletal therapies encompasses the generic work known as therapeutic massage. As a nursing intervention, therapeutic massage has a twofold purpose. First, clients who are on bed rest or immobilized in a wheelchair require the circulatory stimulation that massage brings. Second, massage is a means of relaxation.

During this century, nurses have performed therapeutic massage primarily on the backs of their clients. Back care is not new; for decades, it has been incorporated into the standard bathing and evening care routine of most hospitals. Because of time constraints and traditional neglect of the body therapies in institutions, these patients receive only a portion of the complete range of touch therapies.

Learning full-body massage greatly augments and expands the nurse's basic massage techniques. Most practitioners learn these techniques in continuing education classes, but books on massage are also available that illustrate the techniques.

Because no two clients, either within or outside the institutional setting, have the same needs, the nurse must become skilled at adapting the therapy to the setting and the time available. Massage techniques that can be performed quickly—for example, massage for the hands, feet, or neck and shoulders—may have beneficial results in short time periods.

Other types of therapeutic massage include Swedish massage, Esalen massage, neuromuscular therapy, myofascial release, lymphatic massage/drainage therapy, and Aston-patterning. To use these specific techniques, the nurse must take special courses, which often grant a certificate of completion. Massage licensure laws vary from state to state; some states require that even registered nurses take an additional course to become certified prior to practicing massage therapy.

Eastern, Meridian-Based, and Point Therapies

The category of Eastern, meridian-based, and point therapies includes acupressure, AMMA therapy, Jin Shin Jyutsu, Shiatzu, myotherapy, reflexology, and touch for health. Since the Eastern medical approach is very different from that in our Western training and education, the nurse must study these methods in a program that teaches about meridians, pressure points, reflex points, and Eastern healing philosophy. AMMA therapy is a program in Eastern bodywork endorsed by the American Holistic Nurses' Association; it teaches nurses Eastern medical principles for assessing imbalances in the energy system combined with a Western approach to organ dysfunction.

Energy-Based Therapies

New programs and modalities are being created regularly in the rapidly growing field of energy-based interventions. Some of the more well-known and well-studied methods used by nurses include therapeutic touch, Reiki, polarity therapy, the techniques of Barbara Brennan, and the lightbody work of the Nirvana School in Scottsdale, Arizona.

Therapeutic Touch

A healing modality that involves touching with the conscious intent to help or heal, therapeutic touch decreases anxiety, relieves pain, and facilitates the healing process.[45] The process of therapeutic touch has four phases:

1. centering oneself physically and psychologically; that is, finding within oneself an inner reference of stability
2. exercising the natural sensitivity of the hand to assess the energy field of the client for clues to differentiate the quality of energy flow
3. mobilizing areas in the client's energy field that appear to be nonflowing (i.e., sluggish, congested, or static)
4. directing one's excess body energies to assist the client to repattern his or her own energies[46]

Several factors ensure the safe and successful practice of therapeutic touch: intentional motivation, personal recognition, and acceptance by the practitioner of the reason that he or she has chosen to act in the role of healer.[47] Krieger describes these qualities.

Intention connotes a clear formulation of a goal; it suggests that the TT [therapeutic touch] practitioner should have a lucid concept of how to help heal as well as the mere desire to do so. The practitioner's motivation provides the psychodynamic thrust toward healing and, therefore, it colors the emotional tone of the dyadic relationship between healer and healee. Finally it is important for the practitioner to understand his/her own drives in wanting to play the role of healer. It does not matter what these drives are; what is important is that the practitioner willingly recognizes the personal foundations for his/her involvement in this highly personalized interaction.[48(p.v)]

Therapeutic touch is taught at beginning, intermediate, and advanced levels in continuing education programs, graduate nursing education programs, and intensive summer workshops. Of all the touch therapies, therapeutic touch is the one that nursing regards most highly, for it arises through the natural potential of the process by which the nurse inspires healing in clients through touch. In recent years, many studies and books have explored therapeutic touch and related energy-based therapies from a great variety of nursing and health perspectives.[49–90]

Most of the energy-based touch therapies have certain common tenets, although the methods for applying them may vary. Nurses are becoming increasingly involved in the use of energy-based modalities for inspiring balance and bodymind connection.

Energy Field Disturbance

In the 1995–1996 *Nursing Diagnoses: Definitions and Classification*, by the North American Nursing Diagnosis Association, the definition of "energy field disturbance" made its entry into the world of professional nursing. Energy field disturbance is defined as "a disruption of the flow of energy surrounding a person's being which results in a disharmony of the body, mind, and/or spirit. Defining characteristics include: temperature changes (warmth/coolness); visual changes (image/color); disruption of the field (vacant/hold/spike/bulge); movement (wave/spike/tingling/dense/flowing); sounds (tonewords)."[91(p.37)]

Nursing Intervention Classifications

In addition to including a new nursing diagnosis related to energy healing, the *Nursing Interventions Classification*, which lists therapeutic touch, specifies simple massage as a nursing intervention, and consideration is being given to the addition of simple touch and therapeutic massage as well.[92]

Acupressure and Shiatzu

The Eastern energy system of meridian lines and points is the foundation of acupressure and Shiatzu. The application of finger and/or thumb pressure to energy points along the meridians releases congestion and allows energy to flow.

There are 657 designated points on the human body that can be stimulated or treated in acupuncture, acupressure, or Shiatzu.[93] These points run along 12 pathways, or meridians, that connect the points on each half of the body. In addition to the 12 pairs of body meridians, there are two coordinating meridians that bisect the body. Acupressure is concerned primarily with the 12-organ meridian system.

The word *shiatzu* comes from the Japanese words *shi* (finger) and *atzu* (pressure).[94] The technique is a product of 4,000 years of Eastern medicine and philosophy. Although widely known and practiced in Japan, Shiatzu was virtually unknown in the West until acupuncture began receiving widespread public attention. Shiatzu is based on the same points that are used in acupuncture. Instead of inserting needles, however, the practitioner applies pressure on these points with the thumbs, fingers, and heel of the hand. Another difference between acupuncture and Shiatzu is that the main function of Shiatzu is to maintain health and well-being rather than to treat imbalance, as in acupuncture.

Reflexology

In the early 1900s, William FitzGerald noted that application of pressure to certain points on the hands caused anesthesia in other parts of the body.[95] Another physician, Edwin Bowers, learned of Fitz-Gerald's work and joined him in the exploration and development of this zone therapy. The technique became more specific as it evolved into reflexology, which encompasses many more pressure points.

Reflexology is based on the theory that 10 equal longitudinal zones run the length of the body from the top of the head to the tips of the toes.[96] This number corresponds to the number of fingers and toes. Each big toe matches to a line that runs up the medial aspect of the body through the center of the face and culminates at the top of the head. The reflex points pass all the way through the body within the same zones. Congestion or tension in any part of a zone affects the entire zone running laterally throughout the body. More than 72,000 nerves in the body terminate in the feet.[97] A problem or disease in the body often manifests itself through formation of deposits of calcium and acids on the corresponding part of the foot.

The purpose of this therapy is twofold.[98] First, relaxation alone is an important goal. Good health is dependent on one's ability to return to homeostasis after injury, disease, or stress. From this perspective, reflexology is effective in helping the body-mind restore and maintain its natural state

of health because foot manipulation triggers deep relaxation. The second goal of this therapy is to release congestion or tension along the longitudinal and lateral zones by pressure manipulation at the precise endpoints of the zones. This pressure stimulates the reflexes in the feet to cause a corresponding release. All skeletal, muscular, vascular, nervous, and organ systems are believed to be affected. Manuals with specific diagrams are used to instruct the therapist.

At this time, no documented scientific research exists to validate the effectiveness of reflexology, although it relaxes muscles and causes a simultaneous bodymind connection that results in the relaxation response. This relaxation affects the autonomic response, which is tied into the endocrine, immune, and neuropeptide systems.

Emotional Bodywork

The category of emotional bodywork includes numerous techniques developed by individuals operating in the various fields that combine psychotherapy and bodywork. Some of the specific techniques include Lomi, network chiropractic, Hellerwork, rolfing, structural integration, and psychoenergetic balancing. Some of these methods derive from ancient traditions, others from established health fields such as chiropractic. *Psychoenergetic balancing* is a phrase coined by the nurses who recently authored a book on energy healing and emotional release, *Energetic Approaches to Emotional Healing*.[99]

Manipulative Therapies

Manipulative therapies often involve more invasive bodywork and demand a complete program of education often considered separate from nursing. Some nurses study these techniques to augment their nursing endeavors. Manipulative therapies include chiropractic and osteopathy (which involve manipulation of bones, ligaments, and soft tissue areas, including work on the head and dura). A similar related field of study is physical therapy.

Other Holistic Therapies and Programs Related to Touch

The number of bodywork and somatic therapies and touch-related programs is too extensive to cover completely here. A sampling is included below to awaken nurses to the magnitude and scope of what is available.

- **Alexander technique:** a method using gentle hands-on guidance and verbal instruction to teach simple ways of moving for improved balance, posture, coordination
- **AMMA therapy:** techniques for working with the physical body, bioenergy, and emotions to restore optimal balance
- **Barbara Brennan School of Healing Science program:** a multidimensional healing program based on the teachings of Barbara Brennan; includes chelation work through the layers of the human energy field
- **chiropractic:** an alternative form of medical care involving manipulations to create spinal alignment; requires extensive training
- **Crucible Program:** a multidimensional healing program based on the teachings of the Reverend Rosalyn Bruyere
- **Feldenkrais method:** developed by Moshe Feldenkrais, this technique involves gentle manipulations to heighten awareness of the body; teaches movement reeducation
- **healing touch:** a multilevel energy healing program combining techniques from a variety of sources; endorsed by the American Holistic Nurses' Association
- **Jin Shin Jyutsu:** "the art of compassionate spirit," a gentle acupressure-type self-healing approach
- **Lomi:** a technique that aids the learning of postural alignment to enhance the flow of energies, directing attention to muscle tensions
- **National Association for Nurse Massage Therapists:** for nurses specifically trained in massage therapy
- **Nirvana School of Enlightenment:** a program headed by Mary Bell, RN, based in Scottsdale, Arizona; presents an eclectic 2-year program based on nursing and spiritual principles
- **osteopathy:** an alternative form of medical care that emphasizes soft tissue work, skeletal manipulation, and pulses
- **Reiki:** a therapy that works with "universal life energy" and uses techniques to direct healing to specific sites
- **Robert Jaffe Advanced Energy Healing:** a method that emphasizes "heart-centered awareness" and uses clairvoyant perception and other techniques to transform energy patterns thought to contribute to disease
- **Rolfing®:** a technique developed by Ida Rolf that helps clients to establish structural relationships deep within the body; manipulates muscles for balance and symmetry
- **touch for health:** a method that uses kinesiology (muscle testing) and points to strengthen
- **Trager work:** an approach that involves rhythmic rocking to aid relaxation and optimize energy flow
- **Transformational Pathways:** a comprehensive energy-based healing program that focuses on development of healership; includes nursing theory, communication skills, various modalities, and exposure to the transpersonal perspective

HOLISTIC CARING PROCESS

Assessment

In preparing to use touch interventions, the nurse assesses the following parameters:

- the client's perception of his or her bodymind situation.
- the client's potential pathophysiologic problems that may require referral to a physician for evaluation.
- the client's history of psychiatric disorders. The nurse must modify the approach with clients who have present or past psychiatric disorders. Touch itself may present a problem, and the deeply relaxed, semihypnotic state that a balanced person finds enjoyable may actually frighten or alarm an unbalanced individual.
- the client's cultural beliefs and values about touch.
- the client's past experience with body therapies. The knowledge level of clients varies widely. The approach will differ markedly depending on the client's previous experience. Assisting a client in transferring prior learning, such as from childbirth preparation classes to a new situation, is a valuable nursing intervention.

Patterns/Problems/Needs

The following are the patterns/problems/needs compatible with the interventions for touch that are related to the nine human response patterns of the Unitary Person framework (see Chapter 14):

- *Exchanging:* Altered circulation
  Impairment in skin integrity
- *Relating:* Social isolation
- *Valuing:* Altered spiritual state
- *Moving:* Impaired physical mobility

- *Perceiving:* Altered meaningfulness
- *Feeling:* Altered comfort
  Anxiety
  Grieving
  Fear

Outcomes

Exhibit 24–1 guides the nurse in client outcomes, nursing prescriptions, and evaluation for the use of touch as a nursing intervention.

Therapeutic Care Plan and Interventions

Before the Session

- Wash your hands.
- Wear loose-fitting, comfortable clothing. If you have on street clothes, cover them with a laboratory coat.
- Have the client empty the bladder for comfort.
- Prepare the hospital bed, therapy table, or surface on which you will be working. If you will be using a therapy table, drape it with a cotton blanket and place a sheet over the top. Lay out a large towel for the client to use as a cover when he or she lies on the table. Adjust the height of the table or bed for optimal use of your body mechanics.
- Have small pillows or towel rolls available for supporting the head, back, or lower legs.
- Control the room environment so that the room is warm, dimly lit, and quiet. If you are in a client's hospital room, draw the curtain and turn off the television set. A radio or cassette tape player may be left on for soothing music.
- Use relaxation and breathing techniques, imagery, or music to elicit the relaxation response.
- After you have talked with the client, spend a few moments to quiet and center yourself, focus on your healing intention, and then begin.

Exhibit 24–1 Nursing Interventions: Touch

Client Outcomes	Nursing Prescriptions	Evaluation
The client is relaxed following a touch therapy session.	Encourage the client to receive touch therapy in order to evoke the relaxation response.	The client willingly accepted touch therapy.
	During the touch therapy session, help the client • decrease anxiety and fear • decrease pulse and respiratory rate • recognize a feeling of bodymind relaxation • develop a sense of general well-being • increase effectiveness in individual coping skills • increase a sense of belonging and lessened loneliness • feel less alone and express that feeling	The client • exhibited decreased anxiety and fear • demonstrated a decrease in pulse and respiratory rate • reported muscle relaxation • exhibited satisfied facial expression and expressed inner calmness • reported greater satisfaction in individual coping patterns
The client has improved circulation.	Provide the client with information about how touch therapies improve circulation and tissue perfusion	Clients with white skin had a reddened color in the area where the nurse had used effleurage and pétrissage massage strokes. Skin in the massaged area is warmer than before the therapy.
The client receives touch therapy to maintain and enhance health.	Encourage the client to ask for touch therapy. Suggest that the client seek out the nurse. Recommend that the client accept touch when offered by the nurse.	The client asked for touch therapy.

At the Beginning of the Session

- Explain to the client the steps in the touch process to be used. The first session always takes the most time because of the necessary explanations and adjustment. The remaining sessions may last from 15 to 60 minutes.
- As you progress through the intervention, explain what you are about to do before you actually begin.

- Position the head comfortably. If the client has long hair, pull it up and away from the neckline.
- If you are working on the client's entire body, have the client disrobe completely and cover up with a towel from the chest to the thighs. The client lies on a padded therapy table or hospital bed that is covered with a cotton blanket and sheet. The sides of the sheet and blanket are then wrapped over the cli-

ent so that he or she feels protected and warm. (This procedure is used for physical touch therapies and is not needed for therapeutic touch or other energy-based interventions. However, when the client experiences the relaxation response, the body may undergo cooling.)

- Uncover only the body area that is being massaged or pressed as the therapy proceeds.
- In most cases, begin with the client lying on the back. When therapy on the medial aspect and limbs of the body is complete, lift the wraps and reapply them after the client turns over.
- Encourage the client to take slow, deep, releasing breaths. When he or she lets go of tension through breath, affirm in a soft tone, "Ah, feel the body as it relaxes."
- During the turning process, slide the towel around the client's body to ensure that the client will not be exposed. As the client lies prone, continue the therapy on the dorsal aspect of the body.

During the Session

- Be attuned to the client's responses to therapy. This will help the client build trust and achieve optimal relaxation.
- In initial sessions, continue to explain what the client can expect to happen so that he or she feels comfortable with the continued direction of the touch sessions. After trust has been established and the relaxation response is learned, the client will relax more quickly and move to deeper levels in subsequent sessions.
- In subsequent sessions, proceed the same as in the initial session. Explanations may be shorter, however.
- Remember to use your voice in a soft, soothing manner that enables the client to relax.
- Reassess the client's responses as you proceed.

At the End of the Session

- When you have finished the touch therapy session, verbally let the client know that it is time to return gradually to the here and now, to begin to move around slowly, and to awaken fully.
- Anticipate that the client will take a few minutes to reorient to time and place after being in a deep state of relaxation.
- Allow a period of silence for the client to appreciate fully the wisdom of his or her relaxed bodymind.
- Stay in the room while the client rouses and sits up. Give necessary assistance to ensure a safe transfer to an ambulatory position.
- Allow time to receive the client's verbal feedback about the meaning of the session, if the client feels the need to talk. If this does not occur spontaneously, ask for feedback. The insight gained provides guidelines for further sessions or specific ideas that the client can follow up in daily life.
- When the touch therapy is used for relaxation or sleep induction for hospitalized patients, close the session by softly pulling the bedcovers up over the patient's back and quietly turning off the light as the patient moves into sleep. Let the client know in advance that you will leave quietly at the end.
- Use the client outcomes that were established before the session (see Exhibit 24–1) and the client's subjective experience (Exhibit 24–2) to evaluate the session.
- Schedule a follow-up session.

Specific Interventions: Touch

General Touch (Basic)

Each of the therapies discussed in the text has basic, intermediate, and advanced levels. The complexity of each type depends on the amount of time spent studying the multiple variations of the therapy and whether the therapy is used in conjunction with another therapy, such as music and imagery. A nurse who begins at the basic level and likes the given approach will probably study or take continuing education courses to learn the intermediate and advanced levels.

Therapeutic Massage (Basic to Advanced)

Although they may be called by different names (massage, Swedish massage, massage therapy), the techniques of therapeutic massage are all essentially the same. They involve the use of effleurage, pétrissage, and tapotement: the classic nursing backrub strokes. These strokes are designed to enhance the circulation of both blood and lymph. Therapeutic massage increases the dispersion of nutrients to promote the removal of metabolic wastes by increasing both lymphatic and blood flow.

Therapeutic Touch (Advanced)

Therapeutic touch is generally taught by experienced practitioners in continuing education seminars. The courses include discussion of some or all of the following elements: assessment; hand scanning; intuition; energy field reading, mapping, and recording; pattern comparison; verbal communication of information; stress levels; relaxation levels; meditation experience.

In a therapeutic touch session, the practitioner may ask the client to visualize clearly the part of the body that is to be influenced in order to enhance contact with the energy field of that body part. The practitioner's goal is to ascertain the degree of blockage in the energy field of the muscles or viscera. For practitioners to come in contact with these energies, they must develop an awareness of events that normally occur below the level of consciousness. The imagery and visualization process is one way of tuning into this unconscious process. Therapists can synergistically use one modality (imagery) to affect another (touch).[100]

Figure 24–1 illustrates a 5-year-old child's use of imagery and drawing to describe her self-perception before and after the use of therapeutic touch to treat an

A

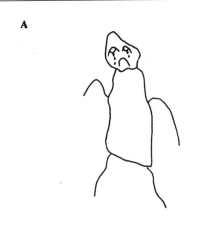

B

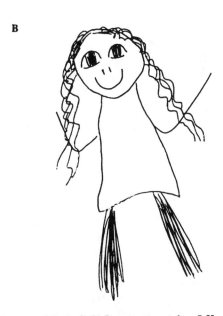

Figure 24–1 Self-Perception of a 5-Year-Old Girl with Asthma before **(A)** and after **(B)** Therapeutic Touch Session.

asthmatic episode. The child said that, when she has an asthma attack, she "feels bald-headed and sad." In drawing A, the disconnected arm is moving up to wipe away her tears. The figure lacks sturdy legs to support it. At the completion of the 15-minute therapeutic touch session, the child felt well and happy and was free of respiratory distress. In drawing B, the child increased the figure size, strengthened the lines, and added long hair that symbolizes strength to the child.

The therapeutic touch process should be halted when there are no longer any differences in body symmetry relative to density or temperature variation. Four commonly observed responses are (1) flushed skin, (2) deep sighs, (3) physical relaxation, and (4) verbalized relaxation. A caution in therapeutic touch is to limit the amount of time spent and/or energy sent in working with the very young, the old, and the infirm. When the client's energy field is full, the energy pushes the nurse away.

Healing Touch (Advanced)

An energy-based therapeutic approach, healing touch combines philosophy with a way of caring and considers healing a sacred art. It uses a collection of noninvasive, energy-based treatment modalities with the purpose of restoring wholeness through harmony and balance. The healing is done through the centered heart, thus establishing a spiritual process.[101] Specific uses of healing touch are

- acceleration of wound healing
- relief of pain and increased relaxation
- reduction of anxiety and stress
- energizing of the field
- prevention of illness
- enhancement of spiritual development
- aid in prevention for and follow up of complications after medical treatments and procedures
- support for the dying process[102]

Acupressure and Shiatzu (Basic to Advanced)

A broad range and depth of techniques are used in acupressure and Shiatzu. Most practitioners receive continuing education in this area; some spend years perfecting these techniques.

Reflexology (Basic to Advanced)

The primary purpose of reflexology is to evoke bodymind relaxation. Some practitioners believe that the areas shown in Figure 24–2 represent the nerve or meridian endings for the specific vital body parts. When a therapist works on these specific areas, a corresponding energy release or relaxation occurs in the internal body system.

Nurses who have not studied reflexology can still use general massage on the client's feet to elicit relaxation. The primary caution in this practice, as well as in other body therapies, is to stop massage in any area that provokes pain. Additional touch therapies not discussed in this chapter are noted in Table 24–1.

Case Studies

Case Study No. 1

Setting:	Oncology unit of a general hospital
Patient:	E.S., a 58-year-old single male
Nursing	1. Anxiety
Diagnoses:	2. Altered comfort
	3. Social isolation
	(All related to terminal cancer)

E.S. knew that he was in the terminal stage of cancer, yet he was ambulatory and in basically good humor. E.S. had grown up in the city in which he now found himself hospitalized. He had never married and had no remaining living family.

A nurse who was knowledgeable about touch therapy and felt comfortable using this modality worked evenings on the unit where E.S. was assigned. After assessing his condition, she felt that E.S. needed

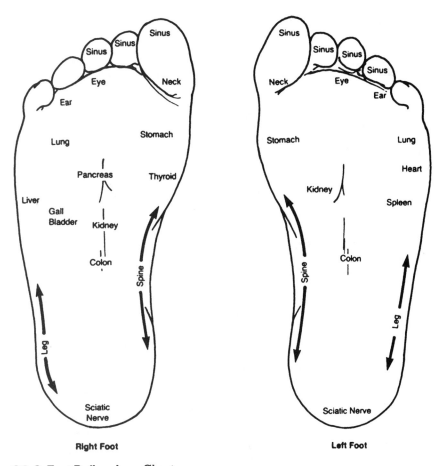

Figure 24–2 Foot Reflexology Chart.

touch to increase comfort and to allay apprehension. Because the unit was continually short-staffed and little time was available for lengthy one-on-one interventions with clients, this intervention had to become a priority in E.S.'s care. Evening back care was entered on his care plan and, despite sometimes hectic assignments, was never omitted when this particular nurse was on duty.

Back care became so important to E.S. that he eagerly greeted the nurse when she came on shift and was ready when she arrived at the appointed time. The touch he received from this nurse was the high point of his hospital stay. During the sessions, he relaxed so deeply that his breathing rate

became slowed; he stated that his perception of pain decreased and that he felt the pleasure of closeness to another caring human being. When the nurse was about to take a few days off after working for 10 consecutive days, E.S. was profoundly saddened that he might have to go without this daily anticipated ritual. The nurse assured him that she had left specific orders for his back care for the oncoming nurse for the next evening. The next evening, however, the regular nurse called in sick, a float nurse was assigned to the unit, and E.S. received no special attention. He died unexpectedly in his sleep during the night.

At this point, we lack the sophisticated tools needed to measure the relationship

Table 24–1 Additional Touch Therapies

Therapy	Originator	Primary Purpose and Function
Applied kinesiology	George Goodheart	Focuses on the relationship of muscle strength and energy flow. The theory is that, if muscles are strong, then circulation and other vital functions are also strong.
Chiropractic	D.D. Palmer	Based on alignment of spinal vertebrae. This therapy involves manipulations to restore natural alignment.
Feldenkrais method	Moshe Feldenkrais	Gives the client gentle manipulations to heighten awareness of the body. As awareness increases, clients can make more informed choices about how to move the body in daily situations.
Jin shin Jyutsu	Master Jiro Murai of Japan in early 1900s	A milder form of acupressure that involves pressure along eight extra energy meridians.
Kofutu touch healing	Frank Homan	Developed in the early 1970s when a series of symbols for use in touch came to the originator during meditation. It is called "Kofutu" for the symbols and "touch" healing because the auras of the healer and recipient must touch. This therapy uses higher consciousness energy symbols to promote self-development and spiritual healing.
Lomi	R.K. Hall, R.K. Heckler	Directs attention to current muscle tension to aid learning of postural alignment to enhance free flow of the body's physical and emotional energies.
Polarity therapy	Randolph Stone	Repatterns energy flow in the individual by rebalancing positive and negative charges. The practitioner places finger or whole hand on parts of the client's body of opposite charge to facilitate energy balancing where it is needed. Through these contacts, with the help of pressure and rocking movements, energy can reorganize and reorder itself.
MariEL	Ethel Lombardi	A 1980s variation of Reiki.
Neuromuscular release		Involves movement of the limbs toward and away from the body by the practitioner to assist the client in learning to let go for the purpose of enhanced circulation and emotional release.
Reiki	2,500-year-old Buddhist practice lost and rediscovered in late 1800s	Term means universal life energy. A touch technique in which the practitioner places hands in one of 12 positions on the recipient's body to direct healing energy to those sites.
Rolfing®	Ida P. Rolf	Helps the client establish deep structural relationships within the body that manifest themselves via a symmetry and balanced function when the body is in an upright position. Technique involves deep muscle manipulation.
Trager work	Milton Trager	Involves rhythmically rocking the limbs and often the whole body to aid relaxation of the muscles and promote optimal flow of blood, lymph, nerve impulses, and energy.

between such deaths and the omission of certain nursing interventions. Consequently, we cannot make any direct correlations. We can only begin to ask research questions and gather anecdotal data about whether the omission of a nursing intervention such as back care can so grieve a client that the resulting physiologic changes can lead to death.

Case Study No. 2

Setting:	Wellness center
Client:	J.S., a 36-year-old married woman
Nursing Diagnoses:	1. Anxiety related to personal and family stress
	2. Altered self-image related to obesity

A psychologist referred J.S. to a nurse in a wellness center for weight management. In addition to enrolling in the weekly counseling program, this client elected to follow each counseling session with a therapeutic massage. She also continued to work with the psychologist for resolution of personality disorder problems. Both the psychologist and the nurse saw J.S. regularly for more than a year until her move away from the area terminated the relationship.

The counseling sessions with the nurse focused on J.S.'s eating disorders, nutritional education, and ways to institute lifestyle changes that would alter the pattern of overweight. These sessions were sometimes emotional but for the most part were straightforward and did not evoke emotional, spiritual, or attitudinal change. In contrast, the elective therapeutic massage elicited a response that allowed J.S. to make connections with a deeper level of herself and finally understand the true nature of her physical problems. While using touch, the nurse also played relaxation music and/or guided J.S. in imagery. In addition, the nurse performed foot reflexology and concluded the sessions with therapeutic touch.

When work with J.S. first began, the client complained of a feeling of a knot in her stomach that had not abated for 15 years. The only time her stomach felt better was after eating. After a few sessions of therapeutic massage, J.S. stated that this stomach pain was relieved during the time that she received the touch therapies.

As J.S. became more trusting of the nurse, she gradually began divulging more of her feelings while in the deeply relaxed state that she experienced during the session. She revealed that she was physically distant from her husband and her 14-year-old daughter. After receiving the massage for approximately 6 weeks, she learned to relax immediately upon reclining on the table—which dissolved her stomach knot. After 8 weeks of massage, the pain stayed away for 2 to 3 days after a session, and weight loss became possible. By the fourth month, she began to hug and touch her daughter at home to dissolve the discomfort she had with their relationship.

The power of touch became so important to her that, by the eighth month, she brought her daughter to the nurse so that her daughter could experience massage firsthand. The daughter, of course, did not have the emotional response or release felt by the mother, for she had not experienced the years of holding tension and withdrawal. The daughter was happy to see how massage was done, however, as she and her mother planned to exchange massage sessions at home between visits to the nurse. Touch had initiated a healing bond between mother and daughter.

Evaluation

With the client, the nurse determines whether the client outcomes for touch therapies (see Exhibit 24–1) were successfully achieved. To evaluate the session further, the nurse may again explore the subjective effects of the experience with the client using the evaluation questions in Exhibit 24–2.

Exhibit 24–2 Evaluation of the Client's Subjective Experience of Touch Therapies

1. Was this a new kind of experience for you? Can you describe it?
2. Did this feel like a comforting, stimulating, or both tactile sensation?
3. Was it pleasurable on all planes—physical, mental, emotional, and spiritual—or more focused in one area than another?
4. Were you aware of your surroundings during the experience, or did you sink into a sense of timelessness?
5. Did emotions surface during the experience? If so, what were they? Can you focus on them now?
6. Did you experience any imagery during the touch session?
7. Did you feel comfortable with the therapist? Is there anything that you want to do to increase your comfort level with the touch therapist?
8. Did you feel relaxed and refreshed after the experience?
9. Would you like to try this again?
10. What would be helpful to make this a better experience for you?
11. Can you develop a plan or strategy to integrate more of the touch therapies into your life on a regular basis?

DIRECTIONS FOR FUTURE RESEARCH

1. Investigate the effects of therapeutic massage on relaxation, pain relief, sleep induction, stress management, relief of sensory deprivation and apprehension, and other parameters.
2. Examine the effects of reflexology on pain relief, relaxation, and/or specific physiologic parameters.
3. Develop valid and reliable tools to measure the effects of touch.
4. Formulate studies to examine the relationship among guided imagery, music, smell, color, taste, and touch.
5. Determine if clients can be taught relaxation techniques by using images of the sensations and emotions evoked during the touch therapy session.
6. Conduct qualitative studies that investigate the meanings of nonprocedural touch throughout the life cycle.
7. Investigate whether periodic touch therapy sessions can increase work performance or productivity.
8. Examine the relationship between the touch therapies and healing.
9. Ask how the results of therapeutic touch on a child at rest compare to the results of therapeutic touch on a child under stress.
10. Examine how the age of the child influences the outcome of therapeutic touch.
11. Investigate how touch can be taught effectively in nursing schools and what methods are best suited to accomplish this.
12. Ask how the nurse's cultural learning, acquired prior to entering nursing school, affects subsequent learning in school.

NURSE HEALER REFLECTIONS

After reading this chapter, the nurse healer will be able to answer or begin the process of answering the following questions:

- How do I feel about using touch as an intervention?
- What do I experience with touch therapy when I touch a client from a place of centeredness?
- When I touch with intention, what is my inner experience?
- When I use touch, what happens to my sense of time?
- How does my touch as a nurse affect the recipient?
- Whom do I know who can be my mentor to help me increase skills with touch?
- What other modalities can be used concurrently to heighten the effectiveness of touch?

NOTES

1. D. Krieger, *The Therapeutic Touch* (Englewood Cliffs, NJ: Prentice-Hall, 1979), 36.

2. Quest for Healing: Massage, Manipulation, Movement, televised program on the Discovery Channel, May 14, 1987.

3. R. Jahnke, The Body Therapies, *Journal of Holistic Nursing* (1985): 7–14.

4. L. Baldwin, The Therapeutic Use of Touch with the Elderly, *Physical and Occupational Therapy in Geriatrics* 4 (Summer 1986): 45–50.

5. C. Guzzetta and B. Dossey, *Cardiovascular Nursing: Holistic Practice* (St. Louis, MO: Mosby–Year Book, 1992), 586–587.

6. R. Jahnke, Body Therapies, *Venture Inward* (March/April 1986): 41–45.

7. S. Burnham, Healing Hands, *New Woman* (March 1986): 72–77.

8. H. Harlow, Love in Infant Monkeys, *Scientific American* 200 (1958): 68–74.

9. R. Spitz, *The First Year of Life* (New York: International Universities Press, 1965).

10. L.L. Roth and J.S. Rosenblatt, Mammary Glands of Pregnant Rats: Development Stimulated by Tickling, *Science* 151 (1965): 1403–1404.

11. B. Grad, Some Biological Effects of the Laying on of Hands: A Review of Experiments with Animals and Plants, *Journal of the American Society for Psychical Research* 59 (1965): 95–127.

12. M.J. Smith, Enzymes Are Activated by the Laying on of Hands, *Human Dimensions* (February 1973): 46–48.

13. J. Khable, Handholding: One Means of Transcending Barriers of Communication, *Heart and Lung* 10 (1981): 1106.

14. C. Schmahl, Ritualism in Nursing Practice, *Nursing Forum* 11 (1964): 74.

15. L. Fisher and D. Hunt Joseph, A Scale To Measure Attitudes about Nonprocedural Touch, *Canadian Journal of Nursing Research* 21, no. 2 (1989): 5–14.

16. J. Bottorff, A Methodological Review and Evaluation of Research on Nurse-Patient Touch, in *Anthology on Caring*, ed. P.L. Chin (NLN Publications, 1991), 303–343. Publication 15-2392.

17. M. Glick, Caring Touch and Anxiety in Myocardial Infarction Patients in the Intermediate Cardiac Care Unit, *Intensive Care Nursing* (February 1986): 61–66.

18. R. McCorkle, Effects of Touch on Seriously Ill Patients, *Nursing Research* (1974): 125–132.

19. D.C. Aguilera, Relationship between Physical Contact and Verbal Interaction between Nurses and Patients, *Journal of Psychiatric Nursing* 5, no. 1 (1967): 5–21.

20. S.J. Weiss, Effects of Differential Touch on Nervous System Arousal of Patients Recovering from Cardiac Disease, *Heart and Lung* 19, no. 5 (1990): 474–480.

21. M. Tovar and V. Cassmeyer, Touch: The Beneficial Effects for the Surgical Patient, *AORN Journal* 49, no. 5 (1989): 1356–1361.

22. S. Schoenhofer, Affectional Touch in Critical Care Nursing: A Descriptive Study, *Heart and Lung* 18, no. 2 (1989): 146–154.

23. S. Simon, Please Touch! How To Combat Skin Hunger in Our Schools, *Scholastic Teacher* (October 1974): 22–25.

24. H. Rozema, Touch Needs of the Elderly, *Nursing Homes* (September/October 1986): 42–43.

25. K. Barnett, A Survey of the Current Utilization of Touch by Health Team Personnel with Hospitalized Patients, *International Journal of Nursing Studies* 9 (1972): 195–209.

26. I.M. Burnside, Touching Is Talking, *American Journal of Nursing* (1973): 2060–2066.

27. E. Duffy, An Exploratory Study: The Effects of Touch on the Elderly in a Nursing Home [Master's thesis, Rutgers—The State University, New Brunswick, NJ, 1982].

28. E. Steuding, Selected Psychosocial Effects of Touch on the Elderly in a Nursing Home [Master's thesis, Rutgers—The State University, New Brunswick, NJ, 1984].

29. S.J. Tobiason, Touching Is for Everyone, *American Journal of Nursing* 4 (1981): 728–730.

30. A Yurick et al., *The Aged Person and the Nursing Process* (New York: Appleton-Century-Crofts, 1980), 298.

31. S. Oliver and S.J. Redrern, Interpersonal Communication between Nurses and Elderly Patients: Refinement of an Observational Schedule, *Journal of Advanced Nursing* 16, no. 1 (1991): 30–38.

32. M. Marx and P. Werner, Agitation and Touch in the Nursing Home, *Psychological Reports* 64 (1989): 1019–1026.

33. M. DeWever, Nursing Home Patients' Perceptions of Nurses' Affective Touching, *Journal of Psychology* 96 (1977): 163–171.

34. N. Kramer, Comparison of Therapeutic Touch and Casual Touch in Stress Reduction of Hos-

pitalized Children, *Pediatric Nursing* 16, no. 5 (1990): 483–485.

35. E. Birch, The Experience of Touch Received during Labor: Postpartum Perceptions of Therapeutic Value, *Journal of Nurse-Midwifery* 31, no. 6 (1986): 270–276.

36. C.A. Estabrooks and J.M. Morse, Toward a Theory of Touch: The Touching Process and Acquiring a Touching Style, *Journal of Advanced Nursing* 17 (1992): 448–456.

37. P. Heidt, Effect of Therapeutic Touch on Anxiety Levels of Hospitalized Patients, *Nursing Research* 30 (1981): 32.

38. E. Keller and V. Bzdek, Effects of Therapeutic Touch on Tension Headache Pain, *Nursing Research* 35 (1986): 101–106.

39. Krieger, *The Therapeutic Touch*, 36.

40. J. Quinn, One Nurse's Evolution as Healer, *American Journal of Nursing* 79 (1979): 662.

41. A. Montagu and F. Matson, *The Human Connection* (New York: McGraw-Hill Book Co., 1979), 89.

42. Montagu and Matson, *The Human Connection*, 90.

43. S. Smoyak, High Tech, High Touch, *Nursing Success Today* 3, no. 11 (1986): 88.

44. S. Hartman, Hug a Patient, P.R.N., *Nursing 86* 16, no. 8 (1986): 88.

45. M. Bogusalawski, The Use of Therapeutic Touch in Nursing, *Journal of Continuing Education in Nursing* (October 1979): 9–15.

46. D. Krieger, *Foundations for Holistic Health Nursing Practices: The Renaissance Nurse* (Philadelphia: J.B. Lippincott Co., 1981), 46.

47. M. Boreli and P. Heidt, *Therapeutic Touch: A Book of Readings* (New York: Springer Publishing Co.), v.

48. Boreli and Heidt, *Therapeutic Touch*.

49. E. Bishop and K.A. Caudell, Reader Questions Discussion of Therapeutic Touch, *Oncology Forum* 23, no. 8 (1996): 1165.

50. K.A. Caudell, Psychoneuroimmunology and Innovative Behavioral Interventions in Patients with Leukemia, *Oncology Nursing Forum* 23, no. 3 (1996): 493–502.

51. D. Cowens, *A Gift of Healing: How You Can Use Therapeutic Touch* (New York: Crown Publishing Group, 1996).

52. B. Daley, Therapeutic Touch, Nursing Practice and Contemporary Cutaneous Wound Healing Research, *Journal of Advanced Nursing* 25 (1997): 1123–1132.

53. R. DuBrey, Therapeutic Touch: A Healing Intervention, *Health Progress* 77, no. 3 (1996): 46–48.

54. A. Easter, The State of Research on the Effects of Therapeutic Touch, *Journal of Holistic Nursing* 15, no. 2 (1997): 158–175.

55. J. Engebretson, Urban Healers: An Experiential Description of American Healing Touch Groups, *Qualititative Health Research* 6, no. 4 (1996): 526–541.

56. B. Fletcher, Rabbit, *Rogerian Nursing Science News* 8, no. 3 (1996): 16–17.

57. P.B. Fryback and B.R. Reinert, Alternative Therapies and Control for Health in Cancer and AIDS, *Clinical Nurse Specialist* 11, no. 2 (1997): 64–69.

58. C. Gehlhaart, Therapeutic Touch as Adjuvant Therapy for Cancer Pain Management, *Cancer Pain Update* 35 (1995).

59. J. Gillman et al., Pastoral Care in a Critical Care Setting, *Critical Care Nursing Quarterly* 19, no. 1 (1996): 10–20.

60. R. Glickman and J. Burns, Speak Up! If Therapeutic Touch Works, Prove It! *RN* 59, no. 12 (1996): 76.

61. C.A. Green, Case Study: A Reflection of a Therapeutic Touch Experience: Case Study I, *Complementary Therapies in Nursing & Midwifery* 2, no. 5 (1996): 122–125.

62. B. Harrigan, Janet Quinn—Therapeutic Touch and a Healing Way, *Alternative Therapies* 2, no. 4 (1996): 69–75.

63. A. Jackson, NT's Monthly Digest of Complementary Medicine Research, *Nursing Times* 91, no. 17 (April 26–May 2 1995): 47.

64. D. Knauer, Therapeutic Touch on the Hot-Seat, *Canadian Nurse* 92, no. 6 (1996): 8,10.

65. D. Krieger, *Therapeutic Touch*, 3 audiocassettes and booklet (Boulder, CO: Sounds True, 1997). ESBN 156455070.

66. D. Krieger, *Therapeutic Touch Inner Workbook* (Santa Fe, NM: Bear & Co, 1997).

67. F. Mantle, Contact Points . . . Barriers to Communication Can Be Reduced by Use of Complementary Therapies, *Nursing Times* 92, no. 18 (1992): 46–47.

68. B. McKern, The State of the Art: Where Are We Up To? Complementary Therapies in Nursing Practice in Australia, *Australian Journal of Holistic Nursing* 3, no. 2 (1996): 30–34.

69. A. Mills, Nursing. Therapeutic Touch—Case Study: The Application, Documentation and Outcome, *Complementary Therapies in Medicine* 4, no. 2 (1996): 127–132.

70. A. Minor, The Use of Therapeutic Touch To Reduce Mind-Body-Spirit Distress, in *Psychosocial Nursing: Care of Physically Ill Patients*

and *Their Families*, ed. P.D. Barry (Philadelphia: Lippincott-Raven, 1996).

71. S.S. Mulloney and C. Wells-Federman, Therapeutic Touch: A Healing Modality, *Journal of Cardiovascular Nursing* 10, no. 3 (1996): 27–49.

72. F. Neilsen, From Your AAON President . . . Therapeutic Touch, *Office Nurse* 9, no. 1 (1996): 56.

73. *Patterns of Rogerian Knowing* (New York: National League for Nursing Press, 1997).

74. S.D.E. Peck, The Effectiveness of Therapeutic Touch for Decreasing Pain in Elders with Degenerative Arthritis, *Journal of Holistic Nursing* 15, no. 2 (1997): 176–198.

75. C. Pert, *Molecules of Emotion, Why You Feel the Way You Feel* (New York: Charles Scribner's Sons, 1997).

76. D. Peters et al., Clinical Forum: Panic Disorder, *Complementary Therapies in Medicine* 4, no. 4 (1992): 247–253.

77. D. Peters et al., Chemotherapy-Induced Nausea, *Complementary Therapies in Medicine* 2, no. 4 (1994): 193–194.

78. H. Porter, Therapeutic Touch Is Part of Windsor's Cancer Care, *Canadian Oncology Nursing Journal* 6, no. 3 (1996): 157–160.

79. J.L. Quinn, Therapeutic Touch: A Home Study Course for Family Caregivers, 3 videocassettes (New York: National League for Nursing, 1996).

80. J.L. Quinn, Therapeutic Touch: Healing Through Human Energy Fields, 3 videocassettes (New York: National League for Nursing, 1996).

81. J.L. Quinn, Therapeutic Touch/Energy Medicine 101, one audiocassette (Boulder, CO: Sounds True Recordings, 1996).

82. D. Smith, Healing through Nursing: The Lived Experience of Therapeutic Touch: Part 2, *Australian Journal of Holistic Nursing* 3, no. 1 (1996): 18–24.

83. C.M. Steckel and R.P. King, Nursing Grand Rounds: Therapeutic Touch in the Coronary Care Unit, *Journal of Cardiovascular Nursing* 10, no. 3 (1996): 50–54.

84. M. Vaga et al., Reiki: An Ancient Touch Therapy, *RN* 59, no. 7 (1996): 9–10.

85. S. Van Boven, Giving Infants a Helping Hand, *Newsweek* Special Issue, (1997), 45.

86. A. Vickers, Psychosocial Care: Complementary Therapies in Palliative Care, *European Journal of Palliative Care* 3, no. 4 (1996): 150–153.

87. S. Wager, *A Doctor's Guide to Therapeutic Touch* (New York: Berkeley Publishing Group, 1996).

88. C.L. Wells-Federman et al., The Mind-Body Connection: The Psychophysiology of Many Traditional Nursing Interventions, *Clinical Nurse Specialist* 9, no. 1 (1995): 59–66.

89. S.J. Whitcher and J.D. Fisher, Multidimensional Reaction to Therapeutic Touch in a Hospital Setting, *Journal of Personality and Social Psychology* 37, no. 1 (1997): 87–96.

90. W. Hill, The Therapeutic Touch Network, *Canadian Nurse* 92, no. 10 (1996): 6, 8.

91. North American Nursing Diagnosis Association, *Nursing Diagnoses: Definitions and Classification 1995–1996*, Philadelphia, PA.

92. J.C. McCloskey and G.M. Bulechek, *Nursing Interventions Classification* [NIC], 2d ed. (St. Louis, MO: Mosby-Year Book, 1996).

93. Y. Irwin, *Shiatzu* (Philadelphia: J.B. Lippincott Co., 1976), 15–19.

94. Irwin, *Shiatzu*.

95. A. Bergson and V. Tuchak, *Zone Therapy* (New York: Pinnacle Books, 1974), 15.

96. K. Kunz and B. Kunz, *The Complete Guide to Foot Reflexology* (Englewood Cliffs, NJ: Prentice-Hall, 1980), 2–6.

97. Krieger, *Foundations for Holistic Health Nursing Practices*, 158.

98. Kunz and Kunz, *Complete Guide to Foot Reflexology*, 46.

99. D. Hover-Kramer and K.H. Shames, *Energetic Approaches to Emotional Healing* (Albany, NY: Delmar Publishers, 1997).

100. K. Shames, *Creative Imagery in Nursing* (Albany, NY: Delmar Publishers, 1996).

101. J. Mentgen and M.J. Trapp Bulbrook, *Healing Touch: Level 1 Notebook* (Carrboro, NC: North Carolina Center for Healing Touch, 1994), 7.

102. Mentgen and Trapp Bulbrook, *Healing Touch*, 1.

VISION OF HEALING

Accepting Ourselves and Others

Wholeness and healing can exist only when we have meaningful relationships. The extent to which we are willing to accept ourselves determines the quality of our relationships, however. If we are unable to accept ourselves, then we are unable to accept others. Without self-acceptance, relationships with an intimate other, family, or community may be confined to the fulfillment of social role obligations and expectations. When we remember that each moment with another is an opportunity to heal and be healed and to share love and forgiveness, we may learn to heal and be healed in a relationship.[1]

Habits, beliefs, assumptions, expectations, judgments, and misconceptions can be major obstacles in relationships. They create conflicts and barriers that block effective communication and sharing of perceptions. The following ten reflective questions are suggested to increase an awareness of patterns in relationships so that the process of healing can occur[2]:

1. Do the important relationships in your life satisfy you? Are your needs met? What do you bring to your relationships? What are the predominant qualities that you experience in your relationships? Do you feel competitive, manipulative, victimized, or rejected? Do you experience joy, vitality, synergy, love, and shared purpose?

2. What are the patterns of your relationships? Do you consistently feel misunderstood or mistreated? Do you think you give more than you receive? Do you experience the universal Self as the source and context of relationships?

3. What beliefs and assumptions do you hold about relationships? After taking an inventory of beliefs, do you recognize any restricted patterns? Did you become aware of any areas that you are unwilling to address?

4. What do you identify with as your true self? Is it your physical, mental, emotional, or spiritual potential, or are all of these areas combined? Are you authentic in your relationships? Do you find that when you are honest with yourself, your relationships are more satisfying?

5. What is the purpose of your important relationships?

6. What relationships in your life have had the most meaning?

7. If you were about to die, would you have any regrets concerning the qualities of relationships in your life? Is there anything that you would have changed?

8. If you could change your relationships unilaterally, what qualities would you want to cultivate in your relationships?

9. Which of your relationships are in need of healing right now? What are you willing to do to bring about that healing?

10. Are you willing to forgive? What part of yourself do you have trouble forgiving?

Relationships help us understand at a profound level our interconnectedness with people, nature, and the universe. When we are in healthy relationships, we exhibit mutual love, sharing, and the ability to forgive ourselves and others. All our lives we search for answers to questions about living and dying. Our relationships can provide us with many aspects of these answers, for they help us recognize blind spots within ourselves. A relationship is healing if it nurtures expression of feeling, needs, and desires and if it helps remove barriers to love.

NOTES

1. J. Achterberg et al., *Rituals of Healing* (New York: Bantam Books, 1994).

2. F. Vaughan, *The Inward Arc* (Boston: Shambhala Publications, 1986).

Chapter 25

Relationships

Dorothea Hover-Kramer

Self-responsibility leads the nurse to greater awareness of the interconnectedness of all individuals and their relationships to the human and global community, and permits nurses to use this awareness to facilitate healing.

American Holistic Nurses' Association[1]

NURSE HEALER OBJECTIVES

Theoretical

- Define three different domains in which nurses are required to develop effective relationships.
- List eight characteristics of effective communication patterns that build and strengthen relationships.
- Identify ways that the humanistic psychologies of Jung and Maslow expand holistic thinking.
- Describe transactional psychology's concept of the three major ego states, distinguishing complementary and uncomplementary transactional patterns.
- Identify four archetypes of human relationships that address physical, emotional, mental, and spiritual domains.

Clinical

- Identify core elements that lead to establishing and maintaining effective relationships.
- Describe and use effective relationship styles that incorporate the four archetypes in a holistic model.
- Analyze human transactions to bring about effective nursing interventions and assist in conflict resolution.
- Implement and evaluate effective negotiating styles that address issues while maintaining a sense of relatedness.

Personal

- Increase your personal use of the eight effective personal relationship characteristics.
- Establish personal time to reflect on relationships in the three different external domains of your practice.
- Develop strategies to incorporate effective assertiveness styles for negotiation and conflict resolution.
- Strengthen intentionality and inner resolve to deal with complex relationship issues through inner focusing and mindfulness practices.

DEFINITIONS

Archetype: Jung's name for specific patterns of human collective awareness that symbolically represent human potentials, such as the Healer, the Warrior, the Mother, or the Wise Person.[2]

Complementary Transaction: an interaction in which the ego states match (e.g., adult-to-adult communication). Complementary transactions support and strengthen relationships.

Defense Patterns: protective mechanisms that justify individual action while detracting from relationship building.

Ego State: an identifiable, understandable part of ourselves that is in conscious awareness. Berne identified at least five ego states that can be brought into awareness for personal change or conflict resolution.[3]

Emotional Intelligence: an awareness and attention to personal emotional needs that allows one to be in a position of equality with others, rather than seeking power and control or becoming overly passive.

Forgiveness: a willingness to acknowledge one's own mistakes and shortcomings and to allow others room to acknowledge their shortcomings as well.

Game: in psychologic terms, a dysfunctional pattern of relationship interaction that is recurring and ends in an emotional payoff or sense of entrapment.

Intimacy: a relationship of deep trust and ability to share oneself fully. Such a relationship may be inappropriate in co-worker and policy-setting environments.

Relationship: a healthy sense of connection in which two or more persons agree to share hurts, failures, learning, successes in a nonjudgmental fashion to enhance each other's life potentials. In the context of professional settings, healthy relatedness encompasses advocacy, influence, and effective assertiveness.

Uncomplementary Transaction: an interaction in which ego states do not match (e.g., critical parent–to–adaptive child communication) that may lead to the formation of a psychologic game; an interaction that reduces relationship formation.

THEORY AND RESEARCH

In recognizing the interconnectedness of individuals in relation to the human and global community, holistic nurses look with care at all aspects of their external, outgoing relationships. Effective awareness requires nurses to look at their daily interactions within three different aspects of professional nursing practice:

1. interactions with their clients, those *for* whom they accept responsibility
2. interactions with their co-workers, those *with* whom they work
3. interactions with persons in authority or leadership, those *to* whom they are accountable. Attention to this aspect may involve interactions with supervisors, administrators, health care policy makers, physicians, the public in general, media, and political figures.

First and foremost, nurses accept responsibility for bringing caring and sensitivity into their relationships with their patients or clients. Because of diminished self-care capacity in physical or emotional domains, clients seek the support, advocacy, and useful interventions that nursing has to offer. In increasingly dehumanized clinical settings, nurses can demonstrate human caring via their creative and insightful relationships. Their active patient advocacy and health education help to build healing environments on a day-to-day basis.

If effective relating to clients were enough, nursing professionals would have an easy task. It is also necessary, however, to address intricate interactions with co-workers who possess a wide variety of backgrounds, skills, and education. Thus, nurses may have ongoing transactions with colleagues ranging from a sophisticated medical specialist, who focuses solely on a single domain, to a nursing aide, who may have little training in interpersonal skills or orientation to human caring. Bringing these various interactions into harmony with holistic ethics, theory, and philosophy is a challenging task. It also offers a grand opportunity for building teamwork through effective relationships.

Finally, and perhaps most demanding, are the issues of accountability in relation to various public sectors. These encompass not only the needs of the clients' families and community of friends, but also the very real requirements and pressures of insurance and/or managed care regulators, public policy setters, and facility administrators. Since many of these individuals constitute an anonymous "they" who may influence a nurse's basic feelings and behavior, it is essential to identify and to deal as directly as possible with these issues. The holistic nursing perspective requires nurses to review their relationship to the entire human community, with all its strengths and pitfalls, to create true healing environments.

The qualities of their relationships essentially determine the experience of nurses' professional lives. Effective relationship skills extend beyond the personal area of listening and counseling to include a practical, psychologically sound, theoretical basis for managing strife, making and keeping agreements, maintaining integrity in confrontations, and holding fast to the essence of holistic nursing philosophy.

With positive and supportive relationships, even the most difficult work situation can become a source of learning and opportunity. If relationships are conflicted or undermining, even a relatively easy work task becomes arduous, a peril to one's self-esteem and self-efficacy.

Relationships may also be viewed as interactive human energy fields. The interaction of two or more human energy fields is always enhanced when at least one person is centered and focused. It is as if the interaction moves to the vibrational frequency of the more mature person. If both persons are in a deficit, energetically speaking, outcomes of an interaction may be quite unsatisfactory and even damaging to the relationship. In psychotherapeutic language, effective relatedness is built on the experience of rapport, the bonding and trust that is required to reach to deeper than social levels of sharing.[4]

Personal Characteristics That Build, Maintain, and Enhance Relationships

Relationship implies connection. We are all interconnected in complex ways—from the subtle interaction of subatomic particles with each other, to the huge impact of political powers that rule and determine the lives of millions of people. Certain defense patterns may undermine or detract from building a sense of connection with others.[5] One of the major personal defense mechanisms that everyone knows and has used is denial, simply refusing to acknowledge what one does not wish to see. Displacement is the mechanism used to shift blame onto another person or situation, rather than taking personal responsibility. Its cousin is projection, the process of ascribing internal conflicts to another person in an effort to diminish personal anxiety or responsibility. Rationalization is the mental justification of feelings and thoughts that are inappropriate to a situation. Individuals may also repress an uncomfortable experience, selectively forgetting unpleasant memories or tasks. They may even regress, reverting to a more primitive style of behavior, such as cursing, yelling, slamming things, or even hitting. Clearly, none of these mechanisms allow for connection with others, nor do they create an environment that would lead to genuine problem solving. Envisioning and developing effective outcomes requires a firm and constant relationship base.

Eight major personal characteristics can be helpful in moving toward effective relationship styles:

1. Willingness to look at personal defenses and "blind spots;" identifying and letting go of defense patterns
2. Correct sense of self-worth, confidence, and self-esteem; having no grandiosity, but not putting oneself down
3. Flexibility; looking at things from different perspectives, "walking in another's shoes"
4. Willingness to take personal responsibility for feelings or actions, emotional intelligence; using "I" statements rather than blaming or using indirect "you" language
5. Intentionality and boundary setting that allow a clear sense of purpose, goal orientation, and direction
6. Motivation to be understood, perserverance to find common ground; seeking and integrating feedback
7. Empathy and mutual respect for others without appeasing, complying, or attempting to be overly pleasing
8. Willingness to re-visit, re-think, re-define previous decisions, accepting the possibility of being wrong and allowing others the space to acknowledge their mistakes as well

These qualities can be seen in skillful negotiators and effective communicators. They bring integrity and balance to the three areas of professional relatedness in nursing.

Well-Known Theorists

Carl Gustav Jung

In the early twentieth century, the great Swiss psychologist Carl Gustav Jung ex-panded the concept of personal consciousness. While Freud's theories focused largely on the nature of the individual, Jung came to believe that vast realms of the personal subconscious mind displayed the pervasive interconnectedness between all human beings.[6] His extensive cross-cultural research showed that humans are aligned with each other through a shared human history and experience, even to the point of having similar dreams and myths despite greatly varying cultural contexts. Long before quantum physics proved the interrelatedness of subatomic particles with each other, Jung posited the idea of a collective unconscious, the intuitive, creative interconnectedness that humans have with each other. This connection through a collective human awareness is the dynamic underpinning of successful, soul-satisfying relationships.

Jung used the term archetypes to describe symbolic representations of human potentials that emerge from the collective consciousness of humanity. Archetypes are broad personality typologies that have been in evidence throughout human history. Among these many patterns are the Healer, the Visionary, the Teacher, the Warrior, the Mother, and the Wise Person.

Abraham Maslow

In the middle of the twentieth century, American psychologist Abraham Maslow moved the study of psychology from its predominant focus on pathology to an increased understanding of healthy human functioning and relationships. This shift opened the way, in the latter part of the twentieth century, for medical practice to become more oriented to the study of human wellness and health maintenance practices. Thus, Maslow prepared the path for the modern holistic emphasis with its blossoming of consumer health awareness and interest in healing partnerships.

Maslow became the founding influence behind modern educational and industrial psychologies by exploring the realm of interpersonal relationships. He identified every individual's hierarchy of needs as:

- safety and security
- sense of belonging
- status
- meaning and significance
- self-actualization
- emergence of transpersonal spirituality[7]

Each level of need builds on the previous one and supports the next. As a more basic need is met, the individual can seek out the next level of understanding. For example, it would be inappropriate (and very frustrating) to discuss creative ideas for patient care in an organization that does not meet safety and security needs, as evidenced by tentative job assignments or irregular pay periods. Under such conditions, confusion and ill will that are destructive to individuals' well-being and their relationships will result. Successful negotiation requires addressing the needs of the lower level of the hierarchy before considering upper level goals.

From his psychologic perspective, Maslow identified health as an ever-expanding human potential for self-actualization. His ideas brought about the birth of the "human potential movement" with the founding of the Association of Humanistic Psychology and the Association of Transpersonal Psychology in the 1970s. His work is evidenced in the modern emphasis on the importance of all human relationships, the need for adequate self-care, and the importance of personal responsibility to bring about global change and healing.

Eric Berne

A psychiatrist, Eric Berne began in the early 1970s to popularize his brainchild, transactional analysis, a practical approach to understanding human interactions. He viewed human relationships as based on a series of understandable transactions between two or more persons, who

each have five powerful ego states.[8] So appealing were his ideas that much of Berne's language has passed into everyday vernacular.

To summarize briefly, the consciously held and acknowledged ego states are the *Parent*, *Adult*, and *Child* with additional aspects in the Parent and Child, giving a total of five different areas of personal awareness:

1. The nurturing parent is the accepting, caring, and supportive aspect of this dimension.
2. The critical parent encompasses the judging, discriminating, or discounting aspects of parental awareness.
3. The adult ego state characterizes the thinking, decision-making capacity of the person. Nursing process ideally comes from the adult, who simultaneously receives input from the other states of awareness.
4. The free child is the lively, creative, and playful part of the personality.
5. The adaptive child is the feeling component of the personality that is less functional, with such emotions as compliance, shame, withdrawal, frustration, or fear.

According to Berne, human relatedness is based on transactions between two or more persons who each can use these five states.

Basically, there are two types of transactions: complementary and uncomplementary. Complementary transactions are those in which the ego states match each other (Figure 25–1). Parent-to-parent communication includes sharing of values or opinions, as demonstrated in a mutual discussion of "how things ought to be." Adult-to-adult complementary transactions are based on mutual exploration of ways of getting things done, decision making, and resultant agreements. Child-to-child communication is about feelings, either playfulness and joking, or the sharing of more adaptive emotions regarding a situation,

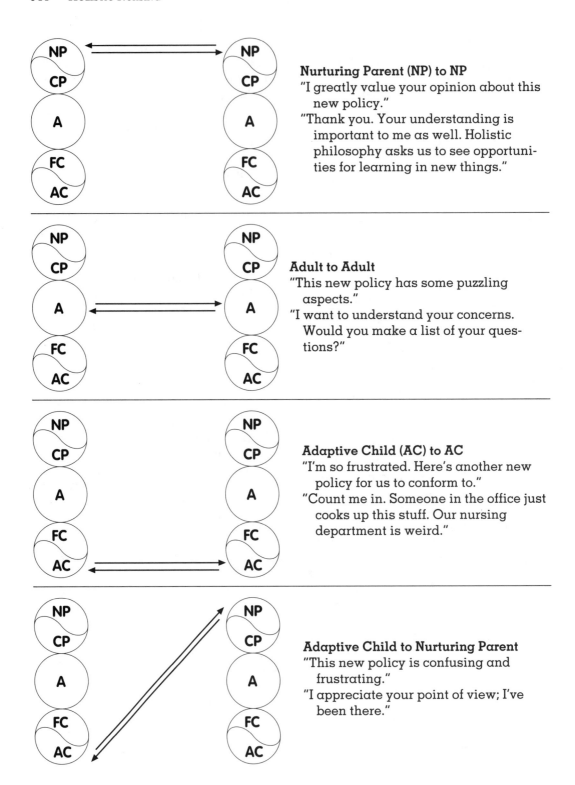

Nurturing Parent (NP) to NP
"I greatly value your opinion about this new policy."
"Thank you. Your understanding is important to me as well. Holistic philosophy asks us to see opportunities for learning in new things."

Adult to Adult
"This new policy has some puzzling aspects."
"I want to understand your concerns. Would you make a list of your questions?"

Adaptive Child (AC) to AC
"I'm so frustrated. Here's another new policy for us to conform to."
"Count me in. Someone in the office just cooks up this stuff. Our nursing department is weird."

Adaptive Child to Nurturing Parent
"This new policy is confusing and frustrating."
"I appreciate your point of view; I've been there."

Figure 25-1 Complementary Transactions That Support Relationship Building

such as frustration or helplessness. Complementary interactions build positive empathy in relationships.

Uncomplementary transactions are those in which the ego states cross in some way (Figure 25–2). In such interactions, agreement is lacking, the outcome is unexpected, or a less than desirable pattern emerges. Berne called dysfunctional patterns, which occur frequently and end with an emotional payoff or a sense of being "had," psychologic games.[9] Uncomplementary interactions and psychologic games detract from a sense of relatedness, bringing in a range of reactions from mild discomfort to overt hostility.

A common psychologic game in nursing practice runs somewhat akin to the following scenario. An insurance regulator (parent) tells home health care nurses via the supervisor (another parent) that they must limit patient visits to 15 minutes and chart on their own time. The nurses comply quietly because they fear the disapproval of the supervisor or the loss of employment (child). Later, there is grumbling and stress among the workers (more child). Someone dares to question the whole process (adult) by which this decision was made and is roundly chastised for questioning authority (critical parent). The nurses become frustrated, experience "burnout," and start to consider other careers (child behaviors) rather than renegotiating with other options (adult capacities).

Another precept from Berne, so simple and profound it is assumed in most interactions, is the idea of mutual respect, captured in the epithet "I'm OK; you're OK." In essence, healthy self-esteem and a sense

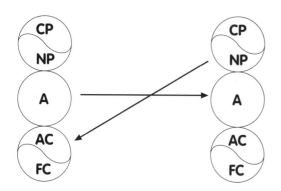

Example 1: Adult Communication with Critical Parent (CP) Response
(A) "Where are the keys to the filing cabinet?"
(CP) "You're so disorganized! Did you ever wonder why your memory is so poor?"
(Communicator's AC is hurt or irritated)

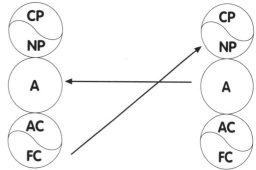

Example 2: Free Child (FC) Communication with Adult Response
(FC) "This new job is fascinating; let me tell you about my visit with the D. family."
(A) "I just don't have time right now for this."
(Communicator may accept response from A or feel offended in the AC)

Figure 25–2 Uncomplementary or Crossed Transactions That Detract from Relationships

of caring toward another is the only relationship style that can succeed. The belief that "I'm not OK; you're OK" results in many of the self-effacing, co-dependent patterns seen in nurses.[10] This belief may be used to justify passivity or a sense of innate helplessness. The opposite, also faulty relationship pattern, is "I'm OK; you're not OK." This belief results in an individual's devaluing others, being aggressive, and subtly or overtly communicating a sense of superiority. The most destructive pattern in this paradigm is the belief that "I'm not OK; neither are you." The essential hopelessness of this position fosters the irrational and unpredictable behaviors seen in passive–aggressive individuals. Caregivers who are passive–aggressive may not express themselves, even when seriously asked to do so, but may later criticize everyone and everything; no sense of collaboration or hopefulness can grow in relationships with these individuals. Steady assertiveness coming from a sense of mutuality and agreement on goals fosters the trust and bonding needed for creativity.

Transactional analysis has been used in hospital and other clinical settings to enhance staff functioning.[11,12] As students of the process learn the tools of accessing different ego states and identifying the nature of transactions, a sense of personal empowerment and self-confidence unfolds. Furthermore, transactions become more positive, supporting stronger relationship bonds for dynamic resolution of problems.

Angeles Arrien

Currently active anthropologist and transpersonal psychologist Angeles Arrien has advanced the concept of four guiding principles, or Jungian archetypes, that manifest in all cultures.[13] These archetypes provide a helpful framework for viewing the physical, emotional, mental, and spiritual dimensions of interactive relationships. The four archetypes can also be effectively used by nurses in giving a holistic perspective to interrelationships.

The Warrior archetype corresponds to the physical aspect of relationship building. Characteristic of the Warrior is the ability to stand firm and be well grounded. The Warrior uses resources effectively; reminiscent of swordsmanship in the past may be the Warrior's ability to use the sharp tools of knowledge, citing facts and statistics, having information, and using it effectively. The Warrior also works with courage to modify behavior in self and others, and translates ideas into action with vitality.

The Healer archetype is more familiar to the nursing profession, as it honors the feeling dimension of relatedness. As a guiding principle, the Healer addresses others with love and compassion. The Healer is highly motivated to bring about emotional easement for others to become whole. In addition, the Healer brings a caring quality to all interactions, valuing self and other with unconditional positive regard.

The Teacher is the metaphorical representation of the mental aspect of relationships. This pattern brings wisdom and knowledge to others and assists learners in developing insight and new perception. The Teacher delights in sharing wisdom and is always willing to learn. Many holistic nurses are presently manifesting the Teacher in their practices and communities.

The Visionary is the archetype that demonstrates the spiritual component of relatedness. A fair and nonjudgmental witness, the Visionary holds the image of greater truth as best as it can be understood. The Visionary uses qualities of clarity and perception to discern conflicts and assist in resolution. Furthermore, the holder of this ideal is intentional and focused. The Visionary acknowledges intuitive knowing, bringing others to the goal of achieving the highest good possible.

Nurses in general have effective interpersonal skills with clients, although relationships with persons in power and leadership may be more confounded. Establishing and maintaining effective relationships with administrative personnel, third-party payers, medical organizations, and communities require conscious skill development. Since every interaction either builds or detracts from a relationship, nurses must enhance their interactive potentials to communicate effectively with these groups, and they must be willing to counter detractors with assertiveness. The language of negotiation and conflict management must become an integral part of nurses' relationship style, along with their well-recognized capacity for caring and compassion.[14,15]

HOLISTIC CARING PROCESS

Assessment

In preparing to use relationship interventions, the nurse assesses the following parameters:

- the ego state most in evidence in the other person's transactions
- the ego state that the nurse is using
- the events that happen repeatedly
- the nurse's feelings (e.g., What is the child part saying?)
- the nurse's values (e.g., What is the parent input?)
- the nurse's options
- respect for self and the other person
- use of power or control
- opportunities for mutuality in this exchange

The inherent qualities of Arrien's four archetypes lead to a more comprehensive, holistic assessment of relationships. The Warrior archetype addresses the physical dimension of relatedness in practical terms to determine the appropriate goal and to define the common ground for interaction. Awareness of the Healer archetype supports the emotional dimension; the caregiver may examine the overall feeling and tone of the interaction in order to bring qualities such as nondefensiveness and positive regard into it. The Teacher archetype allows the nurse to assess specific learning needs of a given situation. The spiritual aspect of relatedness is addressed through the Visionary, who holds a sense of fairness and trust in outcomes for the highest good. In assessment, this archetype is manifest in determining the positive intent of each person and establishing the dimensions of human interconnectedness.

Patterns/Problems/Needs

The following patterns/problems/needs compatible with the interventions for relationships are associated with the nine human response patterns of the unitary person (see Chapter 14):

- *Communicating:* Withdrawal
  Denial
  Repression
  Rationalization
  Regression
- *Relating:* Changes in parenting and family structure
  Human sexual dysfunction
  Lack of social coherence
- *Valuing:* Spiritual disconnectedness and distress
- *Choosing:* Altered family process
  Ineffective coping
- *Moving:* Self-care deficits
  Self-care dysfunction
- *Feeling:* Anxiety
  Grief
  Fear
  Response to trauma

Outcomes

Table 25–1 guides the nurse in client outcomes, nursing prescriptions, and evaluations for effective relationship interventions.

Table 25–1 Nursing Interventions: Relationships

Client Outcomes	Nursing Prescriptions	Evaluation
The client will recognize personal and relationship patterns and how they support or detract from quality of life.	Assist the client in identifying • the importance of relationships • the patterns that increase comfort and effective communication • family relationship patterns and areas that could be improved • sources of emotional stress in his or her relationships • the human needs that are fulfilled by quality relationships • the impact of relationships on health and illness.	The client verbalized the dynamics within the family relationship patterns. The client stated the importance of his or her relationships to quality of life. The client identified areas in which relationships could be improved. The client recognized factors that create stressors in relationships. The client stated understanding of the interconnection between relationships and health or illness.
The client will recognize and identify complementary and uncomplementary transactions in relationships.	Demonstrate examples of complementary and uncomplementary transactions, and help the client to identify such transactions in family and caregiver relationships.	The client identified a complementary transaction and an uncomplementary transaction.
The client will increase awareness of parent, adult, and child ego states.	Demonstrate examples of the differences in the three ego states.	The client identified his or her personal use of parent, adult, and child ego states.
The client will identify personal response patterns to others' ego states.	Assist the client in identifying personal response patterns to others' ego states, and help the client to improve the effective expression of inner feelings. Describe the four archetypes and their applications in communicating physical, emotional, mental, and spiritual perspectives.	The client recognized another person's use of an ego state and his or her personal response.
The client will incorporate new strategies to improve the quality of interpersonal relationships.	Provide the client with techniques to improve relationships, such as making "I" statements ("This is how I feel, . . . My feeling is . . ."), noting ego states in a transaction, and activating the four archetypes.	The client showed interest in the four archetype patterns and willingness to try out new communications from each perspective.
The client will increase awareness of the physical, emotional, mental, and spiritual aspects of relationship interactions.	Teach the client to express awareness of physical needs and take reponsibility for practical aspects of his or her care, such as need for more information and understanding of optimal outcomes.	The client demonstrated the ability to express personal feelings using "I" statements.
The client will recognize opportunities for effective negotiations with willingness to reconsider ineffective aspects.	Assist client to identify arenas where he or she can negotiate, make choices, or reconsider previous decisions; to see the open-ended nature of present relationships, especially with caregivers and family; to view the present disease as an opportunity for learning and change.	The client negotiated effectively after considering options. The client reconsidered relationship interactions that were ineffective. The client expressed interest in the open-ended nature of learning from his or her illness and treatment.

In addition to effective outcomes with clients, it is important to examine possible outcomes in the other areas of nursing interaction. Thus, an expansion of outcomes includes the following:

- The nurse will recognize family and relationship patterns.
- The nurse will use complementary transactions whenever possible and increase awareness of uncomplementary transactions to avoid psychologic games.
- The nurse will demonstrate skill in communicating from the adult ego state whenever possible, with awareness of the personal use of parent and child ego states.
- The nurse will use the child ego state through humor and awareness of feelings when appropriate.
- The nurse will identify healthy boundaries in each interaction, readily confronting any put-downs or defense patterns.
- The nurse will recognize opportunity for effective negotiations and conflict management, using the characteristics of effective communicators.
- The nurse will work from the dimension of mutual respect, valuing both self and others without discounts.
- The nurse will plan for identifiable outcomes in transactions, drawing on the four archetypes as needed, and evaluate outcomes on an ongoing basis.
- The nurse will increase skills in addressing practical, emotional, mental, and spiritual aspects of relationships through the use of the four archetypes.
- The nurse will increasingly see opportunities for new relational patterns in challenging situations.

Therapeutic Care Plan and Implementation

The holistic nurse's careful planning and preparation enhance the effectiveness of relational interactions. The following are guidelines for planning and implementing effective relational patterns.

Before the Session

- Take a moment to set your intent and focus, allowing yourself to breathe fully, to sense your center, and to align with your sense of purpose.
  —Take several deep breaths and relax the body.
  —Rehearse a new pattern in your mind.
  —Imagine the successful outcome.
  —Acknowledge your positive intent.
  —Be willing to learn from each experience.

During the Session

- Notice the ego states that are in evidence, specifically the feelings that are triggered within yourself.
- Be aware of ways that finding common ground enhances rapport.
- Consider options that can achieve the goal of the communication.
- Make "I" statements when speaking about your personal point of view or experience.
- Set limits, such as time frames, topics to be discussed, and the context.
- Be willing to change direction, or reconsider a point, to come to feasible compromises.
- Above all, keep the intent of the communication positive and maintain a relationship of mutual respect, even though specific content areas may be questioned and differing viewpoints are expressed.

At the End of the Session

- Use the client outcomes (see Table 25–1) to assess ways you assisted the client in moving toward goals of understanding relationship patterns.
- Consider alternatives and make concrete plans for future action.

- Evaluate your own relational skills, your use of different ego states, your use of the archetypes.
- Honor your learning process in accepting mistakes or in thinking about what you might have done differently.
- Consider methods to make trying new behaviors safe and enjoyable, such as sharing your process with a friend or mentor.

Specific Interventions

Counseling and Psychotherapy. A client who exhibits normative behavior may seek counseling that focuses on coping behaviors.[16] For example, counseling may involve assistance with smoking cessation or weight reduction. Psychotherapy provides more in-depth interventions, such as working with clients in the struggles and challenges of life roles, individual/family priorities, intimacy, or changing relationship patterns in a marriage. Psychotherapy is definitely indicated when a client exhibits severe personality disorders or pathologic behaviors, although a client need not demonstrate pathologic behavior to begin psychotherapy.

By demonstrating acceptance of the client's intrinsic worth and dignity, the nurse conveys empathy to the client and facilitates the client's disclosure of personal information. Genuineness and congruency convey the nurse's honesty and personal caring to the client.

Counseling techniques can be incorporated into all areas of nursing, although some of the advanced techniques lend themselves better to individual counseling. Even so, the nurse who is aware of the techniques can integrate various levels of the techniques in the acute care setting.

Storytelling. Stories reveal the importance that we assign to our experiences in life and our perceptions of the world.[17] Storytelling technique becomes advanced when parables and metaphors are used.

All stories may be a means of building double descriptions and enabling the perception of higher order patterns.[18] Because we can take our stories from one situation to the next, we establish different contexts and structures for those stories. This creates the potential for opening new dialogue with the self, which can also contain new purpose and meaning. An additional way to enhance storytelling is to incorporate relaxation, imagery, music, life review, and self-reflective interventions.

Nurses are always listening to clients' stories. If they listen with focused attention, they hear stories about stories. These stories are the therapy; they are the basis for the healing event. We should see therapy as conversation, rather than always classifying it in medical terms. The following guidelines enhance the use of stories as therapy.

- Listen for the themes that bridge one story to the next; listen for the threads of information that also weave through one story to the next.
- Train yourself to determine if a client is telling only one side of a story.
- Get the client to talk about what the two sides of any story may be, because clients frequently perceive only one side of a story. Viewing the other side gives new meaning and context, however, and enables one to create double descriptions of stories. For example, it is very easy to identify things and events that are wrong in one's life, but it is more valuable to find the strengths in the current situation and the underlying meaning or message of the present situation.
- Become aware of the importance of the stories that you construct from the client's stories. While listening to a client's stories, the nurse is also constructing a story that guides the therapy. When the nurse tells these stories to the client, the exchange of stories allows the client to see or hear

new patterns and relationships. With this feedback, the client gains new information and can construct a new way of viewing life. All stories are a means of building double descriptions that facilitate change.

Development of Spiritual Understanding. Individuals must recognize that they are the spiritual experts about their lives, that the journey of wholeness and healing requires spiritual understanding, and that this understanding is a developing process.[19,20] Burkhardt and Nagai-Jacobson suggest that, if spirituality is a given and is the essence of one's being, it is useful for individuals to acknowledge their innate qualities.[21] When a person gives these qualities names and tends to them, the qualities are more likely to become healing tools. Ways to increase clients' awareness of opening to their healing potentials include the following:

- connecting: connecting with self, others, higher power, universe; allows individuals to experience being grounded.
- disconnecting: opening to new creative techniques, such as relaxation, imagery, dance, and laughter.
- empowering: challenging one's mind to learn things other than the day-to-day work; exploring personal wisdom; taking a class of a new interest; consulting friends, family, or a therapist when necessary.
- purifying: washing away, not only with water; sitting quietly by a roaring fire or out in nature in the sunshine; "playing in the dirt" without transforming the garden; taking a long bath or shower.
- journeying: traveling in one's imagination; reading a good book; walking or taking a leisurely drive; writing in a journal.
- transforming: using raw materials to restore order and create something

new; painting, weaving, needlepoint, or other craft; gardening or creative cooking; cleaning a closet, drawers, or desk.

Ways To Work through Fear. Individuals often have difficulty making change within the family or in other life situations because of fear. Jeffers suggests that, as individuals learn to identify levels of fear, it becomes much easier to make change and that the best way through the fear is "dare to feel the fear . . . and do it anyway."[22] Fear can be broken down into three levels. Level 1 fears have two subsets—fears of things that happen and fears of things that require action. Things that happen include aging, illness, retirement, being alone, loss of financial security, change, and dying; things that require action include making decisions, changing a career, making or ending friendships, losing weight, going back to school, being interviewed, or giving a speech. Level 1 fears translate into statements such as "I can't handle illness."

In contrast, Level 2 fears are not situation-oriented. These fears involve the ego and have to do with a sense of self and one's ability to handle life's situations. For example, an individual may fear success, failure, rejection, vulnerability, helplessness, loss of image, or disapproval. Level 2 fears translate into such statements as "I can't handle failure."

Level 3 fears keep a person stuck. The biggest fear of all is that the individual will be unable to handle whatever life may bring. Level 3 fears translate into "I can't handle it!" What underlies this level of fear is an individual's idea that, if he or she could handle anything that came his or her way, what would there be to fear? The answer is, Nothing.

In counseling people who are fearful, the strategy is to help them develop more trust in their own ability to handle whatever comes their way. All people feel the different levels of fear many times in life, even when we realize that there is nothing to fear.

Improved Communication. Communication patterns have a direct impact on mind modulation of the autonomic, immune, endocrine, and neuropeptide systems. Because our relationships evoke every conceivable emotion and communication pattern, they have a significant impact on our physiologic state.

Nurses can help clients improve communication patterns by teaching an awareness of the psychophysiologic response that occurs with communication. With an increased awareness of the direct link between body and emotions, the client can learn to recognize and increase healthy dialogue. As a result, there will be more sharing and owning of emotions, and relationships will be healthier.

Communication involves state-dependent learning and the imagery process, so there are an enormous number of variables in communication interventions. Because they facilitate the incorporation of relaxation skills and awareness of bodymind responses with all dialogue, these interventions are helpful for all nurses and clients. Advanced communication interventions incorporate in-depth psychophysiologic therapy and biofeedback training.

Case Studies

Each of the following case studies suggests a variety of situations in which relational options can effect useful outcomes. These case studies demonstrate how evaluation of relationships is an ongoing, moment-by-moment process with long-term results. Review at the end of a working day is also helpful to note which interactions were effective and which ones were not.

Case Study No. 1: Use of Different Archetypes

Setting:	Outpatient cardiac rehabilitation unit
Client:	46-year-old white businessman who is used to having his own way and being in charge

Patterns/ Problems/ Needs:	1. Altered comfort level related to physical distress
	2. Altered relationship patterns caused by loss of usual social status
	3. Ineffective individual coping related to anxiety and stress

Nurse K. was a sweet and gentle person who demonstrated the empathic Healer archetype most frequently. She became tongue-tied and flustered when Mr. B., one of her patients in the cardiac rehabilitation program, suddenly and emphatically refused to comply with his treatment schedule. At first, she attempted to side with his emotional state. She reflected back to him, "You seem upset. Perhaps you could tell me what you are feeling." He retorted, "You have no idea how I feel. I hate this illness and this unit. Don't even try that psychologic stuff on me!" All Nurse K.'s usual interventions caused Mr. B. to become even more defensive.

At first, Nurse K. felt confused and helpless. She centered herself with a few quiet moments away from the treatment area and considered her options. She decided that exploring other archetypes would give her the following alternatives:

1. As a practical Warrior, Nurse K. could bring her knowledge and information into the situation. She could ask with courage and integrity, "What is causing this change? Please tell me what's happening with you. My experience and the statistical research tell me that your medical condition can improve if we implement the cardiac treatment plan developed in this unit on a daily basis."

2. As a manifestation of the Teacher, Nurse K. could educate her client with wisdom to bring more insight. For example, "Our outpatient schedules are designed to accomplish the best results in the shortest amount of time. There are some areas of choice and

some areas that cannot be redesigned. I need to know your goals for being here. The best outcome would be to negotiate a compromise that honors your goals and allows you to learn all you can about your illness."

3. As a Visionary who brings intuition and fair witness to difficult settings, Nurse K. would have the option of allowing time to establish a centered healing presence with Mr. B. She might say, "We seem to be at an impasse here. Let's take a moment to take some deep breaths, going back to the positive intent we both have; yours, to be well; mine, to assist you as best as I can."

Bringing awareness of the archetypes into conflict situations allows the nurse to be more flexible and to consider the relationship from a holistic, integrative perspective. The physical, mental, emotional, and spiritual dimensions of human consciousness enrich interaction and may facilitate problem resolution from the adult ego states. Even if this does not occur, the parties can acknowledge positive intent while they work through differences of opinion.

Thus, Nurse K. re-approached Mr. B. after internally exploring her archetype options and simply asked him, "What can we do today that would honor your desire for healing? We both recognize that it is an ongoing daily commitment, and I'm willing to assist you when you feel ready."

Feeling safe with her nondefensive response, Mr. B. decided to give himself time to "bottom out," to express his feelings about his illness fully. The empathic nurse assisted him by providing him with clay for directly expressing his frustration and with paper for journaling his inner experience. He admitted later, "I was just an awful kid needing to vent and you heard me. Thanks."

He continued the 6-week treatment program and returned to work. He stated to all that would hear that the day of venting was the beginning of a more caring lifestyle

change that would affect his family life, his professional relationships, and his heart.

Case Study No. 2. Use of Different Ego States

Setting:	Medical surgical unit at time of shift change
Clients:	Nurses in relation to each other
Patterns/ Problems/ Needs:	1. Anxiety related to job performance
	2. Ineffective individual coping
	3. Spiritual distress related to professional ideals in conflict with reality situation

The incoming day shift nurse barked at the tired night nurse, "You probably forgot to do X again. It's always the same with you night people" (critical parent). The night nurse bit her tongue, feeling cowed, helpless, and angry (adaptive child).

Alternatives for dealing with such a transaction may be as follows:

1. Activate the adult. The night nurse may respond, "You're right, this is a frequent problem. What could we do about it? Let's sit down and explore options."

2. Admit feelings and acknowledge the child. The night nurse may respond, "I feel bad when you say that. We both have strong feelings here for various reasons" and then (moving to adult) "Let's vent to get feelings out in the open, and invite someone neutral to help us sort this out."

3. Bring in the nurturing parent. The night nurse and day shift nurse may assist each other by affirming their strengths. For example, they may say to each other, "I sense how much you care about your patients. I share with you your concern and support you in finding solutions."

As nurses consider the holistic perspective, they must recognize that their relationships with each other are as vital to professionalism and ethics as their relationship with clients. The quality of interactions in today's hectic clinical settings can help to create a healing environment in which caregivers can grow and thrive, empowering and supporting each other. Without mutual respect and consideration, the work environment can be destructive to the participants as well as to the clients who will surely sense the unresolved tension and pressures.

Case Study No. 3: Negotiation with Co-workers

Setting:	Hospital staff wishing to incorporate holistic ideas
Clients:	Interested co-workers with varying goals
Patterns/ Problems/ Needs:	1. Ineffective individual coping related to job stress and anxiety
	2. Ineffective valuing related to uncharted nature of the discussions and moving into new domains

The nurses in Hospital D. wished to establish an alternative health care clinic. Many of the staff wanted to participate, although only a few could be hired for the project. Those who were truly interested decided to hold a meeting and identify the strengths and resources within the group. Some of those present were interested primarily in their own advancement, while others wanted to collaborate in order to reach the goal of establishing a complementary health care program.

As the group developed over time, those with the knowledge base and practical skills, the empathy toward others, the goals of teaching and learning, and clear intent—in other words, those manifesting the four archetypes—began to be more vocal. Natural leaders emerged from those who could most clearly maintain good relationships while discussing complex issues.

Of course, things did not go smoothly in terms of human relationships. One of the self-oriented people asserted, "I'm not getting what I want." Several of the collaborative-style workers countered with empathy,

facts, and their vision. In essence, they said, "I understand your frustration. We're all in this together, and the nature of negotiation requires each of us to release some of our individual desires so that we can find what is best for most of the group and accomplish our goal. Would you insist on your own way if it were to hurt others or limit our project?" This response allowed for inner reflection on the common goals of the project, which were quite different from the individual's needs for recognition or status. She started learning from the leaders of the group. Later, she decided that she had other goals and would rather open an independent center.

Effective communication requires maintaining mutual respect and recognizing the positive intent behind each person's actions, while addressing very real differences of opinion. A rule of thumb for effective negotiations is to be "hard on the issues and soft on the people" while working to reach an agreement that results in the best outcomes for the most people. This kind of confrontational, yet caring, communication is new to nursing. In truth, there are values higher than individual contentment. Nurses must develop a wide variety of skills to build and maintain relationships in order to bring about the policy changes that will be required in the twenty-first century.

Case Study No. 4: Conflict Management with a Health Maintenance Organization

Setting:	Home health care organization that is part of a health maintenance organization (HMO)
Clients:	Nurses employed by the HMO
Patterns/ Problems Needs:	1. Anxiety related to job insecurity
	2. Ineffective individual coping due to stress and anxiety
	3. Spiritual distress related to professional ideals in conflict with mercenary values of a for-profit corporation

4. Altered comfort related to lack of clarity and lack of enforceable agreements

The management of a large HMO told the staff nurses that costs must be decreased and asked the nurses to choose between reducing the number of staff or accepting lower salaries (i.e., a 10 percent wage cut). The nurses voted for the salary reduction, but 3 months later, half of them were laid off anyway. Feeling abandoned and discounted, they cried, "Foul!"

Unfortunately, such dilemmas are all too common in these days of budget cuts and medical cost overruns. As a professional group, nurses may jump too quickly for short-term advantages (adaptive child) rather than looking at the bigger picture (parent values) and ensuring effective, legally binding negotiations (adult). In this situation, the basic steps of negotiation to define management's relationship with nurses did not take place. If, for example, a tenacious, assertive spokesperson had been able to demonstrate the cost-effectiveness of nurses' services to the organization, agreement about finances might have included a provision for job security for at least 6 months. Then any nurses laid off as quickly as 3 months later would have had legal recourse. Better yet, there should have been a provision for legal monitoring of the pay cut agreement at the outset, bringing in the practical, down-to-earth Warrior archetype.

In another home health care organization, a group of nurses in an almost similar situation worked through their union representative to bring their negotiation points to discussion. At first, management was totally hostile, but because they had signed the union contract, they had to negotiate. After many meetings, which were open to all who could attend, an agreement involving pay cuts was struck for a period of one year. It was not ideal, but at least it gave the nurses the job security that allowed them to move forward and establish good relationships with their clients. As the year progressed, new referrals increased because of the positive nurse–client interactions, and community faith in the agency grew. The next year, management gave pay raises to the nurses and praised the union for their positive participation in the agency's efforts.

Evaluation

With clients or co-workers, the nurse determines whether outcomes for relationship interventions were successfully achieved (see Table 25–1). To evaluate the session or interactions further, the nurse may explore the subjective effects of the experience (Exhibit 25–1). Healthy relationships increase well-being and wholeness. As clients and nurses become more aware of the value of open, effective relationship patterns, they can mutually move in the direction of increased health and healing in the relational context.

It is a truism that "hindsight is always better than foresight." Similarly, it has been said that all good counseling brings today's solutions to yesterday's problems. A belief in these epithets may deter the exploration of new possibilities for healing relationships. It is helpful to recognize that there are no ideal solutions, no perfect relationships. Life, in terms of the important interconnections, is a series of encounters from which individuals gain experience and gradually progress toward more insight. Everyone is in the learning curve for establishing and maintaining relationships. It is wise to remember that hindsight is much, much better than no sight at all. As long as there is willingness to learn, there is hope for relationships, even the most thorny and conflicted.

Human connectedness is an open-ended process of assessing problems, trying out new options, and evaluating outcomes. Martha Rogers, one of nursing's meta-theorists, held that nurses are continually evolving to higher levels of complexity as "our patterns are continually changing, in-

Exhibit 25–1 Evaluating the Nurse's Subjective Experience with Relationship Interventions

1. Can you continue to identify and be aware of the relationship that is troublesome to you?
2. Is it possible for you to be clear about your wants and expectations in this relationship?
3. Have you tried out new patterns, such as making a conscious choice of a different ego state? What was the result?
4. Have you considered the transactions in this relationship to make them more complementary?
5. Is it possible for you to communicate your strengths in this relationship? What are the strengths and intent of the other person that could also be acknowledged?
6. Can you imagine how the Healer in you could approach this relationship? How about the Teacher? The Visionary? The practical, grounded Warrior?
7. What would a healed relationship with this person be? How would you feel?
8. Can you identify the steps you could take to move in this direction?
9. What interventions would be most helpful in moving toward healing this relationship?
10. Do you have any questions about any of the new strategies that you have learned for healing this relationship?
11. What is your next step?

novative and creative."[23] Even in space travel, she asserted, nursing's skills in relationships would be an essential requirement for determining environments in which healing could occur.

CONCLUSION

Inner work with the expressive arts is helpful in understanding personal feelings and clarifying relationship patterns. Ultimately, moving into right relationships with ourselves, each other, and our environment is the healing force for our lives. This poem celebrates the use of the breath to refocus in the day-to-day complexities of nursing practice. It is offered here to be used as a reminder that realigning of thought and action can flow from an integrative, focused intent.

With Every Breath

With every breath
   there's a chance to forget
   to become lost in the brambles
   the entangled pathways of thoughts,
   activities, overdoing,
   losing purpose
      trailing nowhere...
With every breath
   there's a chance to remember
   to bring back the mind
   to its true nature
   simplicity, strength
   loving-kindness
   forgiveness, peace
   to find the direct path
      that leads home.
      —© 1998, Dorothea Hover-Kramer

DIRECTIONS FOR FUTURE RESEARCH

1. Develop valid and reliable tools that help nurses to identify barriers to effective relationships.
2. Evaluate the efficacy of relationships tools, such as Transactional analysis, for analyzing functional and dysfunctional relationship patterns.
3. Develop and evaluate active programs for relationship building in clinical work settings.
4. Demonstrate and evaluate effective relationship interventions through role playing and workshops.
5. Document and evaluate in the nursing literature effective group problem-solving process in dealing with current issues, such as policy changes and complementary modalities.

NURSE HEALER REFLECTIONS

After reading this chapter, the nurse-healer will be able to answer or begin a process of answering the following questions:

- How do I feel at the end of the work-day?
  - Can I acknowledge the child within?
  - What gives me pleasure?
  - What bothers me?
  - Which defenses do I use?
  - What do I wish I had done differently?
- Were there any unpleasant interactions?
  - Who was the critical parent, the adaptive child, the adult?
  - What other options could have been considered?
  - How would I respond to the situation from each of my five ego states?

- Are there repeated patterns in my relationships that indicate "games" or "payoffs"?
  - What belief (such as "I'm not OK, and/or You're not OK") or action on my part maintains this pattern?
  - How could I change the pattern?
- Will I be able to practice new responses with a friend or co-worker?
  - What will I do differently?
  - Will I have support from trusted friends?
  - Will I honor and acknowledge myself as a growing learning being, aligned with inner light and truth?

NOTES

1. American Holistic Nurses' Association, Standards of Holistic Nursing Practice (Flagstaff, AZ: AHNA, 1998), 1.

2. C.G. Jung, *Man and His Symbols* (New York: Doubleday & Co., 1964), 67–69.

3. E. Berne, *Principles of Group Treatment* (New York: Oxford University Press, 1964), 281.

4. D. Hover-Kramer and K. Shames, *Energetic Approaches to Emotional Healing* (Albany, NY: Delmar Publishers, 1997), 25–47.

5. E. Wachtel and P. Wachtel, *Family Dynamics in Individual Psychotherapy: A Guide to Clinical Strategies* (New York: Guilford Press, 1986), 43–64.

6. C.G. Jung, *Man and His Symbols* (London: Aldus Books, 1964).

7. A. Maslow, *The Farther Reaches of Human Nature* (New York: Penguin Books, 1971).

8. E. Berne, *Transactional Analysis in Psychotherapy* (New York: Grove Press, 1961).

9. E. Berne, *Games People Play* (New York: Grove Press, 1964).

10. C. Snow and D. Willard, *I'm Dying To Take Care of You* (Redmond, VA: Professional Counselor Books, 1989).

11. D. Jongeward, *T.A. for Hospitals* (Boston: Addison Wesley, 1976).

12. D. Hover-Kramer, The Evaluation of Learning of a Course in Transactional Analysis for Hospital Personnel (Unpublished doctoral dissertation, Nova University, 1978).

13. A. Arrien, *The Four-Fold Way* (San Francisco: HarperCollins, 1993).

14. R. Fisher and W. Ury, *Getting to Yes* (New York: Penguin Books, 1981).

15. G.I. Nierenberg, *The Art of Negotiating* (New York: Simon & Schuster, 1981).

16. L. Banks, Counseling, in *Nursing Interventions: Essential Nursing Treatments*, 2nd ed., ed. J. Bulechek and J. McCloskey (Philadelphia: W.B. Saunders, 1992), 279–291.

17. M. Sandelowski, We Are the Stories That We Tell, *Journal of Holistic Nursing* 12, no. 1 (1994):23–33.

18. Ibid.

19. M. McKivergin and M.J. Daubenmire, The Healing Process of Presence, *Journal of Holistic Nursing* 12, no. 1 (1994):65–81.

20. M. Burkhardt and M.G. Nagai-Jacobson, Reawakening Spirit in Clinical Practice, *Journal of Holistic Nursing* 12, no. 2 (1994):9–21.

21. M. Burkhardt and M.G. Nagai-Jacobson, Spirituality: The Cornerstone of Holistic Nursing Practice, *Holistic Nursing Practice* 3, no. 3 (1989): 18–26.

22. S. Jeffers, *Feel the Fear and Do It Anyway* (New York: Fawcett Columbine, 1987), 11–18.

23. M. Rogers, *Portraits for Excellence*, video (Oakland, CA: Studio III, Helene Fuld Trust fund, 1987).

SUGGESTED READING

Bass, B.M. From Transactional to Transformational Organizational Dynamics, *Journal of Group Work* 18, Winter 1990: 3.

Benne, K., and Babad, E. *The Social Self* (Beverly Hills, CA: Sage Publishing, 1983).

Corey, G. *Theory and Practice of Counseling and Psychotherapy* (Pacific Grove, CA: Brooks Cole, 1991).

Deluca, P. *The Solo Partner: Repairing Your Relationships on Your Own* (Point Roberts, WA: Hartley & Marks, 1996).

Gottman, J. *Seven Principles for Making Your Marriage Work* (New York: Simon & Schuster, 1999).

Heilveil, I. *When Families Feud: Understanding and Resolving Family Conflicts* (Berkeley, CA: Berkeley Publishing Group, 1998).

Homans, G.C. *The Human Group* (New York: Harcourt, 1982).

Kippner, D.A. Dynamics of Role Satisfaction, *Journal of Group Psychology* 44, Spring 1991: 2.

McCollon, M. The Group Dynamics Instructor as Boundary Manager, *Journal of Management Education* 16, May 1992: 2.

Miller, M.J. Training Issues in Group Work, *Journal for Specialization in Group Work* 18, May 1993:2.

Needleman, J. *A Little Book on Love* (New York: Doubleday, 1996).

Neuman, M.A. *Health As Expanding Consciousness* (New York: National League for Nursing, 1994).

Peplau, H.E. *Interpersonal Relations in Nursing* (New York: Springer, 1988).

Pierrakos, E. *The Pathwork of Self-Transformation* (New York: Bantam Books, 1990).

Roark, A.S., and Sharah, H.S. Factors Related to Group Cohesiveness, *Small Group Behavior* 28, February 1989: 1.

Sheehy, G. *Pathfinders* (New York: William Morrow Co., 1987).

Toffler, A. *The Third Wave* (New York: Bantam Books, 1988).

Weeks, G.R., and Hof, L. (eds.) *The Marital Relationship Therapy Case Book: Theory and Application of the Intersystem Model* (New York: Brunner-Mazel, 1994).

Wheatley, M.J. *A Simpler Way* (New York: Barrett-Koehler Publishing, 1996).

VISION OF HEALING

Releasing Attachment

Nothing prepares us completely for our own death or for the death of a loved one. Although we know that we will die, most people have become so accustomed to their bodies that they fear death or view it as a tragedy. Modern culture emphasizes extending life at all costs, often despite pain and suffering. When we choose to prolong life, however, we may deny death. One's soul may literally die in agony before the physical body dies.

Nouwen tells the story of a trapeze artist who admonished a fan to watch the catcher of the trapeze artist, not the one who jumps from a trapeze to the catcher. "The catcher is the real star. . . . The secret is that the flyer does nothing and the catcher does everything. . . . A flyer must fly, and a catcher must catch, and the flyer must trust, with outstretched arms, that his catcher will be there for him."[1] For Nouwen, the dying person is a flyer who chooses to let go of the bar and trusts that the catcher will pull him safely into the next world. Nouwen suggested that this is what is meant by the words of Luke 23:46, "Father into your hands I commend my Spirit." Dying well, moving to a new existence, requires choice, trust, and the willingness to let go.

Despite the notion that life is a series of episodic events from birth to death, it has been shown that time is very different from the classic Newtonian model that real time flows in a linear sequence and is divisible into past, present, and future (the predominant Western view). We are dependent on an external reality when we think of these events in a linear fashion, but the only way that we can experience birth, health, illness, and death is by our senses, by our own internal experience. Thus, our meaning in life determines our sense of time.[2] Thoughts of death often evoke words such as desperate, panic, final, always, ending, or forever. These words create a constricted sense of time and inflict fear and urgency on our experiences. Because our experience of time is bound to our senses, we can learn to expand time, not constrict it with fear and worries.

We can also gain insight from the Eastern world view, which approaches life and death as complementary dimensions of the same unified experience. To experience one is simultaneously to experience the other. Conscious preparation for the moment of death begins with the little daily deaths that serve to prepare us for the death at the end of our physical lives.[3] These little deaths include changes, losses and disappointments at work or with family and friends, goals not accomplished, or temporary illnesses (e.g., allergies, ulcers, infection). These little deaths can also occur as realizations that we should release old behaviors and relationships that no longer serve us to allow room for new behaviors, relationships, and possibilities.

True healing and dying in peace come from releasing our attachment to the physical body, and to the conflicting emotional and spiritual issues that hold one in bondage to this body and this world.[4] Recognizing our integration in the Divine universe, we must learn to open our body-mind-spirit to healing. The paradox is that, although this healing awareness may seem to be rare, it is a very ordinary and natural event available to each of us at all times. As we practice living in peace, we enter a healing state in which our questions about the complementary nature of living and dying are answered. The insight comes from our own inner wisdom and strength.

Many fears surrounding death have to do with our ego, the separate individual I-ness, our identifying with personal mental images of objects, desires, wants, and needs.[5] The will to live is very strong, and it is hard to give up our individual personalities and bodies. The ego keeps us separate from the grander scheme of totality of beingness, connectedness, and wholeness. We can, however, learn to listen to an inner voice, and experience thoughts, feelings, and images without attachment. Going to the core of our inner wisdom dissolves the ego attachment as we move toward the death moment and know that death is near.

NOTES

1. H. Nouwen, *Our Greatest Gift: A Meditation on Dying and Caring* (San Francisco:Harper, 1995), 67.

2. L. Dossey, *Recovering the Soul* (New York: Bantam Books, 1989).

3. A. Sheikh and K. Sheikh, *Death Imagery* (Milwaukee, WI: American Imagery Institute, 1991).

4. S. Levine, *A Gradual Awakening* (New York: Anchor Press, 1979).

5. K. Wilbur, *Grace and Grit* (Boston: Shambhala Publications, 1991).

Chapter 26

Dying in Peace

Melodie Olson and Barbara Montgomery Dossey

NURSE HEALER OBJECTIVES

Theoretical

- Use theories of grief, self-transcendence, myths, and beliefs to guide the process of helping the dying to experience their deaths peacefully and meaningfully.
- Discuss with colleagues difficult issues surrounding the care of dying people.
- Interview patients who have experienced nearing death awareness.

Clinical

- Explore personal myths and beliefs about death with colleagues.
- Use co-meditation to help a dying patient experience peace.
- Use the life review process to help a person experience a sense of integration.

Personal

- Plan your ideal death.
- Record several imagery scripts and experience "letting go" with these exercises.

DEFINITIONS

Death: a moment in time.

Deathing: the conscious preparation for the moment of death.[1]

Dying: a stage of life that fits into a broader philosophy, giving both death and life meaning.

Grief: a response to loss, characterized as dynamic, pervasive, individual yet normative.

Loss: the absence (or anticipated absence) of someone or something of real or symbolic meaning.

Mourning: the expression of a sadness or sorrow resulting from the loss.

Myth: story lines created by individuals and cultures about meaning and journeying in life.

Nearing Death Awareness: the dying person's knowledge of death and attempts to describe this experience to health care providers, family, and friends.

Self-Transcendence: the ability to move beyond conceptual self-boundaries of time and space.[2]

THEORY AND RESEARCH

To die peacefully, to die with the knowledge that life has had meaning and that one is connected through time and space to others, to God, and to the Universe, is to die well. Helping people to die well requires knowledge and skill, as well as a willingness to be intensely involved in the most intimate phases of another's life. Physical, spiritual, psychologic, and social distress must be addressed with concern and compassion. The nurse, in being present "in the moment" with the patient and family, inevitably confronts her or his own mortality. Care for the caregiver (professional and family) is a requirement, a part of the care of the dying.

Recent studies are beginning to address appropriate ways of easing the burden for those who are caring for the terminally ill.[3] Developing theories to guide end-of-life care are based on standards of care, like "the standard of a peaceful end of life" proposed by Ruland and Moore.[4] Theories related to grief and loss, self-transcendence, myths and beliefs, and nearing death awareness are particularly useful in formulating effective plans of care for the dying.

Grief and Loss

Grief theory links concepts of loss, bereavement, and mourning into a fabric of ideas that help decide action on the part of caregivers, family members, and patients. Several theorists have identified stages of grief, or patterns of grief, as a part of the framework that guides appropriate care. Grief is not only normative, but also dynamic, pervasive, and individual, however. Each individual moves through bereavement at a different pace and copes in a different manner, depending on inner resources, support, and relationships. Society may think that the period of mourning has been long enough (a normative statement), but the individual may need more (or less) time before beginning to take charge of a changed life.

Grief is a necessary process for both the dying person and his or her significant others. The more bonded and intimate two people have been, the more intense the grief. Feinstein and Mayo stated that appropriate grief work has three characteristics.[5] First, it furthers the healthy grieving process by encouraging ventilation, planning, and insight. Second, it does not exploit others; the mourner has a healing team to provide comfort, but does not act as a parasite who feeds on another's energy. Transactions are caring and clear. The mourner continues to recognize the importance of personal inner work. Third, appropriate grief work cannot be rushed. It takes time to accept that death has occurred and to work through feelings. The person who successfully addresses grief and goes through the process may experience a sort of transformation from profound sadness to a comfort with memories and even joy.[6]

Stepnick and Perry linked the stages of spiritual development first identified by Peck with the phases of grief originally identified by Kubler-Ross.[7-9] Nursing care during each of the phases takes into account the spiritual maturity of the griever, whether it is the dying person or those who love that person. A person who is in the early stages of spiritual maturity, whether a child or an adult, needs much external help, information, communication, and developing trust. This person may not achieve acceptance (and transcendence) without moving to a higher level of spiritual development. Persons who have a more formal spiritual practice may use rituals, rites, symbols, and activities that incorporate them for comfort; thus, they may find comfort in planning their own funeral. Skeptics may build on the comfort found in the formal structures, but often add intellectual processes, such as bargaining with medical science (e.g., becoming part of experimental studies), reading books on death and dying, considering their contributions in this life, yet acknowledging a fear of the final moments . . . fear of pain and loss. Those in the last spiritual stage (labeled "mystic" by Peck) believe in a common bond uniting humanity, the world, and the universe. They are attracted to the mystery of faith. Therefore, the dying person in this stage may worry more about others, become angry about the effect the disease or the dying has on loved ones, choose humanitarian goals, become introspective and prayerful, and contact family and friends to say good-bye. Nursing care requires a careful assessment of a dying person's spiritual resources to assist with peaceful death.

The nurse's own developing spiritual maturity can be a useful support, as when one accompanies an acquaintance for a while along a road. The nurse maintains an attitude of being open, listening, and assessing the client's path even when his or her own journey changes directions. Successfully dealing with grief allows the dying client to achieve peace and allows the family and significant others to move on with a changed life, cherishing memories while creating new ones.

Self-Transcendence

Many people have studied self-transcendence, the sense of a temporal integration of self, the feeling that past and future enhance the present. In studying survivors of concentration camps, Frankl discovered that those who survived seemed to transcend (beyond self) either toward other people or toward meaning.[10] Transcendence may occur through creativity, the family, or works of art; through receptivity toward others; or through acceptance of a situation that cannot be changed. People who can be identified as self-transcendent at the end of life tend to have less depression, less self-neglect, and less hopelessness.[11] They have a greater sense of well-being and a greater ability to cope with grief.[12] The self-transcendent person lives in the present and usually sees death as a normal part of life. Encouraging people to seek meaning and connections either in

the present or through the ages helps people move toward self-transcendence to achieve peace.

Measures to support one's movement toward self-transcendence build on the need to look inward for connectedness and a sense of timelessness. Life review—the systematic review of one's life to see that it was meaningful, to remember those who are loved, and to know one's own place in history—is one example of a useful process.[13] Life review is the story of this life, of living in this space on this earth in this time. Studies show that systematic life review helps reduce depression and anxiety, and it promotes a feeling that this was my life, no one else would have done it this way, and I have a unique place in this universe.[14]

Myths and Beliefs

Myths are our story lines, values, beliefs, and images; they are our personal manual about the meaning and the journey of the human spirit.[15] Myths help us seek the unfolding mystery in life. In seeking life's meaning and purpose, personal myths help us manifest hope, learn to accept daily struggles and challenges, and deal with ambiguity and uncertainty. Myths help us recognize strengths, choices, goals, and faith. They also help us to assess our perception of our world, recognize our capacity to pursue personal interests, and demonstrate love of self and self-forgiveness. Myths provide a sense of connection and of oneness with all of life and nature.

Throughout life, we create many myths; some serve us well, while others hinder our healing journey. From their work on rituals for living and dying, Feinstein and Mayo suggested a five-stage program to create empowering mythologies that will evoke courage in deathing and, thus, promote a peaceful death.[16] Each of the five stages has a specific purpose and corresponds with one of the phases in the natural development of personal myths. The first stage deals with recognizing our deepest fears about death. The second stage helps us search for counterforces to our fear of death. The third stage attempts to resolve the natural conflict between the prevailing myth identified in the first stage and the emerging countermyth identified in the second stage by integrating the best of each side into a renewed mythology. In the fourth stage, the deeper solutions to inner conflicts are further articulated, expanded, and anchored in our being. The task in the fifth stage is to weave our renewed mythology into daily life involving three personal rituals: (1) attending to that which will survive us, (2) creating ceremony for the final hour and beyond, and (3) establishing peaceful moments with what we do between now and the final hour.

Twenty years ago, the Senior Actualization and Growth Exploration (SAGE) study began to question society's beliefs about older people and their potential.[17] The researchers taught seniors deep relaxation, biofeedback, breathing exercises, meditation, yoga, and ways to expand creativity through movement, music, art, education, and group discussion. This project not only helped the participants reshape their declining years to an understanding of healthy aging and lifestyles that promote the goal of healthy aging, but also gave them new, practical ways to cope with personal problems and a more confident self-image. With healthier lifestyles, most people can add a vital 30 or more years to their lifespan. There is also more time to practice a new way of living so that dying in peace is a clear choice for each person.

Nearing Death Awareness

During their many years of hospice nursing, Callanan and Kelly have identified several recurring themes in the stories of dying patients and their families.[18] Messages about death awareness from dying persons fall into two categories: (1) attempts to describe what they are experiencing while dying and (2) requests for something that they need for a peaceful death. This awareness is not to be confused with near death experiences that happen as a result of cardiac arrest, drowning, or trauma in which a person feels the self suddenly leave this life, but quickly return. In a state of nearing death awareness, a person's dying is slower, often because of a progressive illness such as acquired immunodeficiency syndrome (AIDS), cancer, or heart or lung disease. The person remains inside the body, but at the same time becomes aware of a dimension that lies beyond, a drifting between this world and another, perhaps a space of transcendence, yet not one that touches "an Ultimate." The slower dying process allows the dying person to have more time to assess his or her life and to determine what remains to be finished before death. Some dying patients try to describe being in two places at once, or somewhere in between. It is a time for a caregiver to respond to their wishes and needs, and to listen to what dying is like for them. This can be a period of challenge for many caregivers. This is also a final gift to prepare each of us for what may happen in our deathing.

Those individuals who are tired of living but do not believe that it is time to die describe the dying process differently from those who are truly ready to depart. The statements of those who are truly ready are different in the clarity with which the words are spoken, the look from their eyes, or their touch. Their statements, looks, or touches are like no others that have been made before or during the deathing process.

HOLISTIC CARING PROCESS

Assessment

In preparing to use interventions for promoting peaceful dying, the nurse assesses both the dying person and the family or significant others in the following areas:

- the different emotions that surface during the process
  - *guilt:* blame of self and others over management of the dying person; distress over inability to decrease pain
  - *anger:* toward God, disease, family/ significant others, doctors, or survivors; over inability to fix things physically, emotionally, and spiritually
  - *ability to laugh:* the shortest distance between two people; relationship between comedy and tragedy (joy and sadness pathways cannot operate simultaneously)
  - *love:* an essential element in living and in deathing; a state of self-giving and presence of beingness of a person, where openness and willingness exist for self or another; the network that brings and weaves families/significant others together to work through the dying process and move into total acceptance of death
  - *fear:* often evocation of separateness and aloneness, but can become a path leading deeper into the present moment; useful in that it reveals areas of resistance; return to unconditional love and a sense of equanimity after release of fear
  - *forgiveness:* essential element for inner peace; an exercise in compassion that is both a process and an attitude
  - *faith:* the larger vision of existence, which is different for each person; helps to harness energy to evoke healing resources and power.
  - *hope:* support of patient or family/ significant others during death's darkness; an inner moment that perceives lightness when in the midst of darkness and has the potential for leading to deeper love; hope for decreased pain and increased physical and spiritual comfort, for a miracle, for peace of mind, for a remission, for peaceful death transition, and for acceptance of a shorter life than expected or the death of a loved one
- the patient's interactions with others and the effect of the patient's emotions on these interactions
- the need for education about what will happen and what can be done to help, for the family and the patient
- comfort needs, assessed according to the patient's wishes for[19]
  - pain control and symptom management
  - hydration
  - nutrition
  - respiratory assistance
  - movement
  - touch
- signs of psychiatric illness, under- or overmedication that may interfere with a patient's ability to cope with dying
  - hallucinations
  - delusions
  - depression
  - denial that interferes with the ability to move toward comfort and peace
  - excessive anxiety
  - confusion, agitation, or memory loss, especially in the aged

Patterns/Problems/Needs

The following patterns/problems/needs compatible with the interventions for dying in peace relate to the nine human response patterns (see Chapter 14):

- *Exchanging:* Altered circulation
  Altered oxygenation
  Altered body systems
- *Communicating:* Altered communication

Effective
communication
(see Nearing
Death Awareness)
- *Valuing:*   Spiritual distress
Spiritual well-being
(see Nearing
Death Awareness)
- *Choosing:*   Ineffective
individual/family
coping
- *Moving:*   Self-care deficit
- *Perceiving:* Body image
disturbance
Powerlessness
Hopelessness
- *Feeling:*   Pain
Anxiety
Death anxiety
Grieving
Fear

Outcomes

Table 26–1 guides the nurse in identifying patient outcomes, nursing prescriptions, and evaluation for assisting patients and their families/significant others during the dying process.

Therapeutic Care Plan and Implementation

The following guidelines are appropriate for both the dying person and the caregivers, whether family, friends, or nurse. They are helpful in all settings. The guidelines apply from the first awareness of a coming interaction with a patient and family who are moving through the dying process, through the deathing process, and afterward.

Before the Interaction

- Spend a few moments centering yourself to recognize and honor your presence there.
- Begin the session with intention to facilitate healing and peaceful dying.

At the Beginning of the Interaction

- Encourage the patient and the family/significant others as the caregiver(s)
  — set realistic goals.
  — identify different behaviors that have surfaced in their interactions with each other during this period.
  — gather a healing team and honor the patient's personal needs and feelings to avoid more suffering.
  — accept current circumstances, and release things that are beyond their control. Accept the fact that release may not be possible at this time, but they can work toward it.
  — take frequent breaks, at least 20 minutes daily, to evoke quality quiet time with relaxation, imagery, music, meditation, prayer, journal keeping, or dreamwork to assist in the letting-go process.
  — exercise, take long hot baths or showers, eat nutritious foods, eliminate excess caffeine or junk food, and ask other people for relief.
- Encourage the patient and caregivers to tell themselves over and over what a good job they are doing and that it is the best job that they can do. Repeating it helps in releasing guilt, anger, and frustration.

During the Deathing Process

- Recognize the one who is dying as the person who is usually the best teacher about what is right. The place of death is not as important as the care, trust, compassion, acceptance, and love that is provided and shared in deathing.
- Determine the care needed. The whole family should consider the following questions and issues:
  — Will the dying person receive better care in a hospital, in a hospice, or at home?

Table 26–1 Nursing Interventions: Dying in Peace

Patient Outcomes	Nursing Prescriptions	Evaluation
The patient will demonstrate an understanding of reasons for ongoing assessment and management of anxiety, including • quiet environment • explanations of all personnel, procedures, and equipment • touch and reassurance by nurse • relaxation skills	Continue to reassess states of anxiety and provide ways to decrease anxiety. • Provide quiet environment. • Explain all interventions. • Offer reassurance. • Teach relaxation and imagery skills.	The patient demonstrated an understanding of the reasons for assessment and management of anxiety.
The patient will verbalize feelings of anxiety and will talk spontaneously about fears. (If the patient is intubated, the patient and the nurse use specific communication codes.)	Provide quality time for the patient to share worries and fears. Use common symbols for communication if the patient is intubated.	The patient verbalized anxiety and fears.
The patient will use effective coping mechanisms during course of illness.	Focus on the patient's strengths.	The patient used effective coping mechanisms during the course of illness. (List specific examples.)
The family will communicate stressors associated with the patient's illness to staff.	Allow time for the family to express worries and fears.	The family/significant others communicated stressors to staff.
The patient will verbalize fears of death.	Be present with the patient and allow time for the patient to talk about fears of dying.	The patient talked of death.
The family/significant others will verbalize fears that the patient may die and what this means to them.	If death seems imminent, be with the patient and family to assist them through the death.	The patient's family/significant others acknowledged the impending death and shared feelings about death.
The family/significant others will receive support from nurses and clergy.	Provide spiritual support for the patient through presence, life review, prayer, talking, and handholding. Allow the family to be with the patient. Call clergy for assistance, if requested.	The family/significant others received spiritual support and talked to nurses and clergy.
The patient, family, and significant others will express fears and other feelings associated with dying and death.	Assist the patient and family to focus on what has been accomplished in life. Provide as much privacy as possible.	The patient and the patient's family focused on life accomplishments.
The patient will experience closure on matters of daily living.	Provide the opportunity to complete "unfinished business." Fulfill the patient's requests to see a member of the family, lawyer, member of the clergy, or a physician.	The patient and the family completed unfinished business.
The patient will be comfortable and participative until death occurs.	Evaluate the procedures and treatments that can be discontinued to make the patient more comfortable. Make provisions for someone to remain with the patient all the time if so desired by the patient.	Procedures and treatments were used for comfort only.

—What kind of medical treatment, technology, and equipment is needed?

—What information is needed to make decisions about care choices (e.g., providing hydration, withholding nutrition)?

—Can a hospice nurse or health care professional assist with treatments and medication?

—Is a parish nurse or congregational nurse available for liaison with the congregation involved?

—What expenses will be involved? What expenses will be covered by insurance? Is the patient eligible for state or federal disability payments, veterans or Social Security benefits, or Medicaid or Medicare?

—Who will assume the care 24 hours a day? Who will provide respite care? Are there children at home who also need continuous care? Can the care of the dying person and young children both be managed?

—Will organs be donated?

• Explore the advantages and disadvantages of dying at home (or alternative sites). Advantages for staying in the home include the freedom of the patient and the family to do anything they wish because they can change or alter routines and schedules at will. In addition, staying in the home makes the continuous support of family, friends, and even pets available; allows meals to be prepared fresh and served with attention to details; eliminates the stress of traveling to and from the hospital or hospice; provides the unique beauty of familiar surroundings; makes quality time available to focus on inner work for the moment of death; and permits the patient and family to experience feelings and emotions in a different way because their closeness is subject to fewer interruptions. Finally, the patient and family can make most of the decisions regarding care, medication, and treatments and can ask advice from professionals when needed. Disadvantages to staying at home may include inadequate support for coping with care needs or competing needs for care by small children, older adults, other sick or disabled family members. Sometimes inpatient hospice units help blend some of the advantages of care in the home with the additional support an individual may need that significant others cannot provide.

• Integrate therapies.

—Does the dying person believe that medical and nonmedical modalities are complementary?

—How motivated is he or she to try nonmedical resources (e.g., acupuncture, aromatherapy, touch therapies)?

—What nonmedical resources are available?

—Does the dying person really want to try different modalities, or is he or she receiving so much advice about therapies that the response is passive rather than active?

—Is the dying person choosing to try therapies to please caregivers? A patient should feel free to choose not to include complementary therapies if they are not wanted.

• Incorporate the senses in rituals.

—*Touching.* Lovingly, freely, and joyfully convey through your hands what your heart is feeling. Touching is a powerful way to break the illusion of separateness, loneliness, fear; it may evoke laughter, calmness, or tears. Create times to give and get hugs. Hold a hand now and then.

—*Smelling.* Use lotions and colognes with mild fragrances, remembering that illness will probably change the types of fragrances that can be tolerated. Use caution, as some odors cause nausea and unpleasant feelings. Try light natural scents like rosemary or vanilla, perhaps as a plant growing in the room or a candle in the bathroom.

— *Tasting.* Remember that taste varies with degrees of illness, but stays with us until the end of life. Tasting and eating have social and symbolic meaning to patient and family. Explain what will happen if the patient stops eating within the progression of terminal illness, that it may be normal and may not cause undue suffering. Provide tastes and foods that are desired.[20]

— *Seeing.* Arrange in a pleasing manner healing objects and different touchstones that have special meaning and symbolize people, places, and events in the patient's life. A room that receives soft, subdued rays from the sun can bring balance to surroundings. Sitting out on the patio in good weather allows one to feel the sun as well as see the sunlight. Light colors are usually more soothing than dark colors.

— *Hearing.* Remember that the sense of hearing is often sharp to the end of life, so special words at death can be heard. Be present in silence also, sitting or holding one another. Music can be nice, but not all the time.

- Practice sitting quietly with relaxation, meditation, or prayer. Gentle sounds from wind chimes or environmental recordings of ocean waves, wind, rain, birds, and music (e.g., harp, flute, stringed instruments) can offer a sense of peace. Music thanatology, referred to as sung prayer, uses the human voice when chanting or singing to bring balance to the dying, dissolving fears and lessening the burden, sorrows, and wounds.[21] Use words ending in *ing* such as releasing, letting, floating, softening, or words ending in *ness* such as openness, beingness, awareness, vastness, to help the patient to relax.

- Recognize the patient's going in and out of awareness. The moment of death itself has no pain, but is a reflex last breath. It opens up very special exchanges of intention, intimacy, and bonding where the patient may share the dying spaces. The patient's eyes can take on a staring, a glazing, a spaciness so different that the patient appears to be going to another realm of knowing or to be focusing on something that the caregiver cannot see; the dying person can return with a smile and possibly share that he or she was in a space of peace.

- Learn about changes in the body during dying. Knowing what body changes to expect as death approaches helps the family anticipate personal healing rituals and removes the fear, shock, and mystery from the moment of death.

- Understand and accept the body's shutting down. The conscious dying person knows that it is time to leave the physical body and can choose to shut physical life down. The caregiver and family journey with the dying person as far as possible and then tell the person it is all right to leave; this can evoke the purest, most special moments for all involved. For those people who wish to experience every morsel of life, even if that morsel is physical agony, respect the choice. For them, it may be inappropriate to suggest that they leave. Tell them that you love them and will stay with them as long as they need you (or a significant other).

At the Moment of Death

- Prepare rituals for the moment of death. The dying person usually has serenity and inner calm, particularly if healing rituals have been carried out prior to death. Before the dying person's eyes close, tight brow muscles may become relaxed; the peace in the face or within the room is often palpable. Trust your inner wisdom for how to touch, hold, talk, and be with the dying one in ways that deepen hope and faith for a peaceful crossing into death and beyond.

- Surround yourself and the dying person with the peace and the light of love, taking the energy of love and light in with each breath; imagine and experience literally going inside the breath, flowing inside the breath with co-meditation (see script Specific Interventions) into the death of each moment.

- Continue to communicate with family caregivers and those there to support the dying patient. Talk to the dying loved one as restlessness or agitation moves to unresponsiveness; give gentle love squeezes, touches, and hugs; play favorite music; read poems, or say mantras and prayers. Shut the half-closed eyes, stroke and hug the physical body, and adjust the loved one's head on the pillow for the last time. Give permission for this special person to be free, to soar, to meet God and others who have died before, if this is appropriate. Say all you need to say, and share your own kind of blessings for the smooth transition.

- If appropriate, when the person has taken a last breath, carry out additional rituals that may be helpful to those present. Holding hands around the bed, saying a blessing or prayer, or anointing with healing oil, for example, may be planned ahead of time for this moment.

- Schedule a follow-up session/visit with family/significant others, if appropriate. If grief support groups are available, a referral may be helpful.

- Take care of yourself. Adequate rest, relaxation, exercise, and nutrition are always important; the person who cares for dying people needs to "go apart for a little while." Center, meditate, celebrate, or plan your own self-renewal times. There are retreat centers and sanctuaries for those who wish to use them. Simply sharing your experience with others, either verbally or in writing (e.g., journaling, writing poetry or narratives), is helpful. Be glad for the opportunity to share such a sacred moment with others, and use those special times for your own growth.

Specific Interventions

Planning an Ideal Death. To help patients and families experience peace in the dying process, it is important to engage them in planning. To be of maximum assistance to someone else in the deathing journey, it is helpful for the nurse to explore this journey as well. The following reflective questions provide enormous insight about death myths, beliefs, problem solving, loving, and forgiving:

- What would an ideal death be like?
- When are you going to die?
- Where are you going to die?
- Who do you want to be with you, or do you want to be alone?
- What legal matters, relationships, or other personal business must be finished?
- What have been and what are the most precious events in your life?
- Who are the important people in your life?
- Have you told them why they are important?
- Are there family or friends who need to be told special things that you have never shared?
- Do you need to forgive or be forgiven?

- Have you written your obituary or your epitaph?
- Have you completed advanced directives, in writing, and shared them with those involved?
- Who do you want to care for your pets?
- What are your assets?
- What treasures do you wish to leave to specific family members or friends?
- What person/s have you appointed to be in charge of your medical decisions? Do they know what you want done?
- Have you planned rituals for your burial, or a funeral, memorial service, or cremation? Are they recorded and available to those who will perform them . . . family, religious institution, funeral home?
- If to be buried, what do you want to be buried in?
- What kind of a coffin or container do you want for your body?
- Who will perform your burial ceremony?
- What kind of a ceremony do you want?
- Do you prefer a wake or another form of ceremony?
- What prayers, passages, poems, or music do you want to have used?
- Who will direct the ceremony? Or do you want a death day celebration for people to celebrate your life during or in place of a funeral, and to be celebrated in subsequent years?

Part of confronting death is deciding how to use medical care and technology. As part of their right to die, individuals can decide whether they want medical treatment; what kind of treatment; and under what circumstances to start, continue, or stop treatment. The American Medical Association has created a document called the medical directive,[22] a three-page form on which an individual can record his or her wishes for four different life situations: (1) mental incompetence, (2) terminal illness, (3) irreversible coma, or (4) persistent vegetative state. It also has a place for the appointment of someone to make medical decisions for the individual, should that become necessary, and a place for information about the individual's wishes regarding organ donation. Most hospital and hospice organizations have similar documents available.

Since states vary in the legislative details of such documents, it is necessary to call the office of the state attorney general or consult an attorney. Furthermore, because these wishes often reflect philosophic, personal, religious, and spiritual desires, individuals should discuss these matters with the family and friends who will function on their behalf should they become incompetent. It is important for those who will be asked to make decisions to understand fully the nature of the request. Withholding of nutrition and fluids is often thought to be a cruel decision and a cause of suffering, yet history suggests that artificially feeding and hydrating a person who is clearly dying is an anomaly and reflects society's denial of death. Some research has indicated that patients who stop taking food and fluids slowly sink into unconsciousness and coma over a period of 5 to 8 days and die several days later.[23] Any discomfort that they experience, such as dry mouth, can be addressed with routine care. Those who make these kinds of decisions need to be fully informed, both about the patient's desires and about the effects of their wishes. Those who cannot do what the patient asks of them should have the choice of withdrawing from the decision-making role.

Learning Forgiveness. Forgiveness is important because it helps us get on with life. Many people are "stuck" in feeling guilt or assigning blame. Self-guilt leads to depression, and blaming others leads to anger. Both of these conditions steal energy and focus, reduce coping ability, and rob a person of precious time that could be used in establishing a positive relationship and attending to end-of-life goals. Borysenko described the steps to forgiving self and others as a parallel six-step process.[24] The six steps to forgiving ourselves are (1) taking responsibility for what we have done; (2) confessing the nature of the wrongs to ourselves, another human being, or God; (3) looking for the good points in ourselves; (4) being willing to make amends where possible, as long as we can do this without harm to ourselves or other people; (5) looking to God for help; and (6) inquiring about what we have learned. Likewise, the six steps to forgiving others are (1) recognizing that we are responsible for what we are holding onto; (2) confessing our story to ourselves, another person, and God; (3) looking for the good points in ourselves and the other person; (4) considering whether any specific action needs to be taken; (5) looking to God for help; and (6) reflecting on what we have done. These steps take time to complete. As the awareness of forgiving self and others is developed, we recognize unconditional love. Because it helps us connect more with our source of joy, not focusing on loss, sadness, or pain, unconditional love helps release us from fear.

Becoming Peaceful: Relaxation and Imagery Scripts. To learn how to let go of attachments, what is right and wrong, what is good and bad requires commitment and practice. Nurses encourage patients to hear their inner voice of judging and to release the judging, just to listen and be ready for the next moment of listening, and to be in the present moment. Centering, meditation, and contemplative prayer are helpful in learning to listen to the inner soul. The skill of opening and releasing ordinary fears allows a person to emerge with awareness in the healing moment and to be more present when assisting another during death.

Patients who are dying and their caregivers may set aside 20 minutes or more several times a day to practice opening to the moment. It may be helpful to create a special relaxation and imagery tape as part of a personal ritual to practice releasing and letting go. The breathing, relaxation, imagery, and music scripts that follow are important experiential exercises to help self and others learn the letting-go experience of calming the mind and creating a sense of spaciousness within the body (see Chapters 21, 22, and 23). Recording one or several of these scripts, after a 5- to 10-minute relaxation exercise, allows the dying patient and caregivers to use them repeatedly, even when professionals are not present. It is important to be sensitive about which scripts are likely to be useful for particular individuals. A person who has suffered from a respiratory disorder such as emphysema for many years may not do well with a script focused primarily on breathing, for example. The following scripts are adapted from the work of Stephen Levine, and Anees and Katrina Sheikh.[25–27]

> ***Script:*** *Introduction. (Name), as your mind becomes clearer and clearer, feel it becoming more and more alert. Somewhere deep inside of you, a brilliant light begins to glow. Sense this happening. The light grows brighter and more intense. Breathe into it. Energize it with your breath. The light is powerful and penetrating, and a beam begins to grow out from it. The beam shines into the core of your spirit.*

> ***Script:*** *Letting Go. Notice the rhythm of the breath . . . becoming more aware of all the sensations that arise from the breath. Watching . . . noticing . . . feeling . . . as the breath begins to breathe you. As you become more*

aware of the breath, let your conscious awareness release the notion of breathing ... becoming more and more aware as the breath arises in each moment. As interfering thoughts arise, let them float on ... dissolving into awareness ... quieting the constant chatter of the ego. ...

Script: *Opening the Heart. Relax into the moment of the awareness of the breath. ... Let the rhythm of the breath just breathe you. Allow a fearful image to emerge in thought ... noticing where it is in the body ... letting the feelings of fear be in the body. In a way that seems right for you ... let the fear move to the center of your chest ... to the center of your heart. There is space within your heart to let the fear be ... noticing the sensations of fear as they rest in the spaciousness of your heart center ... opening and softening ... opening and releasing denial ... letting the fears become what they need to be ... opening and accepting. Within the center of your heart ... your love and compassion are present to let the fear(s) be present.*

Script: *Forgiving Self and Others. Relax into the moment of the awareness of the breath. ... Let the breath just begin to breathe you. Allow yourself to let an image emerge of a person ... alive or dead ... who brings forth feelings of resentment. As that image is forming, ... notice the spa-*

ciousness of your heart ... and the openness of your heart center. Send the image of the person who causes you to feel resentment into your heart center. From the spaciousness of the center of your heart ... hold the image of this person as you repeat, "I forgive you for anything you may have done in the past ... in thoughts, words, or actions that may have caused you or me pain. I forgive you."*

As you do this, ... notice any change in the feelings of resentment ... opening and softening to the moment. If any feelings such as pain ... tightness ... or any other body sensation arise ... just let them be ... watching ... noticing ... all changes ... opening into the moment. Just continue to focus on the image of this person ... speaking from your heart ... releasing resentment ... pain ... forgiving yourself ... forgiving others.

Script: *Releasing Grief and Pain. With one or both thumbs or the palms of your hands, locate the point just at the base of your sternum, and press into this area; feel the point of maximum pressure for you. Notice any sensations of tension, pain, or aches that result from sadness, grief, and loss. Continue to hold the thoughts, feelings of yourself, the loved one you have lost, or any other person or issues that cause you loss. If it seems right, as often as needed, return yourself to the power of the awareness of your own breath as it breathes you.*

Relax into the moment of the awareness of the breath.... Let the breath just begin to breathe you. Within your heart just now may be grief and pain ... the feelings of loss ... the heaviness of sadness. With your thumb(s) or palm(s) of your hand(s), ... press into the area below your sternum.... Become aware of any sensations of pressure, pain, or any aches. Continue to hold the pressure. As you notice the pressure in this area, ... breathe slowly into the sensations as they arise ... emerging through the many levels of protection. Let yourself open into the pain ... being with the feelings that come ... not holding back ... not pushing away ... opening ... softening. Observing and experiencing ... allowing the pain ... the fear ... the sadness ... the loss ... just to be ... not evaluating. Continuing to hold the pressure ... releasing control ... become aware of the fear ... all fears that come as you feel the fear of losing your loved one ... all loved ones. And become aware of your fear of your own death ... any pain, fear ... anger ... sadness.

Let all your feelings now penetrate to the center of your heart ... opening to the moment ... receiving the love ... the caring ... the warmth ... coming from the center of your heart. And now ... let yourself release the physical pressure ... continuing to receive the love and caring from your heart center.

While consciously living, it is possible to experience conscious dying. It is helpful to use a relaxation or imagery technique to become grounded before the exercise. After the exercise, this same technique can facilitate the return to full alertness and readiness to proceed with daily activities. These scripts are intended to be a rehearsal, not an actual shutting down and leaving of the physical body.

Learning to confront our own death helps us be more present to assist others in facing their death. It reaffirms that we really need to do nothing but be present with another and speak with our hearts in dying time. The nurse may begin with an extended head-to-toe general relaxation or other breathing exercise (see the previous scripts). Because the experience of dying can be described as melting or dissolving away at the moment of death, the words dissolving and melting are used in the script. To continue this script, the four elements of the body described by the ancients—earth, water, fire, and air—are used to represent decomposition as the body dissolves.

> **Script:** *Conscious Dying. Relax into the moment of the awareness of the breath. Let the breath just continue to breathe you. As you focus on the breath, ... begin to notice how the breath lets you move from heavy sensations in the body to the lighter ... subtle body of awareness ... all awareness on the breath ... the breath in ... and the breath out.... Let yourself be in the heavy body ... and now all awareness on being in the light body.... The breath is all that there is ... just breathing ... let each thought dissolve into the breath ... melting into the breath ... awareness of the*

light body... and now letting the breath go... this is the final breath... let the breath in... and the breath out... dissolving... opening to death... and let yourself die.

Script: *Earth. The body... solid... heavy... mass... compact... all changing as death comes... the vital body losing its form... weakening and dissolving... becoming thinner like the elements of earth... changing... dissolving... all parts dissolving... organs... extremities... muscles... all senses dissolving... fading away... melting away....*

Script: *Water. All feelings becoming one... dissolving... all sensations dissolving... body fluids that flow through you... drying up... all body organs closing down... dissolving....*

Script: *Fire. The fire of life within you... going out... all body warmth and heat leaving... all organs ceasing to function... your body becoming cooler and cooler... your sense of boundary is dissolving... all senses dissolving... breath is dissolving....*

Script: *Air. Your body is without function.... The air is the element of consciousness... dissolving... all sensation... all feeling... all senses have gone... body boundaries are no more... light... melting... dissolving... no separate body... no separate mind... all separateness dissolving... all in the vastness of oneness....*

Take a few slow, energizing breaths and, as you come back to this awareness, know that whatever is right for you at this point in time is unfolding just as it should and that you have done your best, regardless of the outcome.

Adapted from Levine's work, the following script is useful for someone who is preparing for the death moment or for a family member or friend whose loved one has just died.[28] It can be expanded as needed. The four elements part of the imagery script may also be used to assist one whose death is imminent.

Script: *Moving into the Light. Fill yourself with an awareness of brilliance of clear light... a pure light within you and surrounding you... go forward... releasing anything that keeps you separate... pushing away nothing... spaciousness... releasing... dissolving... all body... dissolving into consciousness itself.... Let go of all distractions.... Listen and be with the transition... what is called death has arrived.... You are not alone... many have gone before you... let yourself go... into the clear light.*

The dying person may move in and out of sleep or comatose states after this script or the conscious dying script. The nurse or family member sits with the person as long as necessary to bring closure to this time. If the person lingers a while longer, the nurse or family member may close with the following phrases.

Script: *Closure. Take a few slow, energizing breaths and, as you*

*come back to this awareness,
know that whatever is right for
you at this point in time is unfolding just as it should, and
that you have done your best,
regardless of the outcome.*

The Pain Process. In 90 to 99 percent of
cases, pain can be managed. Pain medication should be evaluated at least every 72
hours. When giving the medication, the
nurse reminds the patient that the pain
medication is in the body and working.
Nurses should understand and use the
most current pain management strategies
and treatments. These include new medications, methods of administration, physical treatments (e.g., massage, ice, movement), combinations of treatments,
documentation, and evaluation techniques. The administration of medication
should precede activity (e.g., positioning).

Although the physical body can experience pain, the mind's fear of the pain is often
more intense. Acute pain has qualities of
suddenness and surprise that can evoke
anxiety and fear. The best thing to do with
this suddenness is to encourage the dying
person to breathe rhythmically and soften
into the pain to decrease the resistance to
the experience. Relaxation, imagery, or
acupressure may be combined with pain
medication. Even the worst of pain can be
shifted in many ways. For example, shifting
the pain experience by calling it sensations
rather than pain often reduces discomfort. It
also helps to encourage the person to make
decisions over which he or she has control,
such as decisions about medications, treatments, and daily routines.

When guiding the person in pain, the
nurse may suggest allowing pain images
and the different felt experiences to
emerge. Each person enters pain in a way
that opens in the moment, and each person
will know how far to go in exploring the
pain. Common expressions an individual
may have about the pain (e.g., pain attacks,

it has a grip on me and takes my breath
away, it has a loud and deafening pulsa-
tion, it is violent and unrelenting) create
negative images that may interfere with
the emergence of healing images. These
negative images may become positive if
the person focuses on the grip of pain being
released, a deep belly breath coming forth
evenly and effortlessly, or the pulsating
sound becoming like the falling of gentle
raindrops or falling snowflakes. Different
relaxation and imagery exercises help the
person practice letting go of the perception
of the physical body. This letting go helps
ease both physical pain, like difficult procedures, and emotional pain, like conflicts,
and allows the person to experience death
with peace and dignity.

With continued gentle exploration of
opening and releasing into the pain, the
person may begin to experience the pain as
floating and diminishing. This is also a
way of expanding one's sense of time. Another suggestion is to have the patient step
aside in the mind and watch the pain to see
how it might be changed to release some of
the pressure, resistance, and holding on to
the pain. Such guidance and presence over
time will help the person to stay with a focused attention, opening and softening
and expanding into the pain.

Blending Breaths and Co-Meditation.
The simple release of the breath and the
ah-h-h-h sound is an ancient ritual for dying into peace. The practice of sharing the
breath with another is called co-meditation
or cross-breathing.[29] Co-meditation is
based on the principle that respiration
evokes a particular state of mind and
serves as a direct link to the nervous system. There is a direct correlation between
breathing and thinking. At first, the ah-h-h-h
sounds may be like an echoing of words,
but staying with the sounds allows the release of tension, fears, and pain.

Following are the steps for co-meditation:

- Position yourself comfortably close to the patient. A session may last 20 to 30 minutes or longer. Obtain whatever is necessary to make you and the person comfortable, such as pillows or a light blanket.
- Suggest to the person that watching the breath is an ancient method of calming the body and the mind. Let the person first begin noticing the rise and fall of his or her abdomen with each breath in and each breath out.
- Sitting at the person's midsection, focus on the rise and fall of the abdomen with each inhalation and each exhalation. Focus your attention on the person's lower chest area, and observe closely for the natural flow of the exhalation from the person. With this focused attention, you can begin breathing in unison with the person. At the beginning of the exhalation, begin softly and out loud to make the sound ah-h-h-h, matching the respiration of the person.
- Occasionally, say simple, powerful phrases, such as peaceful heart or releasing into the breath. The fewer words spoken, however, the more powerful the breath work. If the person should fall asleep, you may wish to sit with the person for a while or sit until he or she awakes.

Mantras and Prayers. A mantra is the repetition of a word or sound, either aloud or silently. The word may be given by another or discovered. It has meaning to the individual. Repetition moves one toward peace.

A prayer may be special phrases or repeated words, or it may be a unique and spontaneous communication with God. There is considerable evidence for the effectiveness of at least two forms of prayer, the directed and the nondirected.[30,31] In direct prayer, the individual has a specific goal or outcome in mind. In the nondirected

form, the individual takes an open-ended, nonspecific, non–goal-oriented approach. In one form of contemplative prayer, Lectio Divina, one listens for the word of the Divine following a meditative focus on a few words of scripture.[32] In centering prayer, individuals seek "an original place, deep inside themselves, where they live in rich harmony with other people and with God . . . the place of wisdom, of not-wanting and yet having."[33] Every faith group has prayers of the faithful that provide comfort and joy in the last moments.[34]

Saying mantras and prayers can decrease the number of lonely hours at home, as well as in the hospital, although this is not the main reason for the practice. They serve as an affirmation of a deeper faith. In asking the dying person about wishes for prayers or repeated phrases, we may encourage him or her to select phrases that are short, easy to remember, and rhythmic. The personal selection of focus words enhances the faith factor.[35] It may be helpful to pray for the highest good for the dying one or ourselves rather than for what we want. If we are praying for another, we need to hold the person for whom we are praying in our conscious thought, not ourselves. If we are totally focused on the patient, we cause ourselves less grief, frustration, and fear, recognizing that we are not responsible for outcomes. The nurse and the patient should agree on what to pray for before the prayer begins, and the nurse must be sensitive to the individual's formal system of belief.

Reminiscing and Life Review. A process basic to human existence is reminiscing and recounting past events, either alone or with friends. We spend much of our time talking, thinking, or writing about plans, goals, resources, successes, disappointments, and failures. This is especially true when facing death. Life review is a more formal process that involves reviewing present and past experiences. A life review experiencing form

(Exhibit 26–1) is useful in ordering questions related to each stage of life from earliest memories to old age. To conduct a life review, it is best to plan six to eight sessions. Each session requires approximately 45 minutes. During each session, the patient tells the story of that phase of life. Open-ended questions are preferable, and it may be helpful to record the session. The first session is primarily an introduction. The last session is the most important, as it is a summing up or discussion of the meanings of the story. The patient may feel emotions of all kinds during any session, reflecting the emotions that he or she felt during the stage of life being discussed. It is the acknowledgment of emotional content, in part, that facilitates integration. In the summary, perhaps earlier, an individual usually begins to feel a sense of integration with the past and present, a kind of wholeness to life. Unfinished business becomes finished. This is helpful in achieving peace.[36,37] Levine used a meditative approach to the life review, reviewing the life story to honor and heal the past.[38]

Exhibit 26–1 Haight's Life Review and Experiencing Form

Childhood:
1. What is the very first thing you can remember in your life? Go as far back as you can.
2. What other things can you remember about when you were very young?
3. What was life like for you as a child?
4. What were your parents like? What were their weaknesses, strengths?
5. Did you have any brothers or sisters? Tell me what each was like.
6. Did someone close to you die when you were growing up?
7. Did someone important to you go away?
8. Do you ever remember being very sick?
9. Do you remember having an accident?
10. Do you remember being in a very dangerous situation?
11. Was there anything that was important to you that was lost or destroyed?
12. Was church a large part of your life?
13. Did you enjoy being a boy/girl?

Adolescence:
1. When you think about yourself and your life as a teenager, what is the first thing you can remember about that time?
2. What other things stand out in your memory about being a teenager?
3. Who were the important people for you? Tell me about them. Parents, brothers, sisters, friends, teachers, those you were especially close to, those you admired, those you wanted to be like.
4. Did you attend church and youth groups?
5. Did you go to school? What was the meaning for you?
6. Did you work during these years?
7. Tell me of any hardships you experienced at this time.
8. Do you remember feeling that there wasn't enough food or necessities of life as a child or adolescent?
9. Do you remember feeling left alone, abandoned, not having enough love or care as a child or adolescent?
10. What were the pleasant things about your adolescence?
11. What was the most unpleasant thing about your adolescence?
12. All things considered, would you say you were happy or unhappy as a teenager?
13. Do you remember your first attraction to another person?
14. How did you feel about sexual activities and your own sexual identity?

continues

Exhibit 26-1 Continued

Family and Home:

1. How did your parents get along?
2. How did other people in your home get along?
3. What was the atmosphere in your home?
4. Where you punished as a child? For what? Who did the punishing? Who was "boss"?
5. When you wanted something from your parents, how did you go about getting it?
6. What kind of person did your parents like the most? The least?
7. Who were you closest to in your family?
8. Who in your family were you most like? In what way?

Adulthood:

1. What place did religion play in your life?
2. Now I'd like to talk to you about your life as an adult, starting when you were in your twenties up to today. Tell me of the most important events that happened in your adulthood.
3. What was life like for you in your twenties and thirties?
4. What kind of person were you? What did you enjoy?
5. Tell me about your work. Did you enjoy your work? Did you earn an adequate living? Did you work hard during those years? Were you appreciated?
6. Did you form significant relationships with other people?
7. Did you marry?
   (yes) What kind of person was your spouse?
   (no) Why not?
8. Do you think marriages get better or worse over time? Were you married more than once?
9. On the whole, would you say you had a happy or unhappy marriage?
10. Was sexual intimacy important to you?
11. What were some of the main difficulties you encountered during your adult years?
    a. Did someone close to you die? Go away?
    b. Were you ever sick? Have an accident?
    c. Did you move often? Change jobs?
    d. Did you ever feel alone? Abandoned?
    e. Did you ever feel need?

Summary:

1. On the whole, what kind of life do you think you've had?
2. If everything were to be the same would you like to live your life over again?
3. If you were going to live your life over again, what would you change? Leave unchanged?
4. We've been talking about your life for quite some time now. Let's discuss your overall feelings and ideas about your life. What would you say the main satisfactions in your life have been? **Try for three. Why were they satisfying?**
5. Everyone has had disappointments. What have been the main disappointments in your life?
6. What was the hardest thing you had to face in your life? Please describe it.
7. What was the happiest period of your life? What about it made it the happiest period? Why is your life less happy now?
8. What was the unhappiest period of your life? Why is your life more happy now?
9. What was the proudest moment in your life?
10. If you could stay the same age all your life, what age would you choose? Why?
11. How do you think you've made out in life? Better or worse than what you hoped for?
12. Let's talk a little about you as you are now. What are the best things about the age you are now?
13. What are the worse things about being the age you are now?
14. What are the most important things to you in your life today?
15. What do you hope will happen to you as you grow older?
16. What do you fear will happen to you as you grow older?
17. Have you enjoyed participating in this review of your life?

NOTE: Derived from new questions and two unpublished dissertations:

Gorney, J. (1968). *Experiencing and Age: Patterns of Reminiscence Among the Elderly*. (Unpublished Doctoral Dissertation, University of Chicago).

Falk, J. (1969). *The Organization of Remembered Life Experience of Older People: Its Relation to Anticipated Stress, to Subsequent Adaptation and to Age*. (Unpublished Doctoral Dissertation, University of Chicago).

Source: © 1982 Barbara K. Haight, RNC, Dr.PH.

Death Bed Ritual (Basic). At the moment of death and immediately after, it may be helpful to implement a planned ritual. If anointing has not already been done, it may be done at this time. Family, special friends, care staff, clergy may choose to hold hands, surround the bed of the deceased and share a moment of silence, a prayer, a song, or hugs. They may choose to touch the body, prepare the body according to rituals within the faith community involved, and say good-bye. It is important to allow as much time as needed.

Leavetaking Rituals (Basic). A nurse who works with survivors must remember that their grief period is unique for them. Furthermore, grief has no timetable. Healing grief requires a commitment to imagine a fulfilling life without a loved one. Action steps toward continued self-discovery after the death of a loved one may include dreamwork, meditation, movement, drawing, journal keeping, crying, sighing, drumming, chanting, singing, and music, as well as the following rituals.[39]

- *Celebrating Holidays*. Special holidays, birthdays, anniversaries, and other important dates can be a time for creating rituals to ease the pain of loss and acknowledge feelings. For example, a widow fixed a place at the Christmas dinner table for her deceased husband. She and her six children gave him a farewell toast and shared special memories of him before they ate. A young couple who had a stillborn child asked several of the nurses and the attending physician to a memorial service in the hospital chapel before the baby was taken to the funeral home. After her mother died, a woman chose to have her healing team of eight friends with her at a memorial service by the sea. The family of a teenaged girl who died in an automobile accident had a gathering for her class and gave each person an opportunity to say special things about the girl. Her favorite music was played while dancing and singing began in her honor.

- *Rearranging and Giving Away*. If a loved one has died at home, the family member who shared the bedroom must decide what is best to do. Some wish to rearrange the room and remove hospital beds and other equipment quickly after death. Giving away a loved one's possessions, such as special mementos of jewelry, clothes, shoes, makeup, shaving equipment, and other personal possessions, is healing. Some people need a shrine or memorial for a period of time, however.

- *Letting Grief Be Present*. There are periods after death when a person appears brave, in control, or strong to others. Grief will come, however. It is important to share with the grieving person that there is no special way to grieve. When pain, fear, and anger can dissipate, the body-mind-spirit knows the best way to grieve. Grieving allows love to heal the loss one feels for self and the person who has died.

- *Sustaining Faith and Hope*. There are many ways to sustain faith and awareness toward life, meaning, and purpose during grieving time. For example, survivors sometimes have a sense of talking to deceased loved ones, being enveloped in their love, and feeling their presence. People have described experiences such as having a faith in oneness, feeling an energy, vaguely sensing the presence of the deceased person, hearing the voice of the deceased giving guidance, or working on the same problem at different energy levels. One woman said, "My [deceased] husband told me how to finish this business deal." Another woman created a healing ritual after the death of her husband. When the weather permitted, she would get in her truck in the evening and drive to her husband's favorite hill on their big Texas ranch. As she looked out over the prairie and gazed into the Milky Way, she would choose a bright star and carry on a dialogue with the star, experiencing a sense of unity with her deceased husband somewhere in infinity. This provided her with calmness, wisdom, and clarity of thought.

- *Releasing Anger and Tears.* The release of anger, sadness, and tears is a cleansing process of the human spirit that makes a person more open to experience living in the moment. Holding grief in increases the suffering, fear, and separation.
- *Healing Memories.* It is not necessary to stop thinking about the person who has died. Often, a grieving person who feels that the grief process is over finds that a memory, a song, or a meal suddenly evokes a sense of loss so deep that it seems as though it will never heal. The person needs to stay with the pain, sadness, guilt, anger, fear, or loneliness. Love and joy will begin to fill the heart again. The wisdom is to let pain in and to stay open to it, to let the pain penetrate every cell in your body, to trust pain, to know that what emerges from the pain is a new level of healing awareness.
- *Getting Unstuck.* Grieving can bring on suffering; therefore, it may be helpful for survivors to ask for assistance from friends, family, or a health care professional to help them move past the blocks. Some people think, "It's been 6 months since my mother died [or a year since my husband, son, or wife died], why am I still depressed and cry so frequently?"

Case Studies

Case Study No. 1

Setting:	Critical care unit where visiting schedule was one visitor every 2 hours.
Patient:	S.R., a 30-year-old mother of three children
Patterns/ Problems/ Needs:	1. Decreased cardiac output related to end-stage heart failure 2. Grieving related to imminent death 3. Spiritual strength related to dynamic belief systems and family/friend support

S.R. said to the nurse, "I feel death over my right shoulder. Call my husband. I need him to come and bring my children, my parents, and my three friends. Tell them to come as soon as possible." The nurse also had an inner felt sense of the presence of death and began calling S.R.'s family. Four hours before her death, all her family was present. Her friends sang her favorite songs as one played a guitar.

Case Study No. 2

Setting:	Writing thoughts about healthy grief in a letter, 4 years after son's death
Client:	V.D.J., a 45-year-old professional and mother
Patterns/ Problems/ Needs:	Spiritual strength related to ability to deliberate the meaning of life, death, grief, and suffering

There is a holy purpose in grief and nothing should stand in its path. Grief begins with so few words. Sounds take shape traveling from a great distance. Within, a reserve is sensed. Something sacred that holds a luminous darkness which stills the mind even as the heart shudders with waves of deep sorrow. The natural quality of grief is ancient and bone bare. It tolerates nothing false. Grief is unrestrained; conscious effort is not required.

A mother who has lost a child learns what true freedom is. It is being cut free from the knot of habit, customs, rules. It is not being bound by considerations or even fear, for the worst has happened. Your child is dead, and you live. A mother's lament begins.

Your heartbeat creates a tone for your body to hear. It drums and moves you slowly forward with your family even as you weep and prepare to say your last goodbye. Now is not the time to be a bystander. It is crucial that you support and include your other children and family in the vigil, the wake, the funeral and burial or cremation ceremonies. They, too, are in shock and disbelief. And it doesn't end there.

Let nothing be left undone, unsaid, unwritten or unsung in this farewell. This is not the place to lose courage or even your humor, for you will need both to sustain the intense suffering you have yet to bear. Nature provides the exact dosage for dealing with the constant strikes of pain experienced. Usually there is no real need for outside medication. Your body in its perfect wisdom gauges your requirements and numbs you accordingly. You will feel cold, but your mind/body will not allow more pain than you can tolerate. To disrupt the natural safeguards may only postpone the initial pain in your mourning process.

During the vigil and the wake your only thought is to do everything you can do to console your children and other family members. You realize they have the same concern for you. Plan the funeral ceremonies together. In the process, some small consolation may be experienced. The Path of Grief leads inward when you watch and listen. Didn't you bring this spirit child into the world, flesh of your flesh? This last goodbye may enable you to complete the circle; keeping a vigil through the night allows you to be closer to your child.

The vigil with your child provides a place to begin to say goodbye, the goodbye you were both denied, by sudden, unexpected death. You hear yourself talking and reassuring your son. You must now help your child to take the first steps into the Great Mystery, by talking aloud and guiding, much as you did when he was very young. Empty your mind and your heart, and give him all your love and spiritual strength for his journey.

The week following the funeral I moved everything from my bedroom except basic essentials. I felt driven to sleep on a mat and to make a low altar which I filled with family photographs, mementos, and childhood treasures belonging to Sean and my children, family poetry, drawings, vigil candles, prayer fans, fresh flowers and ceremonial sage.

Prayers became conversations and chants and death songs for the son who had no time to create them for himself. Forty-nine days of talking-prayer asking the angelic beings to guide my son on his journey. Each member of the immediate family scattered Sean's ashes in places special to him. A spirit bundle was placed and kept before the altar for him. Always the moving between worlds; letting go of the loneliness through weeping, sound and moving prayer to returning to repose, listening, and sitting. A year goes by.

You find it difficult to speak. Your breathing habits are changing. You become aware of differences in your breath. You sense your heart breathing, your brain breathing. You notice that when you breathe out, you see thought. Some days you don't remember breathing at all.

You keep a journal as an on-going discussion with your child, seeking solace. You somehow deal with daily life, guilt, illness, helplessness, and the grief of your other children.

Four more years go by; four years of dreams, voices and mourning. I begin to understand the innate usefulness of creative work and humor as an antidote to loneliness and pain. My children need me and continually pull me onto the more solid ground where they stand. Dream walks, drumming, chanting, and round dancing lead me to my tribal traditions. My children personify the creative weaving of compassion, intelligence and courage and remind me of how precious each individual life is and the miracle of being together with Sean and with each other in this life and in this time and in this place.

My son Sean has taught me that the true object of death is life. I have learned that a dream can be shaped by the dreamer; that in the act of sacrifice, the sacred is manifested through surrender of all that is.[40]

Case Study No. 3

Setting:	Bedroom at home of daughter (M.L.) who recently brought her ill mother (L.Y.) home to care for her
Patient:	L.Y., a 90-year-old mother of two middle-aged adults, grandmother of two, who has been ill for 4 months. She had lived alone for the last 40 years
Patterns/ Problems/ Needs:	1. Moderate pain related to diagnosis of cancer 2. Decreased cardiac output (including altered oxygen-

ation) related to multisystem organ shutdown
3. Family grieving related to imminent death
4. Spiritual well-being and effective individual coping related to patient desire to care for her grieving family

M.L. checked with her mother to see that she was not in pain or distress prior to going out of the house on a short errand. L.Y. told her daughter to go, adding that she was quite comfortable and would be fine. M.L. noticed her mother's skin was mottled and cool, but her breathing was unlabored and she seemed peaceful. Her husband remained in the home. When M.L. returned, she found that her mother had stopped breathing. The bedclothes were unruffled, and her mother's face was peaceful. Her husband had heard nothing to indicate when the passing occurred. M.L. called the hospice nurse, the nun who was her neighbor and belonged to the same church, and other family members, and they carried out the ritual that they had planned for this moment. They held hands around the bed, prayed together in the ways of their tradition, and played a hymn that had been taped. After this, they informed the doctor, called the funeral director, and took care of legal obligations. A woman who had lived alone for 40 years had chosen to die alone, but cared for, to the end. The family grieving needs were also addressed.

Evaluation

With the patient (family/significant others), the nurse evaluates whether the patient outcomes for planning and implementing a peaceful death (see Table 26–1) were successfully achieved. To evaluate the interventions further, the nurse may explore the subjective effects of the experience with the patient (family/significant others), using questions such as those shown in Exhibit 26–2.

Exhibit 26–2 Evaluating the Patient's (Family's/Significant Other's) Subjective Experience with Deathing Interventions

1. Can you continue to be aware of ways to recognize your anxiety, fear, and grief at this time?
2. Which of your strengths can best serve you as you move through this difficult time?
3. What are the things that you will do to take care of yourself at this time?
4. Do you have any questions that I can help you with just now?
5. Will you call on others to help you?
6. Whom can you ask for help?
7. Were the imagery exercises helpful for you? Do you pray?
8. Are there images, feelings, or emotions that surfaced during the imagery exercises that I can help you with?
9. Can I help you with anything just now?
10. Are there rituals that you can begin to create to help you deal with your grief?

Note: These subjective experiences may be used in helping a patient/family/significant others during the deathing process or with the family/significant others during the grieving process.

Like peaceful living and dying, the care of a dying person and the family/significant others is an art. Preparing for death can be a series of conscious, spirit-filled, light-filled moments that lead to the ultimate peaceful moment of death. It is different for each person. True healing and deathing in peace come from integrating the creative process and the art of healing into our daily lives. The paradox is that, although this healing awareness may appear at first to be rare, it is a very ordinary and natural event that is available to each of us at all times. As each of us seeks to understand and integrate our spirit-filled lives as meaningful and connected with others throughout the ages, we learn about life and death. The more we integrate solitude, inward-focused practice, and con-

scious awareness into daily life, the more peaceful is the deathing process and the moment of death.

DIRECTIONS FOR FUTURE RESEARCH

1. Evaluate the attitudes and stress levels of nurses who work with deathing and death; compare the stress levels in nurses who routinely use self-regulation nursing interventions with the levels in nurses who do not use self-regulation interventions.
2. Determine the effects of using scripts to let go on the patient's physiologic responses, nearing death awareness, and peaceful dying.
3. Evaluate the use of life review in assisting patients with a sense of integration of life.
4. Determine the special needs of nurses who work with dying people who are friends and relatives, or who have special experiences while dying (like negative near-death experiences).

NURSE HEALER REFLECTIONS

After reading this chapter, the nurse healer will be able to answer or begin a process of answering the following questions:

- Do I feel a greater sense of healing intention when I include relaxation, imagery, or music in my life every day?
- What are the effects on me when I guide others in healing modalities to facilitate peace in deathing?
- How do I know that I am actively listening?
- What new death mythologies and skills can assist me in releasing attachment to my physical body, possessions, and people?

NOTES

1. A. Foos-Graber, *Deathing: An Intelligent Alternative for the Final Moments of Life* (York Beach, ME: Nicolas-Hays, 1992).

2. P. Reed, Self-Transcendence and Mental Health in Oldest-Old Adults, *Nursing Research* 40, no. 1 (1991):5–11.

3. R. McCorkle et al., The Effects of Home Nursing Care for Patients during Terminal Illness on the Bereaved's Psychological Distress, *Nursing Research* 47, no. 1 (1998):2–10.

4. C.M. Ruland, Theory Construction Based on Standards of Care: A Proposed Theory of the Peaceful End of Life, *Nursing Outlook* 46, no. 4 (1998):169–175.

5. D. Feinstein and P.E. Mayo, *Rituals for Living and Dying* (San Francisco: Harper San Francisco, 1990).

6. G.G. Fersz et al., Transformation through Grieving: Art and the Bereaved, *Holistic Nursing Practice* 13, no. 1 (1998): 68–75.

7. A. Stepnick and T. Perry, Preventing Spiritual Distress in the Dying Client, *Journal of Psychosocial Nursing and Mental Health Services* 30, no. 1 (1992):17–24.

8. M. Peck, *The Different Drum: Community Making and Peace* (New York: Simon & Schuster, 1987).

9. E. Kubler-Ross, *On Death and Dying* (New York: Macmillan, 1969).

10. V. Frankl, *Man's Search for Meaning*, 3d ed. (New York: Simon & Schuster, 1963).

11. Reed, Self-transcendence and Mental Health in Oldest-Old Adults.

12. D. Coward, Self-Transcendence and Emotional Well-Being in Women with Advanced Breast Cancer, *Oncology Nursing Forum* 18, no. 5 (1991): 857–863.

13. B. Haight, Psychological Illness in Aging, in *Perspectives on Gerontological Nursing*, ed. E.M. Baines (Newbury Park, CA: Sage Publications, 1991): 292–322.

14. Haight, Psychological Illness in Aging.

15. L. Dossey, *Meaning and Medicine* (New York: Bantam Books, 1991).

16. D. Feinstein and P.E. Mayo, *Rituals for Living and Dying* (San Francisco: Harper San Francisco, 1990).

17. G. Luce, *Your Second Life: The SAGE Experience* (New York: Delacorte Press, 1979).

18. M. Callanan and P. Kelly, *Final Gifts: Understanding the Special Awareness, Needs, and Communication of the Dying* (New York: Bantam Books, 1993).

19. J.M. Hoefler, *Managing Death: The First Guide for Patients, Family Members, and Care Providers on Forgoing Treatment at the End of Life* (Boulder, CO: Westview Press, 1997).

20. E.E. Bral, Caring for Adults with Chronic Cancer Pain, *American Journal of Nursing* 98, no. 4 (1998): 26–32.

21. T. Schrodeder-Sheker, Music for the Dying: A Personal Account of the New Field of Music Thanatology. History, Theories, and Clinical Narratives, *Journal of Holistic Nursing* 12, no. 1 (1994):83–99.

22. L.L. Emanuel and E.J. Emanuel, The Medical Directive: A New Comprehensive Advance Care Document, *Journal of the American Medical Association* 261 (1989):3288–3293.

23. Hoefler, *Managing Death.*

24. J. Borysenko, *Guilt Is the Teacher, Love Is the Lesson* (New York: Warner Books, 1990).

25. S. Levine, *A Gradual Awakening* (New York: Anchor Press, 1979).

26. S. Levine, *Healing into Life and Death* (New York: Doubleday, 1989).

27. A. Sheikh and K. Sheikh, *Death Imagery* (Milwaukee, WI: American Imagery Institute, 1991).

28. S. Levine, *Who Dies?* (New York: Anchor Press, 1982).

29. R. Boerstler, *Letting Go* (Watertown, MA: Associates in Thanatology, 1982).

30. L. Dossey, *Healing Words: The Power of Prayer and the Practice of Medicine* (San Francisco: Harper San Francisco, 1993).

31. L. Dossey, *Recovering the Soul* (New York: Bantam Books, 1989).

32. M. Casey, *Sacred Reading: The Ancient Art of Lectio Divina* (Liguori, MO: Liguori Publications, 1995).

33. M.B. Pennington, *The Way Back Home: An Introduction to Centering Prayer* (New York: Paulist Press, 1989).

34. T.J. Craughwell, *Every Eye Beholds You: A World Treasury of Prayer* (New York: Quality Paperback Book Club, 1998).

35. H. Benson, *Beyond the Relaxation Response* (New York: Times Books, 1984).

36. G. Black and B.K.Haight, Integrality as a Holistic Framework for the Life-Review Process, *Holistic Nursing Practice* 7, no. 1 (1992):7–15.

37. M. Olson, *Healing the Dying* (Albany, NY: Delmar Publishers, 1997).

38. S. Levine, *A Year To Live: How To Live This Year As If It Were Your Last* (New York: Bell Tower, 1997), 75.

39. V. Durling Jones, personal communication, 1991; used with permission.

40. J. Achterberg et al., *Rituals of Healing* (New York: Bantam Books, 1994).

VISION OF HEALING

Nourishing Wisdom

Our hurried meals often reflect our hurried lives. Explore for a few minutes how we can experience food as nourishing wisdom. David referred to this awareness as principles of ordered eating.[1]

When we eat with conscious awareness, the true meaning of nourishing wisdom of food deepens. It is an awareness of the food (e.g., its color, texture, aroma), the process of eating (e.g., chewing, swallowing, feeling food in our stomach), and all aspects of the atmosphere and environment (e.g., temperature of the room, the colors and shapes within the room, the table setting).

If we are sharing a meal with others, we are aware of the company and enjoyment of these people. We recognize that the presence of others can be nourishing to us, as well as to them. If we are eating alone, this awareness may provide an intimate experience of being alone, calm, relaxed, and present with each morsel of food. If we smile while we eat, we may experience more joyfulness in the moment of eating. As we reflect on the way that food feels within us and satisfies us, we deepen the experience of the art and ritual of eating.

We acknowledge our connection with the food by recognizing the origin of the food (e.g., the earth, animals, plants, trees) and being thankful for the sun, rain, water, and soil; for the farmers who cultivate the growing, flowering, and harvesting of the food; and for the packaging and delivery of the foods to the store or marketplace. Our awareness of being connected to the food source can also help us to eat in moderation and to eat balanced, healthy foods. This wisdom encourages us to choose from a variety of foods grown locally and to receive the benefit and nourishment of seasonal foods. Then, as we prepare the food, adding our own personalized taste with herbs and spices, we experience the joy of composing a meal of different foods, tastes, and textures that we believe to be right for us—not what another imposes on us as a correct combination of foods.

Nourishing wisdom of food also helps us to increase our awareness of the synergy of the food by combining food with exercise, rest and sleep cycles, relaxed breathing, and our other healing rhythms.

The more we are aware of body-mind-spirit connections while choosing, preparing, eating, and finishing the eating of foods, the greater is our potential for inner satisfaction and personal unfolding in relationship to food.

NOTE

1. M. David, *Nourishing Wisdom: A New Understanding of Eating* (New York: Bell Tower, 1991), 170–173.

Chapter 27

Weight Management Counseling

Sue Popkess-Vawter

NURSE HEALER OBJECTIVES

Theoretical

- Discuss the strengths and weakness of biologic, behavioral, psychologic, and cognitive theories of weight management.
- Describe and explain the theoretical framework for cognitive restructuring based on reversal theory.

Clinical

- Describe three differences between unidimensional and multidimensional interventions for long-term weight management.
- Discuss and adapt the basic principles of the holistic self-care model for long-term weight management to clients in your nursing practice.
- List one positive self-talk statement to replace the three negative self-talk statements most frequently used by your clients; identify in which of the eight metamotivational states these statements originated.

Personal

- Discuss how you base your eating habits on the food pyramid and the American Diabetic Association diet using the EAT for hunger strategy.

- Describe your personal aerobic and strength exercise program using the exercise for LIFE strategy.
- Describe how you deal directly with unpleasant feelings, instead of eating to cope.

DEFINITIONS

Body Mass Index (BMI): weight [kg]/ height squared [m^2] ranging from 25 to 29.

Obesity: body weight greater than 20 percent above ideal or body mass index ranging from 30 to 38.

Overeating: eating when not hungry.

Overfat: percentage of body fat greater than recommended for a client's gender and age (e.g., 28 percent for women and 20 percent for men).

Overweight: body weight 10 percent to 20 percent above ideal or body mass index.

Self-Talk: mental verbalizations that elicit emotional reactions.

Weight Cycling/Yo-yo Dieting: repeated weight loss greater than 10 pounds followed by weight gain three or more times over the past 2 years.

Weight Management: holistic, long-term lifestyle adjustments in clients' bio-psycho-social-spiritual dimensions to promote a high level of individual wellness; caring for and assisting clients to reach sufficient self-acceptance, self-love, and self-responsibility to adjust their lifestyles to support eating for hunger only and exercising regularly.

THEORY AND RESEARCH

The Growing Weight Problem in the United States

Today, more than $33 billion are spent annually on weight loss interventions.[1] During the Great Depression and through war times, however, those in the United States focused on peace and financial security. Times were literally lean because of financial and nutritional shortages. As the economic struggles in the United States began to resolve and its citizens gained greater wealth, they also gained weight. Advances in automation rapidly mechanized a once active society, making it faster paced but paradoxically slowing it down physically. Four key factors can explain the stimulus–response nature of being overweight in the United States: (1) a fast-paced eating style consisting of fatty "fast foods" and large bites, (2) excessive calorie intake, (3) reduced physical activity, and (4) heightened responsiveness to food as a stimulant.[2] People learned to overeat in celebration of their new-found freedom and prosperity, and they used eating as a coping mechanism. From an operant conditioning perspective, food acted as the powerful positive reinforcer that stopped the unpleasant feeling of hunger (the negative reinforcer).[3] Eating to feel better, in the presence or absence of hunger and a wide variety of pleasant and unpleasant feelings, soon became a habit in the U.S. culture as foods (usually those high in fat) became more affordable and convenient.

Classical conditioning theory can further explain weight-gaining habits through the strong association between environmental circumstances before eating (usual times of breakfast, lunch, and dinner or the aroma and/or sight stimulus of food) and the mistaken perception of hunger.

Long-term habits of overeating without hunger and little or no physical exercise in a fast-paced society can explain the growing weight problem among U.S. citizens. To date, most weight loss interventions in the United States have not helped to reduce weight over the long term and perhaps have even contributed to the overweight problem.

Approaches to Weight Management

Most weight management approaches are based on at least one of four categories of theories—biologic, behavioral, psychologic, and cognitive.

Biologic Theories

Interventions based on biologic theories are aimed at correcting excess weight and fat by reducing the numbers of available calories, so excessive fat will not be deposited and fat stores will be used. Four biologic theories explain excess weight gain from genetic and energy balance perspectives.

According to two genetic theories, individuals have a genetic predisposition to an excessive accumulation of fat, either by hypertrophy (enlarged size) or hyperplasia (excessive numbers) of fat cells. Average-sized adults have approximately 30 billion fat cells or adipocytes that store fat synthesized from the diet.[4] One theory focuses on the size of the fat cell as a regulatory mechanism for food consumption; that is, when existing adipocytes have expanded to their size limitation, a signal causes the individual to stop eating.[5] Individuals who have excessive numbers of fat cells could continue eating longer than those who have fewer fat cells, thus maintaining their original size.

Another genetic theory focuses on the number of fat cells resulting from fat cell proliferation, which usually happens during infancy and puberty. According to this theory, individuals are destined to continue their degree of fatness according to the number of fat cells present in childhood and adolescence. The adipocyte hypertrophy theory supports adult-onset obesity, while the adipocyte hyperplasia theory supports child-onset obesity.[6] Neither genetic theory leaves much room for therapeutic interventions.

Set point theory, another popular theory, gained attention in the 1980s and 1990s. Nesbitt, who introduced this theory in 1972,[7] claimed that individuals have but one body weight at which their energy expenditure is normal. Despite changes in the rate of energy expenditure, be they higher or lower, individuals eventually will gain or lose weight to return to their weight to its set point.[8] Thyroid hormone (given in past years to increase metabolism) may facilitate weight loss, but at the cost of normal thyroid function; in some cases, its administration has resulted in permanent damage to the thyroid. Other metabolic stimulants used for weight loss, such as amphetamines and nicotine, involve similar risks. Regular, vigorous exercise is one healthy way to lower the set point. According to the theory, no matter which measure is used to lower the set point, weight returns to its previous level once the measure is withdrawn.

Energy balance theory has been widely used as the basis of weight loss interventions.[9] The chronic positive energy balance version of the theory perhaps is most accepted, to the extent that most believe it to be a law of physiology. Some describe this theory in the opposite view and from a therapeutic perspective as the negative energy balance theory. Simply put, the theory holds that an excessive number of calories ingested, but not required, for metabolic needs results in an excessive body weight. Conversely, fewer calories in the presence of demanding exercise and work create a deficit that allows weight loss to occur. No matter what the source of energy (e.g., carbohydrate, protein, fat), excessive calories are converted to be stored as fat. Excessive body

weight, then, usually is from excessive intramuscular and subcutaneous fat stores.

Behavioral Theories

The primary focus of behavioral theories in weight management is that behaviors such as overeating are learned responses. Interventions such as behavior modification techniques (based on Skinner's stimulus response theory) are aimed at controlling stimuli that result in actions that perpetuate overeating.[10] Some believe stimulus control strategies can permanently change external motivations related to eating. Thus, stimulus control strategies are designed to control eating by restricting calories, choices, locations, and timing, while avoiding environmental or external stimuli that may lead to eating outside those limitations.

Many calorie-restricted diets and food supplements are a type of stimulus control strategy that concentrates on controlling antecedent stimuli (controlling what, when, where, and how much to eat). At one end of a nutritional continuum are extreme, unhealthy diets (e.g., grapefruit diet or high-protein diet); at the other end are balanced healthy diets from the food pyramid. Even healthy diets can be difficult to comply with over the long term when they are aimed at controlling hunger. No matter how healthy they may be, stimulus-controlled diets focus on avoiding or eliminating hunger. When the body's natural, physiologic, internal signals of hunger are erased, individuals are forced to focus on external cues to tell them when they need to eat.

The holistic self-care model for long-term weight management is based on the premise that stimulus control addresses only half of the reasons for weight gain—the external reasons. The other half of the reasons for weight gain are internal. To make long-term lifestyle changes that promote fat loss, it is necessary to emphasize healthy eating for hunger rather than the elimination of hunger.

Clients should be assisted in calculating the number of calories that they require to meet their basic metabolic and exercise metabolic needs, based on American Dietetic Association guidelines (daily calories 1,200). Health-promoting behavioral techniques help clients learn how to distribute calories among the food pyramid groups and record daily intake according to time, place, kinds, amounts, pyramid groups, social situation, and hunger level.

Weight management strategies that concentrate on modifying behavior by differentiating stimuli before, during, and after eating (i.e., identifying stimuli other than hunger that trigger eating, monitoring amounts and conditions during eating, and rewarding appropriate actions) are a healthy start toward lasting weight management. Two health-promoting programs based primarily on behavioral strategies are Weight Watchers and Brownell's LEARN program—Lifestyle, Exercise, Attitudes, Relationships, and Nutrition.[11] Environmental modifications can enhance the effectiveness of dietary restrictions that lead to weight loss.[12] Modifying environmental stimuli before eating includes limiting the place, the amounts and types of available foods, shopping, and food preparation. Techniques for modifying environmental stimuli during eating include using small dishes, eating slowly, chewing multiple times before swallowing, and putting eating utensils down between bites. Modifying after eating includes keeping a food diary, weighing daily, and reinforcing positive actions (losing weight and exercising).

Most behavioral programs require individuals to monitor and record their compliance with prescribed dietary restrictions. They are assisted with setting up a meaningful reward system, such as money, special gifts, and entertainment. Individuals usually are weighed weekly, as weight loss becomes the external indicator of progress. Generally, there is less emphasis on internal indicators of progress, such as

changes in thinking and feelings, than on external indicators, such as weight, body shape, and body size. Behavioral therapy has been effective on a short-term basis for those who have little weight to lose. Researchers have reported greater success when behavioral approaches are paired with cognitive techniques.[13]

Psychologic Theories

Weight management interventions based on psychologic theories usually are directed toward decreasing stress-induced eating and helping to find ways to control eating in the presence of stressful situations. Similarly, negative body image, poor self-esteem, depression, and issues of social discrimination become the focus of psychotherapy, while dietary and exercise prescriptions usually receive less emphasis during therapy. Binge eating disorder, bulimia, and compulsive overeating are treated as relationship disorders that have similar etiologies but are manifested differently. When in therapy, individuals with eating disorders are encouraged to focus on related issues of abandonment and verbal, sexual, and physical abuse rather than the eating problem per se, unless physical well-being is threatened.[14]

Cognitive Theories

Beck explained how unrealistic and negative thinking triggers unpleasant emotional responses that can lead to overeating and not getting regular exercise.[15] Interventions based on cognitive theory are aimed at providing rapid symptomatic improvement and understanding of mood changes, coping strategies for self-management when upset, and guidance for personal growth. Individuals are assisted in assessing their basic values and attitudes that lead to negative feelings, as well as in reevaluating and challenging basic assumptions about their self-worth. Problem solving and coping techniques help clients to deal effectively with major, realistic problems (e.g., low self-esteem, guilt) and minor vague irritations (e.g., frustration, apathy) that seem to have no obvious external cause.

The first principle of cognitive theory is that all moods are created by thinking. Beliefs, perceptions, and mental attitudes make up cognitions, that is, how people interpret their world and what they are saying to themselves at a specific moment in time. Thinking brings about feelings and emotional responses. The second principle of cognitive theory is that negative emotional responses are pervasive and tend to color other perceptions of the world in a negative way. Although people's negative perceptions are very real to them, their perceptions often are illogical in actuality. The final principle is that the negative thoughts that elicit emotional turmoil usually contain gross distortions; most of the time, suffering results from distorted thinking rather than from the actual perceived cause.

Beck offered cognitive restructuring techniques to help identify and eliminate cognitive distortions that elicit irrational emotional responses. Beck's approach to cognitive restructuring uses three steps:

1. Identify automatic thoughts that are self-critical.
2. Identify any cognitive distortions and unrealistic beliefs underlying the thoughts.
3. Provide rational responses that defend the self.

The aim of cognitive restructuring is to substitute objective rational thoughts for illogical, harsh self-criticisms that predominate in response to negative events.

Failure of Traditional Weight Management Interventions

Failure rates for most weight reduction programs have been estimated to be as high as 90 to 95 percent.[16] Many interventions that have been shown to fail to pro-

mote long-term weight management (1) are restrictive in calories, choices, and times to eat; (2) are unidimensional, using only one major means to achieve weight loss and not including regular exercise; (3) do not permit individuals to tailor weight management to their preferences, lifestyles, and humanness; and (4) do not focus on internal motivations for overeating and for not exercising regularly.

Restrictions on Calories, Choices, and Times

Interventions that restrict calories, choices, and times to eat offer a temporary and artificial modification that is unrealistic for the long term. In a 1985 national health survey, 45 percent of women respondents were dieting to lose weight.[17] Almost a decade later, Wing reported that approximately 75 percent of women had attempted to lose weight.[18] Despite dieting attempts, the prevalence of being overweight increased from 25 to 33 percent between 1980 and 1991.[19] Also people are trying to eat less fat, but are getting fatter.[20] In a 1994 Agriculture Department survey of 5,500 U.S. citizens, one in three adults was overweight.[21] In an effort to follow recommendations to reduce fat intake, they reported eating more grains, but in doing so increased their intake of snacks by 200 percent and their intake of ready-to-eat cereals by 60 percent. It seems that their responses to dietary restrictions and deprivation have ultimately resulted in overeating, which may have led to weight gain. When calories and choices are restricted, human beings usually revert to old patterns that led to being overweight in the first place. Finding less restrictive means of reducing caloric intake while providing for human fallibility is necessary for long-term weight management.[22,23]

Use of One Dimension Only

Interventions that use only one major means to achieve weight loss and do not include regular exercise do not address the many reasons that people gained weight in the first place. Brownell and Wadden stressed that the time has come to abandon the societal mentality that a single weight reduction approach will be successful for all people desiring to lose weight.[24] The most successful long-term interventions to date are those that have combined a control of healthy food intake and aerobic exercise.[25,26] Since the 1980s, weight management literature often focused on the very low calorie diets (VLCDs), offered alone, in combination with stimulus control, or in combination with exercise, or on all three interventions at once.[27-30] Once again, while most of these diets led to weight loss, the regain of weight was remarkable across all programs. It seems likely that the long-term failure of these programs can be traced to the food restrictions discussed earlier. Most diets, especially VLCDs, are unnatural and time-limited. Exercise that has been teamed with dieting is often discontinued when the diet is discontinued, possibly because the program was not tailored to individuals' preferences, lifestyles, and humanness.

Similarly, many medical interventions that can yield weight loss in the short term fail in the long term. Such interventions include surgical reduction of the gastrointestinal tract, stomach expansion devices to simulate feeling full, and drugs to suppress the appetite—all aimed at reducing amounts of ingested foods. Appetite suppressants, such as the recently banned dexfenfluramine (Redux) and fenfluramine (PhenFen), promoted weight loss as long as clients continued taking them.[31] There is a dramatic weight regain when the medication is withdrawn and clients have not incorporated lifestyle changes, such as concurrent regular exercise, however. Perhaps equally disconcerting about taking pharmacologic agents are the negative side effects, such as neurotoxicity and pulmonary hypertension.[32]

Regular exercise as part of weight management is controversial. Researchers have found conflicting evidence about the role that exercise plays in weight loss; also controversial is the belief that dietary restrictions decrease the resting metabolic rate. About 60 to 75 percent of daily energy expenditure is accounted for by the resting metabolic rate. Therefore, any reduction in the resting metabolic rate could inhibit weight loss and lead to weight regain. Research findings suggest that exercise can prevent a reduction in the resting metabolic rate, either by elevating it following the exercise or by maintaining or increasing fat-free mass (lean body mass).[33] The results of one recent meta-analysis indicated that, while weight loss was similar between diet only and diet and exercise groups, the diet only groups lost proportionally more weight as fat-free mass or lean body mass (25 percent) than did the diet and exercise groups (17 percent).[34] Greater loss of lean body mass has potential for reducing resting metabolic rate; consequently, daily energy expenditure also is reduced.

Some researchers have demonstrated an elevated resting metabolic rate following exercise.[35,36] These discrepancies may result from variability in research methodologies. Recently, Wadden and associates tested resting energy expenditure and fat-free mass in a 48-week diet and exercise study with four treatment conditions—diet alone, diet plus aerobic exercise, diet plus strength exercise, and diet plus combined aerobic and strength exercise.[37] At 48 weeks, they found no statistically significant differences among conditions in weight or body composition; however, all three exercise conditions had smaller reductions in resting energy expenditure than did the diet alone condition. A combined aerobic and strength exercise program used in long-term weight management appears to maximize individuals' chances of not reducing fat-free mass and resting metabolic rate. Also the combined exercise program offers multiple types of exercise that increase variability and flexibility in exercise routines.

Magical thinking encourages individuals to seek "quick fix" programs with little or no exercise. Some individuals, especially women, hold to the magical thinking that they can rapidly achieve slimmer images and will have lasting results without extended and consistent use of nutritional and exercise strategies. In the author's experience, women who do *not* think magically about weight loss are usually older (35 to 45 years), often have tried many weight loss methods, have failed frequently, and have learned from their experiences that quick-fix weight loss methods lead only to more failures. They can articulate what they want in life and are more willing to expend effort to achieve "a healthier, more energetic body, mind, and lifestyle."

Foster and associates found that obese women who were more dissatisfied with their weight had greater feelings of failure and initially made greater efforts to lose weight.[38] These dissatisfied subjects, however, also felt less success when they reached their goal weight. They expressed less self-acceptance, were less likely to have long-term success, and often regained weight.

Inability To Tailor Weight Management Program to the Individual

Interventions that do not permit individuals to tailor weight management to their preferences, lifestyles, and humanness cannot be lasting. Weight loss interventions fail when program directives are too stringent for individuals to gain a sense of ownership and to accept the weight management strategies as a way of life. Instead, individuals view weight management as something that will happen magically if they can endure program directives long enough. Usually, they do not view "the program" as a long-term lifestyle change and, therefore, do not address their individual preferences (e.g., dislike for certain foods and types of exercise), way of life (e.g., working nights, family versus single), and "being human" along the way (e.g., not feeling guilty or dropping out when they deviate from the plan).

The American Dietetic Association has stated that, to achieve long-term weight management, adults must make a lifelong commitment to healthy lifestyle changes.[39] Both daily physical activity and eating should be *sustainable* and *enjoyable*—terms that imply personal tailoring of healthy, yet livable lifetime habits. Without individualization, a lifelong program is not possible, since life is ever-changing and adaptation is the norm.

Inability To Focus on Internal Motivation for Overeating and Lack of Exercise

Interventions that are not focused on internal motivations for overeating and for lack of regular exercise generally do not uncover the underlying reasons for overweight. Weight management programs that do not assist overweight individuals in understanding their motivations for keeping the weight on have limited long-term success.[40] Perhaps the reason that stimulus control techniques have had limited success is because they seek to control the diet and environment, but do not take into account that eating may be a coping mechanism to manage unpleasant feelings.[41] Researchers have emphasized that weight management should include biologic, psychologic, and social interventions to normalize eating and separate physical from emotional hunger.[42]

New Weight Management Interventions

When overweight individuals first recognize that they often cope with stressors by eating and then learn to manage stressors in healthier ways, controlling intake and environmental influences can gradually lose their importance for long-term weight management. Existing programs that use behavioral approaches, cognitive restructuring, or combinations thereof may not address the effects of negative beliefs about self and irrational perceptions of the world. Self-talk and cognitive restructuring used in most interventions focus on thinking about food, relationships with others around food, and restructured thinking about hunger and satiation. For example, in his popular LEARN Program for Weight Control, Brownell presented a cognitive approach concerning unattainable goals that individuals trying to lose weight tend to set for themselves for eating, exercise, and weight loss. "When the goals are not met, the negative emotional response can send . . . progress into a tailspin."[43] Setting realistic goals is important for a long-term weight loss program; however, the holistic self-care model takes a different approach by first helping individuals set realistic goals for assessing overeating situations and discovering what feelings may have triggered them (instead of goals focused on eating, exercise, and number of pounds lost). Cognitive restructuring based on reversal theory extends the current use of this technique to include self-talk about self and relationships in addition to food and weight-related topics.

Based on reversal theory states as a frame of reference, cognitive restructuring centers on the negative self-statement (probably unrelated to being overweight) that triggered overeating and/or prevented regular exercise. Using cognitive restructuring based on reversal theory worksheets (see Exhibit 27–1), clients are assisted to pinpoint negative self-talk stemming from overeating situations, but they also are assisted to move to a higher level than many weight management programs to identify illogical, unrealistic, and negative self-talk about themselves and their relationships. Traditional stimulus control strategies of-

fer assistance to lose weight by controlling diet and environmental factors. Cognitive restructuring strategies discussed in weight management literature offer assistance only at the first level beyond stimulus control strategies by adding inquiry about self-talk related to being overweight, eating, and dieting. When cognitive restructuring is used in a limited or random way of relating only to weight-related concerns, it may serve as just another stimulus-control strategy.

Reversal theory states provide needed structure for ensuring that the underlying issues related to overeating and lack of exercise can be discovered and managed directly. Cognitive restructuring based on reversal theory offers a higher level of assistance to address negative and faulty thinking about self and relationships that may lead to overeating and skipping exercise. The National Task Force on the Prevention and Treatment of Obesity urged researchers to help overweight individuals make lifelong changes in behavioral patterns, diet, and physical activity.[44] Recently, weight management researchers recommended that interventions should focus on healthy new lifestyle habits that eventually bring about a moderate, permanent weight loss.[45] The holistic self-care model is a multidimensional approach designed to counter each reason that traditional weight management programs fail.

First, reversal theory will be explained and then the combined theoretical framework for cognitive theory based on reversal theory (used as the basis of the holistic self-care model) will be reviewed. Specific cognitive strategies based on reversal theory will be presented.

Reversal Theory

Apter's theory of psychologic reversals, commonly referred to as reversal theory, provides a framework to explain factors related to overeating and lack of exercise in overweight individuals.[46] According to this

Exhibit 27-1 Reversal Theory Sample Self-Talk

About Self and Others

What is my fat self saying to me?   What is my thin self saying to me?

TELIC
(Serious-minded, goal & future-oriented)
(anxious or calm?)

"I keep on task."

"I never seem to get my work done."

PARATELIC
(Playful, emphasizing good feelings, present-oriented)
(bored or excited?)

"I'm active & play often."

"I'm not having much fun these days."

CONFORMIST
(Following rules, agreeable, concerned about what others think) (uncomfortable or comfortable?)

"I know when to play people games."

"I never seem to be able to do the right thing."

NEGATIVISTIC
(Sticking up for what I think, angry, doing my own thing) (trapped or free?)

"I can tactfully say what I think."

"I can't say what I really think."

MASTERY
(Do my best, be strong, be tough, compete)
(out of control or in control?)

"I know when to give it my all."

"I'm out of control."

SYMPATHY
(Want harmony, feel deserved reward, feel tender)
(deprived or cared for?)

"I'm having a good social life."

"I have no social life."

ALLOIC
(Think of others first before myself)
(Feel ashamed or satisfied?)

"I like to give to others."

"I withdraw from giving to others."

AUTIC
(Think of self first before others)
(Feel bad about self or good about self?)

"I'm not afraid to put myself first occasionally."

"I never get what I want from others."

---

phenomenologic theory of arousal, motivation, and action, Apter posits that personality is inherently inconsistent and that individuals reverse between opposing, paired
states called metamotivational states because they are not, in themselves, concerned with motivation, but rather with the
way in which motivation is experienced.
Psychologically healthy individuals experience their motivations and actions in different ways, depending on metamotivational states. Four pairs of opposing states
have been identified: telic/paratelic, con-
formist/negativistic, mastery/sympathy,
and alloic/autic (Exhibit 27–2). At a given
point in time, individuals are in combinations of the different states, consisting of
one state of each of the four pairs, but never
in both states of a pair at the same time.

When in the telic state, individuals are
serious-minded and goal-oriented; when in
the paratelic state, they are playful and
spontaneous (see Exhibit 27–2). When in the
conformist state, people prefer to go along
with rules and regulations; when in the
negativistic state, they prefer to break rules
and want to be rebellious or noncompliant.
When in the mastery state, individuals feel
that being tough and being in control are
important; when in the sympathy state,
they feel that being tender and not competing are important. In the alloic state,
people derive pleasure from thinking of
others before themselves in an altruistic
way; in the autic state, they derive pleasure
from thinking of themselves before others.
Healthy individuals reverse between
states easily and often throughout the day.

Researchers explored reversal theory in
smoking cessation studies as an explanation of behaviors in smoking relapse and
abstinence.[47] Subjects who were more likely
to relapse were in the paratelic, negativistic,
and sympathy states, while those who were
more likely to abstain were in the telic, conformist, and mastery states. Similarly, reversal theory may explain how dieting and resisting overeating are consistent with telic,

conformist, and mastery states. Paratelic,
negativistic, and sympathy states may be
one explanation for the apparent self-sabo-
tage of overweight individuals who can
cope with stressors some of the time without
overeating, but not at other times.

Unpleasant Feelings and Tension Stress.
Each metamotivational state has pleasant
and unpleasant feelings and responses associated with it (indicated by asterisks in
Exhibit 27–2). Pleasant responses, depending on the metamotivational state, include
feeling calm, excited, free, and proud. Unpleasant responses include feeling anxious, bored, angry, trapped, ashamed, humiliated, guilty, and resentful, which
represent tension stress. According to reversal theory, tension stress is the discrep-
ancy between desired and actual feelings.
Individuals can take actions to reduce the
level of tension stress within the same
metamotivational state or may experience
a spontaneous reversal to the opposing
state within the metamotivational pair.

> K.Z., 29 years old, reported how
> she repeatedly used overeating
> as an attempt to reduce tension
> stress within the same reversal
> theory state.[48] "While I'm eating,
> I'm oblivious to everything else.
> I'm not thinking about what is
> hurting me. . . . Its just like an es-
> cape . . . to be able to eat is just an
> escape from everything. . . . The
> only time I can turn myself off is
> when I'm eating." K.Z. spontane-
> ously described a happening re-
> ferred to in the literature as the
> escape phenomenon and in clini-
> cal practice as "numbing out."
> She obtained relief from unpleas-
> ant feelings (tension stress) by
> "numbing out" during eating,
> even though she knew she would
> not feel good later.
>
> On the particular occasion that
> K.Z. related overeating, she had

Exhibit 27–2 Reversal Theory Metamotivational States Pairs and Characteristics

---

EIGHT WAYS OF BEING HUMAN
(Characteristics of Apter's Reversal Theory Metamotivational States Pairs)

TELIC
Serious-minded
Goal-oriented
Plan ahead
Try to accomplish something
Future-oriented
*anxiety **calmness

PARATELIC
Playful
Spontaneous
Emphasize good feelings
Have fun for fun's sake
Present-oriented
*boredom **excitement

CONFORMIST
Don't make waves or disagree with others
Follow the rules
Feel embarrassed/guilty if I break a rule
Compliant
Agreeable
Stay in line
Do what others do
Worry about what others think
*unprotected **protected

NEGATIVISTIC
Stick up for what I think when I disagree
 with others
Bend/break the rules
Feel angry
Stubborn
Rebellious/defiant
Want to be difficult

*trapped **free

MASTERY
Do your best
Give it your all
Be strong & don't show feelings of weakness
Be tough, stay strong
Compete
Be in control
*soft **hardy

SYMPATHY
Let my feelings tell me what to do
Deserve a break
OK to show & tell feelings of weakness
Be tender, OK to not be strong
Don't compete
Be nurturing
*insensitive **sensitive

ALLOIC
Think of others first
Put self last
Others are most important
*shame **modesty
*guilt **virtue

AUTIC
Think of self first
Put others after self
I am most important
*humiliation **pride
*resentment **gratitude

*unpleasant feelings/responses (tension stress) associated with specific metamotivational states
**pleasant feelings/responses associated with specific metamotivational states
Source: From Popkess-Vawter, S. (1997). Chapter 27 Weight Management. In B.M. Dossey (Ed.), *American Holistic Nurses' Association Core Curriculum for Holistic Nursing* (pp. 211–219). Gaithersburg, MD: Aspen.

---

an unpleasant telephone exchange with her mother. She was saying to herself in her mind, "It's always my fault! I'm always the bad guy!" She related that these negative self-talk words represent many old interpersonal conflicts experienced with her mother and family members.

Repeated negative thoughts can evoke negative feelings that, in turn, can evoke negative behavior such as coping by eating favorite foods to feel better. Another client told about a similar unpleasant incident on the telephone with her sister. "Even though I had eaten breakfast and was not hungry, while still on the phone I knew I was going to go get donuts to feel better."

Cognitive Therapy Based on Reversal Theory. Beck described cognitive therapy as helping clients restructure self-statements to be more realistic and positive, which in turn will elicit positive responses.[49] Cognitive theories by themselves cannot explain why people can cope with stressors some of the time (do not overeat to cope) and not at other times (overeat to cope). Reversal theory, a relatively new theory, offers an added dimension to cognitive restructuring by providing the necessary organizing structure to do two things: (1) locate tension stress in the most salient state where negative self-talk originates, and (2) tailor interventions to decrease tension stress. Reversal theory was found in previous studies to explain overeating and lack of exercise in overweight women and served as the basis for cognitive strategies discussed later.[50-52]

Brownell and others emphasized that overweight individuals need help accepting themselves rather than being in relentless pursuit of an unrealistic ideal.[53] When weight management program designers try to address the humanness involved in weight management, it is easy either to oversimplify or to oversaturate the cognitive–behavioral content. Perhaps program designers are simply inexperienced in including cognitive content specifically directed at underlying thinking and feelings that lead to overeating or not exercising. There is growing objective evidence, however, that this critical psycho-social-spiritual portion in the holistic self-care model can contribute to long-term weight management.[54]

The theoretical framework guiding intervention strategies is based on cognitive and reversal theories. Exhibit 27–3 depicts the theoretical framework and the three cognitive restructuring strategies (EAT for hunger, Exercise for LIFE, and STOP emotional eating). Cognitive restructuring based on reversal theory provides a vehicle focused on self and relationships with others in general *and* on hunger, eating, and exercise in particular.

Cognitive Restructuring As a Weight Management Technique

Although cognitive restructuring is not a new technique used in weight management, the applications cited in the literature do not address directly how negative beliefs about self and irrational perceptions of the world can produce negative self-talk that triggers overeating behavior. Instead, cognitive techniques seem to be targeted at feeling better about food, weight, and weight-related relationships. Self-talk *unrelated* to food, weight, and weight-related relationships can reveal repeating, powerful, and caustic messages that lead to overeating and skipped exercise, however.

Cognitive restructuring based on reversal theory is a set of strategies to identify and replace unrealistic, negative self-talk with realistic, positive self-talk. The eight metamotivational states of reversal theory provide the needed structure for tracking three types of salient self-talk statements: (1) self-talk about self and others in general, (2) self-talk about hunger and eating, and (3) self-talk about exercising in particular (Exhibit 27–1). Beliefs about the self, including self-esteem and body image, may be sufficiently negative and unrealistic to evoke negative thoughts and feelings. Overweight clients can learn to recognize negative self-talk, accept their irrationality, and develop new cognitive skills to manage negative motivations. Cognitive restructuring based on reversal theory seems to bring the first level of understanding and healing for overweight individuals. The next level involves the long-term process of self-discovery, values clarification, and self-talk replacement in order to equip clients with internal skills and strategies for dealing directly with emotional upsets.

Subjects in previous study responded to unpleasant feelings by overeating in ev-

Exhibit 27–3 Daily Calendar

HOLISTIC SELF-CARE   *Thought for the Day:* I equally accept my eight ways of being human.

Today's date ___-___-___ positive self-talk _____

Today's planned exercise _____

This week's goals _____

BELIEFS ⟶ COGNITIONS ⟶ EMOTIONS ⟶ ACTIONS
– Self-esteem   – Thinking   – Feelings   – Overeating
& Unrealistic Beliefs   & – Self-Talk   – Exercising

Cognitive Restructuring ⟶ + Feelings ⟶ + Eating for Hunger
Based on Reversal Theory   + Exercising for Life
EAT for hunger
Exercise for LIFE
STOP emotional eating

E at for body or mind hunger↷ ? Paratelic?   starving 1 2 3 4 5 feel nothing 6 7 8 9 10 stuffed
A sk appetite & enjoy each bite Paratelic?
T ell self when hunger is gone Telic goal?
↷ If mind hunger, go to STOP strategy

(Circle)   Low tension stress 1 2 3 4 5 6 7 8 9 10 high tension stress
                    [Go to RT relaxation-affirmation and Self-talk sheets]
S top   RT relaxation-affirmation
T ell   RT state, feelings & self-talk
O ptions   for positive self-talk
P lan   to deal with feelings without eating
          exercise   self-talk strategy   journal   call friend   other _____

Did I do my planned exercise today?   Yes!! ___ No ___ (Why?)

Did I overeat today?   No!! ___ Yes ___ How many times? _____

What is the *underlying trigger* leading me to overeating, no exercise, and feeling bad
about myself?_____

"X" off servings as you eat   How was my nutrition today?

from the Pyramid ⟹   Wow!___ Good ___ OK ___
                        Better luck tomorrow ___

few
fats & sweets
xl   xl

MILK   **MEAT**
xl xl xl   xl xl

VEGGIES   **FRUITS**
xl xl xl xl   xl xl xl xl

GRAINS
xl xl xl xl xl xl xl xl xl

Source: Copyright © 1996, Sue Popkess-Vawter.

eryday situations, including feeling anxious on the job and before examinations, feeling angry after disagreements with family or friends, and feeling bored and tired after getting off work.[55] Most overeating occasions were *unrelated* to being overweight. It follows that long-term weight management may logically focus more of the time on managing responses to everyday emotional upsets (cognitive restructuring based on reversal theory) rather than on manipulating the environment to remove temptations to eat (stimulus control). For example, in the case of K.Z. discussed earlier, a nurse would assist her (alone or in a group) to reflect on a reported overeating situation and would guide her through the EAT and STOP strategies (see Exhibit 27–3).

The nutritional strategy is called "EAT for hunger": *E*at for body or mind hunger?, *A*sk appetite and enjoy each bite, and *T*ell self when hunger is gone. The first step is cognitive, represented by *E* because it asks individuals whether they are experiencing actual physiologic hunger or emotional hunger. The nurse would guide K.Z. in determining whether she was actually physically hungry or emotionally hungry. If actually hungry, clients rate their hunger on a scale of 1 to 10, where 1 represents feeling starved, 5 represents feeling nothing, and 10 represents feeling excessively full. In the second step, *A*, the nurse asks clients what food their bodies are hungry for while encouraging them to make healthy choices and yet not deprive themselves of formerly forbidden foods. They concentrate on enjoying the personal pleasures of tastes, textures, and consistencies of the food as they slowly enjoy every bite. (Paratelic and autic are salient states.) In the last step, *T*, the nurse again asks K.Z. and the group members to think about rating hunger on a continuum from 1 to 10 while eating and to stop when hunger was gone, usually at about a 5 on the scale. Eating smaller amounts is the aim of the last step to assist them to satisfy the body's needs without excess.

Again using K.Z.'s example, if she identified that she was "emotionally hungry," the nurse would assist her with the psychosocial-spiritual strategy, "STOP emotional eating." Negative self-talk involving self and others can trigger desires to eat, often at times when the individuals are not hungry, adding excess calories. Overweight clients may not be aware of the many daily emotional triggers that habitually lead to overeating. Thoughts, memories, and self-talk can lead them to emotional triggers of overeating.

The purpose of the "STOP emotional eating" strategy is to help clients separate emotions from the eating response and learn new, constructive strategies for managing triggers of overeating. K.Z. and the group would learn to Stop for relaxation–affirmation, Tell feelings and self-talk, explore Options for positive self-talk, and Plan to deal with feelings without eating. The first step is the reversal theory relaxation–affirmation exercise, a 10-minute activity that begins a head-to-toe relaxation response (Exhibit 27–4).

After relaxing, clients move to affirmations intended to remind them of their eight ways of being human (i.e., the eight reversal theory states). Emotions stemming from one salient reversal theory state can be traced to discover the faulty self-talk that triggered the desire to eat. "Feeling the Feelings," a cognitive technique consisting of four ordered skills, can facilitate the Tell feelings and self-talk step. With this technique, the nurse helps clients release tension from unpleasant feelings (lower tension stress) and accept negativistic and sympathy state responses by

1. recognizing and experiencing feelings, such as feeling tired, bored, lonely, anxious, tense, angry, and depressed. Often, clients think that feeling negative emotions is undesirable, rather than viewing feelings as natural human responses to illogical thinking patterns.

Exhibit 27–4 Reversal Theory Relaxation–Affirmations Exercise

---

TEN-MINUTE *EIGHT WAYS OF BEING HUMAN**
Relaxation–Affirmations Exercise

Relaxation

Now, seated comfortably, I close my eyes and take three deep, cleansing breaths letting go of all unpleasant feelings. I gently tighten and relax muscles from my head to my toes (face & neck, hands, arms & shoulders, abdominal & back, legs & feet). Remaining relaxed, I choose to go to my most favorite place in the whole world on a one-minute vacation. I experience fully all of the sights, sounds, smells, and feelings of this place.

2'

2'45" (after 1 minute). . . . Now, with my eyes still closed, I choose to listen to my Eight Ways of Being Human affirmations. As I listen, I can feel myself becoming more and more balanced and becoming my real self.

Affirmations

I know when to **1-work** and when to **2-play.** I choose to do both and I accept both parts of me.

I know when to **3-follow the rules** and when to **4-break the rules.** I choose to do both and I accept both parts of me.

I know when to be **5-tough** and when to be **6-tender.** I choose to do both and I accept both parts of me.

I know when to **7-give to others** and when to **8-give to myself.** I choose to do both and I accept both parts of me.

4'30" I will make good choices for myself. I am letting go of all unpleasant feelings and choose to trust that I will make good choices for myself.
I am still very relaxed with my eyes closed. For the next few minutes, I will picture in my mind a figure "8" representing my Eight Ways of Being Human. I will focus only on that figure "8". If thoughts come into my awareness, I will simply go with them rather than resist them, getting back to my figure "8" as soon as I can.

5' I'm now tracing that figure "8" in my mind.

6' (after 1 minute). . . . Very relaxed, still tracing the figure "8."

9' (after 3 minutes). . . . Now, very slowly, I'm coming back to this time and place.

(after 30 seconds). . . . Still very relaxed, I now open my eyes and keep this relaxed and balanced feeling as I go and make good choices.

*Numbers 1 to 8 in the affirmations indicate the eight ways of being human. Times in the left margin may be used to record a personal audiotape for daily use.
Source: Copyright © 1996, Sue Popkess-Vawter.

---

2. accepting their feelings as part of being human.
3. thinking about ways that past conditioning may have caused them to think about issues in irrational or unrealistic ways, which in turn leads them to respond to feelings by overeating.

4. learning new skills to manage feelings, such as the "Fighting Fair" technique used to manage anger, disappointment, and resentment.

The self-talk worksheets are given to clients to help pinpoint emotional triggers of overeating and excuses not to exercise regularly (see Exhibit 27–1). By using the worksheets, they can learn to "hear" negative self statements and then replace them with Options for positive self-talk. The sample worksheets contain eight sets of abstract drawings of an overweight woman and a normal weight woman, one set for each of the reversal theory states. Beside each drawing, respectively, is a line where clients are assisted to identify and write the self-talk statements in response to two questions, "What is your fat self saying to you?" and "What is your thin self saying to you?" The worksheets in Exhibit 27–1 are samples of self-talk frequently used by individuals who gain and lose weight in a cyclic pattern. Clients can complete worksheets monthly to identify their current self-talk and compare worksheets with those in past months. Clients thus can identify progress and problem areas for support and suggestions.

Nurses teach their clients the four ordered skills in the Fighting Fair technique to help them manage most negative emotions. First, the technique assists clients in determining objectively what they thought about the situation that triggered negative emotions. Second, they tell what they did not like about what happened; third, how it made them feel. The fourth step is to ask clients what they need from themselves and/or other person(s) to negotiate a win–win situation in which they and others can get at least part of what they need. This technique is intended to help clients Plan to deal with feelings without overeating.

Holistic Self-Care Model

Designed to assist overweight clients with individualized nutritional, exercise, and psycho-social-spiritual strategies for a long-term pursuit of healthier and happier lifestyles, the holistic self-care model has an individualized focus. Health care professionals help overweight clients become sensitive to their bodies, motivations, self-talk, feelings, and actions. Holistic self-care emphasizes concurrent work in nutritional, exercise, and psycho-social-spiritual dimensions to reduce the percentage of body fat and increase physical fitness.

Externally focused, "quick fix" methods have limited effects and may compound the overweight problem through, for example, a reduction in metabolic rate and serious drug side effects. In contrast, the holistic self-care model takes an internal perspective to seek insight about negative self-talk that obstructs long-term guidance from the body's natural hunger and satiety signals, as well as the positive benefits and sensations of regular exercise. The challenge that faces health care professionals is to design multidimensional interventions aimed at correcting what researchers know causes individuals to drop out of weight programs—namely, feelings of restrictions and deprivations, no time for exercise, and hassles of daily living that habitually send overweight clients to seek relief from stressors by eating.

The holistic self-care model provides a unique plan of weekly face-to-face counseling appointments and continuing support and guidance for individualizing and adjusting lifelong strategies. It is based on the following principles for long-term weight management:

- There is continual feedback among the three dimensions of eating, physical exercise, and self-talk, as in the integration among mind, body, and spirit.
- Both nurses and clients who gain and lose weight in a cycle must give equal consideration to the mind, body, and spirit trinity as they develop permanent life changes.
- Clients are in charge of redesigning lifestyle patterns in these three areas, consistent with self-care tenets.
- Permanent life changes take a very long time. Old habits can be changed

through small steady efforts that lead to greater success, as opposed to drastic changes that lead to feelings of deprivation, burnout, relapse, and eventual failure.

The holistic self-care model emphasizes integrated care and empowerment of clients in mind, body, and spirit. Nurses sometimes find performing interventions for the mind and body more familiar and comfortable, but supporting and intervening for spirituality concerns may be the most important contribution that they can make to promote health. Spirituality can hold all the other parts of individuals together. Religious beliefs are those beliefs in a power greater than that which humans possess—a higher authority and guiding spirit. Existential beliefs include values, meanings, and sense of purpose.

Nurses who address clients' spirituality as part of caregiving can help strengthen clients' sense of meaning, dignity, worth, and identity; healing becomes possible for low self-esteem, feelings of isolation, anger, powerlessness, and hopelessness. Human practices of honesty, love, caring, wisdom, imagination, and compassion can create a flowing, dynamic balance that allows and creates healing. The cognitive restructuring based on reversal theory is the part of the holistic self-care model that addresses clients' spirituality, the glue that can hold together bio-psycho-social-spiritual beings to become greater than the sum of their parts and to make long-lasting lifestyle changes.

HOLISTIC CARING PROCESS

Assessment

In preparing to use weight management interventions, the nurse assesses the following parameters:

- **body composition**—baseline and at least every 6 months
  - —body mass index
  - —percentage of body fat
- **resting heart rate and blood pressure**
- **blood profile**—baseline and at least every 6 months
  - —cholesterol level
  - —high- and low-density lipoprotein levels
  - —blood glucose level
- **physical fitness**
  - —if possible, exercise testing using submaximal bicycle ergometer or maximal treadmill
  - —strength testing using repetition maximum for chest press and leg press (or comparable exercises)
- **psychologic profile**
  - —Life review and dieting history— from clients' stories of their lives and the evolution of their weight problem; identification of lifestyle patterns
  - —BULIT (Bulimia Test) scale to screen for bulimia[56]
  - —body image according to a 10-point visual analog scale (1 being the best)
  - —tension stress scale[57]
  - —personal daily calendar (see Exhibit 27–3)

Patterns/Problems/Needs

The following patterns/problems/needs compatible with weight management interventions related to the nine human response patterns (see Chapter 14) are as follows:

- *Exchanging:* Altered nutrition (more than body requirements)
- *Valuing:* Spiritual distress
- *Choosing:* Ineffective individual coping
- *Moving:* Decreased physical mobility
- *Perceiving:* Disturbance in body image

Disturbance in self-
esteem
Hopelessness
- *Knowing:*   Knowledge deficit
- *Feeling:*   Anxiety

Specific patterns/problems/needs related to the holistic self-care model and reversal theory are

- overeating related to increased tension stress
- decreased aerobic/resistance exercise related to a poor body image and a feeling of being unworthy to take time for self to exercise
- infrequent episodes of play which are related to early modeling and values that consider work to be more important than play
- lack of skills to express anger/disagreement related to belief that it is unacceptable behavior
- lack of skills to express feelings related to early suppression of feelings as a self-protective mechanism
- inability to put self first related to early teaching that others have greater value and worth

Outcomes

Prochaska and DiClemente developed the transtheoretical therapy model to expand the applicability of change theory.[58] Their stages of change have been applied to a wide variety of health care problems, including weight management. They proposed that individuals may move through five stages of motivational readiness when confronted with lifestyle changes: (1) precontemplation, (2) contemplation, (3) preparation, (4) action, and (5) maintenance. Nurses should tailor their assessments, interventions, prescriptions, and evaluations to the individual's stage to attain long-term weight management (Table 27–1).

Most clients will begin sessions at either the precontemplation or the contemplation stage. It is possible for an individual to be in different stages of the nutritional, exercise, and psycho-social-spiritual dimensions of the program. For example, in the case of K.Z., she may be starting to exercise two to three times per week (preparation stage), but refuses to even discuss nutritional interventions (precontemplation stage). She apparently has no insight into her negative self-talk and, therefore, has no intention of changing (also precontemplation state).

Therapeutic Care Plan and Implementation

Before the Session

- Spend a few moments centering yourself to recognize your presence and to begin the session with the intention to facilitate healing.
- Create an environment in which the client will be encouraged to share his or her story.

At the Beginning of the Session

- Show a listing of the stages of change to the client and have him or her explain any differences between his or her stage at the last session and now. Accordingly, proceed with the holistic self-care model as shown in Table 27–1.

At the End of the Session

- Ask the client to review what he or she gained from the session and answer any questions. Give the client a copy of any relevant support materials, and ask him or her to explain how to use them. Ask him or her to complete a copy of the weekly calendar (Exhibit 27–5) and verbalize what he or she has written and the times allotted for the behaviors.

Specific Interventions

Specific interventions used in the holistic self-care model are listed and interpreted according to the five stages of change as described in Table 27–1.[59]

Table 27-1 Nursing Interventions: Long-Term Weight Management According to Prochaska and DiClemente's Stages of Change

Client Outcomes According to Stage of Change	Nursing Prescriptions	Evaluation
Precontemplation (no intention of changing in the next 6 months): The client will verbalize reasons for not wanting to reduce weight and fat, and perform regular exercise.	Measure client's body mass index, body fat, resting heart rate and blood pressure, cholesterol, lipids, and blood glucose. Administer life review and dieting history, BULIT (bulimia test) scale to screen for bulimia, and body image 10-point visual analog scale.	The client received a clinic weight management brochure with written report of her or his physical and psychologic findings. The client verbalized understanding of the report, implied risks, and invitation to learn more about the clinic weight program.
Contemplation (considering changing in the next 6 months, but not active yet): The client will report fewer overeating episodes and less tension stress during daily eating.	Assist the client to apply the EAT for hunger cognitive restructuring nutritional strategy based on reversal theory. Administer Tension Stress Scale.	The client verbalized the three steps of the EAT for hunger strategy and one difficulty with the strategy to work on in the next 6 months. The client was pleased with freedom of eating for hunger.
Preparation (making some changes, but not at goal): The client will report exercising more frequently, resulting in greater muscle strength, less fatigue, and more energy.	Assist the client to apply the Exercise for LIFE strategy based on reversal theory.	The client described aerobic and strength exercises that she or he is willing to do and one difficulty with the strategy to work on in the next 6 months. The client reported lower tension stress.
Action (6 months of active behavior change): The client will have lower levels of total cholesterol and low-density lipoproteins, a higher level of high-density lipoproteins, and blood glucose levels within normal limits.	Assist the client to apply the STOP emotional eating cognitive restructuring psycho-social-spiritual strategy based on reversal theory.	The client verbalized the four steps of the STOP emotional eating strategy and one difficulty with the strategy to work on in the next 6 months. The client is pleased with exercise progress.
Maintenance (sustained change past 6 months): The client will have a lower percentage of body fat, lower weight, lower resting heart rate, and lower blood pressure.	Assist the client to apply the acceptance of obstacles cognitive restructuring psycho-social-spiritual strategy.	The client verbalized the acceptance strategy and one difficulty with the strategy on which to concentrate efforts in the next 6 months. The client is pleased with lipid levels, weight, and blood pressure.

Precontemplation

When clients are not ready to make lifestyle changes, a nurse cannot "motivate" or manipulate them to do so. The nurse can inform them about his or her assessment of their situation, risks involved, and options available to them. Raising their consciousness without demands can do more to move them to the next level of readiness than giving them "pep talks" and trying to force them to see other perspectives. Thus, the nurse should teach the client the basic principles of the holistic self-care model for long-term weight management:

- There is no need to diet, count calories, and weigh daily/weekly. The percent-

Exhibit 27–5 Weekly Calendar

I, [Name], will do the following for the week of _____

My Realistic Goals for This Week:

Last week's major triggers that keep me overeating, not getting exercise, and feeling bad about myself:

1.

2.

Monday through Sunday Exercise Schedule:

Day of the Week	Aerobic Exercise	Resistance Exercise
Monday		
Tuesday		
Wednesday		
Thursday		
Friday		
Saturday		
Sunday		

Source: Copyright © 1996, Dr. Sue Popkess-Vawter.

age of body fat is a more accurate way to determine if clients weigh too much, since weight can be normal but consist of a high percentage of body fat and vice versa.

- Both physical and psychologic reasons that clients are not losing excess pounds must be addressed to be successful for the rest of their lives.
- Most people with weight problems have lost weight successfully at some point in their lives, but regained the weight. Often, they are very knowledgeable about food and exercise, and they may even be somewhat in touch with the psychologic reasons that they "go off" of their weight reduction programs.
- When young, many people learned to eat to feel better when they experienced unpleasant feelings; their active lifestyles kept them from having

an overweight problem until adult years. Greater responsibilities in adult life forced them to be more sedentary, allowing fat to accumulate and reducing lean body mass.

- Increasing pressures, stressors, and short-term bouts of weight gain (e.g., because of pregnancy, loss of a job) put extra pounds on individuals' bodies.
- Eating must be separated and disconnected from emotions and reconnected with naturally occurring hunger. Emotions, then, must be recognized, felt, and acted upon in healthy ways.
- The holistic self-care model for long-term weight management is the combination of stopping overeating, getting challenging exercise four to six times every week, and reprogramming negative, self-destructive self-talk to be realistic and personally valued self-talk.

Contemplation

Clients in the contemplation stage still believe that the reasons for not changing their behaviors (e.g., I am too tired, too hungry, too busy, don't have enough money) overbalance the reasons that they should. When past dieters view a future of dietary restrictions, their negative feelings toward past failures tip the balance of the scales in the negative direction.

EAT for Hunger Strategy. Under the EAT for hunger strategy, clients learn to eat according to their internal control (hunger) with as many food choices as desired; regulation of eating is according to internal satiation of their hunger.

The purpose of this nutritional strategy is to bring physiologic hunger and the pleasure of eating into balance. Clients should weigh only monthly or wait until the nurse weighs them at an appointment to increase the accuracy of true weight fluctuations and avoid unnecessary emotional responses to false readings of temporary

water weight loss and gain. They can be given the audiotape *Diets Still Don't Work* about how to stop overeating.[60] Group exercises, such as participating in a taste-testing exercise or eating a meal together, can reinforce new principles. Topics discussed in group or individual sessions can include why people overeat, why they lose weight, how thin people think and eat, why diets do not work, and why people choose fat over thin. Essential content in this nutritional strategy includes the food pyramid; the fat, cholesterol, and sodium content of foods; and the need for healthy choices.

Before beginning the strategy, the nurse should administer the BULIT and the tension stress scale to determine clients' risk for overeating and tension stress level before overeating, respectively. Scores on these measures serve as evaluation outcomes over time. The nurse should also encourage clients to think about the meaning that hunger has for them. In most cases, feeling hungry is associated with negative feelings of deprivation, past restrictions, and physical discomforts. They can learn to manage negative feelings associated with hunger and begin to think of hunger as a positive signal that tells them to eat.

Ways To Stop Overeating. Schwartz studied naturally thin people and discovered universal eating patterns.[61] Fat people have a different eating style, mainly that of eating certain predetermined foods and usually feeling deprived when these foods are forbidden. The sense of deprivation can lead to binge eating of the forbidden foods.

The three steps to stop overeating are written as positive self-talk (affirmations):

1. I eat only when I'm hungry, after rating my hunger on a scale of 1 to 10.
   a. Ravenously starved = 1
   b. Uncomfortably stuffed = 10
   c. Feeling nothing = 5
   d. Eating to satisfy hunger = between 4 and 6

2. I eat exactly what I want. My body has the natural ability to know what it wants and needs. When I crave "unhealthy, junk, and forbidden" foods, I ask myself if it is truly a physical craving; if so and I am hungry, I can eat it. If the food does not taste good, I don't eat it. I eat slowly, enjoying every bite. Eating slowly helps me fully experience the pleasure of eating the food. Eating slowly allows time for my brain to get the messages of satisfaction and feeling nothing (usually about 20 minutes). Conscious, enjoyable eating satisfies cravings so they will not return for a while.

3. I stop eating when my hunger is gone and I feel nothing (a rating of 5 on the 1 to 10 hunger scale). When I eat to a rating of 5, it is like drinking water until my thirst is gone. If hunger is still present, I take and enjoy three more bites slowly and then stop.

Minimum daily requirements may be met over 2 or 3 days rather than every day. When clients take in all of their calories to meet minimal daily requirements from foods that they "should" eat, extra calories eaten to satisfy natural cravings will be beyond their needs and result in stored fat. The American Diabetic Association Diabetic Diet consists of taking in six small feedings at regular intervals throughout waking hours.[62] The purpose is to keep blood sugar at a relatively stable level, preventing dramatic peaks and valleys. Similarly, the EAT for hunger pattern does not allow dramatic swings between hunger and fullness.

Old overeating habits come from self-talk that clients may need to become aware of and discuss. Later, new positive self-talk replacements can be learned to overcome these overeating habits:

- I always eat a "good breakfast"—even when I'm not hungry.
- I had better eat now, since I may not have time later.

- I always finish off my meals with a little something sweet.
- I always clean my plate (for the starving children).
- I cannot stand to throw away perfectly good food.
- I eat it whether it tastes good or not.
- I can't eat the foods I want until I eat the healthy foods I should eat first.

Preparation

In the preparation stage, clients begin to make lifestyle changes, but they perform the new behaviors sporadically and have not yet incorporated them as a permanent part of their lifestyles. The nurse can play an important supportive role at this time as the clients gradually override their individual reasons not to incorporate new behaviors into their lifestyles. After each success, they will gain confidence in their new behaviors and find ways to adapt daily habits to accommodate them. The nurse should not push clients at this stage, but rather should be available when they have questions and need suggestions. The Exercise for LIFE strategy is introduced at this stage because individuals often need to be at a higher level of change to put forth the effort and time demanded by regular exercise habits.

Exercise for LIFE Strategy. The purpose of the Exercise for LIFE strategy is to introduce regular, challenging exercise as a means to express self-value and love. The **LIFE** stands for *Love* self, *In, Fitness* and *Exercise*. When clients learn to accept exercise as part of their life, they learn to truly love themselves and their bodies. Valuing self enough to schedule and maintain regular exercise is an act of self-love. When they exercise for others (e.g., physician, spouse, friend, child), efforts are usually short-lived and can end in resentment. When they hold to a regular and challenging exercise plan, while at the same time allowing themselves to miss a few days without panic or guilt, they have learned to exercise for LIFE.

Clients can be given the book *Fit or Fat Woman.*[63] Sessions may be divided equally to discuss the book's topics: reasons that women are fatter than men, use of aerobic and strength exercises to reduce fat, design of a personal aerobic and strength exercise program, incorporation of exercise into one's lifestyle. A health care professional should assess risks involved in performing aerobic and strength training before the client begins training. Once the client's safety is ensured, it is time to prescribe beginning, intermediate, and advanced levels of combined aerobic and strength training protocols based on physical exercise pre-testing results. When possible, the assistance of a colleague educated in exercise physiology or physical therapy is helpful for exercise testing. If colleagues cannot assist clients directly, they can assist the nurse in developing a step test that is easily administered in most settings.

To increase cardiovascular fitness, the American College of Sports Medicine recommends exercising 2 to 3 days per week at an intensity equal to 65 to 85 percent of age-predicted heart rate maximum (H R max).[64] Clients may use any mode of aerobic exercise to sustain heart rate within their working heart range for duration according to their fitness levels. To maintain fat-free mass and increase muscular strength and endurance, the American College of Sports Medicine recommends strength training (weight lifting) with 1 to 3 sets of 8 to 12 repetitions using moderate-intensity resistance at least 2 days per week. Clients should receive instruction about exercising all muscle groups using no equipment, minimal equipment, and strength training gym equipment. Muscle group and related exercises include leg press, bench press, leg curl, lateral pull shoulder press, calf raises, arm curls, triceps press, rowing, back extension, pectorals, and abdominals. Clients usually can

begin training for the first month with 1 set of 12 repetitions at a resistance they can perform with ease (to minimize muscle damage and soreness).

By the second month, clients will perform according to beginning, intermediate, and advanced levels. The usual goal by the end of the first year is to participate in aerobic and strength exercises 2 to 3 times per week each, for a total of 4 to 6 exercise days per week (consistent with American College of Sports Medicine recommendations). If clients need regular, anticipated support, they may find it helpful to join a gym.

Ways To Get Regular, Challenging Exercise. To get ready for a regular and challenging exercise program, clients should seek physician approval and should ensure that their risks are minimal. They should wear loose-fitting, environmentally proper clothes and supportive shoes matched for the type of exercise (e.g., walking, jogging, cross-training). Clients should be knowledgeable about and plan for physical and environmental safety. The nurse should educate and help clients design exercise to fit their lifestyles.

- Clients can learn that having a healthy percentage of body fat (22 to 28 percent) is necessary for metabolic rate to be driven by fat-free or lean body mass. Excess fat is metabolically less active than muscle and results in a slow metabolism, making it more difficult to lose weight.
- Clients can learn about differences between aerobic and anaerobic exercise. Aerobic exercises (e.g., walking, slow jogging, swimming, biking) use more oxygen, use large muscle groups, and are at lower intensities and of longer duration. Anaerobic exercises (e.g., running, swimming, stair-climbing, biking, weight lifting at a very fast/vigorous pace) use more glucose stores, usually use isolated

muscle groups, and are at higher intensities and of shorter duration.

- An exercise schedule should address frequency, duration, and intensity. Frequency of aerobic exercises is 3 and 4 times per week; frequency of strength training/weight lifting exercises is 2 and 3 times per week. Duration of an aerobic workout is from 20 to 60 minutes; duration of a strength workout is from 30 to 60 minutes. Intensity of an aerobic workout is from 70 to 80 percent of the maximum heart rate. A quick method to calculate working heart range (the range within which rate should be kept to gain aerobic benefit) is:

(220– Age) × 70 percent (lower end)
and × 80 percent (upper end)
Example: 220 − 40 = 180
             180 × .80 = 144
             180 × .70 = 126
Working heart range = 126–144

Intensity of a strength workout is from 1 to 2 sets of 12 to 15 repetitions of lifting weights.
Sample workout plans may be prescribed in four levels:
1. Level 1: Exercise 3 days, 1 strength day and 2 aerobic days
2. Level 2: Exercise 4 days, 2 strength days and 2 aerobic days
3. Level 3: Exercise 5 days, 2 strength days and 3 aerobic days
4. Level 4: Exercise 6 days, 3 strength days and 3 aerobic days

- An exercise workout should start with stretching the arms and legs in a static stretch without bouncing. Then comes the warm-up, lasting 3 to 5 minutes to increase the heart rate slowly. After the exercise is the cool-down phase, which is slow-paced, continuing aerobic exercise, again followed by stretching the arms and legs in a static stretch without bouncing

- A slight soreness 12 to 24 hours after exercise shows that the muscles have been sufficiently challenged to require energy-expending repair to build muscle and indicates an increased excess post-exercise oxygen consumption (EPOC). Often called afterburn, EPOC helps clients lose excess fat even at rest, particularly with resistance exercise. For maximum benefit, the client should not do the same workout repeatedly, since the body adapts and will not be challenged.

- Scheduling exercise weekly ahead of time will help develop a new habit. Writing workout days and times in the personal calendar can build the commitment to exercise. Great variability in workouts from day to day will prevent boredom and maximize use of different muscle groups. Workouts with friends and family add interest and challenge.

Action

At 6 months, clients usually have their eating and exercise habits well under control and have experienced pride and satisfaction in their lifestyle changes. They still can resume former habits if boredom, illness/injury, life crises, and burnout occur, however. Thus, it is especially important at this stage to introduce the cognitive portion of the intervention to help prevent relapse. They can truly understand that their new eating and exercise habits are for a lifetime. By learning to listen to their self-talk, they can decrease negative self-talk and increase positive self-talk to support long-term, holistic self-care weight management. The STOP emotional eating strategy based on reversal theory can help clients pinpoint and change their most threatening and sabotaging self-talk.

STOP Emotional Eating Strategy. The purpose of the STOP emotional eating strategy is to separate emotions from eating responses and direct actions for managing underlying problems without eating to cope. Clients can be given a copy of the book *Feeling Good,*[65] excerpts from the article "Why Rational People Do,"[66] and detailed description of reversal theory states (see Exhibit 27–2).

Clients can complete homework using self-talk worksheets for identifying and reframing negative self-talk into positive self-talk replacements (see Exhibit 27–1). Discussion topics include how beliefs, thinking, feelings, and actions are related. Individual and group discussions can include real-life examples of each type of irrational thinking:

- *All-or-nothing thinking*—perceiving absolute, black and white categories
- *Overgeneralization*—seeing negative situation as never-ending
- *Mental filter*—dwelling on negatives, ignoring positives
- *Mind reading and fortune telling*—interpreting others/events as negative without the facts
- *Magnification or minimization of importance*—blowing situation out of proportion or shrinking it unrealistically
- *Shoulding and blaming*—saying should, shouldn't, have to and take/don't take too much/not enough responsibility
- *Labeling*—naming self instead of behavior (instead of I made a mistake, I am a mistake)

To counter each type of irrational thinking, clients can review and practice the challenges to irrational thinking:

- Where is the *evidence* that this thought is true/not true?
- Would an informal *survey* of those I trust show that this thought is realistic?
- Would I talk to and treat my *best friend* the way I talk to and treat myself?

- Can I consider *shades of gray* instead of black and white thinking?
- How can "should thinking" be restated with "preferably" and "sometimes"?

Ways To Change Negative Self-Talk Triggers. Helping clients use reversal theory to balance their eight ways of being human begins with an examination of the frequent emotions found to trigger overeating and lack of exercise. At this point, the effort focuses on desensitizing, practicing, and accepting being in the negativistic state. Then the four steps for fighting fair are phrased as positive self-talk (affirmations):

1. I tell objectively the facts about what happened. ("I saw you with Lucy after you told me you didn't have time to get together this evening.")
2. I tell what I didn't like about his or her behavior. ("I didn't like seeing you with another of your friends after you told me you didn't have time for us to get together.")
3. I tell how I feel about it. ("I felt pushed aside for you to be with Lucy instead of me; I felt unimportant; I felt lonely.")
4. I tell what I realistically want him or her to do. ("I would like to spend time with you every week, and I would like you to make some time for me if that's what you want also.")

By knowing the positive and negative feelings associated with each state, clients can pinpoint states in which they repeatedly experience increased tension stress and turn to overeating to deal with the unpleasant feelings. After posing questions for the eight states to help clients understand their personal meanings and beliefs, the nurse can suggest healthy self-talk replacements.

1. *In the telic state,* feeling pleasant is experienced as flow and productivity, while feeling unpleasant is experienced as anxiety. In the paratelic state, feeling pleasant is experienced

as flow and fun, while feeling unpleasant is experienced as boredom.
Questions to raise consciousness and
pinpoint areas of growth include

- What do I believe about work and
  play? About being serious and fun-
  loving?
- To me (work/serious-minded)(play/
  fun-loving) is ____.
- Being serious/playful is different for
  women compared to men in these
  ways: _____.
- I believe (work/seriousness)(play/
  light-heartedness) is important because ____.

New, healthy self-statements about
work and play include:

- It is good for me to work and be serious-minded because ___.
- It is good for me to play and be fun-
  loving because ___.

2. *In the conformist state,* feeling pleasant is experienced as feeling protected, while feeling unpleasant is experienced as feeling unprotected (fear
   people won't like/love me if I don't act/
   perform/dress/etc. ... perfectly). In the
   negativistic state, feeling pleasant is
   experienced as feeling free, while
   feeling unpleasant is experienced as
   feeling trapped (fear that if I express
   my anger or don't act as I should,
   people won't like/love me). Questions
   to raise consciousness and pinpoint
   areas of growth include
   - Do I feel I have unconditional love,
     positive regard, and am I taken seri-
     ously?
   - Do I fear abandonment? I can really
     be ME, and you won't leave me?
   - Have I learned to meet others' nar-
     cissistic needs to provide what they
     never got from their parents out of
     fear of not being loved, disapproval,
     or abandonment?

New, healthy self-statements about
being conformist and negativistic include

- Sometimes I will choose to do things
  less than 100 percent.
- Sometimes I will choose to ask others to do my task.
- Its OK to be angry if I fight fair.

3. *In the mastery state,* feeling pleasant is
   experienced as feeling hardy and
   strong, while unpleasant feelings are
   experienced as feeling soft and wimpy
   (fear of not being liked/respected if I
   appear weak, less than perfect). In the
   sympathy state, feeling pleasant is experienced as feeling sensitive and
   cared for, while feeling unpleasant is
   experienced as feeling insensitive and
   ashamed (fear if I don't act as I should,
   people won't like/love me). Questions
   to raise consciousness and pinpoint areas of growth include
   - When I truly feel like giving myself
     a break and being tender with my-
     self, does it feel good, or do I feel
     guilty?
   - Why can't I feel my real feelings?
     And when I do feel, why do I eat to
     feel better?

New, healthy self-statements about
work and play include

- I choose to feel my true feelings
  even when they hurt.
- I have the knowledge and skills to
  express my feelings effectively.

4. *In the alloic state,* feeling pleasant is
   experienced as feeling modest, useful, and loyal, while feeling unpleasant is experienced as shame and guilt
   (fear of not being liked/loved/re-
   spected if I put myself first). In the
   autic state, feeling pleasant is experienced as feeling satisfied with self,
   grateful, and cared for while feeling
   unpleasant is experienced as feeling
   humiliated, resentful, hurt, and deprived (fear if I don't act as others expect me to act and do what they want,
   they won't like/love/stay with me).
   Questions to raise consciousness and
   pinpoint areas of growth include

- Why can't I give to myself first?
- Are these my beliefs versus those of my parents, teachers, religious leaders?
- Why do I feel undeserving of being first?
- Do I have to earn the right to consider myself before others?

New, healthy self-statements about work and play include

- I choose to put myself first; right now I need my full attention.
- I choose to give to/spend time with this person.
- I choose to omit feeling guilty from my vocabulary and my life.

Maintenance

Beyond 6 months of clients' practicing and refining lifestyle changes, the nurse can be very instrumental in helping them maintain their lifestyle changes by continuing supportive actions such as being available to answer questions, providing resources, and assisting with modifications in eating and exercise routines. By allowing clients to stay "in touch" and approaching them when the nurse has innovative ideas, the nurse may spark their new and continued interest in their programs.

The nurse may help clients to examine their patterns when they overeat and do not exercise to discover ways to reinforce and strengthen areas of deficit. For example, the nurse may suggest that a client examine the last months of daily exercise sheets for the following:

1. What are the total number of days I reported?
2. What is my average number of exercise days per week?
3. What is my major trigger for not exercising?

The client may also examine overeating over the last months of daily sheets for the following:

1. What is my average number of overeating days per week?
2. What is my major trigger for overeating?
3. On the days I overate, did I exercise or not?
4. On the days I exercised, did I overeat or not?
5. On the days I did not exercise and overate, what reversal theory state was I in and how high was my tension stress?
6. What way of being human do I need to work on?

The final key to lasting change is acceptance. When clients fully accept the sadness, anger, bad, irritating things in life, rather than try to change perfectly, manipulate, succumb to, and overpower these things, a peace can settle into their spirits. Acceptance opens new possibilities that can help move them ahead to grow beyond obstacles. The nurse may point out that constantly "fighting it" (like trying to break the door down) actually can keep them in one place stuck in the past. As a key in a locked door, acceptance can move them to places they have never been or even fathomed.

The nurse guides and directs clients to write in a journal the most problematic obstacle in simple succinct statements. Obstacles are the triggers that repeatedly set off negative self-talk that keep them overeating, not exercising, and feeling bad about themselves. Four steps to the acceptance of the obstacles are written as positive self-talk (affirmations):

1. I say aloud the statements about what I am accepting one time with my eyes open.
2. I say aloud the statements about what I am accepting one time with my eyes closed.
3. I pray/meditate for complete acceptance and am silent with my eyes still closed, listening to and accepting whatever comes to mind.

4. I repeat this exercise daily until it feels comfortable and unnecessary to continue on a daily basis.

Case Study

A.W., a single 34-year-old high-school English teacher, experienced all the stages of change over a period of approximately 1 year. At each stage, the client was asked to rate her readiness in response to a listing and descriptions of the stages of change.

A.W. in the Precontemplation Stage

Setting:	Afternoon appointment in a health clinic for Pap smear and breast examination
Patterns/ Problems/ Needs:	Altered nutrition, more than body requirements (167 pounds, 5 feet, 2 inches tall, 31 body mass index, 35 percent body fat)
	Body image disturbance (8 on a 10-point scale, 1 being best)
	Hopelessness related to 17 years of past failures at weight management

After her regular wellness check, Pap smear, and breast examination, A.W. told her story in a brief life review and weight management history. She had a 17-year history of weight cycling that began when she was in high school. She had always been active in sports and aerobic exercise. In high school, she had a muscular build and average weight. When she entered college, she was less active because she studied more to keep her grades above average. She always felt a lot of pressure from her parents to make all A's and become a college professor like her father.

In high school and college, A.W. developed a habit of munching on chips and candy while studying. She continued the habit as she prepared lectures and graded papers as a high-school teacher. As she gradually gained weight and became more self-conscious about her physical appear-

ance, she did not pursue relationships with men. She remained healthy except for occasional sinus headaches. Because she dieted and exercised throughout the 17 years of weight cycling, she was very pessimistic about her ability to lose and maintain a healthy weight. She became tearful when she told of her repeated failures and said that she was much too busy to exercise regularly.

A.W. was in relatively good physical health other than being mildly obese and inactive. She was to return to the clinic for blood work to be drawn within the next 2 weeks. She was rated "at risk" for binge eating on the BULIT scale, and she ranked her body image as an 8 on a 10-point scale (1 being best). She rated herself as being in the precontemplation stage; she was given a brochure that contained a section in which the nurse wrote a report of the physical findings to date, the health risks involved, and a summary of the holistic self-care model weight management program offered at the clinic. The nurse answered questions and encouraged A.W. to call her for more information about the program whenever she was ready.

A.W. in the Contemplation Stage

Setting:	Return appointment of A.W. 1 month later in a health clinic for blood work (blood glucose and lipid levels)
Patterns/ Problems/ Needs:	Altered nutrition, body requirements
	Body image disturbance
	Hopelessness

A.W.'s blood glucose level was within normal range, but her total cholesterol level and cholesterol:high-density lipoprotein ratio were slightly elevated. She said that she had been thinking about the program and wondered if individuals could choose to attend individual or group sessions. She asked for clarification about the fact that the brochure specified no type of diet—only eating according to hunger.

When the nurse asked if A.W. was considering making some changes in eating and exercise, A.W. said that she was intrigued about a "no-diet" diet. The nurse noted A.W.'s interest in attending a group session and gave her the month's schedule of meetings about the EAT for Hunger strategy in the clinic's weight management program.

A.W. in the Preparation Stage

Setting: Last evening group meeting about the EAT for Hunger strategy in the clinic's weight management program (1 month later after four group meetings)

Patterns/ Problems/ Needs: Altered nutrition, more than body requirements
Body image disturbance
Hopelessness
Decreased mobility related to no regular exercise program
Increased tension stress before overeating episodes—"at risk" scores on the tension stress scale

A.W. related that she enjoyed the group meetings about EAT for Hunger and felt great relief not dieting. She said that she realized how much she had been eating when she was not hungry, especially when she felt pressured to complete her teaching responsibilities. She expressed more hope that she could cut down on overeating by using the new EAT for Hunger strategy. Her major difficulty with the strategy was stopping at a "5" when her hunger was gone (preparation stage). A.W. also said that she was planning to attend next month's sessions on the Exercise for LIFE strategy, although she had not changed her activity level to date (contemplation stage for exercise).

A.W. in the Action Stage

Setting: Last evening group meeting about the Exercise for LIFE strategy in the clinic's weight management program (1 month later)

Patterns/ Problems/ Needs: Altered nutrition, more than body requirements—loss of 6 pounds
Body image disturbance—rated 7 on a 10-point scale (1 is best)
Hopelessness—more hopeful to make long-term lifestyle changes in new program with group support
Decreased mobility related to no regular exercise program—attending group meetings regularly and beginning a 3- to 4-day per week workout program
Increased tension stress before overeating episodes—overeating less often, but tension stress still high with overeating

A.W. began walking with a friend twice every week and came early to walk with two group members before meetings once a week. She bought videotapes of combined aerobics and strength exercises and did a 30-minute workout before leaving for work once a week. She lost 3 more pounds at the end of the third month of participating in the program and lost inches in her body proportions almost equal to one dress size.

A.W. began the third month of the program learning how to STOP emotional eating. She describe the pressures in her high-school teaching job that kept her eating when anxious. Others in the group explained how troubled relationships with husbands, friends, and family members often precipitated overeating. A.W. could not relate to their stories, since she almost never had disagreements with her father, mother, and women friends. Gradually, through the use of the self-talk worksheets, she discovered sources of anxiety, boredom, and anger of which she was unaware. Perhaps her most startling discovery was her new awareness of feeling angry with her father's high expectations and her resultant perfectionism. She did not feel comfortable expressing her feelings in the group; she felt guilty and thought she was being a dishonorable daughter.

A.W. announced to her group 3 weeks later that she was so confident in her progress that she was going to continue working on her own and not return to the group. She said that she needed the extra time for her increasing work demands. She expressed sadness about leaving the group, but was excited to live her new lifestyle on her own.

A.W. did not return to the group until 3 months later after she came to the nurse for a bout with the flu and a sinus infection. She said that it was more difficult to continue the EAT, LIFE, and STOP strategies on her own without the group support. She had regained 4 pounds, but continued to exercise two times most weeks. She thought of returning to the group several times, but said that she thought the discussions were too personal at times. When the nurse asked for specifics, she learned about the anger that A.W. felt toward her father and the consequent guilt she experienced.

A.W. and the nurse agreed to have two or three private, individual sessions to learn more about A.W.'s angry feelings and how they relate to overeating and not getting regular exercise. A.W. was able to understand her perfectionistic behaviors and need for others' approval. After 2 weekly individual sessions, she said that she wanted to return to the group to continue work in the program.

A.W. in the Maintenance Stage

Setting:	Last evening group meeting about the Acceptance of Obstacles in the clinic's weight management program (about 11 months after first meeting A.W. attended)
Patterns/ Problems/ Needs:	Altered nutrition, more than body requirements—from 167 to 148 pounds, from 31 to

27 body mass index, from 35 to 32 percent body fat
Body image disturbance—from an 8 to a 6 on a 10-point scale (1 being best)
Hopelessness—diagnosis resolved after individual counseling and continued group work
Decreased mobility related to no regular exercise program—improving; need more strength exercises added to workout to maximize metabolic rate
Increased tension stress before overeating episodes—lowered "at risk" scores (i.e., within normal range on the tension stress scale)

A.W. returned to group meetings at least monthly, but found individual help from a psychologist recommended by the nurse to work on issues of self-esteem, perfectionism, and approval needs. A.W.'s EAT for Hunger and Exercise for LIFE habits were becoming integrated into her lifestyle. She found that writing in her journal was a helpful way to work on her own issues when not in the group or in counseling. Her major focus was on acceptance and love of herself. Although the experience was painful at times, A.W. said that she was thankful to have greater insight into her past overeating and no exercise habits.

Evaluation

With clients, the nurse determines whether their outcomes for weight management were achieved (see Table 27–1). To evaluate clients' progress on goals, the nurse examines with them their weekly and daily calendar sheets. Together, the nurse and a client may explore the subjective effects of their experiences in the program by answering the questions found in Exhibit 27–6.

Exhibit 27-6 Evaluating the Client's Subjective Experience with Weight Management Interventions

1. How am I feeling about myself and my progress right now?
2. Do I have any questions about my eating and exercise programs?
3. What new insights have I gained about my self-talk?
4. What is my next step, and do I need help to take that step?
5. Are my goals realistic for me right now?
6. What pain and joy can I expect in reaching my goals?
7. Am I seeking my Higher Power to accept the things that I cannot change, and am I thinking positively about changing the things I can change?

DIRECTIONS FOR FUTURE RESEARCH

1. Contrast and evaluate discrepancies between nurses' and clients' perceptions of client readiness according to the transtheoretical stages of change for eating, exercise, and psycho-social-spiritual work.

2. Analyze clients' progress toward outcome variables listed in Table 27-1, and describe differences among individuals within and between different stages of change.
3. Analyze clients' progress toward outcome variables listed in Table 27-1 according to whether they received primarily individual, group, or a combination of individual and group counseling sessions.

NURSE HEALER REFLECTIONS

After reading this chapter, the nurse healer will be able to answer or begin a process of answering the following questions:

- How did I accommodate my eating within the food pyramid and the American Diabetic Association diet using the EAT for Hunger strategy?
- How did my personal aerobic and strength exercise program incorporate the Exercise for LIFE strategy?
- How did I deal directly with unpleasant feelings, instead of eating to cope, using the STOP overeating strategy?

NOTES

1. G.A. Colditz, Economic Costs of Severe Obesity, *American Journal of Clinical Nutrition* 55 (1992): 503S–507S.
2. M. Perri et al., *Improving the Long-Term Management of Obesity* (New York: John Wiley & Sons, 1992), 39.
3. C.B. Ferster et al., The Control of Eating, *Journal of Mathetics* 1 (1962): 87–109.
4. R.L. Leibel et al., Biochemistry and Development of Adipose Tissue in Man, in *Health and Obesity*, ed. H.L. Conrt et al. (New York: Raven Press, 1983), 21–48.
5. I.M. Faust et al., Diet-Induced Adipocyte Number Increase in Adult Rats, *American Journal of Physiology* 235 (1978):E279–E286.
6. Perri et al., *Improving the Long-Term Management of Obesity*.
7. D.W. Reiff and K.K. Reiff, *Eating Disorders* (Gaithersburg, MD: Aspen Publishers, 1992).

8. R. Keesey, A Set-Point Theory of Obesity, in *Handbook of Eating Disorders*, ed. K. Brownell and J. Foreyt (New York: Basic Books,1986), 103–123.
9. J.S. Garrow, *Energy Balance and Obesity in Man* (New York: Elsevier, 1978).
10. Perri et al., *Improving the Long-Term Management of Obesity*, 39.
11. K.D. Brownell, *The LEARN Program for Weight Control* (Dallas, TX: American Health Publishing Company, 1997).
12. R.W. Jeffery et al., Strengthening Behavioral Interventions for Weight Loss: A Randomized Trial of Food Provision and Monetary Incentives, *Journal of Consulting and Clinical Psychology*, 61 (1993):1038–1045.
13. R.G. Nunn et al., 2.5 Year Follow-Up of Weight and Body Mass Index Values in the Weight

Control for Life! Program: A Descriptive Analysis, *Addictive Behaviors* 17 (1992): 579–585.

14. R.E. Vath, Psychiatric Factors, in *Eating Disorders*, ed. D.W. Reiff, and K.K. Reiff (Gaithersburg, MD: Aspen Publishers, 1992), 457–462.

15. A.T. Beck, *Cognitive Therapy and the Emotional Disorders* (New York: International Universities Press, 1976).

16. K.D. Brownell et al., The Dieting Maelstrom: Is It Possible and Advisable To Lose Weight? *American Psychologist* 49 (1994):781–791.

17. R.R. Wing, Obesity and Related Eating and Exercise Behaviors in Women, *Annals of Behavioral Medicine* 15 (1993):124–134.

18. Wing, Obesity and Related Eating and Exercise Behaviors in Women.

19. R.J. Kuczmarski et al., Increasing Prevalence of Overweight among U.S. Adults: The National Health and Nutrition Examination Surveys, 1960–1991, *Journal of the American Medical Association* 272 (1994):205–211.

20. R. Green, Americans Eat Less Fat But Are Getting Fatter, *The Kansas City Star* (17 January 1996):A1, A6.

21. Green, Americans Eat Less Fat But Are Getting Fatter.

22. American Dietetic Association, Position on Weight Management, *Journal of the American Diabetic Association* 97 (1997):71–74.

23. J.I. Robison et al., Obesity, Weight Loss, and Health, *Journal of the American Dietetic Association* 93 (1993):445–449.

24. K.D. Brownell, and T.A. Wadden, Etiology and Treatment of Obesity: Understanding a Serious, Prevalent, and Refractory Disorder, *Journal of Consulting and Clinical Psychology* 60 (1992):505–517.

25. J.D. Allan, Women Who Successfully Manage Their Weight, *Western Journal of Nursing Research* 11(1989):657–675.

26. Perri et al., *Improving the Long-Term Management of Obesity*, 103.

27. T.A. Wadden et al., Responsible and Irresponsible Use of Very Low Calorie Diets in the Treatment of Obesity, *Journal of the American Medical Association* 263 (1990):83–85.

28. T.A. Wadden et al., Treatment of Obesity by Very Low Calorie Diet, Behavior Therapy, and Their Combination: A Five Year Perspective, *International Journal of Obesity* 13 (1989):39–46.

29. T.A. Wadden, Treatment of Obesity by Moderate and Severe Calorie Restriction, *Annals of Internal Medicine* 119 (1993):688–693.

30. R.G Nunn et al., 2.5 year Follow-Up of Weight and Body Mass Index Values, 580.

31. M. Weintraub, Long-Term Weight Control, *Clinical Pharmacology and Therapeutics* 51 (1992):619–633.

32. U. McCann et al., Dexfenfluramine and Serotonin Neurotoxicity: Further Preclinical Evidence That Caution Is Indicated, *Journal of Pharmacology and Experimental Therapeutics* 269 (1994):792–798.

33. E. Poehlman et al., The Impact of Exercise and Diet Restriction on Daily Energy Expenditure, *Sports Medicine* 11 (1991):78–101.

34. J. Thompson et al., Effects of Diet and Diet-Plus-Exercise Programs on Resting Metabolic Rate: A Meta-Analysis, *International Journal of Sports Medicine* 6 (1996):41–61.

35. S. Maehlum et al., Magnitude and Duration of Excess Postexercise Oxygen Consumption in Healthy Young Subjects, *Metabolism* 35 (1986): 425–429.

36. E. Poehlman et al., The Effect of Prior Exercise and Caffeine Ingestion on Metabolic Rate and Hormones in Young Adult Males, *Canadian Journal of Physiological Pharmacology* 67 (1989):10–16.

37. T.A. Wadden et al., Exercise in the Treatment of Obesity: Effects of Four Interventions on Body Composition, Resting Energy Expenditure, Appetite, and Mood, *Journal of Consulting and Clinical Psychology* 65 (1997):269–277.

38. G.D. Foster et al., What Is a Reasonable Weight Loss? Patients' Expectations and Evaluations of Obesity Treatment Outcomes, *Journal of Consulting and Clinical Psychology* 65 (1997):79–85.

39. American Dietetic Association, Position on Weight Management, 74.

40. C.M. Grilo et al., The Metabolic and Psychological Importance of Exercise in Weight Control, in *Obesity: Theory and Therapy*, ed. A.J. Stunkard and T.A. Wadden (New York: Raven Press, 1993).

41. Brownell et al., The Dieting Maelstrom: Is It Possible and Advisable To Lose Weight? 791.

42. J.I. Robison et al., Redefining Success in Obesity Intervention: The New Paradigm, *Journal of the American Dietetic Association* 95 (1995):422–423.

43. Brownell, *The LEARN Program for Weight Control*, 94.

44. National Task Force on the Prevention and Treatment of Obesity, Weight Cycling, *Journal of the American Medical Association* 272 (1994):1196–1202.

45. Foster et al., What Is a Reasonable Weight Loss? 79.

46. M. Apter, *Reversal Theory: Motivation, Emotion, and Personality* (London: Routledge, 1989), 18–32.

47. K.A. O'Connell et al., Reversal Theory's Mastery and Sympathy States in Smoking Cessation, *Image* 27 (1995):311–316.

48. S.A. Popkess-Vawter et al., Reversal Theory, Overeating, and Weight Cycling, *Western Journal of Nursing Research* 20 (1998):67–83.

49. Beck, *Cognitive Therapy and the Emotional Disorders*.

50. S.A. Popkess-Vawter et al., Unpleasant Emotional Triggers to Overeating and Related Intervention Strategies for Overweight and Obese Women Weight Cyclers, *Journal of Applied Nursing Research* 11 (1998):69–76.

51. S.A. Popkess-Vawter et al., Development and Testing of the Tension Stress Scale, *Journal of Nursing Measurement* (submitted).

52. Popkess-Vawter et al., Reversal Theory, Overeating, and Weight Cycling, 67.

53. Brownell et al., The Dieting Maelstrom: Is It Possible and Advisable To Lose Weight? 791.

54. S.A. Popkess-Vawter and V. Owens, Use of the BULIT Bulimia Screening Questionnaire To Assess Risk and Progress in Weight Management for Overweight Women Who Weight Cycle, *Addictive Behaviors*, in press.

55. S.A. Popkess-Vawter et al., Unpleasant Emotional Triggers to Overeating and Related Intervention Strategies, 76.

56. Popkess-Vawter and V. Owens, Use of the BULIT Bulimia Screening Questionnaire, 4.

57. Popkess-Vawter et al., Development and Testing of the Tension Stress Scale, 3.

58. J.O. Prochaska and C.C. DiClemente, In Search of How People Change, *American Psychologist* 47 (1992):1102.

59. B.H. Marcus and L.H. Forsyth, The Challenge of Behavior Change, *Medicine and Health* 80 (1997):300–302.

60. B. Schwartz, *Diets Still Don't Work* (Houston, TX: Breakthru Publishing, 1990), 58–62.

61. Schwartz, *Diets Still Don't Work*.

62. The American Diabetes Association and the American Dietetic Association, *Exchange Lists for Meal Planning* (Chicago: ADA Press, 1995).

63. C. Bailey and L. Bishop, *Fit or Fat Woman: Solutions for Women's Unique Concerns* (Boston: Houghton Mifflin, 1989), 25–31.

64. American College of Sports Medicine, *ACSM Position Stand: The Recommended Quantity and Quality of Exercise for Developing and Maintaining Cardiorespiratory and Muscle Fitness in Healthy Adults* (Houston, TX: Breakthru Publishing, 1990), 265–274.

65. D.D. Burns, *Feeling Good: The New Mood Therapy* (New York: Signet New American Library, 1980).

66. K.A. O'Connell, Why Rational People Do, *Journal of Psychosocial Nursing* 29 (1991):11–14.

SUGGESTED RESOURCE

For additional information, see the following website: http://www.nhlbi.nih.gov/nhlbi/cardio/obes/prof/guidelns/sum_evid.htm

VISION OF HEALING

Acknowledging Fear

What is fear, and where does it come from? Fear can surface as we contemplate changes in lifestyle patterns. For example, a person who wishes to stop smoking fears not being able to stop, gaining weight, experiencing nicotine withdrawal, offending other people by asking them not to smoke, among other things. Fear comes only in relation to something else. If this is so, how can we gain freedom from fear? This is the healing journey—learning more about the fear in relationship with all things.

Fear somehow can attach itself to the spirit and lodge somewhere within the physical body. Fear makes us feel separate and alone, but it can become a path that will lead deeper into the present moment. It does not have to be a barrier to the moment. Although fear always creates more fear, its every occurrence can become a moment to learn more about another level of life's journey. Fear is useful in that it alerts us to areas in which we have some resistance. Releasing the fear returns us to our unconditional core of love so that we release the "shoulds." Approaching an event

with the notion that we "should" behave in a certain way further distances us from our core of being present in the moment. The basic human fears—fear of failure, fear of rejection, fear of the unknown, fear of isolation, fear of dying, and fear of loss of self-control—are closely related and may overlap. Any kind of fear is related to our level of self-esteem. When our self-esteem is low, our fears even increase. The negative self-talk intensifies the lack of self-confidence and takes us further from the resolution of the fear. It is helpful to identify our stressors and determine the fears that they evoke. We need to reflect on the following questions:

- How do you usually deal with your fears? Are you the type of person who hopes that circumstances surrounding these fears will go away?
- Does one of these basic human fears tend to dominate your list of stressors? If so, why do you suppose that is the case?
- What are some ways to deal with some of these major fears?

Chapter 28

Smoking Cessation: Freedom from Risk

Christine Anne Wynd and Barbara Montgomery Dossey

NURSE HEALER OBJECTIVES

Theoretical

- Analyze the bodymind responses to nicotine.
- Examine theoretical strategies for successful smoking cessation.

Clinical

- Interview a client who smokes and listen to the reasons that the client gives for smoking. Ask if the client has ever tried to quit smoking or will attempt smoking cessation again.
- Give the Smoking Profile Questionnaire to a client. Discuss the score with the client to gain insight into the meaning of smoking, and explore ways to teach smoking cessation.
- Design interventions that correspond to the stages and processes of change as appropriate to the client.

Personal

- Examine the effect of passive smoking on you.
- If you are a smoker, identify habit breakers to become a successful nonsmoker.

DEFINITIONS

Focused Smoking: a smoking reduction technique done under supervision.

Habit Breakers: new action behaviors that replace old smoke signals.

Nicotine Fading: gradual reduction of the nicotine level in the body to avoid withdrawal symptoms.

THEORY AND RESEARCH

The Prevalence of Smoking and Its Health Consequences

Smoking is the major health hazard as well as the chief preventable cause of death in the United States today. It is responsible for an estimated 430,000 deaths annually, approximately one of every five deaths.[1] Tobacco kills more people than acquired immunodeficiency syndrome (AIDS), car accidents, alcohol, homicides, illegal drugs, suicides, and fires combined.[2,3] There would now be about 11 percent fewer overall deaths if all adult smokers from the 1970s had quit the habit. Of these, 58 percent would have been in men, 41 percent in women.[4]

Cigarette smoking contributes to four of the five leading causes of death per year in the United States, including cardiovascular disease (98,000 deaths), lung cancer (123,000 deaths), stroke (24,000 deaths), and chronic obstructive pulmonary disease (72,000 deaths),[5–7] and the United States spends more than $50 billion each year for smoking-related health care costs.[8] In the international scene, it is estimated that by the year 2020, tobacco will kill more people than any single health problem, including the human immunodeficiency virus (HIV) epidemic.[9]

Smokers constitute 25.5 percent of the U.S. population. Twenty-eight percent of males and 23.1 percent of females smoke cigarettes, and 25.9 percent of white adults and 26.5 percent of African-Americans use tobacco.[10,11] Rates of smoking prevalence continue to be high among certain population groups, especially American Indians/Alaska Natives (39.2 percent), blue-collar workers, and military personnel.[12,13] The most frightening trend is with the nation's youth; there is a significant increase in smoking prevalence among high-school seniors.[14] It is estimated that every day 3,000 young people become regular smokers.[15]

Environmental tobacco smoke (ETS) is a combination of smoke from the burning end of a cigarette, cigar, or pipe and the smoke exhaled from a smoker's lungs.[16–20] It contains more than 4,000 highly toxic chemicals, such as formaldehyde, nitrogen oxide, acrolein, Group A carcinogens (asbestos), cadmium, nickel, and carbon monoxide. In addition, ETS contains a radioactive substance from tobacco leaves that are subjected to high phosphate fertilizers.[21]

Children and adults exposed to ETS have a greater risk for respiratory illness, including lung cancer; higher rates of respiratory tract infections; exacerbation of asthma; otitis media; and sudden infant death syndrome.[22,23] Aligne and Stoddard found that the exposure of children to parental smoking costs the United States $4.6 billion in annual direct medical expenditures.[24] Increased exposure to ETS nearly doubles a woman's risk of heart attack.[25] Measures of cotinine, a metabolite of nico-

tine in the bloodstream, demonstrate that 37 percent of adult nonsmokers, and 43 percent of U.S. children, aged 2 months through 11 years, are exposed to ETS in their homes or workplaces.[26]

In the United States, approximately 70 percent of children live in homes where at least one adult smokes. Because mothers usually spend more time in the home and more time with their children than do fathers, maternal smoking has been linked with childhood respiratory problems. Data available on 4,331 children, aged 0 to 5 years, show that young children whose mothers smoke more than ten cigarettes per day are twice as likely to develop asthma as are children of nonsmokers.[27] These same youngsters are 2.5 times more likely to develop asthma in their first year of life and 4.5 times more likely to need medicine to control asthma attacks. Maternal smoking remains an indicator of childhood asthma even after variables such as gender, race, presence of both biologic parents in the household, and number of rooms in the house were taken into account.

Physiologic Responses to Smoking

Smoking and tobacco contribute directly to death. Yet, deaths from smoking do not receive the same amount of attention from the news media as do airplane crashes, violence, and disease epidemics, situations resulting in far fewer deaths. Smoking causes more deaths, but these deaths take a very long time to develop.

Over time, smoking strips the lungs of their normal defenses and completely paralyzes the natural cleansing processes. The early morning cough associated with smoking results from attempts by the bronchial cilia to clear the thick, yellow or yellow-green mucus that accumulates in the air passage to an abnormal amount because toxic cigarette smoke interferes with the cilias' normal function. This cleansing action triggers the cough reflex. As exposure continues, the bronchi begin to thicken, which predisposes the person to bacterial and viral infections, asthma, emphysema, and cancer.[28,29]

The smoker's heart rate speeds up an extra 10 to 25 beats per minute, with a predisposition to dysrhythmias. The blood pressure increases by 10 to 15 percent, thus exposing the person to risks of myocardial infarction, stroke, and vascular disease.[30–32]

Within seconds after the smoke is inhaled, irritating gases (e.g., formaldehyde, hydrogen sulfide, ammonia) begin to affect the eyes, nose, and throat. With each inhaled breath of smoke, carbon monoxide enters the bloodstream, and its concentration eventually rises to a level 4 to 15 times as high as that of a nonsmoker. The carbon monoxide passes immediately to the bloodstream, binding to the oxygen receptor sites and, thus, depleting the cells of oxygen. Hemoglobin, which normally carries oxygen throughout the body, becomes bound to the carbon monoxide and is converted to carboxyhemoglobin, which is unable to deliver oxygen to the cells. In addition, smoking increases platelet aggregation, allowing the blood to clot more easily.[33,34]

The constriction of tiny blood vessels decreases the delivery of oxygen to the skin and contributes to "smoker's face," where deep lines appear around the mouth, eyes, and center of the brow. There is an established link between nicotine and erection problems in male smokers, and smoking is believed to be the leading cause of impotence in the United States today. Smoking also adversely affects fertility by decreasing sperm count and sperm motility. Female smokers are three times more likely than nonsmoking females to be infertile, and female heavy smokers have a 43 percent decline in fertility.[35]

Nicotine is the drug inhaled from cigarettes that quickly reaches the smoker's brain. As the average smoker takes an estimated 10 puffs per cigarette, a pack-a-day smoker gets about 200 puffs per day.[36] Each nicotine "hit" goes directly to the lungs, and the nicotine-rich blood travels to the brain in approximately 7 seconds. This time is twice as fast as that of an intravenous injection of heroin, which must pass through the body's systemic circulatory system before reaching the brain.[37,38]

As nicotine enters the brain, it acts as a "mood thermostat." It does not necessarily alter mood, but it maintains a steady and pleasant mood of psychologic neutrality. Nicotine stimulates people when they are drowsy and calms them when they are tense; it affects cognitive processes of concentration and emotional states. Unlike other powerful "street drugs," nicotine does not interfere with the capacity to work and create, and it may actually enhance individuals' capabilities.[39]

The action of nicotine causes the brain to release norepinephrine and dopamine.[40,41] The brain then adapts to accept these chemicals by increasing the number of nicotine receptors and becomes physically dependent on nicotine. Thus, the general level of arousal is adjusted up or down by introducing nicotine levels that allow the smoker to feel stimulated or relaxed.[42] The effects of nicotine are reached in a matter of seconds; the smoker experiences drug-induced contentedness, all in a legally sanctioned manner.

Norepinephrine controls arousal and alertness. Beta-endorphin, referred to as the brain's natural analgesic, can decrease pain and anxiety. Dopamine is part of the brain's pleasure center and is also able to decrease pain and anxiety. Smoking's "attention thermostat" effect is mediated through the brain's limbic system, where the major neurotransmitters are adrenaline and dopamine, both of which are influenced by nicotine. It appears that nicotine helps the smoker concentrate by promoting selective attention to important tasks, which increases learning and memory. Continued smoking also prevents the unpleasant side effects of nicotine withdrawal, such as irritability, irrational mood changes, low energy levels, inability to feel stimulated, and increased sensitivity to light, touch, and sound.[43]

The overall effect of smoking is a shift in brain chemistry that creates the mood needed for the situation at hand, that is, increased relaxation, alertness, or pleasure and decreased pain or anxiety. Even though this is true, concerned smokers can create and sustain new behaviors to achieve the same positive effects without the health risk to themselves or to passive smokers. Success in smoking cessation requires a plan of action. Moreover, smoking cessation is a process, not something that occurs in a week or so.

Strategies for Smoking Cessation

Measuring Successful Cessation

Because smoking cessation is not an easy task, success is often measured in small increments. Smoking quit rates vary with the different approaches to cessation. Over the years, research has evaluated a variety of public and private multicomponent cessation programs, physician-directed counseling, and community-based programs.[44-46] Measures of success also vary, and smoking cessation may be defined as point prevalence (a measure taken at one point in time) at the end of a cessation program or long-term abstinence lasting for 1 year or more. Schwartz found cessation rates of 20 to 60 percent in a classic study of popular intervention methods.[47] Quit rates for professionally assisted programs averaged approximately 22 percent in one review of cessation methods,[48] while another study demonstrated 1-year abstinence rates up to 30 to 35 percent.[49] DiClemente and colleagues reported a median 6-month quit rate for self-help interventions at 17 percent and at 24 percent for smokers attending group therapy sessions.[50]

Self-Quitters, Physician Counseling, and Nurse Follow-up Advice

Fiore and colleagues demonstrated that more than 90 percent of successful quitters kicked the habit on their own.[51] Quit rates were twice as high for those who quit on their own as for those who participated in a cessation program. Smokers who quit "cold turkey" were more likely to remain abstinent than were those who gradually decreased their daily consumption of cigarettes, switched to cigarettes with lower tar or nicotine, or used special filters or holders. Smokers who received nonsmoking advice from their physicians were nearly twice as likely to quit smoking. Heavy smokers (25 cigarettes a day) and more addicted smokers were much more likely to participate in an organized cessation program than were people who smoked less.

Physicians and nurses have considerable opportunity to reach all demographic subgroups of the population.[52-54] Seventy percent of smokers see a physician at least once per year. Although the impact of physician advice varies, 70 percent of smokers say that they would quit if urged to do so by a physician.[55] For smoking intervention to become a routine part of medical practice, however, medical education must integrate smoking cessation strategies into the curriculum.[56,57] Since 1990, the National Cancer Institute has worked to train practicing physicians nationwide in techniques to prevent tobacco use and to facilitate smoking cessation.[58] Its goal is to train 100,000 practicing physicians in these techniques. Nursing education must also emphasize these techniques, as follow-up can be most effective if done by a physician–nurse team.

In a telephone survey of 24,296 Californians, Gilpin and colleagues found that 9,796 current smokers, including 5,559 daily smokers, had visited a physician in the preceding year.[59] Thus, simple intervention by a physician at every visit can have an impact. For patients who already have cancer, heart disease, or other tobacco-related diseases, education in smoking cessation is essential. For example, patients with small-cell lung cancer who survive cancer-free for more than 2 years, but continue to smoke, have a significantly increased risk for developing a second primary smoking-related cancer; smoking cessation after successful therapy is associated with a decrease in this risk.[60]

Pharmacologic Therapies in Support of Cessation

Physicians can offer smokers nicotine replacement therapy (NRT) in the forms of gum, transdermal patch, intranasal spray, or inhalation; however, NRT must be used in tandem with a smoking cessation program that addresses behavior/lifestyle change. Although NRT is a means for achieving short-term smoking cessation for nicotine-addicted individuals, it does not substitute for learning new and healthier behaviors.[61] With NRT, the smoker focuses on breaking the emotional ties with the cigarette. Nicotine replacement therapy does not release the client from the bad effects of nicotine, which continue to be present in the gum or patch. Thus, NRT must be discontinued as soon as possible. Because of nicotine's dangerous side effects, NRT is contraindicated with cardiac patients.

Although NRT is expensive, it can be helpful. In one study, nicotine patch therapy showed clinical significance when combined with physician interventions, nurse counseling follow-up, and relapse interventions.[62] Smokers with lower baseline nicotine and cotinine levels had better cessation rates. These results provide indirect evidence that a fixed dose of transdermal nicotine may be less satisfactory for those smokers with higher baseline levels.

Another study identified predictors of smoking cessation success or failure with and without transdermal patch treatment.[63] Smoking status (abstinent or smoking) during the first 2 weeks of nicotine patch therapy, particularly week 2, was highly correlated with clinical outcome and served as a powerful predictor of smoking cessation. Smoking behavior early in the treatment also predicted outcome among placebo patch users.

It is now widely known that cigarette smoking is closely associated with a history of depression that often predicts failure with initial cessation attempts.[64–66] Smoking cessation may also trigger the onset of depression as a serious nicotine withdrawal symptom in otherwise healthy individuals.[67] To counteract potential symptoms of depression and to maintain mental balance during cessation, several assistive pharmaceutical therapies are being explored. Nortriptyline, a tricyclic antidepressant, and buproprion (Zyban), an atypical antidepressant, are used to improve abstinence in smokers independent of a history of depression. Inhaled through smoking or ingested through "spit" tobacco, nicotine binds to receptors in the brain and causes the release of dopamine and norepinephrine. Nortriptyline has adrenergic activity for producing dopamine,[68] and buproprion blocks the uptake of norepinephrine and inhibits the neuronal reuptake of dopamine. These drugs mimic the neurochemical effects of nicotine on noradrenergic and dopaminergic systems in the brain, thus alleviating negative affect and depression.[69]

Behavior and Lifestyle Change for Long-Term Cessation and Abstinence

There are 1.3 million U.S. citizens who quit smoking every year. In 1986, more than 30 percent of persons (approximately 17 million) who had smoked during the preceding year reported that they had tried to quit during that same period. If the 1.3 million ex-smokers are representative of the 17 million who attempt cessation, it seems that less than 10 percent who try to quit are successful each year.[70] The major reason that people find it so difficult to quit smoking is that they do not take the time to learn new behaviors for sustained change.[71]

There is often no effective means for measuring individual readiness to change smoking behavior. Within the dynamics of smoking cessation, there are many issues of resistance to change and recidivism. Smoking cessation is not a dichotomous product of smoking, then nonsmoking, but a process of progress and regression, ups and downs, successes and failures.[72] The transtheoretical model of change provides a theoretical basis for explaining when and how people change behaviors.[73-90] It is useful for comprehending self-initiated as well as professionally facilitated change. The model supports the notion that change occurs in a cyclic rather than linear fashion, often causing certain sequences and phases to be repeated before a change goal is reached. There are also varying rates of change. Some individuals move through the change sequence rapidly, while others never move beyond a particular stage.[91]

Prochaska and colleagues began investigating and developing the transtheoretical model of change by integrating diverse theories of change from the psychotherapy literature.[92,93] They examined the cognitive, affective, and behavioral processes as individuals moved through different levels of change. Specifically, the researchers studied attrition and relapse, which were more the rule than the exception. "Inadequate motivation, resistance to therapy, defensiveness, and inability to relate are client variables frequently invoked to account for the imperfect outcomes of the change enterprise."[94]

Two major constructs organize the framework of the transtheoretical model—the stages and the processes of change. Other important concepts are self-efficacy, pros and cons of decisional balance, and temptations for relapse.[95] Five stages of change provide a temporal structure for monitoring the change process. Applied to smoking cessation, the five stages of change are

1. precontemplation: no intention of quitting within the next 6 months
2. contemplation: seriously considering quitting within the next 6 months
3. preparation: seriously planning to quit within the next 30 days and has made at least one quit attempt in past year
4. action: former smoker continuously quit for less than 6 months
5. maintenance: former smoker continuously quit for greater than 6 months[96]

The stages are important for measuring progress toward quitting and help to predict relapse.[97]

Precontemplators have no intention of changing their behaviors in the near future. They cannot really see that they have a problem. Contemplators are aware that a problem exists and are thinking seriously about changing their behaviors, but they have not yet made a commitment to take action. Individuals in the preparation stage combine intention with preliminary actions to change behaviors in the near future. They may have made a past attempt to change that was unsuccessful. Smokers in the preparation stage may begin with small changes, such as smoking fewer cigarettes in a day, delaying the first cigarette of the morning, and changing some of their smoking habits (e.g., forgoing the "pleasant" cigarette with coffee after a meal). People who move into the action stage actually shift from thinking about the problem to doing something about the problem. They dedicate a considerable amount of commitment, time, and energy to the change. Finally, individuals who make a change and stick with it move into the maintenance stage and work to prevent relapse. They begin to stabilize the behavior change and make it a way of life.[98-103]

The processes of change are activities and events used to change problem behaviors successfully. These processes help to explain and predict change at each stage. Many interventions for promoting change are tailored to the five experiential and five behavioral processes of change (Table 28–1).[104] The experiential processes of consciousness raising, dramatic relief, and environmental reevaluation are most successfully used during movement from precontemplation to contemplation. Behav-

ioral processes are more appropriately used during the later stages of change from preparation to action and maintenance.

The transtheoretical model of change is well-founded in empirical research and provides sound principles for evidenced-based practice.[105] In one study, cardiac patients who smoked were recruited into an intensive action and maintenance-oriented smoking cessation program. Ninety-four percent of the smokers who began the program at the preparation or action stages were successful nonsmokers at a 6-month follow-up. Sixty-six percent of the smokers in a control group receiving tradi-

Table 28–1 Processes of Change

Type	Process	Definition	Possible Interventions
Experiential	Consciousness raising	Increasing information about self and problem	Observations, confrontations, interpretations, education
	Dramatic relief	Experiencing and expressing feelings about one's problems and solutions	Psychodrama, grieving losses, role playing; negative imagery
	Environmental reevaluation	Assessing how one's problem affects the physical environment	Empathy training, documentaries
	Self-reevaluation	Assessing how one feels and thinks about oneself with respect to a problem	Values clarification, positive imagery, corrective emotional experience
	Social liberation	Increasing alternatives for nonproblem behaviors available in society	Advocacy for rights of repressed, empowerment, policy interventions
Behavioral	Reinforcement management	Rewarding one's self or being rewarded by others for making changes	Contingency contracts, overt and covert reinforcement, self-reward
	Helping relationships	Being open and trusting about problems with someone who cares	Therapeutic alliance, social support, self-help groups
	Counterconditioning	Substituting alternatives for problem behaviors	Relaxation imagery, desensitization, assertion, positive self-statements
	Stimulus control	Avoiding or countering stimuli that elicit problem behaviors	Restructure of one's environment (e.g., removing alcohol, cigarettes, fattening foods), avoidance of high-risk cues, fading techniques
	Self-liberation	Choosing and making a commitment to act or to believe in ability to change	Decision-making therapy, New Year's resolutions, commitment-enhancing techniques, positive imagery

Source: Data from J.O. Prochaska, C.C. DiClemente, W.F. Velicer, S. Ginpil, and J.C. Norcross, Predicting Change in Smoking Status for Self-Changers, *Addictive Behaviors,* Vol. 10, pp. 395–406, © 1985.

tional care, but assessed as being in the preparation and action stages of change, were also successful nonsmokers at 6 months. Independent of membership in the treatment or control groups, 22 percent of those in the precontemplation stage, 43 percent of those in the contemplation stage, and 76 percent of individuals in the preparation/action stages were not smoking 6 months after completing the program. These results firmly demonstrate that internal commitment and readiness for change are necessary before any smoking cessation intervention becomes effective. Pretreatment stage is directly associated with outcomes.[106] In other studies, demographics, such as age and gender, socioeconomic status, smoking histories, goals and expectations, and other fairly stable variables, had little influence on smoking cessation outcomes, but stage differences predicted quit attempts and cessation success at 1- and 6-month follow-up checks.[107,108]

Fava and colleagues studied a highly representative sample of 4,144 smokers from the community at large and found that the early stages of change (precontemplation, contemplation, and preparation) were strongly related to processes of change, therefore validating the transtheoretical model of change.[109] Finally, additional research is demonstrating that health care professionals support the use of the transtheoretical model of change because it allows specific processes and interventions to be tailored to the individual client (as determined by stage). This prevents wasted efforts and provides maximum use of resources for greatest success.[110,111]

Prevention As the Best Protection from Smoking

Prevention should focus on today's youth. Smoking prevalence among high-school students is increasing rapidly. In 1991, high-school smoking prevalence was 27.5 percent; by 1993, it had grown to 30.5 percent. Today's high-school students are smoking at a prevalence rate of 34.8 per-

cent.[112,113] Using figures for the population group aged 12 through 17 years, the American Heart Association cited estimates that as many as 3,000 youngsters start smoking each day in the United States.[114]

In one study implemented in 11 junior high schools in San Diego County, California, researchers used a psychosocial intervention that combined refusal skills training, contingency management, and other methodologies, such as telephone and direct mail brochures, to prevent tobacco use.[115] Eleven other junior high schools served as controls. At the end of the third year, the prevalence of tobacco use was 14.2 percent among the intervention students and 22.5 percent among the controls. According to college undergraduates serving as change agents in this study, direct one-to-one telephone interventions appear to provide cost-effective tobacco-related behavior modification.

There is also a movement to discourage smoking through effective role models on television, in magazines, and in all public advertising. In addition, athletes, particularly baseball players, are being urged to stop the use of smokeless tobacco. The American College of Sports Medicine noted that athletes and others will not only set good examples by not using smokeless tobacco products, but also may avoid serious problems for themselves.[116]

HOLISTIC CARING PROCESS

Assessment

In preparing to use smoking cessation interventions, the nurse assesses the following parameters:

- the client's level of addiction to cigarettes
- the client's attitudes and beliefs about successful and sustained smoking cessation
- the client's motivation to learn interventions to become a permanent nonsmoker

- the client's stage of change in terms of smoking cessation
- the client's eating patterns and exercise program
- the client's existing stress management strategies
- the client's support and encouragement from family and friends

Patterns/Problems/Needs

The following patterns/problems/needs compatible with the interventions for smoking cessation related to the nine human response patterns (see Chapter 14) are as follows:

- *Exchanging:* Altered circulation
  Altered oxygenation
- *Valuing:* Spiritual distress
  Spiritual well-being
- *Choosing:* Ineffective individual coping
  Effective individual coping

- *Moving:* Self-care deficit
- *Perceiving:* Disturbance in body image
  Disturbance in self-esteem
  Hopelessness
- *Knowing:* Knowledge deficit
- *Feeling:* Anxiety
  Fear

Outcomes

Table 28–2 guides the nurse in client outcomes, nursing prescriptions, and evaluation for successful smoking cessation.

Therapeutic Care Plan and Implementation

Before the Session

- Spend a few moments centering yourself to recognize your presence and to begin the session with the intention to facilitate healing.

Table 28–2 Nursing Interventions: Smoking Cessation

Client Outcomes	Nursing Prescriptions	Evaluation
The client will demonstrate attitudes, beliefs, and behaviors that indicate the desire to be a nonsmoker.	Determine the client's desire to be a nonsmoker.	The client demonstrated attitudes, beliefs, behaviors, and the desire to be a nonsmoker.
	Assist the client in setting realistic plans for being a nonsmoker by	The client set a realistic plan and became a nonsmoker over 1 week as follows:
	• establishing quit date	• focused on quit date goal
	• drawing up a nicotine withdrawal schedule	• went "cold turkey"
	• cleansing self and environment of nicotine	• cleansed body/environment of nicotine
	• developing habit-breaker strategies	• adhered to habit-breaker strategies
	• keeping a smoking diary	• kept a smoking, exercise, food diary
	• practicing relaxation and imagery	• practiced relaxation/imagery daily
	• integrating behavior changes	• integrated behavior changes daily
	• deciding on rewards for attaining goals	• rewarded self for attaining goals

- Gather teaching sheets to be used during the session.
- Create a quiet place to begin guiding the client in smoking cessation strategies.

At the Beginning of the Session

- Go over the results of the smoking profile, and explore the meaning of these patterns with the client. Elicit insight into changing behaviors.
- Instruct the client in the importance of keeping a smoking diary.
- Establish pre-quitting strategies. Suggest that the client be patient and identify and combine the methods that can work best.
- Encourage the client to take a few days before the quit date to rid the body of toxins and to clean the house, office, and car of any evidence of cigarettes or odors.
- Have the client establish the quit date and sign a contract that specifies the quit date.
- Encourage the client to call on family and friends on the first smoke-free days, particularly when confidence is low. Remind them that their support is very important.

During the Session

- Reinforce the quit date and have the client imagine being smoke-free in 5 days.
- Teach basic relaxation and imagery skills to shape bodymind changes for internal and external smoke-free images. These new images also create a new felt sense and are a major source of the client's success. Rhythmic breathing and muscle relaxation are most helpful in teaching body-centered awareness and effective coping. Relaxation and imagery help the client to recognize and block smoke signals. Combine this practice with a stop smoking video once or twice a day.

- Teach the client to create specific imagery patterns (see Chapter 22).
  1. Active images—cleansing the body of nicotine and other toxins; finding a safe place that establishes a feeling of security and comfort; envisioning a protective bubble that receives what is needed from others and blocks out negative images, such as smoke signals.
  2. Process images—people, events, and situations that make the client smoke. Have the client rehearse being in a situation where smoking normally occurs, but now using a new behavior, such as reaching for a glass of water.
  3. End-state images—being smoke-free; accessing one's inner healer.
- Have the client create strategies to break smoke signals and become smoke-free—waking up and having a glass of water, reading the morning paper in a different room, taking a break and drinking water or juice, talking on the telephone, and practicing relaxation and rhythmic breathing.
- Encourage the client to be patient in making this major lifestyle change and to remember that smoking is about self-protective control. The old unhealthy control must be replaced with a new, healthy control. Identify internal and external experiences as new health behaviors are being shaped. Some are easy to change; others take longer.
- Ask the client to become aware of new opportunities for being with family, friends, and self while being smoke-free.

At the End of the Session

- Suggest that the client create a personal reward after 5 smoke-free days.
- Evaluate with the client the goals of behavior changes—reduction of

smoking urges and development of new habit patterns.

- Encourage the client to make a list of anticipated high-risk situations and decide in advance steps to prevent a relapse. The most frequent high-risk situations are social situations, emotional upsets, home or work frustration, interpersonal conflict, and relaxation after a meal.

- Reinforce the fact that the client can avoid relapse. Having learned to recognize high-risk situations for relapse, the client can be ready to act quickly in using strategies to resist smoking temptations. Successful coping strategies must honor internal responses (body-mind feelings and thoughts) and action-oriented responses (action steps).

- Suggest that the client become a support person for someone else who is trying to become smoke-free to decrease chances of relapse.

- Use the client outcomes (see Table 28–2) that were established before the session to evaluate the session.

- Schedule a follow-up session.

Specific Interventions

Recording Habits. Smoking is such a pervasive, automatic habit that it is essential to keep a smoking diary of when, where, how often, and what moods are associated with smoking. The client records the feelings associated with smoking and begins to think about new habits to replace these urges. Keeping such a record for several weeks before the quit date allows the client to identify patterns, and knowing the smoking triggers leads to permanent changes. To strengthen the new awareness, the client may record thoughts, feelings, urges, and observations about smoking. With each cigarette that is smoked, for example, the client should consider the following questions:

1. What internal cues made me think that I needed a cigarette (e.g., breath-ing patterns, mouth watering, tense muscles, fidgety hands)?
2. What external cues made me think that I needed a cigarette (e.g., talking on the phone, watching television, finishing eating, sitting down with friends)?
3. Now that I've smoked that cigarette, did I enjoy it?

Preparation for Quit Date. The desire to be a nonsmoker should build. Becoming smoke-free requires preparation. The client should take the time to identify personal reasons for quitting, such as to reduce the risk of heart, lung, or circulatory disease; to increase endurance and productivity; to improve sense of smell and taste; to increase self-esteem; to be in control; or to decrease the risk to family health from passive smoking. Once certain that it is time to quit, the client's goal is to be a nonsmoker in 5 days. The nurse may encourage the client to identify family members, friends, or a specific person who may want to join the effort as a quit-smoking partner. The client should tell significant people the quit date.

Preparation for Nicotine Withdrawal. There is no one best way to quit smoking. Some people are successful at just quitting "cold turkey" and going through the nicotine withdrawal, with the worst part usually lasting 5 days or less. Others require a gradual decrease of nicotine with the use of NRT. The client must decide which way is best for him or her.

If the client does not wish to use NRT, nicotine fading is a way to reduce the nicotine level in the body gradually and avoid withdrawal symptoms (e.g., irritability, lack of energy, increased cough). Each week for 3 weeks, the client buys a different brand of cigarette, each containing progressively less nicotine. By the end of the 3 weeks, the level of nicotine in the body has been substantially reduced. While using nicotine fading, it is important to record smoking habits accurately; the nicotine amount, time smoked, place smoked, alone or with others, and mood or feeling. The client should continue to smoke the same number of cigarettes and maintain the same manner of inhaling, because changes here defeat the purpose of this technique.

Another way to quit smoking is called focused smoking or rapid smoking. Clients should try this technique only under supervision, particularly those with heart disease or diabetes. Because this technique is not a pleasant experience, many researchers believe that it should be a last resort. The client needs cigarettes, matches, ashtray, candle and candle holder, wastepaper basket, paper to record responses, and pen or pencil. During a session, the smoker goes to his or her place and arranges the supplies. The wastepaper basket is placed to one side to be available in case vomiting occurs. The smoker lights a candle, then lights a cigarette from the candle flame, and takes a puff every 6 seconds. Immediately upon finishing one cigarette, the client lights the next cigarette. This is continued until the client is nauseated, three cigarettes have been smoked, and more smoking is impossible due to unpleasant body responses. The process is recorded and then repeated.

The client should record unpleasant body responses, such as hot lips, hot mouth, hot tongue, burning throat, burning lungs, dizzy feeling, pounding heart, tingling hands and legs, flushed face, watering eyes, nausea, or headache. The responses should be rated on a scale of 1 (not at all unpleasant) to 10 (extremely unpleasant).

Acupuncture programs that include the use of citrate compound are another means of reducing the body's nicotine level and are a rapid way to quit smoking, but, for sustained success, it is necessary to plan and learn new behavior strategies to bring about new health behaviors to replace smoking habits. This kind of program involves a single acupuncture session and the oral administration of a citrate compound, which causes the urine to become alkaline and retards the urinary excretion of nicotine. This process prevents a sudden fall of nicotine blood level, which reduces the craving for nicotine and the withdrawal symptoms.

Smoke-Free Body and Environment. During the first few nonsmoking days, the client rids the body of toxic waste left from the cigarettes by bathing, brushing teeth, drinking water, exercise, relaxation, imagery, rest, and good nutrition. A fresh nonsmoking living environment can be accomplished by placing clean filters in heating and cooling units and cleaning carpets, drapes, clothes, office, and car. Signs may be placed on the office door: "Thank you for not smoking." The more energy that the client puts into these activities, the more likely that the client will quit on the target date and become a permanent nonsmoker. The client should become aware of how quickly the senses of smell and taste increase and how disgusting the smell and taste of cigarettes become.

Identification of Habit Breakers. Becoming smoke-free is directly related to minor changes in daily routines, referred to as habit breakers. Many ex-smokers report that the first 5 days of being smoke-free are the hardest. Minor or major changes in daily activities can be less stressful if accompanied by a healing state of awareness. If the client should slip and fall back into old routines, these relapses can become learning situations. The client can identify negative self-talk or a stressful situation in which a new habit breaker may not have been used soon enough. The following events are the times when smoking is most likely:

Before starting the day:	• Getting out of bed • Taking a bath or shower • Eating breakfast • Reading the newspaper

Mornings:
- Starting work or driving to work
- Telephone calls
- Office or housework
- Meetings
- Morning breaks
- Before, during, and after lunch

Afternoons:
- Telephone calls
- Office or housework
- Meetings
- Afternoon breaks
- Completing and organizing your work for the next day
- Driving home or resting in late afternoon

Evenings:
- Before, during, and after dinner
- Relaxing, watching television, or out with family or friends
- Preparing for bed

It is helpful to create habit breakers for each of these events. Success with habit breakers requires commitment to identifying them, writing them down, and finding ways to personalize this list. For example, the client can take this list, divide a piece of paper into two columns, and write down new habit breakers.

Routine	*Habit Breaker*
Turning to radio news on awakening	Play relaxing music
Five cups of coffee at breakfast	Hot tea instead of coffee
Frequent lighting of cigarettes	Keep hard candy nearby
Get energy from morning smoke	Eat an apple; drink water

Integration of Exercise. To the person becoming smoke-free, an exercise program serves as a stress manager (as an alternative to smoking), helps with weight management, and increases energy levels. If the client does not have an exercise program, the nurse offers assistance and helps the client decide what lifestyle patterns to approach first. It usually takes about 3

months for an exercise program to become a regular part of life, so the client may look for an exercise partner who is as serious about exercising or being a nonsmoker.

Weight gain can be avoided. It occurs because the nonsmoker eats too much, lacks aerobic exercise, and consumes too much alcohol. If weight management is a challenge, it is helpful to set a target date for establishing and following an exercise program 3 months or longer before the quit date. (Refer to Chapter 27 for specific strategies to maintain healthy weight.) Then, as the client commits to quitting smoking, one component of an effective stress management program has already begun.

Assertion of Bill of Rights. Clients may find it helpful to recite their Bill of Rights. They can be creative and add to this list.

I have a right to

- be smoke-free in any situation.
- review my list of reasons to stop smoking frequently, particularly before any social gathering.
- ask others not to smoke in my home, office, or car.
- sit in nonsmoking sections.
- remind myself that cigarettes actually taste bad and leave toxic substances in my body.
- throw away all objects associated with smoking.
- keep sugarless gum and hard candy close at hand.
- practice my relaxation, imagery, and coping skills anywhere and at any time.
- keep liquids close by at work and at home.
- support legislation to protect nonsmokers from the dangers of passive smoking in public places.

Integration of Rewards. The client should plan a reward at least every 5 to 7 days for having a smoke-free lifestyle. These rewards should continue as long as the client needs to be aware of new lifestyle habits. The client is considered smoke-free when his or her habits are indeed nonsmoking behaviors. Continued use of the listed habit breakers always helps a client anticipate when smoke signals can surface and, thus, quickly take actions to prevent relapse.

Reinforcement of Positive Self-Talk. Feelings, moods, behaviors, and motivation affect physiologic changes. As the client learns to recognize the self-talk that sabotages his or her positive outlook, it is possible for the client to remain in control and not give in to the urge to smoke. Negative rationalization must be recognized, because it can gradually lead to doubt about the ability to change. The client may change "I've become more nervous since I quit smoking" to "I am noticing a change in my moods since quitting and replacing it with relaxation and imagery practice. This makes me feel much better than the short burst of nicotine energy." Similarly, negative thoughts must be identified and replaced with positive thoughts. For example, "I'll never get over this urge to smoke; I'll never be successful at breaking the habit" may be reframed as "Of course, I can get over this urge. I am learning new coping strategies, and I can really imagine myself smoke-free."

Smoking Cessation: Imagery Scripts. To enhance the client's success at becoming smoke-free, the nurse can create a relaxation and imagery tape or provide the following script/s to the client to make his or her own tape. The following scripts help the client form correct biologic images of being smoke-free. They can be modified or expanded, depending on present habits and which new skills the client wishes to develop in order to break the nicotine habit. A relaxation exercise from Chapter 21 may be recorded for 5 to 10 minutes; then the script for smoking cessation is recorded for 15 minutes. The nurse should encourage the client to listen to the tape for 20 minutes several times a day.

Script: *Introduction. (Name), as your mind becomes clearer and clearer, feel it becoming more and more alert. Somewhere deep inside of you, a brilliant light begins to glow. Sense this happening. . . . The light grows brighter and more intense. . . . This is your bodymind communication center. Breathe into it. . . . Energize it with your breath. The light is powerful and penetrating, and a beam begins to grow from it. The beam shines into your body now as you prepare to focus on being smoke-free. . . .*

In your relaxed state, . . . affirm to yourself at your deep level of inner strength and knowing . . . that you can stop smoking. Say it over and over as you begin to see the words and feelings in every cell in your body. Feel your relaxed state deepen. You can get to this space anytime you wish. . . . All you have to do is give yourself the suggestion and stay with the suggestion as you move into your relaxed state. This is a skill that you will use repeatedly as you move into being smoke-free.

Script: *Quit Date. Congratulate yourself for setting your quit date. You are aware of all your resources to quit. With your mind's eye now . . . see your calendar and experience yourself reading your quit date. With full intention to quit, mark your quit date on the calendar. Enlist the help of your family or a friend as you set your quit date.*

Script: *Cleansing Your Body and Environment. It is now time to rid your body of toxins left from the cigarettes. Begin to cleanse your body. . . . Feel the toxins flowing out of your body as you increase the liquids you drink. Practice your deep breathing exercises, remembering to exhale completely . . . enjoying this new awareness of how healthy your lungs will become with the cleansing and clearing of toxins. Experience your breath, skin, hair . . . fresh as a spring breeze. See yourself making your surroundings smoke-free day by day. Notice the pleasant changes in your new, nonsmoking environment. . . . First, begin to notice how you are becoming more sensitive to smells. . . . Enjoy the freshness of your clothes, home, office, and car being free of smoke.*

As you keep your records, become aware of your progress. Reward yourself regularly. Imagine you have had 5 smoke-free days. The worst of any withdrawal is over. What is your first reward going to be? Give yourself a big reward!

As you continue to deepen your relaxation, repeat to yourself the words "I am calm." Let your body experience these words in your own unique way. Register this feeling throughout your body. Begin to increase your awareness of feeling good about being alive, to be conscious of beginning new habits . . . free of smoking.

Script: *Smoke Signals. Starting now, reflect on your wonderful decision to release the habit of smoking . . . a habit that could cause illness and take away your energy and vitality. Get in touch with your smoke signals. Is it a certain time of day, a person, a place, or social gathering? As you bring them into awareness, . . . rehearse in your mind the healthy behaviors you will use to replace the urges. . . . Is it drinking a glass of water . . . chewing sugar-free gum, going for a walk, listening to music, chewing on a toothpick, or taking a hot shower or bath? And as you think about smoking urges . . . those foolish habits . . . you can hear your powerful inner voice repeating clear affirmations, . . . "I have stopped smoking . . . I am free of smoking . . . I feel strong and healthy . . . I can taste, and smell fragrances. My cough has gone."*

Hear your own voice saying, "I no longer crave a habit negatively affecting my health. This habit is diminishing steadily, and I can envision being completely free of this addiction. My mind is functioning in such a manner that I no longer crave tobacco . . . a habit that has affected my lungs and heart. I no longer place unnecessary strain on these organs so vital to life."

When you feel the urge to smoke, hear yourself saying, "Stop! I don't need to smoke any more. I am free." These words will become more powerful the more you say them. Remember this message is always with you . . . and you are no longer a smoker. That is behind you.

Script: *Nutritious Eating and Exercise.* "As I stop smoking, I will not be excessively hungry or eat excessively. Because of the power of my unconscious mind, I am free of my addiction. I am conscious of increasing my exercise to three or four times a week for 20 minutes or longer. I am increasing my fluid intake and chewing sugar-free gum. I am sleeping soundly at night. I am free of smoking. . . . I am free." You can reach this inner wisdom any time that you wish. . . . All you have to do is take the time.

Script: *Closure.* Take a few slow, energizing breaths and, as you come back to full awareness of the room, know that whatever is right for you at this point in time is unfolding just as it should and that you have done your best, regardless of the outcome.

Case Study

Setting: Nurse-based wellness clinic smoking cessation program

Client: J.N., a 48-year-old interior designer, telling her story to the new clients after she has been smoke-free for 5 years

Patterns/ Problems/ Needs: Health maintenance related to engagement in strategies to remain smoke-free

"You can call it midlife crisis or whatever; I just happened to wake up and tell myself that I'm worth a better state of health and mind. How did I do it—lots of determination and reprogramming my mind with successful images. I never dreamed that I could be so successful at quitting smoking. I'd tried to quit on many occasions, but the reason I never was able to sustain change is that I had tried to quit before I really was ready to do so.

"I'd been smoking for 27 years, and I just got tired of my chronic cough and feeling tired. Other things began to happen also. My family and friends began to ask for non-smoking sections in restaurants and gave me 3 months before they declared the house a nonsmoking house. They also placed a disgusting, ugly series of pictures of me smoking with a title on it saying, 'We Love You—Quit Smoking!' The first time I looked at the pictures, I burst into tears and heard their message loud and clear. I got in touch with why I began smoking in the first place as a teenager—I thought I looked important and glamorous. Those pictures certainly didn't convey that image.

"The last straw that really got my attention was when a friend and I were driving along with our windows down on a nice spring day. My friend said to me, 'Who do you think is smoking?' We could see no person smoking, but my friend could smell it. It turned out that our lane of traffic started moving before the one next to us. Sure enough, there was a smoker three cars in front of us in the left lane to us. I was driving, and, as we passed the car, smoke came in our window. I couldn't smell it even though I could see the smoke coming in the window. My friend was able to smell it long after we passed the smoker. I was astounded that I couldn't smell it.

"I really planned a ritual for my quit date for ending smoking—which has changed my life in many ways. I have now been smoke-free for 5 years. Let me begin by saying that, in the previous 15 years, I had tried to quit smoking seven times; each time I was successful for 1 month at the longest, so I knew that it was possible. As I look back on it now, the reason that I didn't have any sustained change was that I didn't shape any new behaviors or thoughts.

"Let me share with you my rituals. I planned a 5-day period to be by myself to focus on shaping new behaviors. The reason I chose to stay at home was the importance of preparation and concentration of new thoughts and behaviors prior to my quit date.

"Prior to that special week, I began my 'detox' process. I decided to buy a new bright blue toothbrush, which I placed in a beautiful small wicker basket. I also placed this on the opposite side of where I usually kept my toothbrush. It just seemed important to change all of my bathing habits. When brushing my teeth gently, frequently followed by a mouthwash, I was aware of repeating words to myself about cleansing and purifying. I used these same thoughts when I bathed. I would stand in the shower and concentrate on the water washing the toxins from my skin. For the internal removal of toxins, I increased my fluid intake of water and herb teas to 6 to 8 glasses a day. Exercise also became part of my ritual. I would get up each day and start my morning with a 30-minute walk. On the walk, I used the time to see myself smoke-free. When I came in from my walks, I would watch a 20-minute video of beautiful images and healing statements about successfully breaking the smoke habit and being free. [See resource list.]

"Well, my home environment reeked of smoke and staleness. My drapes and fabric chairs and couches had not been cleaned in 16 years; my carpets, in 8. I allowed myself the luxury of having them professionally cleaned. Not only did the house smell fresh, but all the colors were very fresh and seemed new. Air conditioning filters were changed. I cleaned clothes that were well overdue. I aired the house.

"The biggest task was to gather all the cigarette packages throughout the house. They were in every room, and I had about three full cartons when I finally gathered them all up. This was really scary for me, because when I saw them all together, the thought that came to me was, 'I'm really addicted. There is no way I can break this habit.' Out of nowhere, this very loud, powerful voice blurted out, 'Yes, you can, and you have already begun.' I have never heard such volume from my own voice. It was as if it was a voice other than my own. Prior to that, I also removed all of the ashtrays and bought a beautiful door sign which read, THANK YOU FOR NOT SMOKING. When I placed it above the door bell, I felt this inner sensation of glee and energy. It was very affirming to me, and, from that moment on, there was no stopping my success. I really believed for the first time that I was going to be successful, and I felt an inner strength that I had never experienced before. I also received so much encouragement from my husband and two children when they came home that evening. I cleaned my car as well as I had the house. Now it was time to sign my contract with the family.

"During this period of 1 week of cleaning my body, house, and car, I recorded my internal and external cues of why I smoked. It was when I was hungry, talking on the phone, when I was putting on my makeup in the morning, and after meals. During this time, I let myself smoke no more than three cigarettes a day—outside standing up. I concentrated on what a disgusting habit smoking was. As I focused on these messages to myself, I not only slowed down the smoking, I also didn't enjoy the cigarettes and found that it was really not as pleasant as in the past. I had tried this before, but my thoughts were also on how much I was going to miss the smoking and pleasure of the buzz from smoking. I was so aware of not really enjoying it as much as I used to.

"I well remember my quit date 5 years ago. It is so clear; it is as if I planned it just yesterday. The reason it seems so recent is that my preparation and commitment to stopping smoking has spilled over into other areas in my life. Do I miss smoking? Frankly, I'll say yes. I have those urges on occasions. However, as I've integrated relaxation, imagery, and positive affirmations in my life, my commitment to being smoke-free is stronger. I honor that inner voice that says, 'Light Up.' For me, what works best is to hear the message, honor that I heard it, but to replace smoking with something that is always with me—the power of relaxed breathing. I also use a saying a friend taught me, which is Avoid H.A.L.T.—Avoid becoming too hungry, too angry, too lonely, or too tired. Time, commitment, and believing in my success is part of every day for me. Quitting smoking is one of the hardest things I've ever done. I can't remember planning so well for any event in my life. I believed I could do it, and that is exactly what continued to happen."

Evaluation

With the client, the nurse determines whether the client outcomes for smoking cessation (see Table 28–2) were achieved. To evaluate the session further, the nurse may again explore the subjective effects of the experience with the client (Exhibit 28–1).

In becoming an ex-smoker, a client must understand that it is a gradual step-by-step process that requires learning new skills. Smoking cessation involves (1) recognizing smoking habits, (2) establishing habit breakers, (3) preparing for detoxification of body and environment, (4) following a good nutrition and exercise program, and (5) modifying behavior. The integration of these five areas helps clients achieve new awareness about being smoke-free with new lifestyle patterns and improved relationships with people at work and at home.

DIRECTIONS FOR FUTURE RESEARCH

1. Determine the nursing interventions that most effectively minimize stress as clients begin a smoking cessation program.
2. Evaluate combinations of smoking cessation content and teaching methods to determine which are most effective in assisting a client in sustained smoking cessation.

Exhibit 28–1 Evaluating the Client's Subjective Experience with Smoking Cessation Interventions

1. Did you gain any new insight today about your smoking patterns?
2. Do you have any questions about preparing for a quit date?
3. Do you have any questions about recording your habits?
4. Can you identify two new habit breakers right now to be smoke-free?
5. Are you aware of your bodymind signals of wanting to smoke?
6. What relaxation exercises are most helpful to you in replacing smoking habits?
7. What will be your exercise program?
8. Do you have any questions about the active, process imagery and the end-state imagery exercises that you experienced today?
9. Did you like the imagery exercises?
10. Did you gain any new insight about your self-talk of being smoke-free?
11. What are three affirmations to help you just now create an image change of being smoke-free?
12. What is your next step?

3. Determine the nursing interventions that are most effective in helping a client cope with fears regarding relapse.

NURSE HEALER REFLECTIONS

After reading this chapter, the nurse healer will be able to answer or begin a process of answering the following questions:

- What rituals can I create or assist others in creating to detoxify and cleanse the body and environment of all traces of nicotine?
- What are my internal cues of reacting to smoke?
- What are my external cues of reacting to smoke?
- What are specific process, end-state, and general healing images for teaching myself or others about releasing attachments to smoking and moving forward in being smoke-free?

NOTES

1. U.S. Department of Health and Human Services, Tobacco, *Prevention Report* (1996, Fall): 4–5.

2. B.S. Lynch and R.S. Bonnie, *Growing Up Tobacco Free: Preventing Nicotine Addiction in Children and Youths* (Washington, DC: National Academy Press, 1994).

3. Centers for Disease Control and Prevention, Cigarette Smoking among Adults—United States: 1994, *Morbidity and Mortality Weekly Report* 45, no. 27 (1996): 588–590.

4. L.B. Russell et al., Modeling All-Cause Mortality: Projections of the Impact of Smoking Cessation Based on the NHEFS, *American Journal of Public Health* 88, no. 4 (1998): 630–636.

5. Centers for Disease Control and Prevention, Cigarette Smoking among Adults, 588.

6. Centers for Disease Control and Prevention, Smoking Related Deaths, *Morbidity and Mortality Weekly Report* 46, no. 26 (1997): 448–451.

7. National Center for Health Statistics, Advanced Report of Final Mortality Statistics—1992, in *Monthly Vital Statistics* (1995).

8. U.S. Department of Health and Human Services, Tobacco.

9. C.J.L. Murray and A.D. Lopez, *The Global Burden of Disease* (Cambridge, MA: Harvard University Press, 1996).

10. Centers for Disease Control and Prevention, Cigarette Smoking among Adults, 588.

11. U.S. Department of Health and Human Services, *Tobacco Use among U.S. Racial/Ethnic Groups—African Americans, American Indian and Alaska Natives, Asian Americans and Pacific Islanders, and Hispanics: A Report of the Surgeon General* (Atlanta: Centers for Disease Control and Prevention, 1998).

12. U.S. Department of Health and Human Services, *Tobacco Use among U.S. Racial/Ethnic Groups.*

13. U.S. Department of Health and Human Services, *Healthy People 2000: Midcourse Review and 1995 Revisions* (Boston: Jones & Bartlett Publishers, 1996).

14. Centers for Disease Control and Prevention, Changes in Cigarette Brand Preferences of Adolescent Smokers—United States, 1989–1993, *Morbidity and Mortality Weekly Report* 43, no. 32 (1994): 577–581.

15. U.S. Department of Health and Human Services, Tobacco.

16. American Nurses Association, Position Statement: Environmental Tobacco Smoke (Washington, DC: ANA, 1997).

17. T. Neslund, *Tobacco, the Planet, and You* (Hagerstown, MD: The Health Connection, 1995).

18. U.S. Department of Health and Human Services, Public Health Service, Office on Smoking and Health, *The Health Consequences of Smoking: Cancer and Chronic Lung Disease in the Workplace* (Atlanta, GA: USDHHS, 1985).

19. U.S. Department of Health and Human Services, Public Health Service, Office on Smoking and Health, *The Health Consequences of Involuntary Smoking: A Report of the Surgeon General* (USDDHS, 1986).

20. U.S. Department of Health and Human Services, *Environmental Tobacco Smoke in the Workplace: Lung Cancer and Other Health Effects,* NIOSH Current Intelligence Bulletin 54 (USDHHS, PHS, Centers for Disease Control and Prevention, National Institute for Occupational Safety and Health, 1991).

21. Environmental Protection Agency, Respiratory Health Effects of Passive Smoking: Fact Sheet (Washington, DC: Environmental Protection Agency, 1993).

22. P.S. Blair et al., Smoking and Sudden Infant Death Syndrome: Results from 1993–1995 Case Control Study for Confidential Inquiry into Stillbirths and Deaths in Infancy, *British Medical Journal* 313 (1996): 195–198.

23. H.S. Klonoff-Cohen et al., The Effect of Passive Smoking and Tobacco Exposure through Breast Milk on Sudden Infant Death Syndrome, *Journal of the American Medical Association* 273, no. 10 (1995): 795–798.

24. C. A. Aligne and J.J. Stoddard, Tobacco and Children: An Economic Evaluation of the Medical Effects of Parental Smoking, *Archives of Pediatrics and Adolescence* 151 (1997): 648–653.

25. I. Kawachi et al., A Prospective Study of Passive Smoking and Coronary Heart Disease, *Circulation* 95, no. 10 (1997): 2374–2379.

26. K. Streenland et al., Environmental Tobacco Smoke and Coronary Heart Disease in the American Cancer Society CPS-II Cohort, *Circulation* 94, no. 4 (1996): 622–628.

27. M. Weitzman et al., Maternal Smoking and Childhood Asthma, *Pediatrics* 85, no. 4 (1990): 505–511.

28. T.J. Roby et al., Discriminant Analysis of Lower Respiratory Tract Components Associated with Cigarette Smoking Based on Quantitative Sputum Cytology, *Acta Cytologica* 34, no. 2 (1990): 147–154.

29. D. Krough, Why Do People Smoke Despite the Evidence?, *Healthline* 4 (1993): 2–5.

30. I. Kawachi et al., Smoking Cessation and Decreased Risk of Stroke in Women, *Journal of the American Medical Association* 269, no. 2 (1993): 232–236.

31. K.B. Keller and L. Lemberg, Smoking: A Burden to Patient and Society, *American Journal of Critical Care* 5, no. 4 (1996): 314–316.

32. Krough, Why Do People Smoke Despite the Evidence?

33. Keller and Lemberg, Smoking: A Burden to Patient and Society.

34. Krough, Why Do People Smoke Despite the Evidence?

35. Krough, Why Do People Smoke Despite the Evidence?

36. H. Aston and R. Stepney, Smoking As a Psychological Tool, in *Smoking: Psychology and Pharmacology*, ed. H. Aston and R. Stepney (London: Tavistock Publications, 1982), 91–119.

37. S.A. Brunton, *Nicotine Addiction and Smoking Cessation* (New York: Medical Information Services, 1991).

38. C. Leccese, Tailored Approach Works Best for Smoking Cessation, *ADVANCE for Nurse Practitioners* (1998, April): 67–69.

39. Krough, Why Do People Smoke Despite the Evidence?

40. J. Addington, Group Treatment for Smoking Cessation among Persons with Schizophrenia, *Psychiatric Services* 49, no. 7 (1998): 925–928.

41. S.M. Hall et al., Nortriptyline and Cognitive–Behavioral Therapy in the Treatment of Cigarette Smoking, *Archives of General Psychiatry* 55 (1998): 683–690.

42. Leccese, Tailored Approach Works Best for Smoking Cessation.

43. Leccese, Tailored Approach Works Best for Smoking Cessation.

44. E. Lichtenstein et al., Introduction to the Community Intervention Trial for Smoking Cessation (COMMIT), *International Quarterly of Community Health Education* 11 (1990–1991): 173–185.

45. J.K. Ockene et al., The Physician-Delivered Smoking Intervention Project: Can Short-Term Interventions Produce Long-Term Effects for a General Outpatient Population? *Health Psychology* 13, no. 3 (1994): 278–281.

46. J.L. Schwartz, *Review and Evaluation of Smoking Cessation Methods* (Bethesda, MD: National Cancer Institute, 1987).

47. Schwartz, *Review and Evaluation of Smoking Cessation Methods*.

48. D.R. Powell, A Guided Self-Help Smoking Cessation Intervention with White-Collar and Blue-Collar Employees, *American Journal of Health Promotion* 7, no. 5 (1993): 325–326.

49. H.A. Lando et al., Public Service Application of an Effective Clinic Approach to Smoking Cessation, *Health Education Research* 4 (1989): 103–109.

50. C.C. DiClemente et al., The Process of Smoking Cessation: An Analysis of Precontemplation, Contemplation, and Preparation Stages of Change, *Journal of Consulting and Clinical Psychology* 59, no. 2 (1991): 295–304.

51. M.C. Fiore et al., Methods Used To Quit Smoking in the United States: Do Cessation Programs Help? *Journal of the American Medical Association* 263, no. 20 (1990): 2760–2765.

52. M.G. Goldstein et al., A Population-Based Survey of Patients' Perceptions of Health Care Provider–Delivered Smoking Cessation Interventions, *Archives of Internal Medicine* 157 (1997): 1313–1319.

53. C. Senore et al., Predictors of Smoking Cessation Following Physician Counseling, *Preventive Medicine* 27, no. 3 (1998): 412–421.

54. M.E. Wewars et al., Smoking Cessation Interventions in Nursing Practice, *Nursing Clinics of North America* 33, no. 1 (1998): 61–74.

55. M. Fiore et al., A Missed Opportunity: Teaching Medical Students To Help Patients Successfully Quit Smoking, *Journal of the American Medical Association* 271, no. 8 (1994): 624–626.

56. R.L. Richmond and C.P. Mendelsohn, Physicians' Views of Programs Incorporating Stages of Change To Reduce Smoking and Excessive Alcohol Consumption, *American Journal of Health Promotion* 12, no. 4 (1998): 254–257.

57. R. Richmond et al., Family Physicians' Utilization of a Brief Smoking Cessation Program Following Reinforcement Contact after Training: A Randomized Trial, *Preventive Medicine* 27, no. 1 (1998): 77–83.

58. Fiore et al., A Missed Opportunity.

59. E. Gilpin et al., Physician Advice To Quit Smoking: Results from the 1990 California Tobacco Survey, *Journal of General Internal Medicine* 8 (1993): 549–553.

60. G. Richardson et al., Smoking Cessation after Successful Treatment of Small-Cell Lung Cancer, *Annals of Internal Medicine* 119, no. 21 (1993): 383–390.

61. C. Silagy et al., Meta-analysis on Efficacy of Nicotine Replacement Therapy in Smoking Cessation, *Lancet* 343 (1994): 139–142.

62. R. Hurt et al., Nicotine Patch Therapy for Smoking Cessation Combined with Physician Advice and Nurse Follow-up, *Journal of the American Medical Association* 271, no. 8 (1994): 595–600.

63. S. Kenford et al., Predicting Smoking Cessation: Who Will Quit with and without the Nicotine Patch, *Journal of the American Medical Association* 271, no. 8 (1994): 589–594.

64. A.H. Glassman et al., Heavy Smokers, Smoking Cessation, and Clonidine: Results of a Double-blind, Randomized Trial, *Journal of the American Medical Association* 259, no. 19 (1988): 2863–2866.

65. A.H. Glassman, Cigarette Smoking: Implications for Psychiatric Illness, *American Journal of Psychiatry* 150 (1993): 546–553.

66. A.H. Glassman, Psychiatry and Cigarettes, *Archives of General Psychiatry* 55 (1998): 692–693.

67. L.S. Covey, Major Depression following Smoking Cessation, *American Journal of Psychiatry* 154 (1997): 263–265.

68. Hall et al., Nortriptyline and Cognitive–Behavioral Therapy in the Treatment of Cigarette Smoking.

69. Addington, Group Treatment for Smoking Cessation among Persons with Schizophrenia.

70. Fiore et al., Methods Used To Quit Smoking in the United States.

71. DiClemente et al., The Process of Smoking Cessation.

72. DiClemente et al., The Process of Smoking Cessation.

73. C.C. DiClemente, Motivational Interviews and the Stages of Change, in *Motivational Interviewing: Preparing People for Change*, ed. W.R. Miller and S. Rollnick (New York: Guilford Press, 1991), 191–202.

74. J.L. Fava et al., Applying the Transtheoretical Model to a Representative Sample of Smokers, *Addictive Behaviors* 20, no. 2 (1995): 189–203.

75. J.L. Kristeller et al., Processes of Change in Smoking Cessation: A Cross-Validation Study in Cardiac Patients, *Journal of Substance Abuse* 4 (1992): 263–276.

76. J.O. Prochaska, *Systems of Psychotherapy: A Transtheoretical Analysis* (Homewood, IL: Dorsey Press, 1979).

77. J.O. Prochaska and C.C. DiClemente, *The Transtheoretical Approach: Crossing Traditional Boundaries of Change* (Homewood, IL: Dorsey Press, 1984).

78. J.O. Prochaska et al., Predicting Change in Smoking Status for Self-Changers, *Addictive Behaviors* 10 (1985): 395–406.

79. J.O. Prochaska and C.C. DiClemente, Common Processes of Change in Smoking, Weight Control, and Psychological Distress, in *Coping and Substance Abuse*, ed. S. Shiffman and T. Wills (San Diego, CA: Academic Press, 1985), 345–363.

80. J.O. Prochaska and C.C. DiClemente, Toward a Comprehensive Model of Change, in *Treating Addictive Behaviors: Processes of Change*, ed. W.R. Miller and N. Heather (New York: Plenum Press, 1986), 4–27.

81. J.O. Prochaska et al., Measuring Processes of Change: Applications to the Cessation of Smoking, *Journal of Consulting and Clinical Psychology* 56, no. 4 (1988): 520–528.

82. J.O. Prochaska, Prescribing to the Stages and Levels of Change, *Psychotherapy* 28 (1991): 463–468.

83. J.O. Prochaska, What Causes People To Change from Unhealthy to Health Enhancing Behaviors? *Cancer Prevention* 2 (1991): 30–34.

84. J.O. Prochaska et al., In Search of How People Change: Applications to Addictive Behaviors, *American Psychologist* 47, no. 9 (1992): 1102.

85. J.O. Prochaska and C.C. DiClemente, Stages of Change in the Modification of Problem Behaviors, in *Progress in Behavior Modification*, ed. R.M. Eisler, M. Hersen, and P.M. Miller (Sycamore, IL: Sycamore Press, 1992), 184–214.

86. J.O. Prochaska et al., Stages of Change and Decisional Balance for Twelve Problem Behaviors, *Health Psychology* 13 (1994): 39–46.

87. J.O. Prochaska et al., Standardized, Individualized, Interactive and Personalized Self-Help Programs for Smoking Cessation, *Health Psychology* 12 (1993): 399–405.

88. J.O. Prochaska and W.F. Velicer, Introduction, *American Journal of Health Promotion* 12, no. 1 (1997): 6–7.

89. W.F. Velicer and C.C. DiClemente, Understanding and Intervening with the Total Population of Smokers, *Tobacco Control* 2 (1993): 95–96.

90. W.F. Velicer et al., Minimal Interventions Appropriate for an Entire Population of Smokers, in *Interventions for Smokers: An International Perspective*, ed. R. Richmond (Baltimore: Williams & Wilkins, 1994), 69–92.

91. A.B. Herrick et al., Stages of Change, Decisional Balance, and Self-Efficacy across Four Health Behaviors in a Worksite Environment, *American Journal of Health Promotion* 12, no. 1 (1997): 49–56.

92. Prochaska, *Systems of Psychotherapy: A Transtheoretical Analysis.*

93. J.O. Prochaska and C.C. DiClemente, Stages and Processes of Self-Change in Smoking: Toward an Integrative Model of Change, *Journal of Consulting and Clinical Psychology* 5, no. 3 (1983): 390–395.

94. Prochaska et al., In Search of How People Change.

95. Prochaska and Velicer, Introduction.

96. Fava et al., Applying the Transtheoretical Model to a Representative Sample of Smokers.

97. E.A. O'Connor et al., Gender and Smoking Cessation: A Factor Structure Comparison of Processes of Change, *Journal of Consulting and Clinical Psychology* 64, no. 1 (1996): 130–138.

98. DiClemente et al., The Process of Smoking Cessation.

99. Prochaska et al., In Search of How People Change.

100. Prochaska and DiClemente, Stages of Change in the Modification of Problem Behaviors.

101. Prochaska et al., Stages of Change and Decisional Balance for Twelve Problem Behaviors.

102. Prochaska et al., Standardized, Individualized, Interactive and Personalized Self-Help Programs for Smoking Cessation.

103. Prochaska and Velicer, Introduction.

104. Prochaska et al., Predicting Change in Smoking Status for Self-Changers.

105. M. O'Donnell, Editor's Notes, *American Journal of Health Promotion* 12, no. 1 (1997): 4.

106. J. Ockene et al., *The Coronary Artery Smoking Intervention Study* (Worcester, MA: National Heart Lung Blood Institute, 1988).

107. DiClemente et al., The Process of Smoking Cessation.

108. Prochaska and DiClemente, Stages of Change in the Modification of Problem Behaviors.

109. Fava et al., Applying the Transtheoretical Model to a Representative Sample of Smokers.

110. Richmond and Mendelsohn, Physicians' Views of Programs.

111. R.G. Boyle et al., Stages of Change for Physical Activity, Diet, and Smoking among HMO Members and Chronic Conditions, *American Journal of Health Promotion* 12, no. 3 (1998): 170–175.

112. Centers for Disease Control, Tobacco Use and Usual Source of Cigarettes among High School Students—United States, 1995, *Morbidity and Mortality Weekly Report* 45, no. 2 (1995): 412–418.

113. U.S. Department of Health and Human Services, *Preventing Tobacco Use among Young People: A Report of the Surgeon General* (Bethesda, MD: National Institutes of Health, 1994).

114. P. Gunby, Health Experts to Youth: Don't Give Tobacco a Start, *Journal of the American Medical Association* 271, no. 8 (1994): 580.

115. J. Elder et al., The Long-Term Prevention of Tobacco Use among Junior High School Students: Classroom and Telephone Interventions, *American Journal of Public Health* 83, no. 9 (1993): 1239–1244.

116. P. Gunby, Sports, Medical Officials Call "Spit" Tobacco "Out," *Journal of the American Medical Association* 271, no. 8 (1994): 580.

RESOURCE

Positive Harmonic Imagery: Stop Smoking
    Program (video)
New Era Media
P.O. Box 410685-BT
San Francisco, CA 94141
Telephone: 415-863-3555

VISION OF HEALING

Changing One's World View

A world view is that set of beliefs each of us holds about the way that the world operates, the reasons that things happen as they do, and the rules that they follow. We seldom give a thought to our world view, but it is a powerful, guiding force in all of our lives. We cannot escape the effects of our world view. It begins to operate the very moment we begin each day. The moment we walk into work or into a social gathering, we put our world view into action. Do we have control over our life, or do things happen by accident? Is there some purpose or meaning behind the events with which we are dealing (e.g., stress level, interactions when dealing with clients and families)? Do people with addictions have any control over their illness, or is it only a function of the physiologic processes occurring in the body? Does choice exist in health and illness, or is the body entirely "on automatic"? Our world view gives us answers to difficult questions like these. The more conscious we become of the assumptions that we make in our world view, about "how things work," the more effective we will become in our interactions with self and others.

How can we become more conscious about our world view and our choices in life? To be present for ourselves or others, we must honor our personal needs or we will be physical and emotional wrecks. What are the current circumstances in our lives? We must accept them, releasing efforts to control things over which we have no control. We must honor ourselves each day with relaxation, imagery, music, meditation, or prayer. We can create an exercise program; take long, hot baths or showers; eat nutritional foods; eliminate excess caffeine or junk food; and ask other people for help if needed. We need to tell ourselves over and over that we are doing a good job.

Caring for ourselves each day requires simple things. When waking up in the morning and before getting out of bed, we should say to ourselves, "The part of me that is most in need of healing right now is . . ." and "The things that I can do to bring about my healing are . . ." The answers are usually simple, such as "I need to take a morning break and a lunch break, have a massage, or ask a friend to meet me for a chat." We can repeat this as often as necessary during the day. This increases our awareness of basic assumptions and life choices. By honoring ourselves, we allow fear, depression, loneliness, suffering, feelings of discouragement, crisis, or tragic moments to be released so that being with ourselves or others is quality time. Recognizing one's world view and learning how to care for oneself are at the core of helping a person with addictions move toward healing and spiritual transformation.

Chapter 29

Addiction and Recovery Counseling

Bonney Gulino Schaub and Barbara Montgomery Dossey

NURSE HEALER OBJECTIVES

Theoretical

- Discuss factors leading to addiction.
- Identify patterns of thinking and behavior associated with addictions.
- Identify the reasons that spiritual development is important in long-term recovery.

Clinical

- Develop your skills in assessing clients' relationships to drugs and alcohol and to addictive patterns of behavior.
- Learn to recognize the patterns of denial that perpetuate and protect addictive behaviors.
- Become knowledgeable about the long-term issues in recovery and relapse prevention.
- Identify support systems within the community for the person in recovery, such as support groups, psychotherapists knowledgeable about issues in recovery, meditation and prayer groups, or other resources for spiritual development.

Personal

- Take the Problem Drinker Self-Assessment, and determine if drinking is a problem in your life.

- Assess your responses to stress from the perspective of addictive patterns of behavior (e.g., alcohol use, smoking, excessive sugar consumption), and learn more effective stress management strategies.
- Recognize your own feelings of vulnerability and your characteristic responses to these feelings.
- Assess your environment, and determine whether there are any people with addictions in your personal or work life; notice if you have any patterns of enabling.

DEFINITIONS

Addiction: a physiologic or psychologic dependence on a substance (e.g., alcohol, cocaine) or behavior (e.g., gambling, sex, eating).

Denial: a major dynamic in the process of addiction in which the person willfully refuses to accept the reality of his or her behavior and its effect on self and others.

Detoxification: the physical process of withdrawing from use of drugs or alcohol.

Dry Drunk: referring to alcoholism (dry = not drinking) where a person has stopped drinking but not extended this change to developing mentally, emotionally, and spiritually.

New Consciousness: a concept used in Alcoholics Anonymous that refers to a movement away from addictive thinking and toward an understanding of one's life purpose or spiritual purpose.

Recovery: the mental, emotional, physical, and spiritual actions that support conscious living and freedom from addictive behaviors.

Relapse: a return to addictive behavior, even if on only one occasion.

Spiritual Awakening: an expansion of awareness that results in a realization that the isolated individual is, in fact, participating in a universe of divine intention and order.

THEORY AND RESEARCH

In the United States today, there are 90 million social drinkers who enjoy alcohol and have a habit of using it. There are many theories about the amount that someone can drink and remain healthy. For the majority of people, alcohol seems to be a relatively safe relaxant. For at least 11 million U.S. citizens, however, the use of alcohol leads to an addiction to alcohol.[1]

Alcoholism leads to approximately 200,000 premature deaths a year; it disrupts the lives of some 40 million family members.[2] In 1992, alcoholism's economic cost to society was estimated to be $148 billion in medical bills, property damage, and lost time and productivity.[3] Because of the prevalence of alcoholism and other addictions, nurses in every practice setting will inevitably be working with individuals who are addicted, who are in recovery, or whose lives are affected by the addiction of a friend or family member.

Addiction Defined

Alcoholics Anonymous (AA), in its basic book (referred to by people in AA as the "Big Book"), describes alcoholism as a "mental obsession and a physical compulsion."[4] This description of a pattern of thinking and behaving applies to many things besides alcohol, most obviously the use of other substances such as cocaine, heroin, and marijuana. This pattern is also visible in a broad range of behaviors that are recognizable as addictive processes. The element of obsession and compulsion is evident in the actions of people with unhealthy relationships to food, exercise, work, gambling, sexual behaviors, Internet use, television viewing, shopping, and other activities.

Certain elements distinguish the process of addiction from the healthy or recreational use of any of these substances or behaviors. The key difference is in the individual's relationship to the substance or behavior. In the addictive process, the element of choice is absent. A woman no longer chooses to relax with a glass of wine at a dinner party—she goes to the party because it will be an opportunity to drink a great deal. A man no longer enjoys watching a sporting event—he only watches it because he has a bet on it. A young college student no longer takes up running as part of a healthful regimen—she goes for a run, despite the heat advisory warnings, because she will be depressed and obsessing about her weight without a run of at least 5 miles a day. The mental obsession has overruled any ability to reflect on behavior and bypassed any self-awareness that could lead to alternative behaviors. The addictive use of any of these activities serves the same purpose as alcohol or drugs. The person is seeking relief and distraction from painful, unsafe, and vulnerable feelings.

Cycle of Addiction

All addictions have a basic cycle. Understanding this cycle makes it possible to understand the specific kinds of help that a person with an addiction needs to facilitate the healing process. In the early stage of addiction, people use a substance or substances as a means of changing unsafe or vulnerable feelings. Some commonly heard descriptions of these feelings are "I feel like I don't have any skin," "Everything gets to me," and "Everything is just too much." Typically, there are physical signs of anxiety such as light-headednesss, palpitations, painful levels of self-consciousness and social discomfort, and generally heightened degrees of agitation or irritability.

Vulnerability is a normal human emotion that everyone has experienced. The person vulnerable to addiction feels it more intensely and more frequently. Characteristics such as a low frustration tolerance, a low pain threshold, and a need for instant gratification go along with this vulnerability. These characteristics have the potential to become a problem for nurses in caring for addicted clients.

Most people who have become addicted to a substance have a vivid memory of their first experience of relief from this vulnerability as a result of using the substance. This first encounter typically occurs in early adolescence, a time of normal emotional turmoil and struggle for social identity and acceptance. Thus, the stage is set for dependence and progression to addiction. The process of building emotional and social skills, which is a major developmental task of adolescence, stops because an instant solution has been found. Picking up where they have left off in this process of emotional and social skill building is one of the major challenges for people in recovery.

In the early stage of addiction, the person has some awareness of seeking relief from discomfort. It may simply be an awareness of feeling stressed, anxious, or self-conscious.

Early Stage of Addictive Cycle

1. unsafe feelings
2. mental focus on the feelings
3. a desire to get rid of the feelings
4. using chemicals to get rid of the feelings

5. nervous system disturbance because of the chemicals
6. unsafe feelings[5]

In the middle stage of addiction, the unsafe feeling is not experienced as a thought. It is experienced only as danger or discomfort. The person knows that immediate relief comes with use of the substance.

Middle Stage of Addictive Cycle

1. unsafe feeling
2. using chemicals to get rid of the feelings
3. nervous system disturbance because of the chemicals
4. unsafe feelings[6]

People in the depths of addiction rarely talk about feeling high. The need is more frequently described as a desire to feel "normal." The impulse is to escape a feeling that is intolerable. At the late stage of addiction, physical instability replaces the emotional vulnerability. The addiction has come full circle. What was initially used as an answer to unsafe feelings has become the source of unsafe feelings. Mental instability and confusion, mental terrors and paranoia, hallucinations or feelings of unreality are all possible results of the neurologic damage from the substances.

Late Stage of Addictive Cycle

1. nervous system disturbance
2. using chemicals
3. nervous system disturbance[7]

Models of Addiction

There have been many models put forth to explain why a person develops an addiction. Any nurse who has worked with addicted patients can recognize recurring themes such as familial and environmental patterns of addiction or early childhood trauma and loss. Clearly, addiction defies simple explanations. Each of the different models offers a piece of a complex puzzle.

Medical Model

In the medical model, the emphasis is on the physiologic effect of the substance itself. The body's tolerance for the drug leads to the need for greater and greater amounts in order to achieve the desired effect and results in addiction. The absence of the drug leads to cravings and then to a withdrawal/abstinence syndrome characterized by symptoms such as fever, nausea, seizures, chills, hallucinations, or delerium tremors. In this model, the progression toward addiction is a property of the drug's effect. Those in the media often demonstrate this attitude toward addiction when they describe a celebrity who has attended a 30-day alcohol or drug rehabilitation program as "free" of drugs. In fact, 30 days is the beginning of treatment.

Genetic Disease Model

Much research points to strong patterns of alcoholism within families. People with close relatives who are alcoholic are at a three to four times greater risk for alcoholism. The closer the genetic tie and the higher the number of affected relatives, the greater the risk. Adoption studies show a three times greater incidence of alcoholism in children of alcoholics, even if they have been raised in a nonalcoholic family.[8] This risk factor is also seen with drug addictions across a wide range of substances, including cannabis, cocaine, and opioids.[9,10] The genetic disease model suggests that genetically based differences in biochemistry alter the processing and metabolism of alcohol and other substances, making the affected individuals more susceptible to addiction.

Dysfunctional Family System Model

The frequent appearance of addictions within the families of addicts may indicate that substance abuse can be a learned behavior. In effect, the child learns through daily close observation of the adults in the environment that conflicts and stressors are to be dealt with by drugs and alcohol. Children usually do not have a conscious awareness of this message. They may not have a full understanding of the role that addiction played in their home life until they reach adulthood and begin their own recovery.

Self-Medication Model

According to the self-medication model, the addict has an underlying psychiatric disorder and is, in effect, self-prescribing to alleviate symptoms. Addicts characteristically have tried a variety of substances and have found that they have a strong preference for a particular category of drug and drug effect. For example, a strong relationship has been documented between exposure to traumatic events and alcohol abuse.[11] It is not unusual for addicts to say their preferred substance makes them feel "normal."

Psychosexual Psychoanalytic Model

Emerging from Freud's conceptualization of psychosexual stages of development,[12] addiction appears to be a fixation at the oral stage of development. In the psychosexual psychoanalytic model, an infant or child whose basic needs are unmet becomes focused on seeking gratification of those unmet needs. Emotional development becomes fixated at the age of this early trauma.

Oral gratification is the most basic need of the infant, as seen in the way an infant receives nourishment and pleasure through sucking. In adulthood, people continue to seek comfort and pleasure from gratification of oral needs through behaviors such as eating, smoking, talking, touching their mouth, and various chewing behaviors. While healthy human activity includes some seeking of oral gratification, the addict is fixated at this developmental phase. The compelling need for comfort derived from oral gratification then becomes focused on the consuming of substances.

Ego Psychology Model

Also emerging from Freudian theory,[13] ego psychology suggests that, when an infant's or child's environment does not provide an adequate degree of nurturance and acknowledgment, the child grows into adulthood with an impaired sense of self. This results in feelings of emptiness and hypersensitivity that lead to a self-absorbed and narcissistic relationship with the world. The addict's behaviors are then seen as self-soothing attempts to relieve the basic feelings of emptiness.

Cultural Model

Our culture may be a major contributing factor in addiction because it teaches us to seek materialistic answers outside ourselves in order to experience well-being. People in the United States confront a relentless message of consumerism and quick fixes. This then leads to a society of impulse-disordered consumers who seek instant gratification and believe that there is a pill for every ill.

Character Defect Model of AA

Alcoholics and other addicts are seen as different in character and morals from nonaddicts in the character defect model of AA. Although the idea of a "moral" defect is not used extensively in addiction treatment settings, it is a concept that pervades the AA literature. A person in recovery may explain "my character defect" as the reason for his or her difficulty in making behavioral and attitudinal changes.

Trance Model

Derived from learning theory and the principles of hypnosis, the trance model proposes that the memory of the intense pleasure experienced in response to a substance is never forgotten. The experience is recorded by the pleasure-seeking, pain-avoiding part of the brain and remains as a deeply planted, in effect, posthypnotic suggestion that repeatedly seeks expression. The addict essentially falls in love with the feelings that the addictive behaviors produce.[14] The AA literature speaks to this idea in stating, "The urge to repeat the experience of becoming 'high' is so strong that we will forsake ... our responsibilities and values ... our families, our jobs, our personal welfare, our respect and integrity ... to satisfy the urge."[15]

Transpersonal Intoxication Model

According to the transpersonal intoxication model, the desire to break free of a limited, time-bound, socially defined sense of self and the desire to expand consciousness are the driving forces in addiction. Many people have experimented with lysergic acid diethylamide (LSD), marijuana, and other psychedelic substances and experienced expanded states of awareness that have resulted in spiritual and creative breakthroughs. The challenge then is to integrate these insights into daily life.

There is a significant degree of substance abuse and addiction among artists, writers, performers, and musicians. This model suggests that their desire to break free of mental and emotional limitations is at the heart of their substance use. One part of the artistic process is about finding a way to express the most intimate, subtle, and spiritual aspects of human experience. Artists often mention a fear of loss of this creative capacity, of becoming "ordinary," as they enter recovery. They have given the creative power to the substance rather than trusting that it resides within themselves. The ability to practice their creative endeavor while sober then becomes a major milestone in the recovery process.

Transpersonal–Existential Model

In the transpersonal–existential model, the human condition is such that humans are inherently anxious because they have knowledge of their mortality. Everyone finds ways to bypass or deny this awareness of reality. Becker, in a book authored when he was dying of cancer, wrote that a person "has to protect himself against the world, and he can do this only as any other animal would: by . . . shutting off experience, developing an obliviousness both to the terrors of the world and to his own anxieties. Otherwise he would be crippled for action . . . some people have more trouble with their lies than others. The world is too much with them. . . ."[16] This heightened awareness and sensitivity to the human condition then leads to addiction as a solution to the existential pain.

VULNERABILITY MODEL OF RECOVERY FROM ADDICTION

As a holistic nursing model of the recovery process, the vulnerability model of recovery honors the biologic, emotional, social, familial, neurochemical, and spiritual aspects of addiction. It focuses on the lived experience of the addict, which is that of essential vulnerability. The model points to specific ways that the holistic nurse can facilitate the healing journey of full bio-psycho-social-spiritual recovery. The basic points are presented in Exhibit 29–1.

The vulnerability model points directly to emotional education of children as a key intervention in preventing substance abuse. Children need to learn, in a safe and nonjudgmental setting, about the normalcy of difficult and vulnerable feelings. Learning to identify and then articulate feelings relating to peer approval, self-esteem and self-acceptance, performance anxiety, family conflict, trauma and loss are important tools for healthy living. Self-care skills and stress management skills should be part of children's basic education if they are to be protected from the unhappiness of addiction.

Nurses often have contact with children during one of the most traumatic experiences they can experience, the serious illness or death of a family member or close friend. Oftentimes, the adults involved try to "protect" a child from their own pain and stress by withholding information or offering simplistic or euphemistic explanations. The profound vulnerability that children experience at such a time can be the root of future susceptibility to substance abuse.

Recognition of Addiction

Given the prevalence of alcoholism and other addictions, it can be assumed that nurses in every clinical area are working with people whose lives are affected by this problem—even when the issue is never directly addressed. Therefore, it is essential that all nurses become skilled in assessing the possibility of addiction and recognizing risk factors and behaviors suggestive of problems with substance abuse. Nurses must first examine any preconceived notions that they may have about what an addict or alcoholic looks like. Addiction is a problem that occurs in every profession, in every educational and socioeconomic group, in every ethnic group, and in every age group from early adolescence through senescence.

There is a great opportunity for early intervention in trauma centers, which have largely ignored alcohol abuse. Nearly half do not screen patients for alcohol abuse, and those that do only rarely refer patients found to be alcoholics to treatment programs. Researchers at Seattle's Harborview Medical Center tested 2,378 trauma patients for intoxication on admission (blood alcohol count higher than 100 mg/dL) and chronic alcohol abuse (abnormal levels of the liver enzyme gamma-glutamyl-transferase) and followed these patients for an average of 28 months after discharge. Even after other factors had been accounted for, patients who were drunk at the time of the trauma or chronic abusers were 50 to 60 percent more likely than others to return. This research suggests that

Exhibit 29-1 The Vulnerability Model of Recovery

- Addiction is a repetitive, maladaptive, avoidant, substitutive process of getting rid of vulnerability.
- This addictive process is triggered by an experience of vulnerability that is believed to be intolerable.
- Vulnerability is anxiety ultimately rooted in the human condition of being conscious, separate, and mortal. As such, this vulnerability is a normal emotion, an elemental aspect of our actual human situation.
- People who have a greater degree of vulnerability (explanations for which range from genetic to biochemical to characterlogical to familial to cultural to spiritual) have a greater degree of need to get rid of it.
- Getting rid of vulnerability is accomplished by trying to feel powerful or by trying to feel numb. Trying to feel powerful is an act of willfulness. Trying to feel numb is an act of will-lessness. Drugs are selected to help produce these results. Trying to feel powerful or numb are both choices. Made repeatedly, they become addictive, producing predictable but brief episodes of relief from vulnerability.
- People in recovery from addiction begin to heal their feelings by recognizing and respecting their vulnerability.
- Continued recovery is based on developing new, non-avoidant responses to vulnerability.

- This vulnerability, however, cannot be effectively responded to on a long-term basis by the separate, ego level, temporary sense of self, since it is that sense of self which is at the very root of the vulnerability.
- Advanced recovery therefore requires the development of an expanded sense of self that is communal and spiritual in awareness. Such spiritual development is a normal aspect of adult development, despite the fact that it is ignored by most western psychology.
- Communal awareness is provided by Alcoholics Anonymous and other 12-Step programs through fellowship and service to others in recovery. Spiritual awareness requires development that has been studied by the world's wisdom traditions and, more recently, by transpersonal psychology.
- Many people in recovery do not experience spiritual awareness because this aspect of human nature has been neglected and poorly understood in modern culture. Pioneering transpersonal psychiatrist, Roberto Assagioli, referred to this issue as "repression of the sublime."
- Transpersonal approaches offer insights and practices that can: a) lift repression of the sublime, b) energize spiritual awareness and increase inner peace, c) work at the deepest root of the addictive process.

Source: Reproduced by permission. *Healing Addictions* By Schaub. Delmar Publishers, Albany, New York, Copyright 1997.

trauma can be used to motivate the patient and his or her family to confront alcohol or drug problems.[17]

In another study, 4,663 adult emergency department patients were screened over a 6-month period, using a standardized alcoholism questionaire. Of the 22 percent of the people screened who were judged to be drinking excessively, only 41 percent were offered help for their drinking problem. Of these, 88 percent declined the help.[18]

The most challenging and potentially frustrating aspect of working with people at the stage of active addiction is their per-

vasive denial of the problem, even when confronted with blatant evidence of his or her addiction. Alcoholics Anonymous uses the phrase "self-will run riot" in describing this behavior. It is the key obstacle to entering into the healing process of recovery. (See Exhibit 29-2 for descriptions of denial.)

The addicts' loyalty to their substance is profound. It surpasses loyalty to family and friends and is the cause of the addicts' manipulations. The nurse should not personalize these manipulations. Attempts to be of help often meet outright rejection or failure. The root of the addicts' behaviors is an

Exhibit 29–2 Definitions of Denial

- Continuous negative behavior in the face of obvious negative physical, emotional, and social consequences

  "My girlfriend is constantly bugging me and threatening to break up with me because of my drinking. She's really got hang-ups about drinking because her father is an alcoholic."

- Prideful insistence the person has control of behaviors that are out-of-control

  "I didn't get into that car accident because of the coke. I actually am a better driver when I've done a few lines. It keeps me alert and my reflexes are better."

- A maladaptive strategy for achieving security

  "I don't really have a problem with alcohol, I just need a few drinks when I get home from work because I work the evening shift. My job is very stressful and it's hard to relax enough to fall asleep."

- The energy used to maintain a destructive lie

  "I only use drugs because my girlfriend does. I can stop whenever I want."

- A narrowing of awareness to shut out anything that makes the person vulnerable

  "When I get high I just don't give a damn. All this crap just fades away."

- An unwillingness to experience the feelings the truth provokes

  "My boss was a total hypocrite. He was always on my case. All the guys have a few beers at lunch time. He fired me because he never liked me."

Source: Reproduced by permission. *Healing Addictions* By Schaub. Delmar Publishers, Albany, New York, Copyright 1997.

intense fear of living without the mood-altering effects of the alcohol and/or drugs. The behaviors are attempts to control the world and avoid painful feelings. The first step of recovery is relinquishing this control effort and admitting to self and others that the addictive process is not working, that it is actually making everything worse, that he or she does not know what to do, and that he or she must learn a new way to be in the world. This new way means a change in attitude to recognize that people who want to help stop the addictive behaviors are acting from a place of caring.

Detoxification

The simplest, most straightforward aspect of the recovery process is detoxification. When medical management of the detoxification is necessary, brief inpatient or outpatient treatment is available in many hospitals and addiction treatment centers. Acupuncture has been successfully used in detoxifying people from alcohol, heroin, nicotine, and other drugs. Its use was pioneered in the 1970s by Dr. Michael O. Smith in New York City. In recent years, it has gained wider acceptance and has been found to be a powerfully effective, natural treatment that is simple, safe, and inexpensive. It can be used in either inpatient or outpatient settings.[19,20]

Alcoholics Anonymous

With its 12-step self-help treatment approach, AA offers one of the most important, effective, and widely accepted interventions in addiction treatment. The 12 Steps of Alcoholics Anonymous put forth a systematic progression of actions to take that, when followed, will assist the person in recovery to find a new way to be in the world (Exhibit 29–3).

Enabling

A person in the addictive process has fears about change, but the people closest to him or her also have fears. It is in the nature of the addictive process that the people living and working closest to the person with the addiction have made accommodations to compensate for and cover

Exhibit 29–3 The Twelve Steps of Alcoholics Anonymous

1. We admitted we were powerless over alcohol—that our lives had become unmanageable.
2. Came to believe that a power greater than ourselves could restore us to sanity.
3. Made a decision to turn our will and our lives over to the care of God as we understood Him.
4. Made a searching and fearless moral inventory of ourselves.
5. Admitted to God, to ourselves, and to another human being the exact nature of our wrongs.
6. Were entirely ready to have God remove all these defects of character.
7. Humbly asked Him to remove our shortcomings.
8. Made a list of all persons we had harmed, and became willing to make amends to them all.
9. Made direct amends to such people whenever possible, except when to do so would injure them or others.
10. Continued to take personal inventory and when we were wrong promptly admitted it.
11. Sought through prayer and meditation to improve our conscious contact with God as we understood Him, praying only for knowledge of His will for us and the power to carry that out.
12. Having had a spiritual awakening as the result of these Steps, we tried to carry this message to others, and to practice these principles in all our affairs.

Source: The Twelve Steps of Alcoholics Anonymous have been reprinted with permission of Alcoholic Anonymous World Services, Inc. (A.A.W.S.). Permission to reprint the Twelve Steps does not mean that A.A. is in any way affiliated with this publication, or that it has read and/or endorses the contents thereof. A.A. is a program of recovery from alcoholism *only*—inclusion of the steps in this publication, or use in any other non-A.A. context, does not imply otherwise.

up the addicted person's behaviors. The nurse who takes on the role of working with a person in recovery will find it necessary to help the people closest to the person to change their behavior as well. They need to look at their own patterns of enabling the addicted person's behavior and be willing to keep the focus on their own process of growth and change.

Al-Anon is a self-help program for the friends and family members of alcoholics and other substance abusers. Family members, particularly spouses and partners, who have undoubtedly expended much energy in trying to help the addicted person, learn in Al-Anon how to accept their powerlessness to control others. The emphasis is on reorienting priorities and supporting the group members in focusing energy on making positive life changes for themselves.

Early Recovery

Detoxification, the initial step in early recovery, is just the beginning of a moment-by-moment, hour-by-hour, day-by-day process of making new choices. The nurse can help the person in recovery to make healthy choices by intensive questioning about old patterns of substance abuse and other behaviors. This information can then be used in planning for new ways of responding. Because behaviors associated with addiction are totally integrated into the person's life, he or she needs help in recognizing them and accepting the fact that they are no longer possible. Following are some important questions for the nurse to ask:

- Where did the addictive behavior take place? Some people stay isolated in their home or car when using drugs, while others prefer social settings such as bars, clubs, or work environment.
- What special rituals were a part of the addictive behavior? People typically have a routine associated with their substance use. A marijuana abuser may purchase her favorite foods before using the drug, for example.
- What places serve as cues for the addictive behavior? For the alcoholic,

particular liquor stores or bars may have strong memories and pulls. A particular street sign or exit on the expressway may trigger the desire to go to the neighborhood where drugs were bought and shared.

- What people in the environment are associated with addictive behavior? The person in recovery may come to realize that everyone he or she knows is associated with the drug use. People in recovery often cannot name a single person they can count on to be drug-free. The sense of loss of family and friends associated with this realization can be profound.

Nutritional Issues

Alcohol has high caloric content, but is useless as a source of nutrients. Malnutrition is common in those who are alcoholic because drinkers often fail to consume adequate amounts of food. In addition, alcohol interferes with the absorption of vitamins and minerals. Alcoholics are typically deficient in B vitamins, especially thiamine, pyridoxine, and vitamins B_{12} and folate. There is also some evidence that the B vitamin deficiency itself may increase alcohol cravings.[21]

Some studies have indicated that alcoholics who followed healthful dietary plans that included both nutritional and vitamin supplementation, along with nutrition education, were more successful at maintaining sobriety.[22] The effectiveness of this approach may be attributable not only to the actual physiologic impact of improved nutrition, but also to the individual's commitment to making significant lifestyle changes. As stated earlier, recovery is a process of repeatedly choosing healthy, life-affirming actions.

For the recovering alcoholic or other addict, working with a holistic nurse to develop a nutritious eating plan may be an important first step on the path to health.

As with any treatment plan, the key to its success will depend on compliance. Having a variety of approaches helps to develop personalized care and increase the likelihood of acceptance.

Body Work and Energy Work

In the early phase of recovery, shortly after cessation of use and resolution of any primary withdrawal symptoms, the person in recovery may experience difficulty sleeping, general agitation, and irritability. Acupuncture has been found to be very effective in the reduction of withdrawal symptoms and in the overall rebalancing of the physical system. Other types of body work such as reiki, therapeutic touch, massage, and reflexology can be of help in calming the body. Modalities offering direct physical touch or energy work are of value in the very early stages of recovery. Techniques requiring concentration, such as meditation and imagery for self-care, may be too difficult in the early phase of recovery. Relaxation exercises that focus on very simple breath awareness and counting may be all the person can handle. Avoiding caffeine, drinking plenty of water and soothing herbal teas, exercising, and taking warm baths or showers are all helpful during this period when the body is literally releasing and cleansing itself of a build-up of toxins.

Relapse

A person can achieve abstinence and still not make life changes at the level of emotions and spirit. A person can, in fact, stop drinking and continue to be hostile, rageful, blaming, and irresponsible. These people are controlling their behavior through force of will. Alcoholics Anonymous calls these people "dry drunks." The person functioning in recovery in this way is at greater risk for relapse.

Relapse is an ongoing issue in every stage of recovery. Many people stop without treatment, or with very brief intervention, but others relapse repeatedly.[23] In AA, there is a saying: "The further you are from your last drink, the closer you are to your next." Some addiction specialists have begun differentiating between someone who very briefly returns to drinking and then returns to abstinence, versus someone who resumes heavy drinking. The brief episode is referred to as a "lapse" rather than a full relapse.[24] This distinction may be in response to the "all-or-nothing," black-and-white thinking that can sabotage the process of recovery.

It is estimated that up to 75 percent of people in recovery relapse within the first year. It is significant to note that the figure is estimated to be even higher, up to 90 percent, for women with a history of sexual abuse and trauma.[25] This information points back to the vulnerability model. If sexual abuse and trauma exacerbate the person's unbearable feelings of vulnerability leading to the addiction, then abstaining from the substances that served as the emotional anesthesia results in a return of these feelings. It becomes important to connect the painful feelings to the trauma rather than to attribute them all to the absence of the substance. This opens the door to the need for a second recovery process—the treatment and recovery from trauma. This issue is not addressed in Alcoholics Anonymous, or in basic addictions treatment. It is addressed in the literature and treatments that focus on Inner Child work.

Alcoholics Anonymous has a helpful acronym that is referred to in identifying the times that a person in recovery may be most vulnerable to drinking. It is H.A.L.T. This is shorthand for *Hungry, Angry, Lonely, Tired.* The advice is, if the person in recovery notices the impulse to drink, he or she should stop and take time to determine if any of these factors are creating this feeling. The advice is also to avoid, whenever possible, letting these situations develop.

This simple advice is a very helpful tool to offer a person in recovery.

Gorski and Miller outlined the signs that lead back toward addiction.[26] Nurses can use this list to evaluate a relapse trend in the person's recovery process. Paraphrased from Gorski and Miller, the signs leading to relapse include

- active denial in many areas of life
- efforts to convince others of the need for sobriety, referred to in AA as taking someone else's inventory
- defensiveness
- compulsive behaviors
- impulsive behaviors
- tendencies toward isolation and bitterness
- failure to see the big picture
- idle daydreaming with wishful and magical answers to complex problems
- helplessness and hopelessness
- an immature wish to be happy always
- frequent episodes of confusion
- tendency to judge other people
- quick anger
- irregular eating habits
- listlessness
- irregular sleeping habits
- progressive loss of daily structure
- irregular attendance at treatment meetings
- development of an "I don't care" attitude
- open rejection of help
- self-pity
- opinion that social drinking is manageable
- conscious lying
- complete loss of self-confidence

These are warning signs, not inevitable signs of relapse, and constructive responses are possible. These thoughts and feelings will be with the person in recovery, to one degree or another, on a recurring basis throughout his or her life. Each time the person lives through the experience and finds that it passes, each time the person tolerates the feeling effectively and responds to it in a healthy manner, recovery and satisfaction in living deepen.

Deepening of the Recovery Process

Choosing to take new actions in response to vulnerability is the key to recovery. If the element of choice is absent in the obsession and compulsion of addiction, then reclaiming the ability to make life-affirming choices—reclaiming free will—is the essence of recovery. The use of will can be considered the use of one's life energy. If someone is "willing" to do something, he or she is choosing to give energy to the task at hand. If he or she is "unwilling" to do something, he or she is withholding life energy. There are three different ways to use energy: willfully, will-lessly and willingly. "Willingness and willfulness become possibilities every time we truly engage life. There is only one other option—to avoid engagement entirely [will-lessness]."[27]

Behaviors that reflect willfulness are seen energetically in the use of force, exertion, strain, contraction, constriction, violence, manipulation, controlling actions, and drivenness. It is the fight aspect of the fight-or-flight response to perceived danger. Will-lessness, the withdrawal of energy, is seen in behaviors reflecting withdrawal, escape, giving up, immobilization, collapse, and numbness. Will-lessness is the flight response to fear and vulnerability.

Every person tends to favor one of these patterns of behavior. Typically, a person who is predominantly willful eventually becomes exhausted and collapses into will-less behaviors. A person following a very restrictive and rigid weight loss diet for example, ultimately binges. In contrast, a person who has fallen into a pattern of total will-lessness (e.g., has gone on an extended alcohol binge) suddenly becomes scared, vows to stop drinking, and goes on a "health kick." This grasp of control cannot be sus-

tained because it is not grounded in any deeper changes. Consequently, the person swings back to the will-less behavior.

The array of behaviors that can be identified as willful and will-less are shown in Figures 29–1 and 29–2. These models are useful in teaching a person in recovery about patterns of behavior. People readily recognize and identify with these descriptions, and they generally appreciate the nonjudgmental presentation. As can be seen in these charts, the behaviors can be observed in every aspect of a person's life—in the physical, mental, emotional, and spiritual realms.

Willfulness and will-lessness are extreme uses of energy. They each represent an energetic state of imbalance. The goal in recovery from addictions is to lead a life of balance, harmony, and increasing serenity. Willingness is the active state of living life from the place of dynamic balance, as opposed to the extremes. It can be likened to the ideal of many of the world's wisdom traditions. It is spoken of in the Buddhist path of the middle way, in the Taoist concept of balance of yin and yang energies, in the Greek ideal of the golden mean, and in the common sense of moderation in all things. The qualities of life lived from this ideal are depicted in Figure 29–3.

Spiritual Development and Transformation

Spiritual development is an innate evolutionary capacity of all people. As indicated in Chapter 5, spirituality is not a concept, but a process of learning about love, caring, empathy, and meaning in life. This process leads a person to connect with his or her psyche, soul, or spirit and to have a lived experience of inner peace and harmony that allows access to inner wisdom.

Participants in AA and other 12-step programs are encouraged to seek spiritual growth and connection with their Higher Power. Green and associates explored the

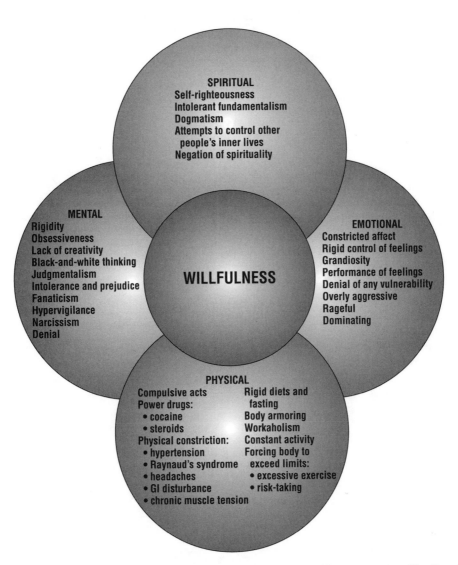

Figure 29–1 The Spectrum of Willfulness. Source: Reproduced by permission. *Healing Addictions* By Schaub. Delmar Publishers, Albany, New York, Copyright 1997.

process of spiritual awakening experienced by a number of people in recovery.[28] They described the life-changing transformations that these people experienced as a result of their intense spiritual journey and embrace of a power higher than themselves. This spiritual awakening appeared to be a significant factor in their sustained abstinence.

In a qualitative phenomenologic study conducted by Bowden,[29] eight recovering alcoholics described the importance of integrating spiritual practices into their daily lives. In addition to developing self-acceptance, those who were doing well in recovery were also participating in an ongoing search for connections with the transpersonal realm. This information confirms

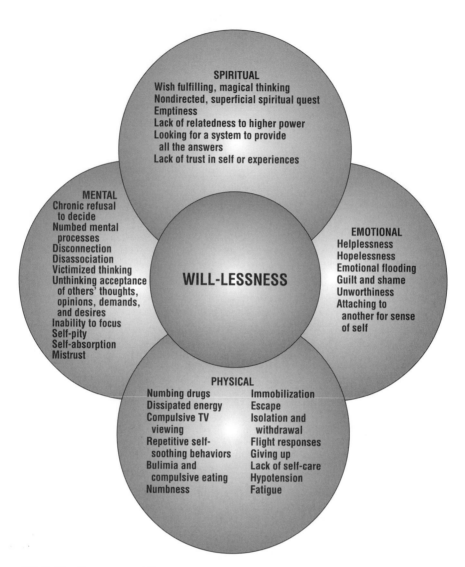

Figure 29–2 The Spectrum of Will-lessness. *Source:* Reproduced by permission. *Healing Addictions* By Schaub. Delmar Publishers, Albany, New York, Copyright 1997.

that it is important to encourage the person in recovery to explore his or her spiritual nature (see Exhibit 29–1).

Bodymind Responses

In a study of 1,862 persons, Benson and Wallace found that those who used prescription and illicit drugs began reducing their intake of drugs as they learned to enter a deep state of relaxation. After 21 months of regular meditation, most had stopped using drugs completely. The investigators looked closely at alcohol use in these same subjects. They classified drinkers as light users (three times a month or less), medium users (once to six times a week), and heavy users (once a day or more). After 21 months of

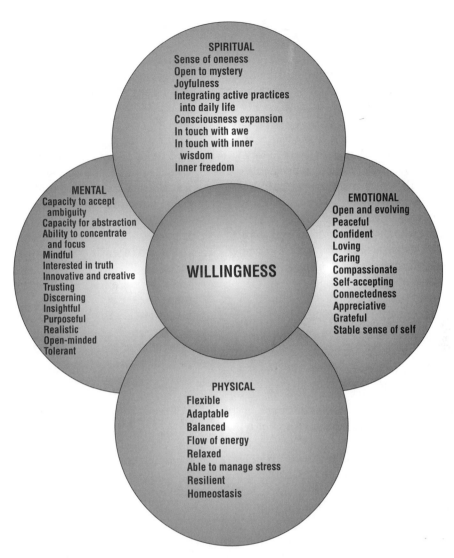

SPIRITUAL
Sense of oneness
Open to mystery
Joyfulness
Integrating active practices
   into daily life
Consciousness expansion
In touch with awe
In touch with inner
   wisdom
Inner freedom

MENTAL
Capacity to accept
   ambiguity
Capacity for abstraction
Ability to concentrate
   and focus
Mindful
Interested in truth
Innovative and creative
Trusting
Discerning
Insightful
Purposeful
Realistic
Open-minded
Tolerant

WILLINGNESS

EMOTIONAL
Open and evolving
Peaceful
Confident
Loving
Caring
Compassionate
Self-accepting
Connectedness
Appreciative
Grateful
Stable sense of self

PHYSICAL
Flexible
Adaptable
Balanced
Flow of energy
Relaxed
Able to manage stress
Resilient
Homeostasis

Figure 29–3 The Spectrum of Willingness. *Source:* Reproduced by permission. *Healing Addictions* By Schaub. Delmar Publishers, Albany, New York, Copyright 1997.

meditation, heavy use of illicit drugs had dropped from 2.7 to 0.6 percent, medium use from 15.8 to 3.7 percent, and light use from 41.4 to 25.8 percent. The percentage of nonusers of alcohol rose from 40.1 to 69.9 percent. Most participants in this study, 61.1 percent, reported that meditation was "extremely important" in helping to reduce their alcohol consumption. The more these people meditated, the less they drank.[30]

In another study, 20 male drug users between the ages of 21 and 38 began a meditation program. Over several months, the men reported that they were no longer taking drugs because drug-induced feelings became extremely distasteful when compared to those experienced during the practice of meditation.[31]

At the University of Washington in Seattle, Marlett and Marques found that college students who were heavy drinkers were able to reduce their alcohol use by 50 to 60 percent when they exercised and meditated regularly.[32] Exercise and meditation are effective because they offer an alternative method of reducing daily stress, confusion, discomfort, and fear.

Brain wave biofeedback has also been used successfully with people in recovery. It is a process in which electroencephalographic feedback helps participants go into deep states of relaxation. This heightened awareness also assists clients in recognizing their feelings of tension and then learning that deep relaxation can replace the chemically induced relief from addictive substances.[33,34]

HOLISTIC CARING PROCESS

Assessment

In preparing to use strategies to assist clients in overcoming alcoholism, the nurse assesses

- the client's characteristics that may suggest alcoholism
  - restlessness, impulsiveness, anxiety
  - selfishness, self-centeredness, lack of consideration
  - stubbornness, irritability, anger, rage, ill humor
  - physical cruelty, brawling, child/ spouse abuse
  - depression, isolation, self-destructiveness
  - aggressive sexuality, often accompanied by infidelity, which may give way to sexual disinterest or impotence
  - arrogance that may lead to aggression, coldness, or withdrawal
  - low self-esteem, shame, guilt, remorse, loneliness
  - reduced mental and physical function; eventual blackouts
  - susceptibility to other disease
  - lying, deceit, broken promises

  - denial that there is a drinking problem
  - projection of blame onto people, places, and things
- the client's current drinking patterns (Exhibit 29–4 provides a self-scoring test that can be taken by a client or by a family member or friend concerned about the client's drinking.)
- the client's attitudes, beliefs, and motivation to learn interventions to become nonaddicted
- the client's available family and friends
- the client's eating and exercise patterns
- the client's existing stress management strategies
- the client's willingness to join a support group

Patterns/Problems/Needs

The following patterns/problems/needs compatible with interventions for addictions related to the nine human response patterns (see Chapter 14) are as follows:

- *Exchanging:* Altered nutrition (more/less than body requirements) High risk for trauma
- *Communicating:* Impaired verbal communication
- *Relating:* Altered social interaction Altered family processes Altered sexuality patterns
- *Valuing:* Spiritual distress
- *Choosing:* Ineffective individual/family coping Noncompliance Health-seeking behaviors

Exhibit 29–4 Are You a Problem Drinker?

---

1. Have you ever tried to stop drinking for a week (or longer), only to fall short of your goal?
2. Do you resent the advice of others who try to get you to stop drinking?
3. Have you ever tried to control your drinking by switching from one alcoholic beverage to another?
4. Have you taken a morning drink during the past year?
5. Do you envy people who can drink without getting into trouble?
6. Has your drinking problem become progressively more serious during the past year?
7. Has your drinking created problems at home?
8. At social affairs where drinking is limited, do you try to obtain "extra" drinks?
9. Despite evidence to the contrary, have you continued to assert that you can stop drinking "on your own" whenever you wish?
10. During the past year, have you missed time from work as a result of your drinking?
11. Have you ever "blacked out" (had a loss of memory) during your drinking?
12. Have you ever felt you could do more with your life if you did not drink?

Did you answer YES four or more times? If so, chances are you have a serious drinking problem or may have one in the future.

Source: The preceding twelve questions have been adapted from questions appearing in the pamphlet, "Is A.A. For You?", and has been adapted with permission of Alcoholics Anonymous World Services, Inc. Permission to use this material does not mean that Alcoholics Anonymous has reviewed and/or endorses this publication. A.A. is a program of recovery from alcoholism only—use of A.A. material in any non-A.A. context does not imply otherwise.

- *Moving:*   Decreased physical mobility
                Sleep pattern disturbance
- *Perceiving:* Disturbance in self-esteem
                Disturbance in personal identity
                Hopelessness
                Powerlessness

- *Knowing:*   Knowledge deficit
                Altered thought processes
- *Feeling:*   Anxiety
                Potential for violence
                Fear

Outcomes

Table 29–1 guides the nurse in client outcomes, nursing prescriptions, and evaluation for overcoming addictions.

Therapeutic Care Plan and Implementation

Before the Session

- Spend a few moments centering yourself, connecting with your inner wisdom and intention to facilitate healing.
- Create a quiet place to begin guiding the client in strategies to overcome addiction/s.

At the Beginning of the Session

- Review the results of the self-assessment.
- Reinforce the concept that overcoming addictions is a process requiring commitment, new behavioral skills, and support from family and friends.
- Get the client to tell his or her personal story.
- Assist the client in identifying the steps necessary for overcoming addictions. If necessary, assist the client in going through detoxification.

During the Session

- Teach the client general relaxation and imagery exercises with a focus on awareness of body sensations and their connection to feelings.
- Teach the client how to create specific imagery patterns (see Chapter 22) and to practice and integrate the following:
  1. active images—cleansing the body of impurities, such as by a gentle water fall; creating a safe place where the client can feel secure and

Table 29-1 Nursing Interventions: Overcoming Addictions

Client Outcomes	Nursing Prescriptions	Evaluations
The client will demonstrate attitudes, beliefs, and behaviors that result in overcoming addictions.	Determine the client's intention to overcome addiction by • seeking support from healthy family and friends • attending AA meetings • seeking support of a sponsor • detoxifying self and environment of alcohol/drugs • practicing relaxation and imagery • integrating behavioral changes • selecting ways to reward self for attaining goals	The client demonstrated attitudes, beliefs, and actions that reflect an intention to overcome addiction. The client set realistic plans for overcoming addiction as evidenced by • accepted support of healthy family or friends • attended AA daily • contacted AA sponsor regularly • detoxified self and environment of drugs and alcohol • practiced relaxation/imagery daily • integrated behavioral changes on a daily basis • rewarded self for attaining set goals

comfortable; using a protective shield to let the client receive what is needed from others and to block out negative images, such as drink or drug signals, places, or events.

2. end-state images—of feeling healthy, of living with a sense of accomplishment and satisfaction, of having healthy supportive relationships.

3. healing images—connecting with inner healer, inner wisdom and with spiritual resources.

4. process images—imagining successfully overcoming drink or drug signals and making healthy alternative choices.

• Teach the client to reframe current situations and problems. For example, instead of the client saying, "I can't admit publicly that I'm an alcoholic," help the client rehearse being at a 12-step meeting and saying, "Thank you for letting me share my story with you. I have been an alcoholic for 10 years, and I am ready to quit."

• Teach the client to use H.A.L.T., checking to notice if being *Hungry, Angry, Lonely,* or *Tired* is a contributing factor when experiencing drink or drug signals. Encourage the client to avoid these conditions whenever possible.

• Encourage the development of creative skills as a means of working with strong emotions and experiences. Some of these areas are actively working with dreams, journal keeping, letter writing (see Chapter 17); using artistic expressions by drawing, painting, sculpting with clay; playing evocative music to enhance images or to dance with the emotions (see Chapter 23).

• Have the client identify his or her habit breakers (see Chapter 28).

• Have the client learn forgiveness (see Chapter 5).

At the End of the Session

• Encourage the client to explore the value of a 12-step program as an adjunct to treatment.

- Emphasize the value of selecting someone in the program as a sponsor so that a support person is available to be contacted on a daily basis.
- Reinforce the idea that the client can outwit relapse by learning how to recognize high-risk situations. Reinforce the value of using H.A.L.T. when experiencing signals for substance use. Is *Hunger*, *Anger*, *Loneliness*, or *Tiredness* contributing to these feelings? Encourage the client to make a list of particular high-risk situations and decide in advance quick action steps to prevent relapse.
- Reinforce the importance of integrating healthful habits into daily life. Encourage the client to select one or two practices to which he or she is willing to make a commitment to include in daily life. Imagery, breathing exercises, meditation, yoga, jogging or other physical activities, and dietary changes are all of value.
- Use the client outcomes (see Table 29–1) that were established before the session to evaluate the session.
- Schedule a follow-up session.

Specific Interventions

Support from Family and Friends. The best gift that a family can give an addicted member is to affirm that the person is loved unconditionally, but that the addicted behavior can no longer be tolerated. The family must decide the best approach to help that member and the whole family with recovery. Each family is unique. It is helpful for the spouse to get professional help, as many husbands and wives are blamed or blame themselves for a spouse's addiction. Professional counseling for the family is advisable even if the addicted person chooses to join a support group.

If the addicted person's behavior is unmanageable, a team of people will be necessary to intervene to get the addicted person admitted into a residential treatment program. An "intervention" is a process in which the significant people in an addict's life join together to confront the individual with the truth of his or her behavior and insist on the need for treatment. Specific information on treatment options is an important component of the intervention. The intervention must also include specific actions that the family is going to take if the person with the addiction fails to cooperate with treatment.

Support Groups and Professional Help. The client needs to continually assess personal and work life stressors. Because group support is vital to success, the client should become actively involved in a local support group for those with his or her specific addiction. Group support programs based on the 12-step programs—Alcoholics Anonymous (AA), Narcotics Anonymous (NA), OverEaters Anonymous (OA), CoDependency Anonymous (CODA), for example—are helpful. These groups are listed under the specific types of addiction in the telephone directory. Alcoholics Anonymous is the best known support program, with a success rate that studies show is on a par with, or better than, expensive inpatient programs. The client should also seek out a professional who is knowledgeable about addictions.

Few individuals successfully achieve freedom from addiction on their own. Addictive behaviors have been established and repeated over many years. Even if a client stays free of alcohol and drugs or stops the binge–purge cycle of bulimia or other addictions without help, the data show that the odds of relapse are high if the person has not learned any new attitudes or health behaviors. Those who stop an addictive behavior often replace it with a new addiction, develop physical symptoms or illness, or begin other destructive behaviors that lead to further dysfunctional patterns. For this reason, it is very important for people in recovery to seek out counseling that can address the tasks of emotional and transpersonal education. Alcoholics Anonymous views recovery as a lifelong issue. The addicted person must be "working the program," according to AA terminology, which means that the individual must explore inner psychologic work. Any resistance to "working the program" is seen as a danger signal in the abstainer's recovery process.

Learning To Tell a Personal Story. Support groups provide clients with an opportunity to tell their unique stories in an environment that is open and accepting. This helps the participant to get past the feelings of shame and self-hatred that are uncovered as the person begins to view past behaviors, and abuse of self and others with sober eyes. Taking full responsibility for past actions is a part of the "fearless moral inventory" that people in 12-step programs are advised to take. One of the most painful and challenging parts of this process is learning to forgive oneself and also those who may have caused the addicted person harm.

Listening to other individuals' stories, as well as being listened to while telling a personal story, allows the client more opportunities to restore self-esteem, meaning, and purpose in life, and to develop a deeper insight into what is life-affirming or self-destructive. The action of bearing witness to others' stories, without offering advice or judgment, allows an inner awareness to develop. This awareness helps in reaching and trusting inner sources of guidance and hope. This process of self-observation can lead to the ability to alter and challenge the self-defeating inner dialogues that cause suffering and threaten recovery.

Resistance to Spirituality. There is much cynicism and discouragement in addictions treatment because professionals in rehabilitation and treatment centers often see the "revolving door syndrome." Yet, un-like so many other conditions that nurses work with, an addiction is completely reversible. There is a real possibility for a person to transform his or her life dramatically and to begin living a healthy and sane life.

Because of the compability with 12-step programs and AA philosophy, spiritually oriented therapies and psychotherapy are important components of care. Addictions treatment is also one of the few areas in health care where spiritual development and exploration are not only openly addressed, but recognized as an integral aspect of care. As nurses and other health care professionals interested in addictions counseling explore their own spirituality, they can serve as role models for grounding spirituality in real, human terms.[35] Furthermore, it is genuinely difficult for spiritually repressed nurses or psychotherapists to assist clients who are working through AA's 12-step program.[36]

No single nurse or therapist can provide enough support and reinforcement for the recovery process. Thus, the nurse must be aware of a client's degree of participation in AA and any resistance to the spiritual aspect of the AA meetings. A person who feels alienated by the spiritual components of AA is unlikely to participate in meetings. Some individuals hear the word "God" or "Higher Power" in meetings and begin to reject AA's "God talk." If this is the case, the nurse can find out if there is a way the person can translate the concepts into personally acceptable ideas to facilitate a broader approach to spirituality. For some people, the idea of a Higher Power can be translated into Mother Nature, or the healing energy and intention of the people in their AA group. Clients may benefit from developing a more open view of spirituality by seeking out books on different spiritual philosophies or exploring spiritual practices such as yoga, t'ai chi, or meditation that offer people ways to experience expanded awareness (see Chapter 5).

Relaxation and Imagery. As previously noted, addicted individuals are not in touch with their bodies or feelings. Basic relaxation and imagery training can help them to experience themselves with new awareness. The daily practice of relaxation and imagery exercises not only reverses stress and depression, but also increases clients' recognition of inner knowledge. People who have been addicted have lost trust in themselves because of all the poor choices that they have made while in their addiction. In addition, there is a deep shame when thinking of all the people they have hurt or disappointed. There is a harsh, condemning, inner voice with which these clients must contend.

Clients must become aware of their physical responses to stress (e.g., heart palpitations, muscle tightness, headaches, or stomach aches). The abuse of alcohol, drugs, food, or other substances or behaviors numbs awareness of body responses, short-circuiting body–mind communication. Clients must learn to practice stress management skills daily rather than waiting until a vulnerable moment occurs. For example, the nurse can teach diaphragmatic breathing as a very basic skill. Shallow, chest–shoulder breathing is a common stress response, one that often becomes chronic. Simply breathing diaphragmatically can bring about significant physiologic and psychologic responses. Changing to this breath pattern efficiently slows the heart rate, increases oxygenation of the blood, strengthens weak intestinal and abdominal muscles, and can bring about a sense of well-being and inner calm.[37]

Teaching a client the concept of "constant instant practice" is a way of linking a new behavior to an activity that is done repeatedly during the course of the day. For example, if the person spends a great deal of time on the telephone, he or she can let the telephone be the reminder to take a few deep, cleansing breaths. If the telephone is ringing, the person can let it ring a few ex-

tra times and take a deep breath before answering. This practice can be linked with any activity that occurs frequently during the client's day.

The mind responds best when it is given positive images about new ideas and new behavior patterns. A nurse may start by guiding clients in rhythmic breathing exercises. When the clients are in a quieted state, they can be guided to imagine being clean and sober and walking down a street where they went to use drugs or alcohol with friends, now experiencing this place from a sober perspective. The image of experiencing their world from a new perspective can then be practiced and reinforced, resulting in the breakdown of addictive responses and the strengthening of positive coping strategies.

Healing Addictions: Imagery Script. To assist in the client's recovery process, the nurse can take time to create special relaxation and imagery tapes that the client can listen to several times a day. The following three imagery scripts focus on substance abuse, but they can be modified for other addictions. A relaxation exercise from Chapter 21 may be recorded for 5 to 10 minutes; then one or several of the scripts for overcoming addictions may be recorded for 15 minutes or longer.

It is best to use these scripts as suggestions. The most effective imagery tapes take advantage of the nurse's creativity, intuitions, and clinical insights—in combination with words and images the client has used—to create an imagery script that is designed for a particular person (see Chapter 22).

Script: **Introduction.** *(Name), as your mind becomes clearer and clearer, feel it becoming more and more alert. Somewhere deep inside of you, a brilliant light begins to glow. Sense this happening. The* *light grows brighter and more intense. This is the body-mind communication center. Breathe into it. Energize it with your breath. The light is powerful and penetrating, and a beam begins to grow out of it. The beam shines into the core of your spirit.*

Script: **Affirming Strengths.** *In your relaxed state . . . affirm to yourself at your deep level of inner strength and knowing . . . that you can stop drinking [or taking drugs]. Say it over and over as you begin to image the words and feelings in every cell in your body. Feel your relaxed state deepen. You can get to this space anytime that you wish. . . . All you have to do is give yourself the suggestion and stay with the suggestion as you move into your relaxed state. This is a skill that you will use repeatedly as you move into your new healthy life patterns.*

You have gone through detox . . . you are sober. Notice what you are feeling. Increase your awareness of deepening your relaxation. You have come a long way and are on your path toward healing.

The client provides affirmations and repeats them several times. For example, "I am at peace," "I am totally relaxed," "I feel safe and calm," "I can drink water or other kinds of liquids that will satisfy my oral needs," "I am secure in my inner knowledge that I have the strength for recovering."

Script: **Overcoming Drink/Drug Signals.** *Get in touch with your drink [or drug] signals. Is it a building, a time of day, a cer-*

tain person, a social gathering? As you bring them into awareness, rehearse in your mind changing one of those signals. For example, if a certain bar is your signal, . . . imagine you are walking down the street and you approach that favorite bar. But see yourself doing something different . . . as you pass by, you take a deep relaxed breath . . . and on the exhale . . . you have walked by the front door of the bar. Consciously affirm to yourself the choice that you have made. You feel confident, excited, pleased with your new patterns.

Imagine that you are with people who are drinking at a party. You have water or another nonalcoholic beverage in your hand. You are enjoying your friends, but in a new way. Experience how well you can talk and share some stories without alcohol [or drugs]. If any tension arises, . . . once again, access your skills of relaxation and images of confidence . . . in control of your life and free of addiction. Notice these new, sensation-rich images of awareness and responsibility.

Script: **AA Meeting Rehearsal.** *See yourself attending an AA meeting. You have opened your body and mind to receive many positive messages and support from others about being sober. Imagine now that you have entered the meeting room and are pleased with yourself for being there. Look around the room. Is there any one person that you might like to meet? If yes, see yourself go-*

ing over to meet this person, and hear your voice as you introduce yourself. If there is no one you wish to meet, that is OK. See yourself finding a place to sit, and continue to focus on your relaxed breathing. With your relaxation you are able to be more present during the meeting . . . to be open to hear other people share their stories.

Imagine that you are ready to share part of your story. Remember, there are many ways to share your story . . . sharing with a friend . . . a counselor . . . or your AA sponsor. Listen to your inner wisdom . . . you will know what is right for you. Can you imagine sharing something special about your journey? What would it be? How would you like to feel? The meeting is now over. Is there anyone that you wish to greet? If so, see yourself doing so.

Script: **Closure.** *Take a few slow, energizing breaths and, as you come back to full awareness of the room, . . . know that whatever is right for you at this point in time is unfolding just as it should . . . that you are willing to enter on this healing journey . . . and that you have done your best.*

Case Study

Setting: AA meeting
Client: S.W., a successful, married professional with two children. At the time he told us his story, he had been free of alcohol and amphetamines for 3 months and had begun his path toward recovery.

| *Pattern/ Problem/ Need:* | Health maintenance related to engagement in strategies to remain free of addiction |

"My healing began when I finally admitted to myself, family and friends I was addicted to alcohol and drugs. I began to explore and own my dark side. I've created some wonderful healing rituals, which include getting the nerve up to attend my first AA meeting—which gave me the opportunity to hear other people tell their story. I've been regularly attending AA meetings and have a sponsor who I've called several times when I felt myself slipping. I realized I didn't know how to do anything to relax except drink. If I needed energy, I didn't know any way to get it but to take speed. So I've learned relaxation and imagery skills, started an exercise program, and am taking time for myself.

"Here I was at 45 feeling lost and wondering if this was all life had to offer. How could I feel lost? I had so much. My career was going well. I had good kids, a loving and supportive wife, good looks, and I was involved in several civic projects. Everyone was always telling me how wonderful I was and stressing my contributions to the community. But I was searching for more to fulfill my life. I had been a secret drinker and had taken speed off and on since college in order to do all that I needed to accomplish. Everybody saw me as perfect, but I could feel my world falling apart. I got scared.

"For the past 5 years or so my wife had said that she thought I was drinking too much—which had recently become a source of tension between us. I told my wife to take the kids and go on a holiday while I worked at home alone. As soon as they left, I got drunk. When I fractured my ankle from a fall in my own house the first day they were gone, I really began to look at my life. I had a month of deep depression. During that time, my inner voice was screaming at me about all the abuse I was into. It was as if I was having a conversation with a part of myself that I had never heard. The message was so clear I couldn't turn it off.

"I'm not like many addicts who lose family, money, jobs, and friends. During a month of struggling to perform and continuing to hear my inner dialogue, one day my depression lifted enough for me to find a local AA meeting and hear myself say,' I've had it; I need help.' I finally admitted in public that I was addicted to alcohol and drugs and used them to be successful. I began educating myself about addictions. I asked for help. What I recognized was that previously I sought ways to connect with sources outside of myself to make me feel good. The real healing came when I learned to connect with the core of my spirit, which awakened my inner resources for feelings of wholeness."

Evaluation

With the client, the nurse determines whether the client outcomes for overcoming addictions (see Table 29–1) were achieved. To evaluate the session further, the nurse may explore the subjective effects of the experience with the client (Exhibit 29–5).

DIRECTIONS FOR FUTURE RESEARCH

1. Determine the effectiveness of imagery and breathing techniques in assisting clients in managing cravings.
2. Determine the effectiveness of cognitive strategies (e.g., teaching about willfullness and will-lessness, using H.A.L.T.) in helping clients to manage feelings of vulnerability.
3. Study the role of spiritual perspective and practice in long-term recovery.

NURSE HEALER REFLECTIONS

After reading this chapter, the nurse healer will be able to answer or begin a

Exhibit 29–5 Evaluating the Client's Subjective Experience with Overcoming Addictions

1. What new awarenesses have you had today?
2. Do you understand how to keep a journal of your habits?
3. Can you identify two habit breaker strategies that you are planning to utilize?
4. Are you aware of your bodymind's signals of wanting a drink?
5. Which relaxation exercises are you finding most beneficial?
6. Do you have any questions on how best to practice your imagery and meditation?
7. What physical activities are you including in your daily routine?
8. Have you been monitoring the pattern of your craving by using H.A.L.T.?
9. What affirmations are you working with to reinforce your intentions to be conscious and sober?
10. What have you observed about your patterns of response to vulnerability? Do you tend toward willfulness or will-lessness?
11. What have you discovered is your preferred way of connecting with your spiritual nature?
12. What is your next step?

process of answering the following questions:

- What addictive patterns do I recognize in my own life?
- What patterns of response to vulnerability do I observe in myself?
- What practices and changes am I willing to bring into my life to encourage my own healing?
- Who are the people in my life who would support me in making healthy changes?
- Can I allow an image to emerge that represents my inner wisdom?
- Can I identify what interferes with my connection to my inner wisdom?
- How do I connect with my spiritual nature and how do I support this in my daily life?

NOTES

1. A. Luks and J. Barbato, *You Are What You Drink* (New York: Villard Books, 1989), 146.

2. K. Blum and J. Payne, *Alcohol and the Addictive Brain* (New York: Free Press/Maxwell Macmillan, 1991).

3. H.J. Harwood et al., Economic Costs of Alcohol Abuse and Alcoholism, *Recent Developments in Alcoholism* 14 (1998):307–330.

4. Alcoholics Anonymous, *Alcoholics Anonymous* (New York: AAWorld Services, 1976).

5. B. Schaub and R. Schaub, *Healing Addictions* (Albany, NY: Delmar Publishers, 1997), 5.

6. Schaub and Schaub, *Healing Addictions*, 8.

7. Schaub and Schaub, *Healing Addictions*, 11.

8. American Psychiatric Association, *Diagnostic and Statistical Manual of Mental Disorders*, 4th ed. (Washington, DC: APA, 1994).

9. K.R. Merikangas et al., Familial Transmission of Substance Use Disorders, *Archives of General Psychiatry* 55, no. 11 (1998): 973–979.

10. L.J. Bierut et al., Familial Transmission of Substance Dependence: Alcohol, Marijuana, Cocaine, and Habitual Smoking. A Report from Collaborative Study on the Genetics of Alcoholism, *Archives of General Psychiatry* 55, no. 11 (1998):982–988.

11. S.H. Stewart, Alcohol Abuse in Individuals Exposed to Trauma: A Critical Review, *Psychology Bulletin* 120, no. 1 (1996): 83–112.

12. Schaub and Schaub, *Healing Addictions*, 23.

13. Schaub and Schaub, *Healing Addictions*, 24.

14. R.L. DuPont, Addiction: A New Paradigm, *Bulletin of the Menninger Clinic* 62, no. 2 (1998): 231–242.

15. Hazelden Foundation, *The Twelve Steps of Alcoholics Anonymous* (New York: Harper/Hazelden, 1987), 2.

16. E. Becker, *The Denial of Death* (New York: Free Press, 1973), 178.

17. Blum and Payne, *Alcohol and the Addictive Brain*.

18. J. Peters et al., Problems Encountered with Opportunistic Screening for Alcohol-Related Problems in Patients Attending an Accident and Emergency Department, *Addiction* 93, no. 4 (1998): 589–594.

19. E. Nebelkopf, Drug Abuse Treatment, *Journal of Holistic Health* 6 (1981): 95–102.

20. NIH Consensus Conference. Acupuncture, *Journal of the American Medical Association* 280, no. 17 (1998): 1518–1524.

21. M.R. Werbach, *Nutritional Influences on Mental Illness* (Tarzana, CA: Third Line Press, 1991), 15.

22. Werbach, *Nutritional Influences on Mental Illness*, 22.

23. W.R. Miller, Why Do People Change Addictive Behavior? The 1996 H. David Archibald Lecture, *Addiction* 93, no. 2 (1998): 163–172.

24. M.J. Meyers, The New Neurochemistry of Recovery, *Professional Counselor* vol. 10, no. 4 (1995):29.

25. Schaub and Schaub, *Healing Addictions*.

26. T. Gorski and M. Miller, *Counseling for Relapse Prevention* (Independence, MO: Independence Press, 1982).

27. G. May, *Addiction and Grace* (San Francisco: Harper, 1991).

28. L.L. Green et al., Stories of Spiritual Awakening: The Nature of Spirituality in Recovery, *Journal of Substance Abuse Treatment* 15, no. 4 (1998): 325–331.

29. J.W. Bowden, Recovery From Alcoholism: A Spiritual Journey, *Issues in Mental Health Nursing* 19, no. 4 (1998):337–352.

30. H. Benson and K. Wallace, Decreasing Drug Abuse with Transcendental Meditation, *Drug Abuse—Proceedings of the International Drug Abuse Conference* (Boston: 1972), 369–375.

31. Benson and Wallace, Decreasing Drug Abuse.

32. G.A. Marlett and J.K. Marques, Meditation, Self-Control and Alcohol Use, in *Behavioral Self-Management: Strategies, Techniques, and Outcomes*, ed. R. Stuart and B. Stuart (New York: Brunner/Mazel, 1977), 117–153.

33. E. Saxby and E.G. Peniston, Alpha-theta Brainwave Neurofeedback Training: An Effective Treatment for Male and Female Alcoholics with Depressive Symptoms, *Journal of Clinical Psychology* 51, no. 5 (1995): 685–693.

34. S.L. Fahrion et al., Alterations in EEG Amplitude, Personality Factors, and Brain Electrical Mapping after Alpha-theta Brainwave Training: A Controlled Case Study of an Alcoholic in Recovery, *Alcohol Clinical and Experimental Research* 16, no. 3 (1992): 547–552.

35. B. Schaub and R. Schaub, Alcoholics Anonymous and Psychosynthesis, in *Readings in Psychosynthesis: Theory, Process, and Practice*, Vol. 2, ed. J. Weiser and T. Yeomans (Toronto: Ontario Institute for Studies in Education, 1988), 55–59.

36. Schaub and Schaub, Alcoholics Anonymous and Psychosynthesis.

37. P. Parks, Psychophysiologic Self-Awareness Training: Integration of Scientific and Humanistic Principles, *Journal of Humanistic Psychology* 37, no. 2 (1997): 67–113.

RESOURCES

Alcoholics Anonymous: World Services, Inc.
P.O. Box 459
Grand Central Station
New York, NY 10163
Telephone: 212-870-3400
www.alcoholics-anonymous.org.

Al-Anon
Family Group Headquarters
P.O. Box 862
Midtown Station
New York, NY 10018-0862
Telephone: 212-254-7230

Children of Alcoholics Foundation
555 Madison Avenue
New York, NY 10022
Telephone: 212-949-1404

National Nurses Society on Addiction (NNSA)
5700 Old Orchard Road Specialty
Skokie, IL 60077
Telephone: 708-966-5010

National Clearinghouse for Alcohol and Drug Information
P.O. Box 2345
Rockville, MD 20847-2345
Telephone: 800-729-6686

New York Psychosynthesis Institute
2 Murray Court
Huntington, NY 11743
Telephone: 516-673-0293

VISION OF HEALING

Recovering and Maintaining the Self

The great majority of us are required to live a life of constant, systematic duplicity. Your health is bound to be affected if, day after day, you say the opposite of what you feel, if you grovel before what you dislike and rejoice at what brings you nothing but misfortune. Our nervous system isn't just a fiction, it's a part of our physical body, and our soul exists in space and is inside us, like the teeth in our mouth. It can't be forever violated with impunity.[1]

The client who has endured abuse or violence has had to live a life of distortion and lies. The choice to move beyond the duplicity and into the truth impacts the physical and emotional health of the individual as well as the family system. The journey toward healthy relationships may expose secrets whose effects ripple out into the client's present family as well as back through generations of abuse.

Working with survivors of abuse and violence is one of the most difficult nursing experiences, but it is also one of the most rewarding Because of a reluctance to inquire, it is possible to work with a client over a long period of time without knowing that he or she has been or may even still be involved in a violent situation. At the other end of the continuum, a nurse may be called upon to provide immediate care for a rape victim in an emergency room. In addition to caring for the client, the nurse must be sure to stay grounded and clear about his or her own needs and issues.

Survivors of abuse may move in and out of the medical–psychologic care system over a period of several years as they process the effects of their abuse. The recovery of the self moves in cycles and layers. Both client and caregiver must be prepared for this circuitous journey to wholeness, taking each new stage as reassurance of progress.

NOTE

1. B. Pasternak, *Doctor Zhivago* (New York: Pantheon, 1958), 483.

Chapter 30

Incest/Child Sexual Abuse Counseling

E. Jane Martin

NURSE HEALER OBJECTIVES

Theoretical

- Trace the history of child sexual abuse from antiquity to the present, identifying the current incidence rates.
- Discuss the repressed memories/false memories controversy.
- Discuss the physical, emotional, and behavioral consequences of child sexual abuse.

Clinical

- Initiate direct questions about abuse into the client interview format as part of routine nursing history taking.
- As appropriate, incorporate teaching about normal physiology and child development in counseling.
- Know the counselors, support groups, and other sources in the community for referral of survivors and perpetrators of abuse whom you counsel.
- Try the intervention techniques on yourself before recommending them to your clients.

Personal

- Do a genogram of your family, noting episodes of abuse or violence over three generations.

- Identify any personal experiences of abuse and, if indicated, seek resolution with a trained counselor.
- Carefully assess your readiness to function as a counselor when abuse/violence are the concerns, referring clients as appropriate.

DEFINITIONS

Child Sexual Abuse: exploitive psychosexual activity that goes beyond the developmental level of the child, to which the child is unable to give informed consent, and that violates social taboos regarding roles and relationships.[1]

Dissociation: the experience of one's mind temporarily splitting off from one's body—a feeling of separation from the body.[2]

Flashback: a nonpsychotic episode in the present in which the person actually relives the abuse as it originally happened.

Grounding: staying oriented in the present, rather than being engulfed by memory.

Incest: any type of exploitive sexual experience between relatives (or surrogate relatives) before the person is 18 years old.[3]

Trigger: any sight, sound, smell, or other sensory experience that stimulates recall of a memory.

Violence: a component of all incest/child sexual abuse, regardless of the intent of the perpetrator.

THEORY AND RESEARCH

History of Incest/Child Sexual Abuse

A request to name one universal cultural belief is likely to elicit mention of the incest taboo. If asked whether this universal prohibition on incest were effective, many would no doubt answer, "Yes." Most educational programs for health care professionals include information about the universal incest taboo and the result—a virtual absence of incest in nearly all societies. Levi-Strauss, a prominent anthropologist said, "The prohibition of incest can be found at the dawn of culture . . . [it] is culture itself."[4] Few questioned this pronouncement. Any discussion appeared to be more focused on explaining why incest is a universal taboo than on identifying if, in fact, it is a taboo. Many reasons have been offered to explain why incest should not, or does not, occur. There are biologic arguments (e.g., to prevent genetic defects arising from inbreeding), economic arguments (e.g., to broaden the family base of power and wealth), sociologic arguments (e.g., to solidify society through a wide network of connections and relationships), and psychologic arguments (e.g., to prevent collapse of the family due to sexual rivalries).[5]

In spite of the universal taboo against it, incest/child sexual abuse has existed since antiquity in every, or nearly every, known culture. In ancient Eastern cultures, the practice of pedophilia was common. In India, according to Mayo,[6] whose extensive investigations there led to the first child marriage laws, childhood began with the child being regularly masturbated by the mother. Children slept in the family bed for several years and regularly observed sexual relations between the parents. By

the time they were 4 or 5 years of age, they were usually taken to bed by others in the extended household. Child marriage was commonplace. Mayo noted that of the nine volumes of testimony published by the Age of Consent Committee in 1929, most defended child marriage, pointing out that children, especially girls, were so oversexed that by the time they were 7 years old, marriage was their only salvation. Historical data from ancient China support institutionalized practices of pederasty of young boys, child concubinage, castration of young boys so they could be eunuchs, child marriage, boy and girl prostitution, and foot binding to break the bones of the foot and facilitate shaping it to become a penis substitute, a practice that continued well into the twentieth century.[7]

In Western cultures, since antiquity, incest/child sexual abuse has been commonplace. In ancient Greece, the frequent practice of pederasty of young boys is well documented on pottery and in poetry from the period. Although these young boys, many of whom had been sold as sexual slaves, were described in loving words, the Greeks' cruelty to their children, including the practice of infanticide, is historically established.[8] Inspired by Greek culture, the Romans adopted many of their practices, including the loss of interest in the boys when they began to sprout facial and body hair. For example, in the Epigrams of Martial, one finds the following verse:

> Before your mouth was fringed
>   with hair:
> All pricks might find a haven
>   there.[9]

Incest and child/sexual abuse were rampant at the courts of the Roman emperors.

In ancient Egypt, practices were similar to those of the Greeks and Romans. Although more enlightened, even the Hebrews saw sexual violation of a young boy under 9 years of age as deserving of only a whipping, because boys under 9 were not considered sexual beings. Violation of a boy over 9 years old was punishable by stoning to death, however.[10]

As Christianity emerged as a force in their lives, people began to associate feelings of shame and guilt with all sexual behavior, reaching a peak in the Medieval Period. It appears that, although they did not eliminate incest and abuse, there were attempts to control the behaviors. The years of the Enlightenment and Victorian Periods were characterized by public nonacceptance of incest and child abuse, so it was carefully hidden. The major evidence of incest and child abuse emerged first in popular literature; as sensibilities became even more acute in Victorian times, such topics appeared in pornographic literature, a vast industry in that period.

Freud's early writings showed his acceptance of the stories of abuse that he heard from his women clients with "hysterical illness," resulting in the publication of his conclusions in the *Ideology of Hysteria* in 1886. His colleagues rejected this revolutionary theory of mental illness (i.e., that sexual experiences in childhood were the major cause of neurotic behavior in adults), however, and excluded Freud from their membership. In less than 2 years, he radically revised his thinking and the Oedipal Complex, which he posited and published in *The Interpretation of Dreams* in early 1899, was the result. The stories of his clients' sexual abuse at the hands of their parents became wishful fantasies of a sexual relationship with the parent that the patients created. This new theory was acceptable to the Vienna Psychoanalytic Society, and Freud was soon an active member.[11]

As Freud's new theory gained wide acceptance, public knowledge that child abuse by parents in their homes was not uncommon was lost again and only rediscovered in 1962 with the publication of "The Battered Child Syndrome" in *The Journal of the American Medical Association*.[12] Since 1962, child sexual abuse has been a subject of continued concern and interest, and the reported incidence rates have risen steadily. From an estimated 7,000 incidents in 1976, the number had increased to an estimated 113,000 by 1985. Careful studies with sufficiently large samples began to be reported in the 1980s, and the ratios climbed alarmingly to one in four for girls and one in seven for boys. More current research suggests that the rates are even higher. DeMause estimated that 60 percent of girls and 45 percent of boys have been victims of incest and/or child sexual abuse.[13]

Over the last decade, with the national attention being paid to the apparent increase in or at least awareness of the alarming incidence of incest and child sexual abuse, the striking increase in self-disclosure in the popular press and on radio and television talk shows, and the greatly increased frequency of legal action on the part of the survivors, it is no surprise that a backlash response has occurred.[14] Many date this response from 1991, when Marilyn Van Derbur (Miss America of 1958) broke years of silence and publicly told the story of her years of abuse by her (then deceased) prominent, highly respected father to a prestigious audience in Denver, Colorado. Van Derbur related that for many years she had no "daytime" memory of the events that occurred at night in her home. The memories were repressed. The media coverage of her speech seemed to open the floodgates; hotlines and women's shelters were deluged with calls for help from other survivors, and many other public figures were moved to disclose their similar histories.[15]

Public response to these disclosures has been mixed. Although many have been deeply touched, offering help and support, others have expressed disbelief, anger, and even condemnation. Among the most troubled and angry have been some of the accused parents. In 1992, they formed a support and advocacy organization that they called the False Memory Syndrome Foundation (FMSF). These parents question the whole concept of repressed memories, and while refusing to blame their children, who made the accusations, they vehemently blame those who have taken on their cause, calling them "New Age healers, self-help movement promoters, political activists, radical feminists, social service providers, and mental health professionals."[16]

Whitfield described the FMSF defense as simply the most recent in a long line of organized resistance against increasing public awareness of child sexual abuse. He systematically addressed the accusations of the FMSF that repression has not been "scientifically proven" and does not exist, and that most delayed memories of abuse are false. Citing eight recent (1987–1995) research studies that examined the memories of 1,091 abuse victims, he noted that from 16 to 78 percent of the survivors, depending on the study, had delayed memories of having been sexually abused.[17] One of the strongest studies, in which the childhood sexual abuse of all 129 women in the study was documented through prior medical records, found that when interviewed 17 years later, 38 percent had forgotten the abuse and another 10 percent had forgotten it in the past, but had recovered the memory in treatment, for a total of 48 percent.[18]

In 1995, an entire issue of *The Journal of Psychohistory* was devoted to the experimental and clinical evidence that recovery of repressed memories not only is common, but also forms a reliable, scientific basis for trusting the childhood memories of traumatic events that are the cause of most mental and social problems. In introducing the issue, the editor, Lloyd deMause, made it clear that he was responding to the backlash atmosphere in the United States and Europe and intended this issue to serve "teachers, students, attorneys, psychotherapists, patients and scholars as a central source for refuting the current widely-repeated notion that no scientific evidence exists for the recovery of repressed memories."[19]

Emotional, Behavioral, and Physical Consequences of Child Sexual Abuse

Adult survivors of incest/sexual abuse suffer a wide array of emotional disorders that manifest themselves in behavioral symptoms.[20] The most common diagnoses are depression, anxiety, personality disorders, dissociative disorders (multiple personality disorders), and post-traumatic stress disorder. The severity of the illness appears to correlate with the duration of the abuse, the type of abuse the person has experienced, the relationship of the perpetrator to the victim (the greatest severity of mental illness occurs when a trusted caregiver is part of the abuse), and the presence of violence.

Depression may occur either intermittently or constantly through adolescence into adulthood. Associated with the depression are low self-esteem, feelings of worthlessness and hopelessness, an inability to trust, passivity, lethargy, feelings of helplessness, inability to concentrate, inability to take control of one's life, confusion, and guilt. Impulsive behavior is common in depression and may include mood swings, rage, inappropriate spending, self-mutilation, accidents, and suicide gestures and attempts.

Dissociation also occurs frequently and may be manifested by nightmares or night terrors, with resultant sleep disorders, amnesia (especially for segments of childhood), feelings of depersonalization, fainting spells, panic attacks, hyperventilation, flashbacks, denial (of incest/abuse), and splitting or multiple personalities.

Relationships are frequently problematic; interpersonal skills are often impaired, and the survivor may seem to seek out those who revictimize him or her and to run from those who offer positive regard and nurturance.

Equally noteworthy is the wide range of physical symptoms that survivors suffer, many times affecting several organ systems and challenging precise medical diagnosis. Survivors rate their general health lower than do non–sexually abused women, and survivors use health care more throughout their lives.[21,22]

Gastrointestinal symptoms are very common. They include nausea, gagging, vomiting, "nervous" stomach, stomach pain, ulcers, and irritable bowel syndrome. Other general physical symptoms include headaches, insomnia, seizures, back pain, and chronic tension. Multiple hospitalizations and multiple surgeries are also common.

Survivors often develop eating disorders, including anorexia nervosa, bulimia, and obesity. Some perceive food as the only area in which they feel in control. Others hope to alter body appearance (becoming very fat or painfully thin) in an attempt to appear unattractive and, thus, sexually unappealing. Substance abuse is a frequent pattern, as survivors learned early that alcohol and drugs would temporarily numb the pain of their existence; it is a kind of chemical dissociation.

Sexual dysfunction of all kinds commonly results from incest/sexual abuse. Manifestations include a range of behaviors, from sexual promiscuity to the point of sexual addiction all the way to sexual abstinence and phobic behaviors. In addition, survivors may experience pain and discomfort, particularly in the anogenital and/or pelvic areas, whether they are sexually active or not. Intolerance, or even fear, of physical touch is another manifestation of sexual dysfunction, further adding to the difficulty with interpersonal relationships.

HOLISTIC CARING PROCESS

Assessment

In preparing to use abuse interventions, the nurse assesses a variety of parameters. Nurses must first

- be personally comfortable with discussions of incest/child sexual abuse and aware of their attitudes toward it

- be aware of their personal history regarding incest/child sexual abuse, and seek resolution of any unresolved issues or concerns
- increase their knowledge base about this serious problem

Nurses then must

- take the responsibility for asking about incest/child sexual abuse as part of their routine nursing history taking
- initiate a discussion rather than wait for the client to offer information
- use good communication techniques
- allow sufficient time for the client to tell his or her story
- provide psychologic support during the interview

Nurses should also assess

- the client's history of dissociative behaviors, which may be manifested by flashbacks, sleep disorders, and splitting or multiple personality
- the client's present level of safety, as well as the current period of safety (i.e., how long since the last abuse?)[23]

If more information is needed, nurses may ask a client to describe his or her perception of the effects of the incest/sexual abuse on eight life domains:

1. Social (e.g., Do you feel isolated, different from others, or unable to interact with others?)
2. Psychologic/emotional (e.g., Are you unable to feel anything, or do you have too many feelings?)
3. Physical (e.g., Do you have pain, headaches, or muscle tension, or do you feel sick when certain activities are mentioned?)
4. Sexual (e.g., Do you engage in sexual behavior or avoid it? Do you have sexual fears?)
5. Familial (e.g., Has your family life changed, for example, through divorce, estrangement, increased closeness?)

6. Sense of self (e.g., Do you feel strong, powerless, worthwhile, ashamed?)
7. Relation to men (e.g., Do you trust them, feel hostile to them, avoid them?)
8. Relation to women (e.g., Do you trust them, feel hostile to them, avoid them?)[24]

Patterns/Problems/Needs

The following patterns/problems/needs compatible with the interventions for incest/child sexual abuse survivors are related to the nine human response patterns of Unitary Person (see Chapter 14):

- **Relating:**   Social isolation
  Impaired social interaction
  Ineffective parenting
  Sexual dysfunction
- **Valuing:**   Altered spiritual state
- **Choosing:**   Altered participation in family
  Impaired adjustment
  Ineffective coping
- **Perceiving:**   Altered self-concept
  Disturbance in body concept
  Disturbance in self-esteem
  Disturbance in self-identity
  Powerlessness
- **Feeling:**   Pain
  Grief
  Anxiety
  Fear
  Post-traumatic response
- **Moving:**   Sleep disturbance
  Self-care deficit

Outcomes

Table 30–1 guides the nurse in outcomes, nursing prescriptions, and evaluation of selected incest/child sexual abuse interventions. Outcomes should flow from the assessment data and problem list, and the client should participate in their development. There should be one or more measurable outcomes for each problem.

Before the Session

- If it is the first session, prepare to be open and receptive to the client.
- If it is not the first session, prepare by reviewing your records, reminding yourself of the "homework" the client was asked to do and the goals for the present session.
- Be sure the environment is comfortable and therapeutic.
- Take time to center yourself and create a space within to be with the client.

At the Beginning of the Session

- After appropriate introductions or greetings, be still and listen to the client.
- Support the client nonverbally and nonintrusively as you listen to the client's story or report of the week's events.
- Keep questioning to a minimum until the client has had the time needed to speak.
- Assess the verbal and nonverbal behavior of the client to evaluate the present situation.

During the Session

- Using the assessment data, validate your impressions with the client.
- Identify both the strategies that have worked well and those that have not.
- Explore them with the client to gain an understanding of the outcomes.
- Hear the client's suggestions for next steps or new directions.
- Work with the client to develop a plan, including goals and interventions to achieve the desired outcomes.

Table 30-1 Nursing Interventions: Incest/Child Sexual Abuse

Client Outcomes	Nursing Prescriptions	Evaluation
The client will attend a social activity three times a week.	Help the client identify feelings of being socially isolated and find ways to move out of social isolation through relating to others; assist the client to choose activities in which he or she can engage comfortably.	The client reports attending social activities of his or her choosing and is comfortable in those social situations.
The client will be comfortable with altered participation in the family of origin.	Help the client understand that altered relationships with the family of origin are a common outcome when incest/child sexual abuse has occurred. Support the client in defining the parameters of relating that are within his or her sphere of comfort.	The client is able to set limits and define the level of relating with the family of origin that supports comfort and healing. This is a recurrent dynamic and will require ongoing support from and teaching by the nurse.
The client will no longer feel powerless.	Help the client identify the goal of empowerment, and support the client in the belief that he or she has the right to make decisions about his or her life.	The client reports that he or she has the right to make decisions about his or her own life.
	Support and facilitate disclosure at the client's level of comfort.	The client discloses the past trauma.
	Provide psychologic support and teach, as appropriate, principles of normal physiology and child development.	The client reports feelings of support and now understands that the body responses felt during the incest/child sexual abuse are "normal physiologic responses" and not evidence of "bad" behavior.
	Explore new behaviors, and teach those of interest to the client.	The client reports attending assertiveness training at the local YMCA.

At the End of the Session

- Summarize the session, including the gains and roadblocks.
- Have the client validate or modify the summary.
- Assign "homework," gaining the client's agreement to carry it out.
- Provide a copy of the plan for the client as well as for the client's record.
- Schedule the next session.
- Document the care provided.

Specific Interventions

Nurses do not need to be experts in working with survivors to be helpful. Many helping techniques decrease the guilt and the shame associated with the long-kept "dirty" secret.

Empowerment

The nurse supports the client while empowering him or her, which enables the client to increase self-esteem and feel more in control of life events. The client goals and outcomes are a result of a joint planning effort, and the treatment plan builds on the client's strengths. With the nurse's support, the client comes to believe that he or she can and should make the decisions about his or her life.

Disclosure is the first step for the survivor, but the client must feel that he or she has the nurse's permission to "tell the story." Thus, the nurse facilitates the disclosure whenever and however the client chooses. The nurse should never express shock or horror at the details of the story. Furthermore, the nurse should be comfortable with the client's silence if it occurs during the disclosure, should follow the client's lead, and should help the client strategize when he or she is ready. The nurse should provide psychologic support if the client experiences flashbacks during the disclosure. The nurse can help the survivor realize that self-disclosure takes great courage and is a real strength.

The nurse should teach basic principles of normal physiology and child development. It may be necessary to help the client forgive himself or herself for any sexual pleasure experienced during the abuse. Reinforcing that the adult is always the responsible party is critical. It is also important to explain that current negative habits and traits such as hyperventilation, somatization, dissociation, denial, and substance abuse can be linked to the incest/abuse and may have been adaptive and even creative when the survivor developed them, but they are no longer helpful and may even be destructive. Finally, the nurse should assist the client in exploring new behaviors and teach those of interest to the survivor, such as assertiveness, anger control, journaling, imagery, and relaxation. It may also be helpful to point out the many books, journal articles, conferences, and self-help organizations that support recovery.[25]

Grounding Skills

Many clients have developed their own ways of staying in the present, and the nurse may observe grounding behaviors during the history taking; for example, clients may consistently touch a piece of jewelry or hold a small object in their hand. It is important for the nurse to verify that it is a grounding object, however, rather than assume that it is. Asking clients to share their most useful grounding techniques can be an effective icebreaker in a group situation.

The nurse should teach clients to assess and monitor their own current level of awareness in order to stay grounded in the present. Grounding is especially helpful when clients experience flashbacks or dissociate. The first step is to teach the survivors to identify and verbalize when they are having a flashback. During a flashback, the nurse should (1) ask the client to describe what he or she is experiencing in the present, (2) tell the client that he or she is safe and not actually in the situation that is being experienced, and (3) encourage the client to reorient self in the present (grounding). This approach enables the client to achieve a sense of control and to distinguish the present from the past. The client learns to recognize that the flashback is in the mind and that it is not an actual experience. It can be useful to teach clients the signs of dissociation, such as losing track of thoughts, stopping in the midst of talking, or staring into space. Additional grounding skills to help clients stay oriented in the present include maintaining eye contact or keeping their eyes moving, looking around the room or at other people in the room, stating aloud the day or the date, or saying the names of the people in the room. Repeating "I am safe" can help the client separate the memory from the present reality.

Since survivors are often revictimized, or their children become victims, grounding skills can help the survivor become empowered to prevent either situation. Therefore, grounding is useful not only in the therapeutic situation, but also in day-to-day activities.

Relaxation

Survivors of abuse often find that relaxation exercises reduce anxiety, promote grounding, and discourage dissociation. Although the nurse may find them to be reluctant to take part in relaxation exercises at first, the skills can be very helpful. Some survivors may not feel "worthy" to take time away from their recovery to relax, whereas others may equate relaxation with vulnerability and, in fact, may experience flashbacks when in a relaxed state. Sometimes, survivors need to relearn the skill of relaxation, which can help them achieve more restful sleep, clearer thought processes, and more pleasant physical sensations.

The nurse can teach clients progressive relaxation, which involves the controlled tensing and relaxation of specific muscle groups. This technique can allow the clients to feel more fully in control of their bodies, thus alleviating feelings of helplessness and vulnerability. If progressive relaxation is joined with systematic desensitization, the survivor can gain some comfort in regard to anxiety-inducing people or events. (See Chapter 21 for in-depth relaxation strategies.)

Writing

An expressive technique, writing can enable the exploration of feelings inaccessible through conventional talk therapy. Clients can be encouraged to use various writing techniques such as journaling, writing a detailed autobiography, developing a detailed lifeline, and writing letters (even if they choose not to send them).

Keeping a journal, writing in it each day, and recording thoughts, feeling, dreams, nightmares, flashbacks, and memories can be very helpful to survivors, both while they are in treatment and as a daily exercise throughout their lives. They may include poetry and stories as well. The journal can help clients regain forgotten memories, see improvements in behaviors, and recall strategies that were useful in earlier difficult times. They may bring their journal to the treatment session for the nurse's review and suggestions. Since the content of the journal is so personal and sensitive, it is wise to discuss with clients the importance of keeping the journal in a secure place that protects their privacy.

Writing a detailed autobiography can help the survivor acknowledge details about the past and can work against reforgetting, a not uncommon occurrence. Even when repression is strong and memory sketchy, the survivor can be encouraged to write what he or she does remember, and this can serve as a general framework for added memories. It is often useful for survivors to ask relatives and friends for information about their childhood. This information may jog their memory or at least add to the store of information.[26]

A detailed lifeline can supplement an autobiography with its graphic portrayal of important family and life events. A lifeline can reveal a previously undetected pattern in the survivor's childhood, adolescence, and adulthood. If the lifeline becomes a focus of discussion in the treatment, the nurse may ask the client to bring in family photographs to assist in telling the story and prompting memory recall. Such photographs can make childhood less remote and hazy, while making the reality of the family situation and the abuse more vivid.

To facilitate full, uncensored expression of thoughts and feelings, the nurse can encourage the survivor to write letters to either or both of the parents, other family members, or significant others. Initially, the letter is not to be sent. It is written to a particular person (e.g., the abuser or the nonprotective parent) without regard for style, tone, emotional censorship, or guilt. The survivor should freely express all thoughts and feelings. The letter can be brought into treatment to facilitate verbal expression of feelings. If the survivor later decides to send the letter, it can be reworked until the form is satisfactory. The value of this technique lies in the survivor's uncensored full expression of feelings toward the person addressed. One note of caution, however: if the survivor wants to send the letter in the hope that the letter will "make a difference" (i.e., the person addressed will finally understand the survivor's suffering and beg for forgiveness), it is better not to send the letter. Such an outcome almost never occurs.

Anger Expression and Management

Both the expression of anger and management of anger are common challenges for the adult survivor of incest/child sexual abuse. It is critical for the nurse to teach survivors first to recognize their anger and then to express and manage it in appropriate ways. Survivors have usually learned early that only the perpetrator of the abuse is allowed to express anger in the home without punishment; as a result, they learn that anger equals power. Since all survivors have experienced anger and been unable to express it openly, they have usually internalized it and expressed it only in disguised form, such as passive–aggressive behavior, manipulativeness, depression, anxiety, and somatic complaints (e.g., headaches, colitis, ulcers). It can also be expressed as self-blame, self-contempt, and self-defeating and self-abusive behaviors.

When the survivor begins to get in touch with his or her anger, it is the ideal time in treatment to explore appropriate anger management techniques. The survivor must learn that feelings of anger and rage are appropriate in view of what happened, but that indirect and aggressive expression of anger will not promote healing. It is helpful for the survivor to learn to "dose" anger (i.e., express it in small, manageable amounts). The use of a 30-second to 3-minute timer can guide the expression of anger for a safe amount of time. Also, recording a verbal expression of anger on an audiotape can be useful if the tape is played in the presence of a nurse or supportive friend who can help validate and justify the anger. Physical exercise (e.g., running) or other techniques (e.g., throwing "softballs at a wall," hitting a punching bag with a plastic pipe, hitting sofa cushions or a bed with a tennis racket) can reduce anger. Workouts to reduce anger should be appropriate to the lifestyle and the comfort level of the survivor.

Imagery

Because imagery, a very private experience, has not usually elicited punishment in the past, the survivor is less likely to censor it in the present. An effective guided imagery technique can help a survivor remember experiences from the past and connect with lost emotion associated with the abuse.

The nurse assists the client to relax deeply and then asks the client to close his or her eyes and imagine the face of the abuser (or some other significant person in the client's past). The nurse may suggest that the face appear on a television screen to protect the client from overwhelming emotion. The client is then asked to describe the facial expression of the person on the screen and describe his or her somatic response to it (e.g., "knots in my stomach"). Next the client is asked to interpret the image, to say what the face represents, and to identify the intensity of the somatic response. Then the client is asked what the face is saying and what the somatic response is. The nurse and the client together determine how far to go with this exercise. Finally, the client is given an opportunity to respond to the abuser by releasing lost emotions.

The nurse can vary this technique to help clients connect with long-buried feelings such as pain, anger, sadness, or pleasure. If the client has never felt or cannot recall ever feeling safe or nurtured, for example, imagery can provide the means to present the possibility. Since acting "as if" produces the same biochemical response as the actual experience, the possibilities for healing in this way are limitless.[27] (See Chapter 22 for more information on imagery.)

Case Study

Setting:	Nursing Center (College of Nursing)
Client:	J.K., a 35-year-old man
Patterns/ Problems/ Needs:	1. Disturbance in self-identity 2. Grief 3. Social isolation 4. Altered participation in family

J.K. called the Nursing Center in response to a radio announcement about group therapy for men who were adult survivors of incest/child sexual abuse that was being offered for the first time at the Center. He had recently moved to the community and was more isolated than usual. His partner of 14 years was employed (they had moved to town for his new position), but J.K. was currently unemployed and feeling at loose ends. He reported that making the call was very difficult; he almost hung up when I answered, but he thought that he recognized my voice. He asked if I had ever lived in X [the city he had just moved from], and I replied that yes, I, too, had recently moved to the community. He asked if I was a season ticket holder at the local theatre in X and, if I had ever called to change tickets for a performance. I said yes to both. He had worked at the theatre ticket office, had liked my voice then, and recog-

nized it now. He saw this as a good sign, a sign that he should follow through with the interview.

At the screening interview, J.K. was very apprehensive, ill at ease, anxious, and seemingly very sad. He described a history of sexual abuse by an older brother beginning at age 6 years and continuing for 10 years until the brother left home to marry. He identified unresolved anger at his mother, questions about his self-identity, and sadness at the loss of his childhood as issues he would like to address in group sessions. He met the screening criteria, and although he reported that he was not generally comfortable in groups and did not relate well to men, he was determined to make the commitment.

J.K. joined a group in progress, along with three other new members, and found the group to be supportive and helpful in resolving the conflicts and concerns that he had carried alone for so many years. He participated fully and appropriately, taking his turn at telling his story (disclosing) to the group. He found disclosure, both his own and that of the other men, to be a powerful healing experience. It helped him realize that he was not alone, that his story was not so different from those of other men, and that he had not somehow brought the abuse on himself because of his behavior or because he was "bad" and deserved to be abused.

One of the activities of the group, writing a letter to the perpetrator, proved to be a pivotal experience for J.K. He stated that it took him the better part of 16 hours to write what turned out to be a page and a half letter. In those 16 hours, he said, he relived his life; he identified the chain of events that had followed one after another from the first episode of abuse, and he realized the losses he had experienced—the choices he had never been allowed to make. He understood his life in a way that he never had before, and he grieved for all that might have been and never would be. He put all this in the form of a story-letter and sent it to his brother, who is a writer. He told the group, "Let him [the brother] use it [the story] if he wants." The important thing was that J.K. felt it "go from him," and his burden was lifted.

Evaluation

With the client, the nurse determines whether the client outcomes for incest/child sexual abuse (see Table 30–1) were achieved. To evaluate the session further, the nurse may explore the subjective effects of the experience with the client (Exhibit 30–1). Because the accomplishment of these interventions may take place over a period of days or weeks, they must be reviewed and reevaluated periodically. Continuing support and encouragement are necessary.

In the process of evaluation, the nurse evaluates outcomes based on the client's attainment of goals, assesses the effectiveness of nursing and self-care measures in meeting outcomes, and revises the plan on an ongoing basis. It is essential for the nurse to document evaluation and outcomes in the client record.

Although counseling with incest/child sexual abuse survivors can be among the most challenging work a nurse will ever do, it is likely to be among the most, if not the most, rewarding. If the nurse has first prepared himself or herself through personal assessment and self-reflection and has taken the steps, if indicated, for personal resolution of any abuse issues, he or she should be ready to function effectively with these most deserving clients.

DIRECTIONS FOR FUTURE RESEARCH

1. Determine if one-to-one counseling or group counseling is most effective for adult survivors of incest/abuse in terms of length of treatment.
2. Determine the impact of disclosure or nondisclosure on treatment effectiveness.

Exhibit 30–1 Evaluating the Client's Subjective Experience of Sexual Abuse Interventions

1. Was this the first time you have ever disclosed the abuse?
2. Can you describe what you felt like before you began to disclose?
3. Did you experience physical or emotional sensations during the disclosure? Can you describe them?
4. Were you able to stay grounded during the disclosure? If not, do you know what triggered your dissociation?
5. Did you feel safe during the disclosure?
6. What did you feel immediately following the disclosure?
7. Would you be willing to disclose to another person at another time?
8. What could I have done to be more helpful to you during the disclosure?
9. Is there anything I can do right now to be helpful?
10. What is your next step or plan to integrate this disclosure experience?

Source: Data from E. Jane Martin and L. Gooding Kolkmeier, Sexual Abuse: Healing the Wounds, in *Holistic Nursing: A Handbook for Practice*, B.M. Dossey et al., eds., p. 423, © 1995, Aspen Publishers, Inc.

3. Compare the effectiveness of a closed group model of treatment versus an open group model.
4. Explore the impact of therapist gender on all-women groups, all-men groups, and mixed groups.

NURSE HEALER REFLECTIONS

After reading this chapter, the nurse healer will be able to answer or begin a process of answering the following questions:

- Are any patterns of abuse evident in my own family genogram?
- What issues are triggered in my own relationships as a result of my work with adult survivors of incest/child sexual abuse?
- Am I comfortable treating clients when sexual abuse and violence are the concerns?
- Do the interventions I use with clients work for me?

REFERENCES

1. L.G. Kolkmeier, Sexual Abuse: Healing the Wounds, in *Holistic Nursing: A Handbook for Practice*, 2d ed., ed. B.M. Dossey et al. (Gaithersburg, MD: Aspen Publishers, 1995), 404.

2. C. Courtois, *Healing the Incest Wound: Adult Survivors in Therapy* (New York: W.W. Norton & Co., 1988), 154.

3. J.C. Urbanic, Intrafamilial Sexual Abuse, in *Nursing Care of Survivors of Family Violence*, ed. J. Campbell and J. Humphreys (St. Louis: Mosby, 1993), 133.

4. C. Levi-Strauss, *The Elementary Structures of Kinship* (London: Eyne and Spottiswoode, 1969), 41.

5. M. Lew, *Victims No Longer* (New York: Harper & Row, 1988), 19.

6. C. Mayo, *Mother India* (New York: Harcourt Brace and Co., 1927), 25–26, 68.

7. L. deMause, The Universality of Incest, *Journal of Psychohistory* 19, no. 2 (1991): 123–164.

8. B. Kahr, The Sexual Molestation of Children: Historical Perspectives, *Journal of Psychohistory* 19, no. 2 (1991): 191–214.

9. Kahr, The Sexual Molestation of Children.

10. Kahr, The Sexual Molestation of Children.

11. J. M. Masson, *The Assault on Truth: Freud's's Suppression of the Seduction Theory* (New York: Farrar, Straus and Giroux, 1984).

12. C. Kempe et al., The Battered Child Syndrome, *Journal of the American Medical Association* 18, no. 1 (1962): 17–24.

13. deMause, The Universality of Incest.

14. E.J. Martin, Incest/Child Sexual Abuse: Historical Perspectives, *Journal of Holistic Nursing* 13, no. 1. (1995): 7–18.

15. L. Terr, Day Child/Night Child, *Family Therapy Networker* 18, no. 5 (1994): 54–63.

16. M. Wylie, The Shadow of a Doubt, *Family Therapy Networker* 17, no. 5 (1993): 18–29, 70, 73.

17. C. Whitfield, *Memory and Abuse: Remembering and Healing the Effects of Trauma* (Deerfield Beach, FL: Health Communications, 1995).

18. L.M. Williams, Recovered Memories of Abuse in Women with Documented Child Sexual Victimization Histories, *Journal of Traumatic Stress* 8, no. 4 (1995): 649–673.

19. L. deMause, Trusting Childhood Memories, *Journal of Psychohistory* 23, no. 2 (1995): 118–190.

20. Courtois, *Healing the Incest Wound*, 98–99.

21. Courtois, *Healing the Incest Wound*.

22. J. Lesserman et al., Sexual and Physical Abuse History and Gastroenterology Practice: How Types of Abuse Impact Health Status, *Psychosomatic Medicine* 58, no. 4 (1996): 4–15.

23. Kolkmeier, Sexual Abuse, 407–408.

24. Courtois, *Healing the Incest Wound*, 368–369.

25. J. Campbell and J. Humphreys, *Nursing Care of Survivors of Family Violence*, 2d ed. (St. Louis: Mosby, 1993), 152–153.

26. Courtois, *Healing the Incest Wound*, 195.

27. Kolkmeier, Sexual Abuse, 412–413.

Index

N